Rotatory Knee Instability

Volker Musahl • Jón Karlsson
Ryosuke Kuroda • Stefano Zaffagnini
Editors

Rotatory Knee Instability

An Evidence Based Approach

Springer

Editors
Volker Musahl
Department of Orthopaedic Surgery
UPMC Center for Sports Medicine
Pittsburgh, PA
USA

Ryosuke Kuroda
Orthopaedic Surgery
Kobe University School of Medicine
Kobe
Japan

Jón Karlsson
Departement of Orthopardics
Sahlgrenska Academy
Gothenburg University
Gothenburg
Sweden

Stefano Zaffagnini
Istituto Ortopedico Rizzoli
University of Bologna
Bologna
Italy

Associate Editors
Christopher Murawski
Department of Orthopaedic Surgery
UPMC Center for Sports Medicine
Pittsburgh, PA
USA

Yuichi Hoshino
Orthopaedic Surgery
Kobe University School of Medicine
Kobe
Japan

Kristian Samuelsson
Departement of Orthopardics
Sahlgrenska Academy
Gothenburg University
Gothenburg
Sweden

Nicola Lopomo
Istituto Ortopedico Rizzoli
University of Bologna
Bologna
Italy

ISBN 978-3-319-32069-4 ISBN 978-3-319-32070-0 (eBook)
DOI 10.1007/978-3-319-32070-0

Library of Congress Control Number: 2016949033

Printed on acid-free paper

This Springer imprint is published by Springer Nature
The registered company is Springer International Publishing AG Switzerland

Foreword I

Rotational stability is crucial for the knee joint. For anterior cruciate ligament (ACL) injuries, evaluating rotational stability is both a diagnostic tool and a postoperative outcome measure. In fact, the pivot shift test is the single most important objective outcome after ACL reconstruction correlating with patient satisfaction.

Rotational stability of the knee has always been of interest to researchers and clinicians alike. However, this has recently increased since the renewed focus on individualized surgery and restoration of native anatomy. In addition to the ACL, various other anatomic structures have been suggested to play an important role in rotational stability of the knee such as the medial and lateral meniscus, the medial and lateral capsular structures, and the bony morphology of the femur and tibia.

Although the importance of the pivot shift as a diagnostic test for rotational laxity is undeniable, the test in its current form has limitations. It is a high variability among users, it is subjective, and the results are inconsistent. There is a strong need to more objectively measure rotatory laxity, and this has led researchers to attempt to standardize and quantify the pivot shift test, measuring aspects like acceleration and lateral compartment translation. This had led to a variety of interesting new measurement devices with very promising prospects for the future.

In the present time, where the interest in rotational stability of the knee is at an all-time high and the consensus regarding the responsible structures, diagnostic tests, and reconstructive methods is lacking, the timing of this book could not be better. *Rotatory Instability of the Knee: An Evidence-Based Approach* by Drs. Karlsson, Kuroda, Musahl, and Zaffagnini is an excellent book which objectively presents all available evidence with regard to rotational instability of the knee including the anatomy and function of the structures involved, injury mechanisms, in vivo biomechanics, physical examination tests, imaging, surgical management, and rehabilitation. Furthermore, it covers important history on this topic explaining the different schools of thought responsible for inspiring innovation. The author list includes some of the most well-known researchers and clinicians from all over the world who have dedicated their career to better understand and treat rotational instability of the knee. It concludes with an outstanding discussion of future directions.

Congratulations to the editors for a job well done. This book is a must-read, and I am certain it will be considered one of the benchmark publications of its time.

Freddie H. Fu, MD, DSc, DPs

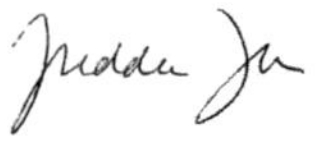

Distinguished Service Professor
David Silver Professor and Chairman
Division of Sports Medicine
Head Team Physician
Department of Athletics
Professor of Physical Therapy
School of Health and Rehabilitation Sciences
Professor of Health and Physical Activity
School of Education
Professor of Mechanical Engineering & Materials Science
Swanson School of Engineering

Foreword II

It is all about rotation!

It is in the 1970s of the last century that rotational instability was described by several surgeons who all were fascinated by the study of knee anatomy and who then influenced modern ligament surgery of the knee. Donald Slocum described anteromedial instability, which made us believe to be able to treat anterior instability of the knee just by doing a "pes transfer" and thus by increasing the mechanical action of pes anserinus. Independently, Marcel Lemaire in Paris and David MacIntosh in Toronto and others believed that the *primary* problem *took* place in the lateral femorotibial compartment, and they individually developed their concepts and drew our attention to a newly discovered subluxation event. While Lemaire had been working in private and his discovery had not immediately been taken up by his own French compatriots and other European knee surgeons, MacIntosh was surrounded by residents and fellows, among them Robert Galway. They called the knee sign the "lateral pivot shift phenomenon" which, by the way, had also been independently observed by Ron Losee in Ennis, Montana, who made major headway toward understanding and surgically repairing the "trick knee." Incidentally, I. MacNab, famous Torontonian spine and shoulder surgeon, with whom I had a chance to work during 6 months in 1975, rightly would say that in his experience nothing was new that had not already been described by a "crazy" German (forgive him the term!) in the last century. Truly in 1936, Felsenreich had described as the first German surgeon the same phenomenon… But even before him, Jones and Smith in 1913 and, shortly after, Hey Groves in 1920 had clearly described that crucial symptom of rotational knee laxity. But these authors seem to have become largely forgotten by many of these reports from the 1970s, the fate of much historical science, during the revolution of modern knee surgical approaches. In fact, referring back to Lose, he had corresponded about this strange dynamic sign, observed in a patient in 1969 with John C. Kennedy from London, Ontario, who himself was not easily convinced of this new entity. I spent 2 years in Toronto 1973–1975, also visiting David MacIntosh regularly in the Athletic Injury Clinic at Hart House, University of Toronto, and was taught by the master himself how to elicit the pivot shift. I also participated at surgery where he performed his lateral extra-articular repair putting the patient thereafter in a plaster of Paris cast (as it used to be called at that time) with the knee flexed to 90° and the lower leg externally rotated. And probably by anchoring the strip of the iliotibial tract under the proximal origin of the lateral collateral ligament, he was not at such a bad spot as modern anatomical and biomechanical data regarding anterolateral ligament function would confirm today. I witnessed intense public debates and discussions during meetings among the two Canadian knee experts MacIntosh and Kennedy. David, a humble person, but very astute scientist, was convinced that the lateral tibial plateau traveled more importantly anteriorly than the medial and that this should be addressed correspondingly, describing a surgical technique that was exclusively based on the principle of controlling anterolateral instability where it was at its advantage with extra-articular repairs by a sling, but leaving the central pillar untouched, similar to Lemaire in Paris. Coincidentally, this occurred without the two knowing of each other's work. Only later did he then also guide the strip into the joint in an over the top manner to reconstruct a missing ACL. Hughston and Andrews in the late 1970s and early 1980s followed on these principles, equally addressing techniques to minimize the dynamic shift event that so badly destroyed the articular cartilage and meniscus of the lateral compartment. In the 1980s, rightly and because of insufficient possibility to control the Lachman displacement with these extra-articular techniques, the pendulum swung away from the periphery to the center with numerous proponents for mere direct reconstruction of the central pillar, leaving the periphery untouched, even when it was very lax, thus allowing for too much anterolateral rotation and secondary loosening of the reconstruction.. Following roughly 30 years, there seemed to rein reluctance to consider the lateral extra-articular problem with the exception of the Lyon School and some surgeons internationally, me included, who in their practice always maintained the traditional thinking of combining intra- and extra-articular reconstruction. Since a few years, it has been more generally but still only slowly accepted to pay attention to this issue again, stressing the importance of accurate examination and analysis of the pivot shift, even "going as far" as trying to grade it, which we attempted in a study in a paper with J. Deland. As a small detail, in this continuum and review of history, our description of the reversed pivot shift sign in 1980 may be quoted where the inexperienced examiner may fall in a trap in the presence of posterolateral instability which then could easily be mixed with a true pivot shift and lead to erroneous surgical reconstruction (Jakob, Hassler, Stäubli).

Later then, the concept of rotational laxity, by which we seniors today got once stimulated during our best years of research and science (Müller, Stäubli, Noyes, Grood, Butler, and many others), went now through an almost forgotten period. And the term envelope of motion by Frank Noyes and others that so well described this interaction between primary and secondary restraints was not used any more.

"Those who cannot remember the past are condemned to repeat it," attributed to W. Churchill, but already stated before by Santayana, is valid as well here and fulfills us with a certain satisfaction *that it may be right:*

- *To learn that chronic anterior or posterior instability of the knee even when initiated by an isolated ligament tear always slowly loosens up the periphery and reflects itself in an increased freedom of rotation*

- *To always respect rotational instability when the amount of anterior instability is marked*
- *To consider combined intra- and extra-articular reconstruction with refining gestures or formal reconstruction of the ligamento-capsular structures in an aim to decrease the volume of the envelope of motion*

Certainly, once these principles are accepted, there remains plenty of room, to find out which is the best way to achieve that goal. Nothing stimulates science as much as a new discovery or a rediscovery of anatomy. There is, however, more to learn, as we just witnessed over the past 12 months, regarding the rediscovery of the true anatomy of the "anterolateral ligament" or even the ACL. We may now all accept that the intelligent central and peripheral ligamentous and capsular structures work in concert, those reconstruction techniques that we propose to a patient must consider both of them, and it may require more than an arthroscope to serve the suffering patient adequately. Too many operated ACL ruptures have been unable to prevent the development of osteoarthritis so that insurers in some countries ask serious and "threatening" questions regarding the indication for too frequently performed ACL surgeries. If we are able to better understand and learn more, we may hopefully achieve superior results!

It is the perfect time for this book to appear shedding more light on the specific scientific topic in an attempt to contribute new knowledge on these concepts. We are sure that the editors and authors understand the work that they stimulated and achieved as a milestone to which, certainly, many more shall follow. I feel honored having been asked to write this foreword on a topic that has kept me busy during all my life as a clinician and modest scientist.

Roland P. Jakob

Contents

Part I

Introduction

In Vitro Biomechanical Analysis of Knee Rotational Stability

1

Amir Ata Rahnemai-Azar, Masahito Yoshida, Volker Musahl, and Richard Debski

Contents

A.A. Rahnemai-Azar • M. Yoshida
Department of Orthopaedic Surgery, Department of Bioengineering, Orthopaedic Robotics Laboratory, University of Pittsburgh, Pittsburgh, PA, USA

Department of Orthopaedic Surgery, UPMC Center for Sports Medicine, University of Pittsburgh, Pittsburgh, PA, USA

V. Musahl
Department of Orthopaedic Surgery, UPMC Center for Sports Medicine, Pittsburgh, PA, USA

R. Debski (✉)
Department of Orthopaedic Surgery,
Department of Bioengineering, Orthopaedic Robotics Laboratory, University of Pittsburgh,
408 Center for Bioengineering, 300 Technology Drive Pittsburgh, Pittsburgh, 15219 PA, USA
e-mail: genesis1@pitt.edu

Department of Orthopaedic Surgery, UPMC Center for Sports Medicine, University of Pittsburgh, Pittsburgh, PA, USA

1.1 Introduction

In vitro biomechanics uses engineering sciences to analyze the movement and structure of biological systems outside of a living subject. These studies advance evidence-based medicine by generating knowledge to improve clinical decision-making and generate significant basic knowledge about joint and tissue structure–function. Although in vitro studies do not consider some of the factors that play a role in living subjects, they have several advantages over clinical trials. The advantages include opportunities to analyze characteristics such as tissue properties and kinematic response to various loading conditions that cannot be done in living humans, being less time-consuming, and being less expensive.

Despite abundant research in the field of anterior cruciate ligament (ACL) injuries, there is still no "gold standard" treatment option for these patients. Residual rotational laxity after recon-

V. Musahl et al. (eds.), *Rotatory Knee Instability*, DOI 10.1007/978-3-319-32070-0_1

struction surgery is one of the main reasons that patients do not return to previous levels of activity [56, 64]. Recent advances in the field of biomechanics have enabled scientists to perform more comprehensive analyses of knee function. This understanding fueled scientists to design the so-called individualized ACL reconstruction surgery with the goal to improve outcomes in these patients [73].

This chapter will review methods applied during in vitro biomechanical studies and then present the role of each knee structure in providing rotational stability as demonstrated by in vitro studies. This knowledge is needed in the management of patients with knee ligamentous injuries and can help clinicians to understand the functional importance of each structure.

1.2 Methods of Biomechanical Studies In Vitro

1.2.1 Models Applied in In Vitro Studies

Human cadaveric specimens are the best models for biomechanical studies. However due to limited availability and related costs, animal models have commonly been used as an alternative. Although no animal model perfectly mimics the human knee, large animals like pigs, sheep, goats, and dogs have been used as a platform for biomechanical studies [11, 22, 28, 32, 33, 72]. It is important that the selected model have as many similarities to the human knee as possible; for instance, porcine knees are a suitable alternative for in vitro studies in terms of anatomical and biomechanical characteristics of the ligaments and mimicking sex-specific characteristics [32, 33, 72].

1.2.2 Methods Applied During In Vitro Studies

1.2.2.1 Devices In Vitro Studies

Electromagnetic tracking devices [1, 4, 5] or surgical navigation systems (with optoelectronic tracking devices) [12, 18, 50] are commonly used to measure joint kinematics while clinicians perform physical examinations on cadaveric knees rather than subjective grading of joint laxity. However, due to variability in performing physical examinations, more attention is directed toward utilization of standardized devices to simulate physical examinations and thus yield more consistent results [55]. At the same time, the mechanical devices used in biomechanical studies to simulate clinical examinations on cadaveric knees include a wide variety of robotic technology. Custom-designed mechanisms and industrial robotic manipulators (Fig. 1.1) enable researchers to standardize rate of loading as well as the magnitude and direction of forces and moments applied to the knee [15, 47, 52, 53, 55]. These devices have a wide range of capabilities such as applying complex loading conditions, measuring joint motion, and determining the force in tissues. Robotic systems are electromechanical machines that have complex control systems using feedback from load cells and motion measurement systems to guide that application of loads to a knee or reproduce joint motion. These systems are either developed specifically for biomechanical studies [23] or were originally developed for industrial purposes and customized to be used in biomechanical studies [15, 52]. Most of these systems can apply loading conditions to a cadaveric specimen and then reproduce the resultant joint motion to examine changes in forces and moments that might occur during alterations to the state of the joint.

1.2.2.2 Pivot-Shift Simulation

Physical examinations can be part of the rotational laxity assessment during in vitro studies [4, 50]. The pivot-shift test is highly valued in assessment of rotational laxity for patients with ACL injury [35]. Application of individual rotational loads and the combined rotational loads that simulate the pivot-shift test is commonly used in in vitro studies to assess rotational laxity. The in vitro simulation of the pivot-shift test typically includes application of valgus and internal rotation torques to the knee, and the resulting

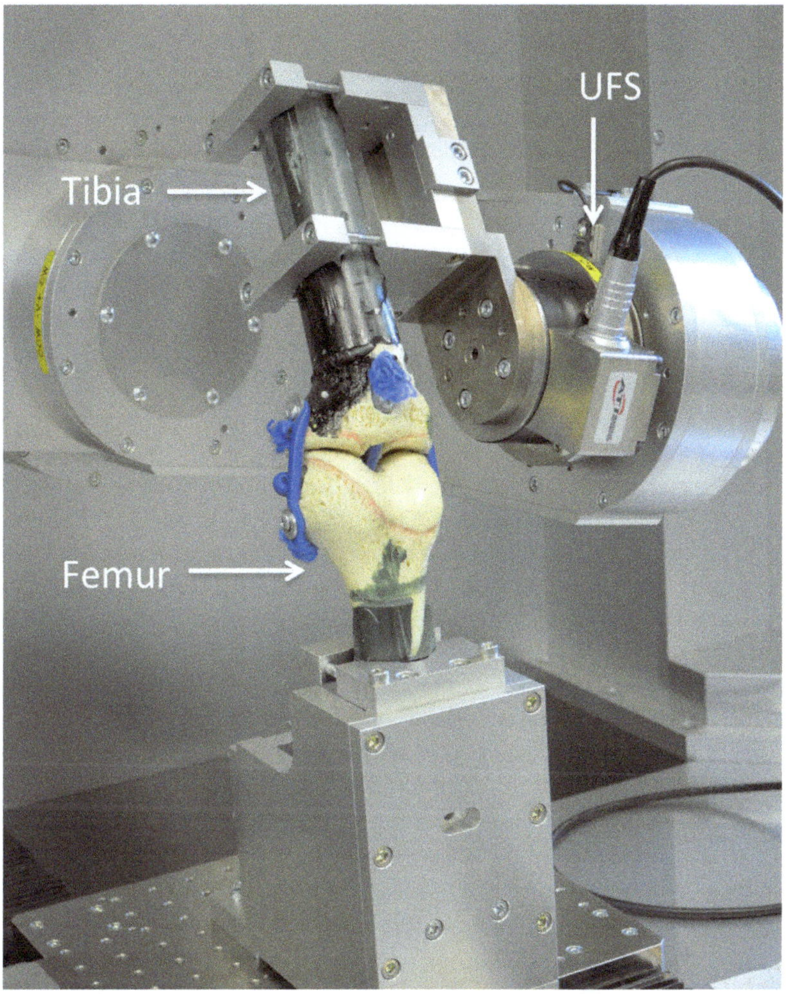

Fig. 1.1 Six degree of freedom robotic manipulator testing a human knee model. The robotic system applies determined loads and records kinematics. *UFS* universal force-moment sensor

anterior tibial translation is reported as the primary outcome [31, 55, 77]. This is justified by studies that showed translation of the tibia relative to the femur is correlated with the clinical grading of the pivot shift [9]. The loading devices can apply these loads at either discrete flexion angles or continuously throughout a range of flexion. Application of the loads at discrete flexion angles narrows the quantity of data obtained which could negatively affect the interpretation of the results. Moreover there is an ongoing debate regarding the clinical utility of static tests versus dynamic tests [54]. Therefore, analyzing knee kinematics continuously throughout the range of flexion is favored compared to static tests [46].

Fact Box 1
Dynamic rotational laxity tests tend to better reproduce complex loads and motions that the joint experiences during activity; therefore they are a better tool for predicting long-term results. Static rotational laxity tests can be easily performed; however, they may not be predictive when compared to dynamic rotational tests.

1.2.2.3 In Situ Force

The in situ force in a structure determines its contribution to joint stability. In addition, relative contributions to joint stability can be compared utilizing this data [63]. The two methods currently utilized to determine the in situ force in a structure are implantable transducers (contact method) [29] and estimation by noncontact methods [14, 43].

1.2.2.4 Contact Method Measuring Tensile Force

In the contact method, the sensors are attached to the ligament to measure tensile force (e.g., buckle transducers) [41] or to measure the strain in the ligament and then estimate the force using a stress-strain curve and cross-sectional area (e.g., liquid metal strain gage and hall-effect transducer) [7, 20]. Measurement of the tensile force directly better estimates the in situ force in a structure since it eliminates potential debate associated with converting strain to force due to variation of cross-sectional area, shape, and material properties along with the length of the ligament. However, contact methods are limited since it is not always feasible to implant sensors in all structures due to technical limitations (e.g., joint capsule, posterolateral bundle (PL) of ACL). Moreover these methods depend on knee flexion angle as well as location and angular orientation of the sensor within the tissue [21, 48].

1.2.2.5 Noncontact Method to Determine In Situ Force

A direct, noncontact method to determine in situ force in a ligament utilizes a universal force-moment sensor (UFS), which measures three forces and moments along and about a Cartesian coordinate system. For a rigid body attached to the UFS, the three forces measured by the sensor define the magnitude and direction of the external force applied to the body. The point of application of the force can also be determined based on evaluation of the three moments measured.

The in situ force in knee structures can also be calculated in a non-direct, noncontact manner without dissection of the joint using the principle of superposition [14, 43]. The principle of superposition requires three fundamental assumptions: (1) there is no interaction between the structures of interest, (2) the bony tissue is rigid relative to the ligaments, and (3) the position of each bone is accurately reproduced [62]. In this method, in situ force is determined by measuring the forces at the knee before and after removing a structure in the joint while reproducing the identical path of motion. Robotic manipulators are typically used to repeat the path of motion before and after removing a structure. The difference in forces before and after removal of the structure represents the in situ force in that structure. Furthermore, this methodology has been used to determine the forces in knee structures during previously recorded in vivo kinematics of the ovine knee joint [30–32]. Optical motion tracking systems were used to obtain the in vivo kinematics of the joint, and after sacrifice of the animals, a robotic system was utilized to reproduce the joint motion during serial resection of multiple knee structures. In the future, better methods of simulation of in vivo activities need to be developed with a special focus on rotational instability.

1.2.2.6 Simulation of In Vivo Study

Although simulation of clinical examinations in vitro provides significant insight to the biomechanical function of the knee structures, these analyses may not generate insight into activities of daily living. Moreover, the interpretation of the results might be limited by ignoring the effect of neuromuscular function during in vivo activities. Thus, in vitro simulation of in vivo activities is also needed. Customized knee simulators have been used to reproduce the function of these structures during daily activities like walking [2, 8, 74, 79, 80, 83]. To reproduce dynamic and active motions, a complex series of forces and torques need to be applied to simulate the combination of muscle tensions and external loads [51, 59, 66].

One example simulator is the Oxford rig (Fig. 1.2) that consists of an ankle unit and a hip unit and allows six degrees of freedom of motion at the knee [16, 45, 87]. Spherical movement of the tibia about the ankle center results in three clinically relevant motions (flexion/extension, abduction/adduction, and internal/external tibial rotation), while the hip unit allows abduction/adduction and flexion/extension. Vertical loads

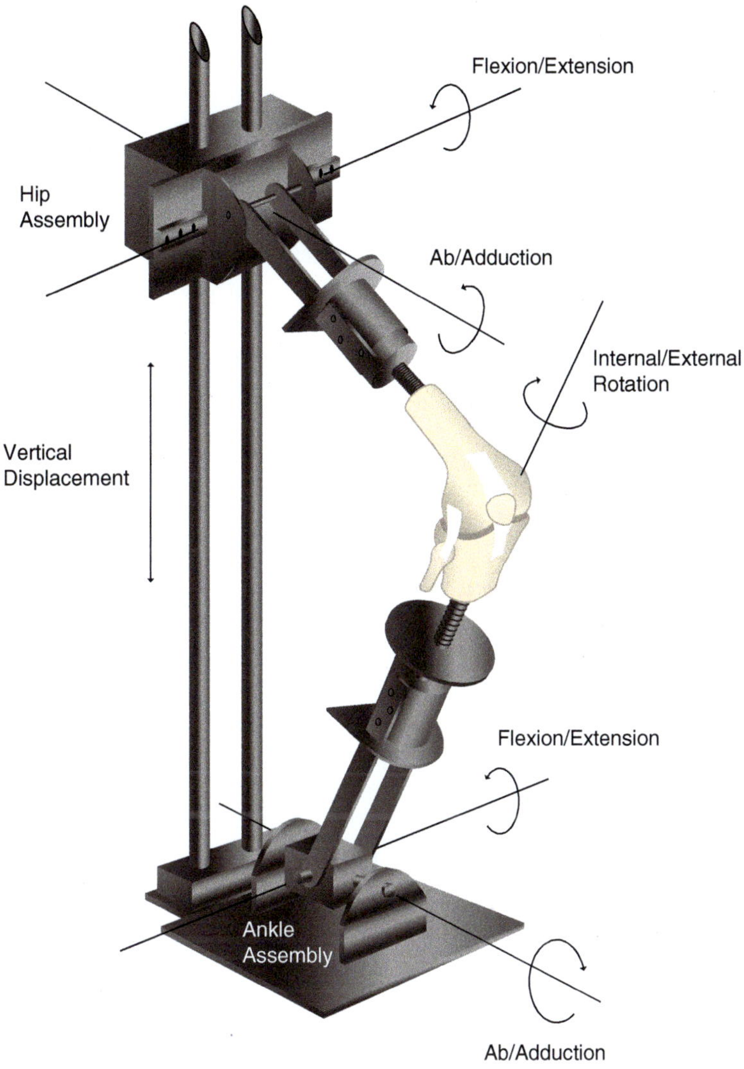

Fig. 1.2 Oxford knee testing rig can make the ankle assembly allow flexion/extension, abduction/adduction, and internal/external tibial rotation. The hip assembly is allowed flexion/extension and abduction/adduction. In addition, the hip assembly can move vertically relative to the ankle assembly

can be applied to simulate body weight by holding assemblies from the hip unit. The rig is used to simulate stance activities with knee flexion, such as the motion during riding a bicycle, rising from a chair, or climbing stairs [87].

1.3 Knee Structures During In Vitro Assessment of Rotational Laxity

Knee motion is mechanically complex with displacements in multiple planes and stability provided by several structures. The relative contribution of these structures to knee stability is described by the concept of primary and secondary restraints [58]. For every plane of knee motion, a primary restraint provides the greatest relative contribution to joint stability, while secondary restraints are engaged to a lesser degree.

1.3.1 ACL

The ACL is one of the most frequently injured structures in the knee joint. This ligament plays a critical role in physiological kinematics of the knee joint, as its disruption eventually causes functional impairment and osteoarthritis [44]. Owing to its unique complex fiber organization, the ACL has a key role in providing both anterior stability and rotational stability.

The ACL restrains internal rotation moments during application of anterior tibial loads, which results in coupled internal rotation of the tibia during anterior tibial translation [24]. Sectioning of the ACL results in a significant increase of rotational laxity [42, 86]. The ACL is generally considered the primary restraint for rotational laxity of the knee. This is supported by studies that demonstrated in presence of an intact ACL, sectioning of the menisci, LCL, posterolateral complex, or anterolateral capsule results in no change in internal or external rotation [42].

The ACL consists of two functional bundles, anteromedial (AM) bundle and posterolateral (PL) bundle, named according to their attachment on the tibia [60]. Both AM and PL bundles work synergistically as a unit to provide knee stability in response to complex loads. More specifically, the PL bundle has a prominent role in controlling rotational and anteroposterior laxity, especially in lower flexion angles (Fig. 1.3) [25, 60, 85]. Increases in anterior tibial translation in response to combined rotational loads after cutting the PL bundle are significantly higher compared to resection of the AM bundle [85]. These facts have implications for the management of patients with ACL injury when ACL reconstruction surgery needs to be designed to restore function of both AM and PL bundles with respect to the patient's native anatomy. The optimal reconstruction would ideally include but not be limited to placement of the tunnels within the native insertion site of the ACL with tunnel aperture area and graft size restoring the native ACL footprint size and the tension replicating the native ACL. A constant technique such as single- or double-bundle ACL reconstruction is not recommended anymore due to variation of anatomy between individuals.

1.3.2 Anterolateral Structures

The role of the anterolateral structures in stability of the knee has been suggested for many years. Dissection of the anterolateral capsule or iliotibial band (ITB) or both results in increased rotational laxity in ACL-deficient knees, indicating a secondary role of these structures in rotational stability [50, 71, 82, 84]. However resection of the ITB may diminish reduction of the tibia during the pivot-shift test [49]. In addition, the ITB acts as an ACL agonist, suggesting that using an ITB graft for extra-articular reconstruction may

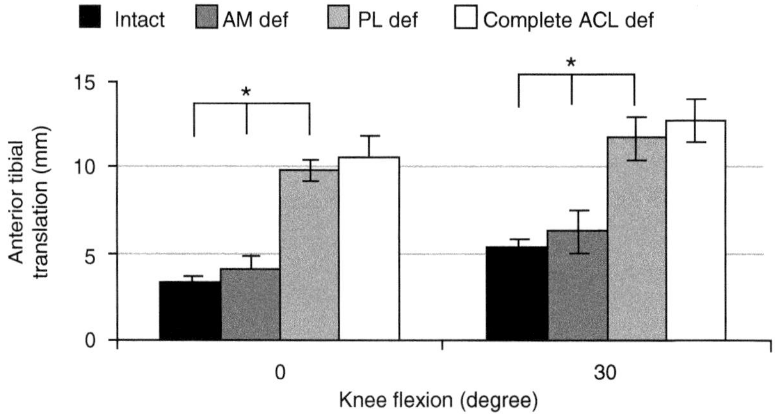

Fig. 1.3 Anterior tibial translation in response to simulated pivot-shift test performed with robotic system. To simulate pivot-shift test, a combined rotational load of 10 Nm valgus and 4 Nm internal tibial torque were applied. Dissection of the posterolateral (*PL*) bundle of the anterior cruciate ligament (*ACL*) resulted in significantly increased in anterior tibial translation when compared to cutting anteromedial (*AM*) bundle

result in hindering its function as a restraint to the knee [84].

Recently there was a resurgence of interest in terms of the role of the anterolateral capsule in rotational stability of the knee with studies reporting a distinct ligament exists in this area [13, 17, 76]. However, the function of this ligament is questionable when considering its dimensions [69]. Despite claims with regard to the primary role of the mid-lateral region of the knee capsule in rotational laxity, the presence of an intact ACL results in no increase of rotational laxity after cutting this structure [42]. However, more quantitative data from biomechanical studies is needed to substantiate the role of this structure.

1.3.3 Lateral and Medial Menisci

Menisci transfer the load from the tibia to the femur and also stabilize the knee during motion. The lateral meniscus has less capsular attachment and posterior wedge effect compared with the medial meniscus [39]. The combined injury of either medial or lateral meniscus in ACL-injured patients is reported to be present in 47–68 % of ACL-injured patients [34, 36, 67]. Concomitant injury to the meniscus significantly increases the risk of future osteoarthritis [44], which can be due to loss of load distribution function of menisci as well as associated increased rotational laxity [3, 6].

Unlike the medial meniscus that is a restraint to anterior translation of the tibia, the lateral meniscus has been shown to control rotational laxity; however, in either case, increased laxity (rotational laxity due to lateral meniscus injury or anterior laxity due to medial meniscus injury) occurs only after the ACL is injured [39, 40, 53]. Therefore the lateral meniscus appears to play a greater role in rotational laxity of ACL-injured patients, especially considering that concomitant injury to the lateral meniscus occurs more commonly with ACL injury [36]. Therefore, during management of patients with ligamentous injury, clinicians should try preserve or repair menisci in order to maintain its functions.

Fact Box 2
Several structures contribute to provide complex multi-planar stability of the knee joint. The ACL is the main restraint to rotational instability during the pivot-shift test. Combined injury to all other structures needs to be appropriately addressed to yield best outcome.

1.3.4 Other Soft Tissue Structures

Injuries to the posterolateral corner do not occur independently, but are often associated with a tear of the ACL [30, 37]. The posterolateral corner structures of the knee consist of the iliotibial tract, the lateral collateral ligament, the popliteus complex, posterior horn of the lateral meniscus, and other soft tissues [70, 75]. The failure rate following ACL reconstructions is thought to be increased [38] when injuries to the posterolateral corner are missed since sectioning of posterolateral corner structures has shown a significant increase of the varus load on the ACL graft. In an ACL-injured knee, internal rotation increases after sectioning the lateral collateral ligament or posterolateral complex, and external rotation increases after cutting the posterolateral complex [42, 86]. Moreover, at 90° of knee flexion, following popliteus complex resection, internal and external rotation was not controlled by the isolated ACL reconstruction. Combined with a complete posterolateral corner lesion, ACL reconstruction was not able to control the rotation at 30 and 90° of knee flexion [10].

The medial collateral ligament (MCL) is the primary stabilizer to valgus rotation [81] and also a secondary stabilizer to anterior translation [61, 65]. In terms of rotational laxity, both MCL and ACL resist internal tibial rotation [65], but MCL also resists external tibial rotation [27]. Dissection of the MCL increases the total rotational laxity of the knee by increasing internal and external rotation [12]. In addition, the MCL plays a significant role during the pivot-shift test when it limits medial movement of the tibia when valgus torque is applied. Therefore in an ACL-deficient knee, the lateral tibial plateau subluxes anteriorly and the tibia rotates internally while the axis of rotation lies close to the MCL [49]. Accordingly, rupture of the MCL decreases the pivot-shift grade of the ACL-deficient knee due to elimination of the tension on the medial compartment [12]. Although these structures may not be the primary restraints, they play a role in rotational stability of the knee. Accordingly, clinicians need to assess injury to all structures and manage them properly.

1.3.5 Bony Morphology

Several studies attempted to investigate the role of bony morphology related to rotational laxity of ACL-deficient knees [19, 26, 57, 78]. Increasing the lateral tibial plateau slope caused anterior translation of the tibial resting position and increases in external rotation of the tibia [19, 26]. In addition, an increase of tibial slope is associated with a decrease in internal rotation in response to an internal rotation torque [57]. In one study when a mechanized device was used to simulate the pivot-shift test, an increase in tibial slope was associated with increased rotational laxity of ACL-deficient knees [78]. Based on current evidence, it seems that the bony morphology of the lateral tibiofemoral compartment, particularly lateral tibial plateau slope, contributes to the grade of the pivot-shift test [49]. However, it is not clear if the slope of the tibial plateau is correlated with residual rotational laxity after ACL reconstruction surgery.

1.3.6 Clinical Significance

Taken together, the ACL plays a primary role in rotational stability of the knee. Injury to the ACL will cause increased abnormal loads to joint cartilage and the secondary restraints, which will result in an increased degeneration of these structures and osteoarthritis [3, 6]. On the other hand, due to load sharing of the structures in the knee, concomitant injuries to secondary restraints can increase the in situ force in the ACL graft tissue after reconstruction surgery and thereby increase failure rate [38]. Thus, concomitant injuries to other knee structures should be addressed with ACL injury in order to restore joint kinematics and yield favorable long-term outcomes.

1.4 Simulation of Activities of Daily Living

Human cadaveric studies have simulated dynamic walking and evaluated kinematics, focusing on the anterior–posterior translation or the contact between the femur and tibia [2, 80]. In these studies, the rotational range of motion and change of contact area were compared between ACL-injured and intact knees during the gait cycle. However, the rotational laxity of the ACL-injured knee could not be assessed due to combined anterior–posterior translation. Stance activities were also simulated to study interaction of quadriceps muscle and ACL on the joint kinematics [68]. The quadriceps muscle was significantly found to control tibial rotation regardless of the ACL status. Moreover, activation of quadriceps will result in increased tension of the graft between 0 and 80° of knee flexion with little effect on full extension. These data can help to design appropriate rehabilitation protocols after ACL reconstruction surgery.

Conclusions

In vitro studies provide insight to the contribution of the knee structures to joint stability by simulation of clinical examinations and activities of daily living. Simulation of pivot-shift test by applying internal rotation and valgus tongues is among the common methods of rotational laxity assessment, whereas activities of daily living are simulated by application of force to the muscles. The function of the ligamentous and bony structures at the knee are complex. However, the ACL is the primary restraint to rotational laxity, and its two-bundle structure needs to be considered during reconstruction surgery. In addition, concomitant injuries to other structures need to be properly addressed to achieve promising outcome. Overall, significant advancements in the understanding of rotational stability and treatment protocols have been made using in vitro studies, and they must be coupled with in vivo studies in the future to further improve clinical care for the knee.

In vitro studies provide feasible way to assess contribution of various factors in knee rotational stability. Based on current evidence, ACL is the main restraint to rotational stability during simulated pivot-shift test and gait analysis: however, other structures play role as well. Accordingly, injuries to other structures and individual inherent characteristics should be considered in the treatment of ACL-injured patients.

References

1. Ahlden M, Araujo P, Hoshino Y, Samuelsson K, Middleton KK, Nagamune K, Karlsson J, Musahl V (2012) Clinical grading of the pivot shift test correlates best with tibial acceleration. Knee Surg Sports Traumatol Arthrosc Off J ESSKA 20(4):708–712
2. Ahmed AM, McLean C (2002) In vitro measurement of the restraining role of the anterior cruciate ligament during walking and stair ascent. J Biomech Eng 124(6):768–779
3. Ajuied A, Wong F, Smith C, Norris M, Earnshaw P, Back D, Davies A (2014) Anterior cruciate ligament injury and radiologic progression of knee osteoarthritis: a systematic review and meta-analysis. Am J Sports Med 42(9):2242–2252
4. Anderson CJ, Westerhaus BD, Pietrini SD, Ziegler CG, Wijdicks CA, Johansen S, Engebretsen L, Laprade RF (2010) Kinematic impact of anteromedial and posterolateral bundle graft fixation angles on double-bundle anterior cruciate ligament reconstructions. Am J Sports Med 38(8):1575–1583
5. Araujo PH, Ahlden M, Hoshino Y, Muller B, Moloney G, Fu FH, Musahl V (2012) Comparison of three non-invasive quantitative measurement systems for the pivot shift test. Knee Surg Sports Traumatol Arthrosc Off J ESSKA 20(4):692–697
6. Atarod M, Frank CB, Shrive NG (2015) Increased meniscal loading after anterior cruciate ligament transection in vivo: a longitudinal study in sheep. Knee 22(1):11–17
7. Bach JM, Hull ML, Patterson HA (1997) Direct measurement of strain in the posterolateral bundle of the anterior cruciate ligament. J Biomech 30(3):281–283
8. Bedi A, Chen T, Santner TJ, El-Amin S, Kelly NH, Warren RF, Maher SA (2013) Changes in dynamic medial tibiofemoral contact mechanics and kinematics after injury of the anterior cruciate ligament: a cadaveric model. Proc Inst Mech Eng H 227(9):1027–1037
9. Bedi A, Musahl V, Lane C, Citak M, Warren RF, Pearle AD (2010) Lateral compartment translation predicts the grade of pivot shift: a cadaveric and clinical analysis. Knee Surg Sports Traumatol Arthrosc Off J ESSKA 18(9):1269–1276
10. Bonanzinga T, Signorelli C, Lopomo N, Grassi A, Neri MP, Filardo G, Zaffagnini S, Marcacci M (2015) Biomechanical effect of posterolateral corner sectioning after ACL injury and reconstruction. Knee Surg Sports Traumatol Arthrosc Off J ESSKA 23(10):2918–2924
11. Bozynski CC, Kuroki K, Stannard JP, Smith PA, Stoker AM, Cook CR, Cook JL (2015) Evaluation of partial transection versus synovial debridement of the ACL as Novel Canine Models for Management of ACL injuries. J Knee Surg 28(5):404–410
12. Cavaignac E, Carpentier K, Pailhe R, Luyckx T, Bellemans J (2015) The role of the deep medial collateral ligament in controlling rotational stability of the knee. Knee Surg Sports Traumatol Arthrosc Off J ESSKA 23(10):3101–7
13. Claes S, Vereecke E, Maes M, Victor J, Verdonk P, Bellemans J (2013) Anatomy of the anterolateral ligament of the knee. J Anat 223(4):321–328
14. Darcy SP, Kilger RH, Woo SL, Debski RE (2006) Estimation of ACL forces by reproducing knee kinematics between sets of knees: a novel non-invasive methodology. J Biomech 39(13):2371–2377
15. Debandi A, Maeyama A, Lu S, Hume C, Asai S, Goto B, Hoshino Y, Smolinski P, Fu FH (2011) Biomechanical comparison of three anatomic ACL reconstructions in a porcine model. Knee Surg Sports Traumatol Arthrosc Off J ESSKA 19(5):728–735
16. Didden K, Luyckx T, Bellemans J, Labey L, Innocenti B, Vandenneucker H (2010) Anteroposterior positioning of the tibial component and its effect on the mechanics of patellofemoral contact. J Bone Joint Surg 92(10):1466–1470
17. Dombrowski M, Costello J, Ohashi B, Murawski C, Friel N, Arilla F, Rothrauff B, Fu F, Musahl V (2015) Macroscopic anatomic, histologic, and magnetic resonance imaging correlation of the lateral capsule of the knee. Paper presented at the Orthopaedic Research Society; Las Vegas
18. Feng H, Song GY, Shen JW, Zhang H, Wang MY (2014) The "lateral gutter drive-through" sign revisited: a cadaveric study exploring its real mechanism based on the individual posterolateral structure of knee joints. Arch Orthop Trauma Surg 134(12):1745–1751
19. Fening SD, Kovacic J, Kambic H, McLean S, Scott J, Miniaci A (2008) The effects of modified posterior tibial slope on anterior cruciate ligament strain and knee kinematics: a human cadaveric study. J Knee Surg 21(3):205–211

20. Fleming BC, Beynnon BD, Tohyama H, Johnson RJ, Nichols CE, Renstrom P, Pope MH (1994) Determination of a zero strain reference for the anteromedial band of the anterior cruciate ligament. J Orthop Res Off Pub Orthop Res Soc 12(6):789–795
21. Fleming BC, Peura GD, Beynnon BD (2000) Factors influencing the output of an implantable force transducer. J Biomech 33(7):889–893
22. Frank CB, Beveridge JE, Huebner KD, Heard BJ, Tapper JE, O'Brien EJ, Shrive NG (2012) Complete ACL/MCL deficiency induces variable degrees of instability in sheep with specific kinematic abnormalities correlating with degrees of early osteoarthritis. J Orthop Res Off Pub Orthop Res Soc 30(3):384–392
23. Fujie H, Sekito T, Orita A (2004) A novel robotic system for joint biomechanical tests: application to the human knee joint. J Biomech Eng 126(1):54–61
24. Fukubayashi T, Torzilli PA, Sherman MF, Warren RF (1982) An in vitro biomechanical evaluation of anterior-posterior motion of the knee. Tibial displacement, rotation, and torque. J Bone Joint Surg Am 64(2):258–264
25. Gabriel MT, Wong EK, Woo SL, Yagi M, Debski RE (2004) Distribution of in situ forces in the anterior cruciate ligament in response to rotatory loads. J Orthop Res Off Pub Orthop Res Soc 22(1):85–89
26. Giffin JR, Vogrin TM, Zantop T, Woo SL, Harner CD (2004) Effects of increasing tibial slope on the biomechanics of the knee. Am J Sports Med 32(2):376–382
27. Haimes JL, Wroble RR, Grood ES, Noyes FR (1994) Role of the medial structures in the intact and anterior cruciate ligament-deficient knee. Limits of motion in the human knee. Am J Sports Med 22(3):402–409
28. Hensler D, Illingworth KD, Musahl V, Working ZM, Kobayashi T, Miyawaki M, Lorenz S, Witt M, Irrgang JJ, Huard J, Fu FH (2015) Does fibrin clot really enhance graft healing after double-bundle ACL reconstruction in a caprine model? Knee Surg Sports Traumatol Arthrosc Off J ESSKA 23(3):669–679
29. Howe JG, Wertheimer C, Johnson RJ, Nichols CE, Pope MH, Beynnon B (1990) Arthroscopic strain gauge measurement of the normal anterior cruciate ligament. Arthroscopy J Arthroscopic Related Surg Off Pub Arthroscopy Asso N Am Int Arthroscopy Asso 6(3):198–204
30. Hughston JC, Jacobson KE (1985) Chronic posterolateral rotatory instability of the knee. J Bone Joint Surg Am 67(3):351–359
31. Kanamori A, Zeminski J, Rudy TW, Li G, Fu FH, Woo SL (2002) The effect of axial tibial torque on the function of the anterior cruciate ligament: a biomechanical study of a simulated pivot shift test. Arthroscopy J Arthroscopic Related Surg Off Pub Arthroscopy Asso N Am Int Arthroscopy Asso 18(4):394–398
32. Kato Y, Ingham SJ, Linde-Rosen M, Smolinski P, Horaguchi T, Fu FH (2010) Biomechanics of the porcine triple bundle anterior cruciate ligament. Knee Surg Sports Traumatol Arthrosc Off J ESSKA 18(1):20–25
33. Kiapour AM, Shalvoy MR, Murray MM, Fleming BC (2015) Validation of porcine knee as a sex-specific model to study human anterior cruciate ligament disorders. Clin Orthop Relat Res 473(2):639–650
34. Kilcoyne KG, Dickens JF, Haniuk E, Cameron KL, Owens BD (2012) Epidemiology of meniscal injury associated with ACL tears in young athletes. Orthopedics 35(3):208–212
35. Kocher MS, Steadman JR, Briggs KK, Sterett WI, Hawkins RJ (2004) Relationships between objective assessment of ligament stability and subjective assessment of symptoms and function after anterior cruciate ligament reconstruction. Am J Sports Med 32(3):629–634
36. Krinsky MB, Abdenour TE, Starkey C, Albo RA, Chu DA (1992) Incidence of lateral meniscus injury in professional basketball players. Am J Sports Med 20(1):17–19
37. Krukhaug Y, Molster A, Rodt A, Strand T (1998) Lateral ligament injuries of the knee. Knee Surg Sports Traumatol Arthrosc Off J ESSKA 6(1):21–25
38. LaPrade RF, Resig S, Wentorf F, Lewis JL (1999) The effects of grade III posterolateral knee complex injuries on anterior cruciate ligament graft force. A biomechanical analysis. Am J Sports Med 27(4):469–475
39. Levy IM, Torzilli PA, Gould JD, Warren RF (1989) The effect of lateral meniscectomy on motion of the knee. J Bone Joint Surg Am 71(3):401–406
40. Levy IM, Torzilli PA, Warren RF (1982) The effect of medial meniscectomy on anterior-posterior motion of the knee. J Bone Joint Surg Am 64(6):883–888
41. Lew WD, Lewis JL (1982) The effect of knee-prosthesis geometry on cruciate ligament mechanics during flexion. J Bone Joint Surg Am 64(5):734–739
42. Lipke JM, Janecki CJ, Nelson CL, McLeod P, Thompson C, Thompson J, Haynes DW (1981) The role of incompetence of the anterior cruciate and lateral ligaments in anterolateral and anteromedial instability. A biomechanical study of cadaver knees. J Bone Joint Surg Am 63(6):954–960
43. Livesay GA, Fujie H, Kashiwaguchi S, Morrow DA, Fu FH, Woo SL (1995) Determination of the in situ forces and force distribution within the human anterior cruciate ligament. Ann Biomed Eng 23(4):467–474
44. Lohmander LS, Englund PM, Dahl LL, Roos EM (2007) The long-term consequence of anterior cruciate ligament and meniscus injuries: osteoarthritis. Am J Sports Med 35(10):1756–1769
45. Luyckx T, Didden K, Vandenneucker H, Labey L, Innocenti B, Bellemans J (2009) Is there a biomechanical explanation for anterior knee pain in patients with patella alta?: influence of patellar height on patellofemoral contact force, contact area and contact pressure. J Bone Joint Surg 91(3):344–350
46. Markolf KL, Jackson SR, Foster B, McAllister DR (2014) ACL forces and knee kinematics produced

by axial tibial compression during a passive flexion-extension cycle. J Orthop Res Off Pub Orthop Res Soc 32(1):89–95
47. Markolf KL, Park S, Jackson SR, McAllister DR (2008) Simulated pivot-shift testing with single and double-bundle anterior cruciate ligament reconstructions. J Bone Joint Surg Am 90(8):1681–1689
48. Markolf KL, Willems MJ, Jackson SR, Finerman GA (1998) In situ calibration of miniature sensors implanted into the anterior cruciate ligament part II: force probe measurements. J Orthop Res Off Pub Orthop Res Soc 16(4):464–471
49. Matsumoto H (1990) Mechanism of the pivot shift. J Bone Joint Surg 72(5):816–821
50. Monaco E, Ferretti A, Labianca L, Maestri B, Speranza A, Kelly MJ, D'Arrigo C (2012) Navigated knee kinematics after cutting of the ACL and its secondary restraint. Knee Surg Sports Traumatol Arthrosc Off J ESSKA 20(5):870–877
51. Morrison JB (1970) The mechanics of the knee joint in relation to normal walking. J Biomech 3(1):51–61
52. Musahl V, Burkart A, Debski RE, Van Scyoc A, Fu FH, Woo SL (2002) Accuracy of anterior cruciate ligament tunnel placement with an active robotic system: a cadaveric study. Arthroscopy J Arthroscopic Related Surg Off Pub Arthroscopy Asso N Am Int Arthroscopy Asso 18(9):968–973
53. Musahl V, Citak M, O'Loughlin PF, Choi D, Bedi A, Pearle AD (2010) The effect of medial versus lateral meniscectomy on the stability of the anterior cruciate ligament-deficient knee. Am J Sports Med 38(8):1591–1597
54. Musahl V, Seil R, Zaffagnini S, Tashman S, Karlsson J (2012) The role of static and dynamic rotatory laxity testing in evaluating ACL injury. Knee Surg Sports Traumatol Arthrosc Off J ESSKA 20(4):603–612
55. Musahl V, Voos J, O'Loughlin PF, Stueber V, Kendoff D, Pearle AD (2010) Mechanized pivot shift test achieves greater accuracy than manual pivot shift test. Knee Surg Sports Traumatol Arthrosc Off J ESSKA 18(9):1208–1213
56. Nakamura S, Kobayashi M, Asano T, Arai R, Nakagawa Y, Nakamura T (2011) Image-matching technique can detect rotational and AP instabilities in chronic ACL-deficient knees. Knee Surg Sports Traumatol Arthrosc Off J ESSKA 19(Suppl 1):S69–S76
57. Nelitz M, Seitz AM, Bauer J, Reichel H, Ignatius A, Durselen L (2013) Increasing posterior tibial slope does not raise anterior cruciate ligament strain but decreases tibial rotation ability. Clini Biomech 28(3):285–290
58. Noyes FR, Grood ES, Butler DL, Raterman L (1980) Knee ligament tests: what do they really mean? Phys Ther 60(12):1578–1581
59. Patriarco AG, Mann RW, Simon SR, Mansour JM (1981) An evaluation of the approaches of optimization models in the prediction of muscle forces during human gait. J Biomech 14(8):513–525
60. Petersen W, Zantop T (2007) Anatomy of the anterior cruciate ligament with regard to its two bundles. Clin Orthop Relat Res 454:35–47
61. Piziali RL, Seering WP, Nagel DA, Schurman DJ (1980) The function of the primary ligaments of the knee in anterior-posterior and medial-lateral motions. J Biomech 13(9):777–784
62. Rudy TW, Livesay GA, Woo SL, Fu FH (1996) A combined robotic/universal force sensor approach to determine in situ forces of knee ligaments. J Biomech 29(10):1357–1360
63. Sakane M, Livesay GA, Fox RJ, Rudy TW, Runco TJ, Woo SL (1999) Relative contribution of the ACL, MCL, and bony contact to the anterior stability of the knee. Knee Surg Sports Traumatol Arthrosc Off J ESSKA 7(2):93–97
64. Scanlan SF, Chaudhari AM, Dyrby CO, Andriacchi TP (2010) Differences in tibial rotation during walking in ACL reconstructed and healthy contralateral knees. J Biomech 43(9):1817–1822
65. Seering WP, Piziali RL, Nagel DA, Schurman DJ (1980) The function of the primary ligaments of the knee in varus-valgus and axial rotation. J Biomech 13(9):785–794
66. Seireg A, Arvikar (1975) The prediction of muscular lad sharing and joint forces in the lower extremities during walking. J Biomech 8(2):89–102
67. Sharifah MI, Lee CL, Suraya A, Johan A, Syed AF, Tan SP (2015) Accuracy of MRI in the diagnosis of meniscal tears in patients with chronic ACL tears. Knee Surg Sports Traumatol Arthrosc Off J ESSKA 23(3):826–830
68. Shoemaker SC, Adams D, Daniel DM, Woo SL (1993) Quadriceps/anterior cruciate graft interaction. An in vitro study of joint kinematics and anterior cruciate ligament graft tension. Clin Orthop Relat Res 294:379–390
69. Stijak L, Bumbasirevic M, Radonjic V, Kadija M, Puskas L, Milovanovic D, Filipovic B (2014) Anatomic description of the anterolateral ligament of the knee. Knee Surg Sports Traumatol Arthrosc Off J ESSKA. doi:10.1007/s00167-014-3422-6
70. Sudasna S, Harnsiriwattanagit K (1990) The ligamentous structures of the posterolateral aspect of the knee. Bull Hosp Jt Dis Orthop Inst 50(1):35–40
71. Suero EM, Njoku IU, Voigt MR, Lin J, Koenig D, Pearle AD (2013) The role of the iliotibial band during the pivot shift test. Knee Surg Sports Traumatol Arthrosc Off J ESSKA 21(9):2096–2100
72. Tantisricharoenkul G, Linde-Rosen M, Araujo P, Zhou J, Smolinski P, Fu FH (2014) Anterior cruciate ligament: an anatomical exploration in humans and in a selection of animal species. Knee Surg Sports Traumatol Arthrosc Off J ESSKA 22(5):961–971
73. van Eck CF, Widhalm H, Murawski C, Fu FH (2015) Individualized anatomic anterior cruciate ligament reconstruction. Phys Sportsmed 43(1):87–92
74. van Houtem M, Clough R, Khan A, Harrison M, Blunn GW (2006) Validation of the soft tissue restraints in a

force-controlled knee simulator. Proc Inst Mech Eng H 220(3):449–456
75. Veltri DM, Deng XH, Torzilli PA, Maynard MJ, Warren RF (1996) The role of the popliteofibular ligament in stability of the human knee. A biomechanical study. Am J Sports Med 24(1):19–27
76. Vincent JP, Magnussen RA, Gezmez F, Uguen A, Jacobi M, Weppe F, Al-Saati MF, Lustig S, Demey G, Servien E, Neyret P (2012) The anterolateral ligament of the human knee: an anatomic and histologic study. Knee Surg Sports Traumatol Arthrosc Off J ESSKA 20(1):147–152
77. Voos JE, Musahl V, Maak TG, Wickiewicz TL, Pearle AD (2010) Comparison of tunnel positions in single-bundle anterior cruciate ligament reconstructions using computer navigation. Knee Surg Sports Traumatol Arthrosc Off J ESSKA 18(9):1282–1289
78. Voos JE, Suero EM, Citak M, Petrigliano FP, Bosscher MR, Citak M, Wickiewicz TL, Pearle AD (2012) Effect of tibial slope on the stability of the anterior cruciate ligament-deficient knee. Knee Surg Sports Traumatol Arthrosc Off J ESSKA 20(8):1626–1631
79. Walker PS, Blunn GW, Broome DR, Perry J, Watkins A, Sathasivam S, Dewar ME, Paul JP (1997) A knee simulating machine for performance evaluation of total knee replacements. J Biomech 30(1):83–89
80. Wang H, Chen T, Koff MF, Hutchinson ID, Gilbert S, Choi D, Warren RF, Rodeo SA, Maher SA (2014) Image based weighted center of proximity versus directly measured knee contact location during simulated gait. J Biomech 47(10):2483–2489
81. Woo SL, Young EP, Ohland KJ, Marcin JP, Horibe S, Lin HC (1990) The effects of transection of the anterior cruciate ligament on healing of the medial collateral ligament. A biomechanical study of the knee in dogs. J Bone Joint Surg Am 72(3):382–392
82. Wroble RR, Grood ES, Cummings JS, Henderson JM, Noyes FR (1993) The role of the lateral extraarticular restraints in the anterior cruciate ligament-deficient knee. Am J Sports Med 21(2):257–262; discussion 263
83. Wunschel M, Muller O, Lo J, Obloh C, Wulker N (2010) The anterior cruciate ligament provides resistance to externally applied anterior tibial force but not to internal rotational torque during simulated weight-bearing flexion. Arthroscopy J Arthroscopic Related Surg Off Pub Arthroscopy Asso N Am Int Arthroscopy Asso 26(11):1520–1527
84. Yamamoto Y, Hsu WH, Fisk JA, Van Scyoc AH, Miura K, Woo SL (2006) Effect of the iliotibial band on knee biomechanics during a simulated pivot shift test. J Orthop Res Off Pub Orthop Res Soc 24(5):967–973
85. Zantop T, Herbort M, Raschke MJ, Fu FH, Petersen W (2007) The role of the anteromedial and posterolateral bundles of the anterior cruciate ligament in anterior tibial translation and internal rotation. Am J Sports Med 35(2):223–227
86. Zantop T, Schumacher T, Diermann N, Schanz S, Raschke MJ, Petersen W (2007) Anterolateral rotational knee instability: role of posterolateral structures. Winner of the AGA-DonJoy Award 2006. Arch Orthop Trauma Surg 127(9):743–752
87. Zavatsky AB (1997) A kinematic-freedom analysis of a flexed-knee-stance testing rig. J Biomech 30(3):277–280

2 Anatomy and Function of the Anterolateral Capsule Structures

Daniel Guenther, Sebastián Irarrázaval, Chad Griffith, Volker Musahl, and Richard Debski

Contents

D. Guenther
Department of Orthopaedic Surgery, University of Pittsburgh, Kaufman Medical Building, Suite 1011, 3941 Fifth Avenue, Pittsburgh, 15203 PA, USA

Trauma Department, Hannover Medical School (MHH), Carl-Neuberg-Str. 1, Hannover, 30625, Germany
e-mail: guenther.daniel@mh-hannover.de

S. Irarrázaval • C. Griffith • R. Debski
Department of Orthopaedic Surgery, University of Pittsburgh, Kaufman Medical Building, Suite 1011, 3941 Fifth Avenue, Pittsburgh, PA 15203, USA
e-mail: sirarraz@gmail.com; cjgriffith@gmail.com; genesis1@pitt.edu

V. Musahl (✉)
Department of Orthopaedic Surgery, UPMC Center for Sports Medicine, Pittsburgh, PA, USA
e-mail: vmusahl@gmail.com

2.1 Introduction

The interplay between the static and dynamic stabilizers of the knee joint is complex. The lateral side of the knee is especially reliant on these stabilizers due to inherent bony instability from the opposing convex surfaces [45]. The joint capsule is a dense, fibrous connective tissue that is attached to the bones via attachment zones. Injuries frequently occur via avulsion of a bone fragment beneath the attachment zone or by tearing of the tendon, ligament, or capsule above it [46]. The capsular attachment can be described with four zones: pure fibrous tissue, uncalcified fibrocartilage, calcified fibrocartilage, and bone [10]. It can vary in thickness according to the stresses to which it is subjected and can be locally thickened to form capsular ligaments and may even incorporate tendons [38].

Biomechanically and anatomically, the structures of the anterolateral capsule have held multiple names throughout history. While there is disagreement in terms of anatomical descriptions,

V. Musahl et al. (eds.), *Rotatory Knee Instability*, DOI 10.1007/978-3-319-32070-0_2

the majority of past and present articles state that a ligamentous structure is present, whose origin is close to the lateral femoral epicondyle and whose insertion is slightly inferior to the tibial articular surface posterior to Gerdy's tubercle. However, there is still a broad variation in the literature regarding both the frequency with which the ligament can be identified and its morphology as a capsular thickening or distinct ligament. There is a lack of biomechanical studies in terms of the function of this structure. Despite the paucity of biomechanical studies, some researchers propose surgical treatment for anterolateral capsular injuries.

2.2 Anatomy of the Anterolateral Capsule Structures

2.2.1 Historical Descriptions

The earliest known descriptions of a pearly, resistant, fibrous band in the anterolateral compartment were made by Segond [39]. Hughston later described a lateral capsular ligament as a thickening of the capsule, which is divided into anterior, middle, and posterior thirds. He also divided the structure into menisco-femoral and menisco-tibial components [22]. Other studies described an anterior oblique bundle, which originated from the lateral collateral ligament and inserted at the lateral midportion of the tibia, blending with posterior fibers of the iliotibial tract [7, 23]. The intimate relationship between the anterolateral capsule and the iliotibial band was frequently mentioned in the previous literature. In fact, the capsulo-osseous layer has been called the "true knee anterolateral ligament" [43]. Attachments between the capsulo-osseous layer of the iliotibial band and the ACL create an inverted horseshoe sling (Fig. 2.1) around the posterior femoral condyle, preventing the anterolateral tibial subluxation that occurs during the pivot-shift test [42, 43]. Despite the different historical descriptions, there is no clear consensus in terms of the anatomy of the anterolateral capsule structures.

Fact Box 1

Anatomy of the Anterolateral Capsule Structures

1. There is no clear consensus in terms of the anatomy of the anterolateral capsular structures.
2. An anterolateral ligament has not been discovered in human fetal dissections to date.
3. Histologically, the collagenous organization of the anterolateral capsule structures is not as aligned as the collagenous organization of the lateral collateral ligament.

2.2.2 Development of Anterolateral Structures

Development of the anterolateral capsule has been observed in the fetus as early as 8 weeks. During O'Rahilly stage 22 and 23, the articular capsule becomes visible and densification of the condylo-patellar ligaments is evident. From the lateral margins of the patella, the articular capsule surrounds the femoral condyles and becomes attached to the peripheral surface of the menisci [29, 30]. The fetal appearance of intracapsular structures is poorly described in the current literature, and a distinct anterolateral ligament has not been discovered in human fetal observation to date.

2.2.3 Histology

Histological studies have shown that parts of the anterolateral capsule are organized into individual bundles, most likely a combination of multiple thickenings of the capsule and not a homogenous ligamentous entity, such as the

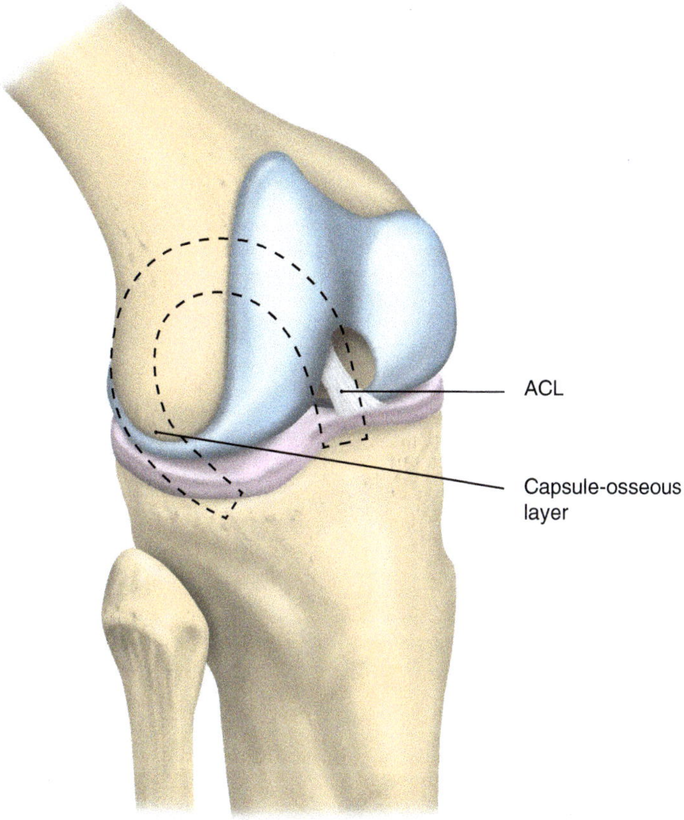

Fig. 2.1 Attachments between the capsulo-osseous layer of the iliotibial band and the *ACL* create an inverted horseshoe sling around the posterior femoral condyle, preventing anterolateral tibial subluxation that occurs during the pivot-shift test [42, 43]

ACL [8]. However, the femoral and tibial attachments of this structure contain a consistent collagenous pattern. Histologically, the transition between the anterolateral capsule, mineralized cartilage, and bone indicates a ligamentous tissue. Immunohistochemistry indicates that this part of the capsule has peripheral nervous innervation and mechanoreceptors [8]. Other studies describe a distinct fibrous structure in contact with the synovium [44] or dense connective tissue with arranged fibers and little cellular material [18]. A more recent study [12] described the histology of the thickenings of the anterolateral capsule, as identified by MRI (Fig. 2.2). The thickening appeared as a transition from loose connective tissue, similar to the capsule, to an organized structure similar to ligamentous tissue. In the area of the thickening, elongated nuclei were positioned between aligned collagen. Histologically, the collagenous organization of the anterolateral capsular structures was not as aligned in the same manner as the collagenous organization of the lateral collateral ligament (Fig. 2.3).

2.2.4 The Anterolateral Ligament

In the early twenty-first century, studies presented several new approaches to evaluate the anterolateral capsular structures. In one study, after resection of the skin, subcutaneous fat tissue, and the iliotibial band, the knee was flexed to 60°, and an internal tibial torque was applied. All

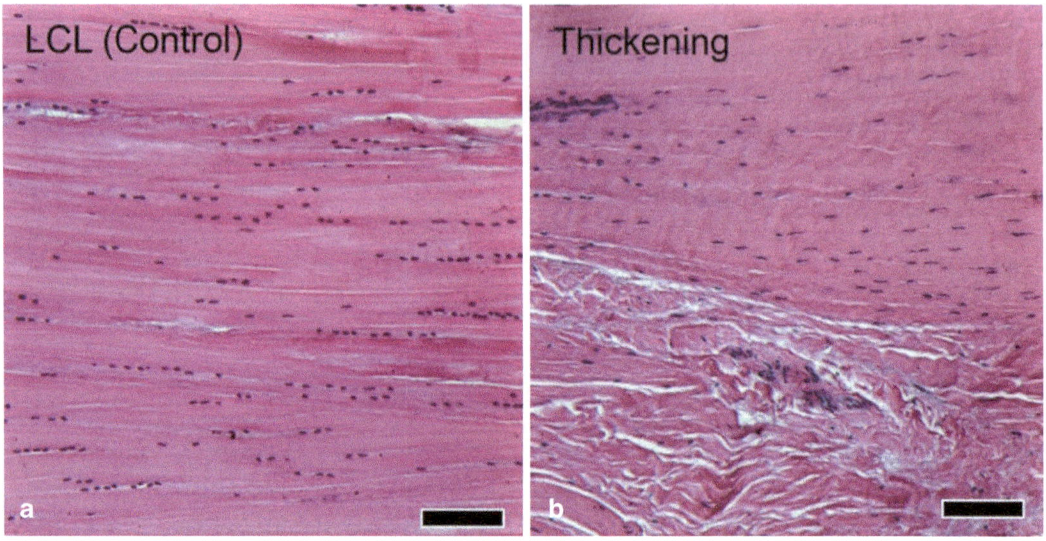

Fig. 2.2 MRI with (**a**) and without (**b**) thickening of the lateral capsule (t2 fat sat sequence). The arrows indicate the anterolateral capsule

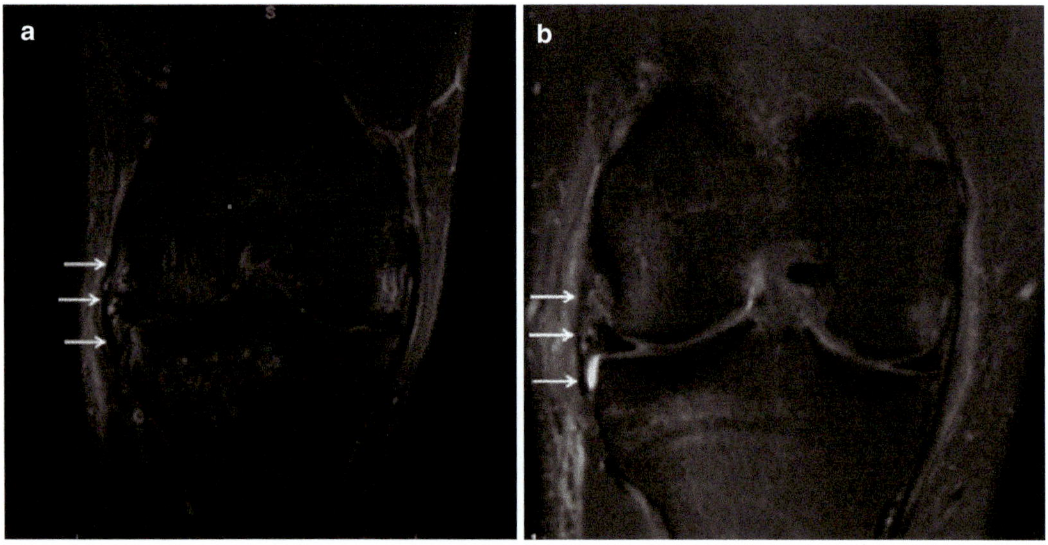

Fig. 2.3 Histologic comparison of the lateral collateral ligament (LCL) (**a**) and a thickening of the anterolateral capsule (**b**), which was confirmed by MRI prior to the dissection (scale = 100 μm)

visible distinct fibers were isolated at the proximal tibia, posterior and proximal to Gerdy's tubercle, and on the lateral femur [9]. In another approach, varus and internal rotational forces were applied between 30° and 60° flexion to highlight any structure coming under tension. Any tissue in the anterolateral region of the knee that did not come under tension was resected, leaving only a ligamentous structure intact [8]. Other authors tightened the lateral joint capsule until a ligament became visible. In addition, they examined 30 patients undergoing knee arthroplasty. In all 30 cases, they identified and dissected a ligamentous structure free from the lateral joint capsule [44]. Dodds et al. [11] studied disarticulated knees with only the anterolateral capsular structures remaining intact. Then, using transillumination, they identified a potential capsular thickening above and below the lateral meniscus. Another study described the structure as a variable thickening of the knee joint capsule [41]. The authors found a continuation of the iliotibial band, a broad, translucent fibrous band connecting the lateral femoral epicondyle to a point on the proximal tibia centered between Gerdy's tubercle and the fibular head.

The soft tissue attachments of the anterolateral ligament are controversial in the literature. Some studies describe an attachment between the ligament and the lateral meniscus [8, 9, 18, 41]. Other studies claim that the structure does not insert into the rim of the lateral meniscus, although there were branching attachments to it [11]. Still others mention that the majority of fibers came close to the meniscal tissue, but continued without interruption toward the tibial plateau [44]. Despite a plethora of anatomical descriptions of the anterolateral ligament in the literature, there is no consensus in terms of its structure and biomechanical function (Fig. 2.4).

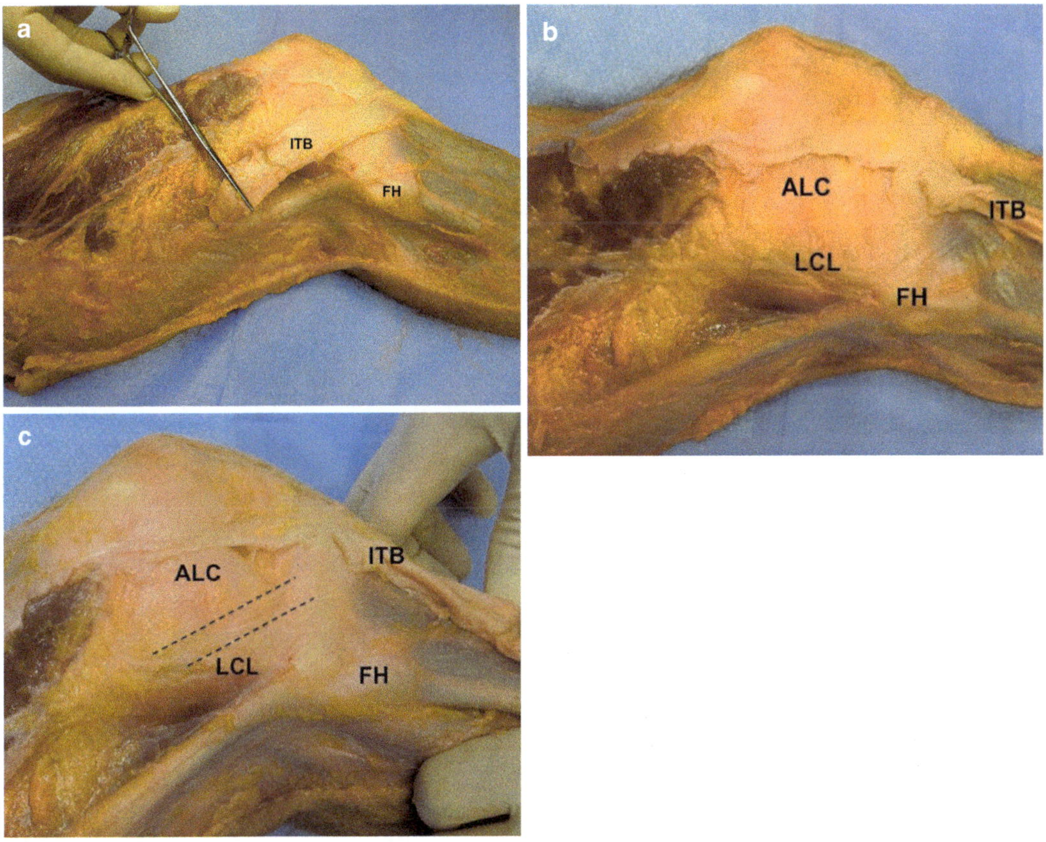

Fig. 2.4 Dissection of the anterolateral capsule structures of the knee. The iliotibial band is carefully detached from the underlying tissue (**a**). In neutral tibial rotation, no clear anterolateral ligamentous structure is present (**b**). When the tibia is manually internal rotated, fibers of the capsule come under tension and a ligament seems to be present (indicated by the dashed lines). However, macroscopic differentiation between a ligament and a thickening of the capsule seems to be impossible (**c**). *LCL* lateral collateral ligament, *FH* fibula head, *ITB* iliotibial band, *ALC* anterolateral capsule.

2.2.5 Anatomic Considerations in Surgical Treatment of Anterolateral Instability

Clinical interest exists as to whether anterolateral capsular injuries in ACL-deficient knees should be surgically addressed at the time of ACL surgery. Some have postulated that a combined intra- and extra-articular reconstruction can restore postoperative laxity and decrease the incidence of posttraumatic arthritis [15, 32]. Multiple techniques and grafts have been described [6, 24, 28, 40]. Mechanical and structural properties of the capsule must be determined to prevent over-constraint of the knee due to non-anatomical graft stiffness and placement. In 2001, Anderson et al. failed to demonstrate benefit of extra-articular tenodesis over intra-articular ACL reconstruction [1]. However, studies have shown excellent long-term results with high satisfaction and few signs of osteoarthritis [27, 37]. One randomized study reported better clinical results and faster return to sport at 5 years' follow-up in patients treated with single-bundle ACL reconstruction plus lateral capsuloplasty compared with single-bundle four-strand hamstrings or patellar tendon [48]. More research is, however, required to establish treatment algorithms based on the individual's anatomy.

2.3 Function of the Anterolateral Capsule Structures

2.3.1 Rotational Stability

Similar to the menisci, the anterolateral capsule is a secondary stabilizer of anterior translation and rotation of the lateral knee compartment [31]. Combined injury to the ACL and anterolateral structures causes increased anterior translation in flexion, as well as in extension, and increased internal rotation at 90° of flexion [47]. Moreover, cadaveric navigation studies showed an increase in pivot-shift grade after sectioning the antero lateral capsule or anterolateral ligament compared with isolated ACL sectioning, suggesting its importance in the control of dynamic rotational laxity [31].

A recent study measured changes in the length of a ligamentous structure in eight knees from 0° to 90° of flexion during application of neutral, internal, and external rotation torques. Small metal eyelets were screwed into the bone at the origin and the insertion of the structure, and the changes in the distance between eyelets were measured using a monofilament suture and a linear variable displacement transducer [11]. Another study measured the strain in the anterolateral complex using polydimethylsiloxane gauges [49]. Recently, a study evaluating the biomechanical function of the capsular structures using robotic technology suggested that these structures are important stabilizers of internal rotation at higher knee flexion angles [35]. The biomechanical studies are a subject of current controversy [17, 36].

Fact Box 2

Function of the Anterolateral Capsule Structures

1. Despite a plethora of anatomical descriptions of the anterolateral ligament in the literature, there is no consensus in terms of its structure and biomechanical function.
2. The published biomechanical studies are a subject of current controversy.
3. The anterolateral capsule becomes an important restraint to anterior tibial load and internal rotation torque in the ACL-deficient knee.
4. Increased strain may lead to plastic deformation and, in rare cases, to tears of the fibrous tissue.
5. More research is required to establish treatment algorithms based on individual anatomy.

2.3.2 Injury Mechanisms to the Anterolateral Capsule

The first description of an injury to the lateral capsular ligament was an avulsion fracture [39]. The Segond fracture is said to result from an avulsion of the lateral proximal tibia due to the insertion of a ligamentous structure. The fact that the anterolateral capsule becomes an important restraint to anterior tibial load and internal rotation torque in the ACL-deficient knee leads to the assumption that in the majority of cases capsular structure injuries appear secondary to chronic ACL tears. Studies on the human glenohumeral joint have shown that, even under physiologic circumstances, strain up to 50 % or more can be present in the joint capsule [33]. Even if the thickness and stiffness of the anterolateral capsule of the knee are different, a rough comparison to the glenohumeral joint capsule is reasonable. Increased strain may lead to plastic deformation and in rare cases to tears of the fibrous tissue.

Fact Box 3

Quantification Tools for Anterolateral Laxity (Fig. 2.5)

1. Image analysis to track markers on the lateral knee (tablet application)
2. Inertial sensor strapped noninvasively to the anterior tibia

2.3.3 Quantification of Rotational Stability

Quantification of injuries to the anterolateral capsule is of paramount importance. Rotatory laxity is mainly based on subjective grading using the pivot-shift test. Even though a standardized pivot-shift test has been proposed [19], the clinical grading and the tibial translation still vary between examiners. A better method to test rotatory knee laxity is via quantitative pivot-shift testing. In this regard, an image analysis method that tracks markers on the lateral knee was found to accurately calculate lateral compartment translation during the pivot shift [2, 5, 21]. Subsequently, a computer tablet application was developed to aid in the processing of the image capture as well as in the calculation of translation (Fig. 2.5) [20, 34]. An inertial sensor strapped noninvasively to the anterior tibia is another quantitative pivot-shift tool (Fig. 2.5) [26]. This device is able to calculate acceleration of the proximal tibia during the reduction movement of the pivot-shift test and is sensitive to ACL injuries [25]. The importance of quantitative pivot-shift testing does not only provide objective laxity parameters but more importantly provides side-to-side comparison of the healthy and injured knee (Fig. 2.6) [4].

2.3.4 Biomechanics Considerations in Surgical Treatment of Anterolateral Instability

Lateral instability of the knee is less frequent, but more disabling than a comparable amount of medial instability [4]. In an in vitro experiment using cadaveric knees, the pivot-shift test was performed preoperatively and postoperatively in ACL-injured knees with or without an anterolateral capsular injury. Surgical treatment included ACL reconstruction with or without an extra-articular tenodesis. Tibial motion relative to the femur was measured by an electromagnetic tracking system during the pivot-shift test. This study showed that either an isolated ACL reconstruction or a combined ACL reconstruction and extra-articular tenodesis restored intact knee kinematics in isolated ACL injury. However, an extra-articular tenodesis was necessary to restore intact kinematics when a lateral capsule lesion was present [3].

Combined intra- and extra-articular reconstruction may provide a more efficient normal restoration of knee kinematics after ACL injury with concomitant anterolateral capsular injury. Some surgeons advocate extra-articular tenodesis due to the longer lever arm of the lateral reconstruction, which may allow efficient control of tibial rotation [13]. Further, extra-artic-

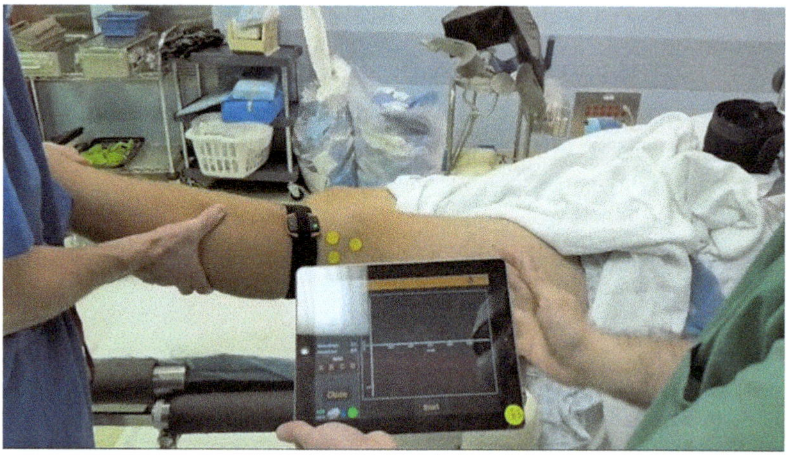

Fig. 2.5 Screen of the tablet application during testing of the tibial anterior translation during the pivot-shift examination and inertial sensor strapped noninvasively to the anterior tibia to quantify the pivot-shift test

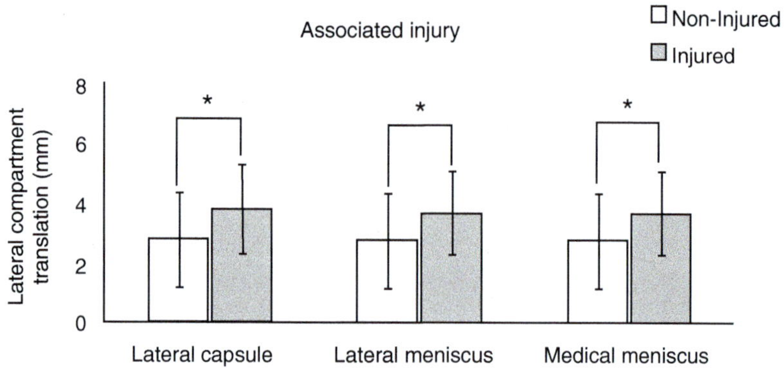

Fig. 2.6 Lateral compartment translation during a quantitative pivot-shift test in ACL-related injuries (*$p \leq 0.05$) [4]

ular tenodesis has been found to decrease the stress on the intra-articular graft by more than 40 %, lending credence to the possible load-sharing role of the native structure [13, 14]. Critics cite the higher pressure on the lateral compartment and the restricted range of motion due to the anterior position of the femoral insertion as disadvantages of extra-articular tenodesis. It should be noted that the majority of ACL injuries can be successfully treated with ACL reconstruction alone. However, in knees with large pivot shifts and anterolateral laxity despite ACL reconstruction, the addition of extra-articular tenodesis might be considered [16]. Individualized ACL surgery is the goal to maximize the patient's outcome and functional return.

Conclusions

Despite various anatomical descriptions of the anterolateral capsular structures, the evidence of a distinct anterolateral ligament and its biomechanical function is still not well understood. Further research is required to evaluate the influence of the anterolateral capsule on rotatory laxity of the knee. The role of additional procedures, such as an extra-articular tenodesis or lateral plasty, requires definition based on severity of the injury.

The standardized pivot-shift test enables the determination of rotatory knee laxity and can be quantified using different customized tools. Based on the results of such tests, treatment algorithms can be established. Moreover, rotatory laxity is not only dependent on the anterolateral capsule structures. The influences of the ACL, the medial and lateral collateral ligaments, generalized joint hyperlaxity with hyperextension of the knee, and bony morphology are currently the focus of intense research.

Based on robotic testing, isolated ACL injuries do not require additional extra-articular tenodesis procedures. The current literature remains unclear in terms of the more complex situation of chronic ACL tears, combined injuries, athletes with generalized joint hyperlaxity, and revision surgeries. The overall goal when treating athletes with high-grade rotatory knee laxity is restoring knee kinematics and joint function as closely as possible to the native knee in order to return the athlete to sport safely and with long-term joint health in mind.

When an extra-articular tenodesis is performed, over-constraining of the lateral compartment of the knee can be an issue, and restricted range of motion and higher pressure on the lateral compartment leading to early posttraumatic arthrosis are concerns that should be recognized.

References

1. Anderson AF, Snyder RB, Lipscomb AB Jr (2001) Anterior cruciate ligament reconstruction. A prospective randomized study of three surgical methods. Am J Sports Med 29(3):272–279
2. Araujo PH, Ahlden M, Hoshino Y, Muller B, Moloney G, Fu FH, Musahl V (2012) Comparison of three non-invasive quantitative measurement systems for the pivot shift test. Knee Surg Sports Traumatol Arthrosc 20(4):692–697. doi:10.1007/s00167-011-1862-9
3. Arilla FV, Rahnemai Azar AA, Guenther D, Yacuzzi C, Engel B, Fu FH, Debski RE, Musahl V (2015) Effects of anterolateral capsular injury and extra-articular tenodesis on knee kinematics. Paper presented at the ISAKOS Biennial congress, Lyon
4. Azar AARA JW, Costello J, Irrgang JJ, Hoshino Y, Samuelsson K, Fu FH, Musahl V (2014) The influence of the anterolateral capsular injury on knee laxity. Paper presented at the AOSSM annual meeting. Seattle, WA, USA
5. Bedi A, Musahl V, Lane C, Citak M, Warren RF, Pearle AD (2010) Lateral compartment translation predicts the grade of pivot shift: a cadaveric and clinical analysis. Knee Surg Sports Traumatol Arthrosc 18(9):1269–1276. doi:10.1007/s00167-010-1160-y
6. Bertoia JT, Urovitz EP, Richards RR, Gross AE (1985) Anterior cruciate reconstruction using the MacIntosh lateral-substitution over-the-top repair. J Bone Joint Surg Am 67(8):1183–1188
7. Campos JC, Chung CB, Lektrakul N, Pedowitz R, Trudell D, Yu J, Resnick D (2001) Pathogenesis of the segond fracture: anatomic and MR imaging evidence of an iliotibial tract or anterior oblique band avulsion. Radiology 219(2):381–386. doi:10.1148/radiology.219.2.r01ma23381
8. Caterine S, Litchfield R, Johnson M, Chronik B, Getgood A (2014) A cadaveric study of the anterolateral ligament: re-introducing the lateral capsular ligament. Knee Surg Sports Traumatol Arthrosc. doi:10.1007/s00167-015-3517-8
9. Claes S, Vereecke E, Maes M, Victor J, Verdonk P, Bellemans J (2013) Anatomy of the anterolateral ligament of the knee. J Anat 223(4):321–328. doi:10.1111/joa.12087
10. Cooper RR, Misol S (1970) Tendon and ligament insertion. A light and electron microscopic study. J Bone Joint Surg Am 52(1):1–20
11. Dodds AL, Halewood C, Gupte CM, Williams A, Amis AA (2014) The anterolateral ligament: anatomy, length changes and association with the segond fracture. Bone Joint J 96-B(3):325–331. doi:10.1302/0301-620X.96B3.33033
12. Dombrowski ME, Costello JM, Ohashi B, Murawski CD, Rothrauff BB, Arilla FV, Friel NA, Fu FH, Debski RE, Musahl V (2015) Macroscopic anatomical, histological and magnetic resonance imaging correlation of the lateral capsule of the knee. Knee Surg Sports Traumatol Arthrosc. Springer, Berlin, Heidelberg doi:10.1007/s00167-015-3517-8
13. Duthon VB, Magnussen RA, Servien E, Neyret P (2013) ACL reconstruction and extra-articular tenodesis. Clin Sports Med 32(1):141–153
14. Engebretsen L, Lew WD, Lewis JL, Hunter RE (1990) The effect of an iliotibial tenodesis on intraarticular graft forces and knee joint motion. Am J Sports Med 18(2):169–176
15. Ferretti A, Conteduca F, Monaco E, De Carli A, D'Arrigo C (2006) Revision anterior cruciate ligament reconstruction with doubled semitendinosus and gracilis tendons and lateral extra-articular reconstruction. J Bone Joint Surg Am 88(11):2373–2379. doi:10.2106/JBJS.F.00064
16. Guenther D, Griffith C, Lesniak B, Lopomo N, Grassi A, Zaffagnini S, Fu FH, Musahl V (2015) Anterolateral rotatory instability of the knee. Knee Surg Sports Traumatol Arthrosc. doi:10.1007/s00167-015-3616-6
17. Guenther D, Rahnemai Azar AA, Fu FH, Debski RE (2015) The biomechanical function of the anterolateral

ligament of the knee: letter to the editor. Am J Sports Med 43(8):NP21–NP22. doi:10.1177/0363546515597217
18. Helito CP, Bonadio MB, Tirico LEP, Gobbi RG, Pecora JR, Camanho GL (2013) Anatomy and histology of the knee anterolateral ligament. Orthop J Sports Med 1(7):2325967113513546
19. Hoshino Y, Araujo P, Ahlden M, Moore CG, Kuroda R, Zaffagnini S, Karlsson J, Fu FH, Musahl V (2012) Standardized pivot shift test improves measurement accuracy. Knee Surg Sports Traumatol Arthrosc 20(4):732–736. doi:10.1007/s00167-011-1850-0
20. Hoshino Y, Araujo P, Ahlden M, Samuelsson K, Muller B, Hofbauer M, Wolf MR, Irrgang JJ, Fu FH, Musahl V (2013) Quantitative evaluation of the pivot shift by image analysis using the iPad. Knee Surg Sports Traumatol Arthrosc 21(4):975–980. doi:10.1007/s00167-013-2396-0
21. Hoshino Y, Kuroda R, Nagamune K, Araki D, Kubo S, Yamaguchi M, Kurosaka M (2012) Optimal measurement of clinical rotational test for evaluating anterior cruciate ligament insufficiency. Knee Surg Sports Traumatol Arthrosc 20(7):1323–1330. doi:10.1007/s00167-011-1643-5
22. Hughston JC, Andrews JR, Cross MJ, Moschi A (1976) Classification of knee ligament instabilities. Part I the medial compartment and cruciate ligaments. J Bone Joint Surg Am 58(2):159–172
23. Irvine GB, Dias JJ, Finlay DB (1987) Segond fractures of the lateral tibial condyle: brief report. J Bone Joint Surg Br 69(4):613–614
24. Lemaire M, Combelles F (1980) Plastic repair with fascia lata for old tears of the anterior cruciate ligament (author's transl). Rev Chir Orthop Reparatrice Appar Mot 66(8):523–525
25. Lopomo N, Signorelli C, Bonanzinga T, Marcheggiani Muccioli GM, Neri MP, Visani A, Marcacci M, Zaffagnini S (2014) Can rotatory knee laxity be predicted in isolated anterior cruciate ligament surgery? Int Orthop 38(6):1167–1172. doi:10.1007/s00264-014-2287-0
26. Lopomo N, Zaffagnini S, Signorelli C, Bignozzi S, Giordano G, Marcheggiani Muccioli GM, Visani A (2012) An original clinical methodology for non-invasive assessment of pivot-shift test. Comput Methods Biomech Biomed Engin 15(12):1323–1328. doi:10.1080/10255842.2011.591788
27. Marcacci M, Zaffagnini S, Giordano G, Iacono F, Presti ML (2009) Anterior cruciate ligament reconstruction associated with extra-articular tenodesis: a prospective clinical and radiographic evaluation with 10- to 13-year follow-up. Am J Sports Med 37(4):707–714. doi:10.1177/0363546508328114
28. Marcacci M, Zaffagnini S, Iacono F, Neri MP, Loreti I, Petitto A (1998) Arthroscopic intra- and extra-articular anterior cruciate ligament reconstruction with gracilis and semitendinosus tendons. Knee Surg Sports Traumatol Arthrosc 6(2):68–75. doi:10.1007/s001670050075
29. Merida-Velasco JA, Sanchez-Montesinos I, Espin-Ferra J, Merida-Velasco JR, Rodriguez-Vazquez JF, Jimenez-Collado J (1997) Development of the human knee joint ligaments. Anat Rec 248(2):259–268
30. Merida-Velasco JA, Sanchez-Montesinos I, Espin-Ferra J, Rodriguez-Vazquez JF, Merida-Velasco JR, Jimenez-Collado J (1997) Development of the human knee joint. Anat Rec 248(2):269–278
31. Monaco E, Ferretti A, Labianca L, Maestri B, Speranza A, Kelly MJ, D'Arrigo C (2012) Navigated knee kinematics after cutting of the ACL and its secondary restraint. Knee Surg Sports Traumatol Arthrosc 20(5):870–877. doi:10.1007/s00167-011-1640-8
32. Monaco E, Labianca L, Conteduca F, De Carli A, Ferretti A (2007) Double bundle or single bundle plus extraarticular tenodesis in ACL reconstruction? A CAOS study. Knee Surg Sports Traumatol Arthrosc 15(10):1168–1174. doi:10.1007/s00167-007-0368-y
33. Moore SM, Ellis B, Weiss JA, McMahon PJ, Debski RE (2009) The glenohumeral capsule should be evaluated as a sheet of fibrous tissue: a validated finite element model. Ann Biomed Eng 38(1):66–76
34. Muller B, Hofbauer M, Rahnemai-Azar AA, Wolf M, Araki D, Hoshino Y, Araujo P, Debski RE, Irrgang JJ, Fu FH, Musahl V (2016) Development of computer tablet software for clinical quantification of lateral knee compartment translation during the pivot shift test. Comput Methods Biomech Biomed Engin 19(2):217–228. doi:10.1080/10255842.2015.1006210
35. Parsons EM, Gee AO, Spiekerman C, Cavanagh PR (2015) The biomechanical function of the anterolateral ligament of the knee. Am J Sports Med 43(3):669–674. doi:10.1177/0363546514562751
36. Parsons EM, Gee AO, Spiekerman C, Cavanagh PR (2015) The biomechanical function of the anterolateral ligament of the knee: response. Am J Sports Med 43(8):NP22. doi:10.1177/0363546515597218
37. Pernin J, Verdonk P, Si Selmi TA, Massin P, Neyret P (2010) Long-term follow-up of 24.5 years after intra-articular anterior cruciate ligament reconstruction with lateral extra-articular augmentation. Am J Sports Med 38(6):1094–1102. doi:10.1177/0363546509361018
38. Ralphs JR, Benjamin M (1994) The joint capsule: structure, composition, ageing and disease. J Anat 184(Pt 3):503–509
39. Segond P (1879) Recherches cliniques et expérimentales sur les épanchements sanguins du genou par entorse. Progrés Méd 7:297–299, 319–321, 340–341
40. Sonnery-Cottet B, Thaunat M, Freychet B, Pupim BH, Murphy CG, Claes S (2015) Outcome of a combined anterior cruciate ligament and anterolateral ligament reconstruction technique with a minimum 2-year follow-up. Am J Sports Med. doi:10.1177/0363546515571571
41. Stijak L, Bumbasirevic M, Radonjic V, Kadija M, Puskas L, Milovanovic D, Filipovic B (2014) Anatomic description of the anterolateral ligament of the knee. Knee Surg Sports Traumatol Arthrosc. doi:10.1007/s00167-014-3422-6

42. Terry GC, Hughston JC, Norwood LA (1986) The anatomy of the iliopatellar band and iliotibial tract. Am J Sports Med 14(1):39–45
43. Vieira EL, Vieira EA, da Silva RT, Berlfein PA, Abdalla RJ, Cohen M (2007) An anatomic study of the iliotibial tract. Arthroscopy 23(3):269–274. doi:10.1016/j.arthro.2006.11.019
44. Vincent JP, Magnussen RA, Gezmez F, Uguen A, Jacobi M, Weppe F, Al-Saati MF, Lustig S, Demey G, Servien E, Neyret P (2012) The anterolateral ligament of the human knee: an anatomic and histologic study. Knee Surg Sports Traumatol Arthrosc 20(1):147–152. doi:10.1007/s00167-011-1580-3
45. Wahl CJ, Westermann RW, Blaisdell GY, Cizik AM (2012) An association of lateral knee sagittal anatomic factors with non-contact ACL injury: sex or geometry? J Bone Joint Surg Am 94(3):217–226. doi:10.2106/JBJS.K.00099
46. Woo SL-Y, Maynard J, Butler D, Lyon R, Torzilli P, Akeson W et al (1988) Ligament, tendon, and joint capsule insertions to bone. In: WSL-YBJ A (ed) Injury and repair of the musculoskeletal soft tissues. American Academy of Orthopedic Surgeons, Park Ridge, pp 133–166
47. Wroble RR, Grood ES, Cummings JS, Henderson JM, Noyes FR (1993) The role of the lateral extraarticular restraints in the anterior cruciate ligament-deficient knee. Am J Sports Med 21(2):257–262; discussion 263
48. Zaffagnini S, Marcacci M, Lo Presti M, Giordano G, Iacono F, Neri MP (2006) Prospective and randomized evaluation of ACL reconstruction with three techniques: a clinical and radiographic evaluation at 5 years follow-up. Knee Surg Sports Traumatol Arthrosc 14(11):1060–1069. doi:10.1007/s00167-006-0130-x
49. Zens M, Ruhhammer J, Goldschmidtboeing F, Woias P, Feucht MJ, Mayr HO, Niemeyer P (2014) A new approach to determine ligament strain using polydimethylsiloxane strain gauges: exemplary measurements of the anterolateral ligament. J Biomech Eng 136(12):124504. doi:10.1115/1.4028837

3 ACL Injury Mechanisms: Lessons Learned from Video Analysis

Hideyuki Koga, Takeshi Muneta, Roald Bahr, Lars Engebretsen, and Tron Krosshaug

Contents

H. Koga, MD, PhD (✉) • T. Muneta
Department of Joint Surgery and Sports Medicine, Graduate School of Medicine, Tokyo Medical and Dental University, 1-5-45 Yushima Bunkyoku, Tokyo 113-8519, Japan
e-mail: koga.orj@tmd.ac.jp

R. Bahr • L. Engebretsen • T. Krosshaug
Department of Sports Medicine, Oslo Sports Trauma Research Center, Norwegian School of Sport Sciences, Oslo, Norway

3.1 Introduction

Anterior cruciate ligament (ACL) injuries occur mostly during sporting activities, and the incidence remains high, especially in young athletes. ACL injuries most commonly occur as a result of a noncontact mechanism, predominantly during cutting or one-leg landing maneuvers [1–3]. In the past decade, various effective prevention programs for noncontact ACL injuries have been developed [4–8]; however, how the different elements in these multicomponent programs play particular roles in preventing the injury is not well understood. Furthermore, the interplay between different components is not entirely understood. Therefore, to develop more targeted injury prevention programs, an improved understanding of the mechanism(s) of noncontact ACL injuries is needed.

3.1.1 Previously Proposed ACL Injury Mechanisms

A number of different methodological approaches have been used to investigate the detailed injury mechanisms in order to develop specific prevention methods for ACL injuries. These include athlete interviews, clinical studies, laboratory motion analysis, video analysis, cadaver studies, and mathematical simulations [9]. Several theories have been proposed based on such studies; however, a matter of controversy remains, with different research groups arguing for either sagittal or

V. Musahl et al. (eds.), *Rotatory Knee Instability*, DOI 10.1007/978-3-319-32070-0_3

non-sagittal plane knee joint loading. DeMorat et al. and Yu and Garrett proposed that aggressive quadriceps loading was responsible, based on a cadaver study which demonstrated that aggressive quadriceps loading could take the ACL to failure [10, 11]. In contrast and based on a mathematical simulation model, Mclean et al. argued that sagittal plane loading alone could not produce such injuries [12, 13]. A small prospective cohort study among female athletes that suggested an association between high valgus load and increased injury risk led Hewett et al. to propose valgus loading as an important component [14, 15]. Moreover, video analyses have also shown that valgus collapse appears to be a main component of the injury mechanism among female athletes [2, 3]. However, cadaver studies and mathematical simulations have shown that pure valgus motion would not produce ACL injuries without first tearing the medial collateral ligament (MCL) [16, 17].

Other simulation studies have suggested that valgus loading would substantially increase the ACL force in situations where an anterior tibial shear force is applied [18]. Based on MRI findings, Speer et al. reported that bone bruises of the lateral femoral condyle or posterolateral portion of tibial plateau occurred in more than 80 % of acute ACL noncontact injuries. The authors concluded that valgus in combination with internal rotation and/or anterior tibial translation (ATT) occurred at the time of ACL injuries [19]. Moreover, it has been shown that valgus loading induces a coupled motion of valgus and internal tibial rotation [20, 21].

Although both cadaver studies and MRI studies have suggested that internal rotation is present in ACL injury situations, video analyses have suggested that valgus in combination with external rotation may be the most frequent motion pattern [3, 22].

In this chapter, a more detailed description of the mechanism(s) of noncontact ACL injuries is outlined in an effort to develop more targeted injury prevention programs.

3.1.2 Development of Model-Based Image-Matching Technique

Of the different approaches available to investigate the ACL injury mechanisms mentioned above, video analysis of injury tapes is the only method available that allows systematic extraction of kinematic data from actual injury situations. Thus far, however, video analyses have been limited to simple visual inspection [1, 3, 23], and the accuracy of these methods has been poor, even among experienced researchers [24]. In addition, it is not possible to extract a time course for joint angles, velocities, and accelerations through simple visual inspection. It is therefore difficult to determine the exact point of ACL rupture.

In order to extract joint kinematics from video recordings using one or more uncalibrated cameras, model-based image-matching (MBIM) technique has been developed as an alternative to simple visual inspection [25–28]. This technique works by matching a model to the background video sequences in order to provide an estimate of the actual three-dimensional (3D) body kinematics. This is achieved by using a commercially available software called Poser® and Poser® Pro Pack (Curious Labs Inc., Santa Cruz, California, USA). This technique has been validated, using 3D motion analysis as the gold standard. The MBIM technique proved far more accurate than simple visual inspection, and the validation study showed that root mean square (RMS) differences for knee flexion, abduction, and rotation with two or three cameras were less than 10°, 6°, and 11°, respectively [24, 25]. Another study found this technique to be feasible for use in actual ACL injury situations [28]. Therefore, videotapes of noncontact ACL injury situations were analyzed using the MBIM technique to describe their kinematics and obtain a more accurate description of the injury mechanisms.

Fact Box 1

- A detailed description of noncontact anterior cruciate ligzament (ACL) injury mechanisms is crucial to develop ACL injury prevention programs.
- Noncontact ACL injury mechanisms are a matter of controversy, with either sagittal or non-sagittal plane knee joint loading being favored.
- The MBIM technique has been developed for detailed video analysis of injury situations, a process previously limited to simple visual inspection.

3.2 Biomechanics of Noncontact ACL Injuries

Recorded with at least two analogue cameras during TV broadcasts, ten ACL injury situations from women's team handball and basketball were analyzed using the MBIM technique (Fig. 3.1), all of which occurred during game situations [26]. All players were handling the ball in the injury situation; seven were in possession of the ball at the time of injury, two had shot, and one had passed the ball. In six cases, there was player-to-player contact with an opponent at the time of injury, all resulting in the torso being pushed or held. There was no direct contact to the knee in any case. The injury situations could be classified into two groups: seven cases occurred when cutting and three during one-legged landings.

3.2.1 Knee Kinematics

The knee kinematic patterns were remarkably consistent across the ten cases studies (Fig. 3.2). The knee was relatively straight at initial contact (IC), with a flexion angle of 23° (range, 11–30°) and had increased by 24° (95 % CI, 19–29°, p <0.001) 40 ms later. The knee abduction angle was neutral, 0° (range, −2° to 3°) at IC, but had increased by 12° (95 % CI, 10–13°, p <0.001) 40 ms later. As for knee rotation angle, the knee was externally rotated 5° (range, −5° to 12°) at IC, but abruptly rotated internally by 8° (95 % CI, 2–14°, $p=0.037$) during the first 40 ms. From 40 to 300 ms after IC, however, we observed an external rotation of 17° (95 % CI, 13–22°, p <0.001). In addition, the estimated peak vertical ground reaction force (GRF) occurred at 40 ms (range, 0–83) after IC.

However, these analyses had limitations. The relatively low frame rate (50 or 60 Hz) and limited picture resolution (768 × 576 pixels) prevented assessment of anterior translation of the tibia. In another noncontact ACL injury situation, a 26-year-old male elite football player was recorded using four high-definition (HD) cameras including two high-speed recordings (100 and 300 Hz) [27]. In this case, the player suffered a noncontact ACL injury to his right knee when he tried to stop after having passed the ball with his right leg. This case was analyzed using the MBIM technique, including an assessment of tibial translations (Fig. 3.3). Knee kinematics were strikingly consistent with the previous analyses of the ten cases (Fig. 3.4). The knee was flexed 35° at IC, with initial extension (26° of flexion) until 20 ms after IC, after which the flexion angle continued to increase. The knee abduction angle was neutral at IC, but increased by 21° 30 ms later. The knee (tibia) was externally rotated 11° at IC, but abruptly rotated internally by 21° during the first 30 ms before subsequently changing to external rotation. In addition, ATT was quantifiable; this movement started at 20 ms after IC where the knee was maximally extended and, by approximately 30 ms after IC, a 9 mm increase in anterior translation was detected. The translations plateaued by 150 ms and then shifted back to a reduced position between 200 and 240 ms after IC.

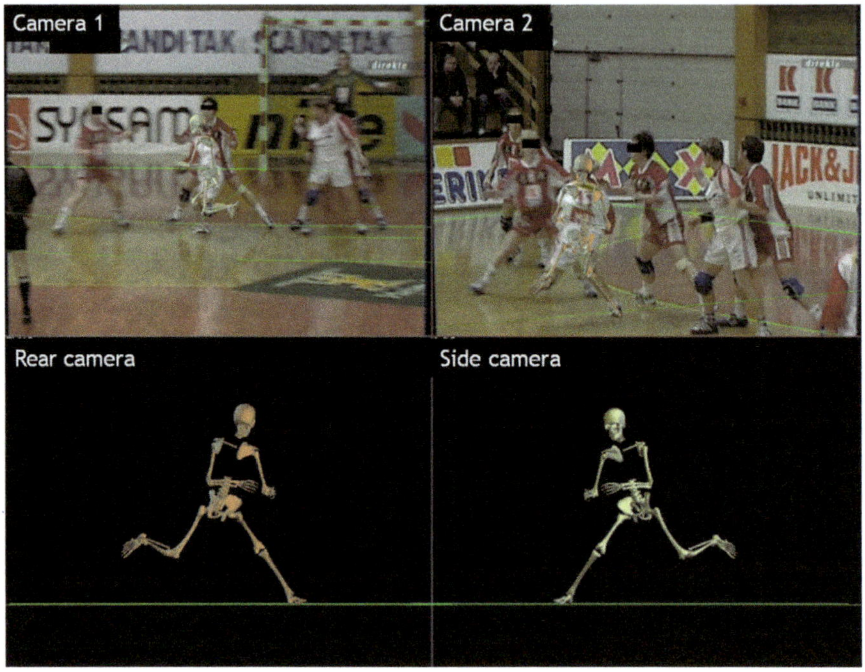

Fig. 3.1 An example of a video matched in poser, two-camera handball injury situation 40 ms after initial contact (*IC*). The two top panels show the customized skeleton model and the handball court model superimposed on and matched with the background video image from two cameras with different angles. The two bottom panels show the skeleton model from back and side views created in Poser

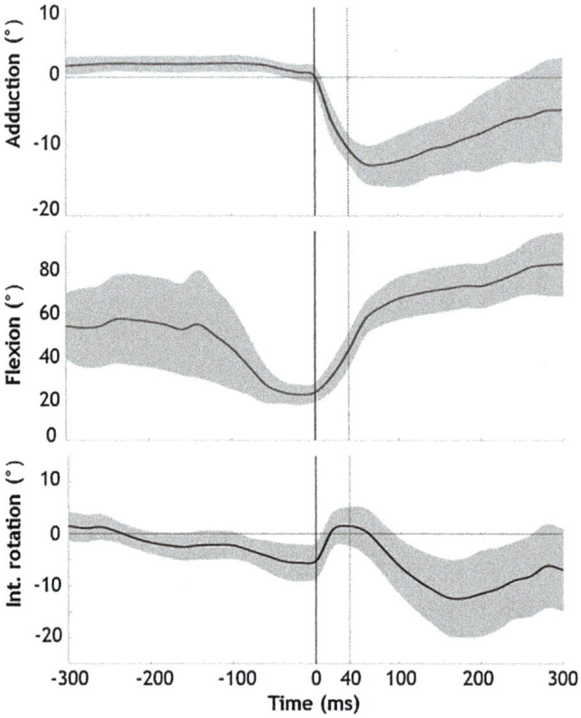

Fig. 3.2 Time sequences of the mean knee angles (°) (*black line*) of the ten cases with 95 % confidence intervals (*CI*) (*gray area*). Time 0 indicates IC and the *dotted vertical line* indicates the time point 40 ms after IC

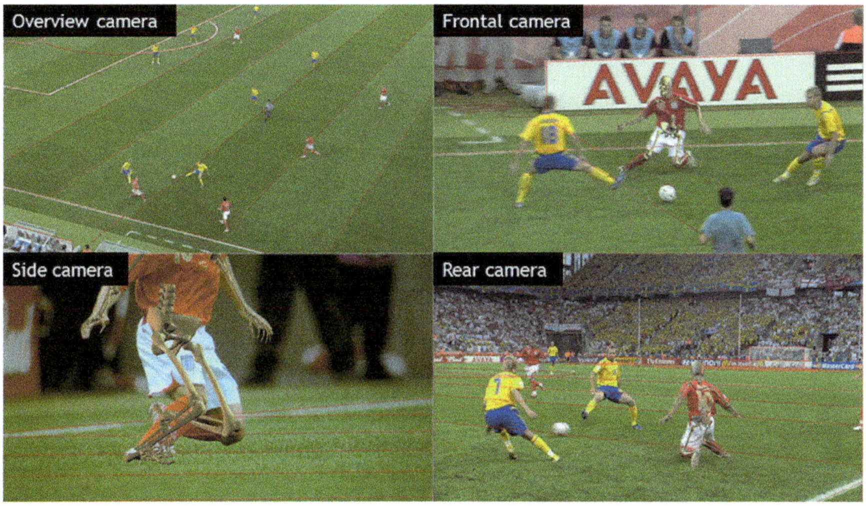

Fig. 3.3 A football injury situation recorded using HD cameras. Each panel shows the customized skeleton model and the football pitch model superimposed on and matched with the background video image from each camera. Overview camera and rear camera had an effective frame rate after being deinterlaced of 50 Hz, frontal camera 100 Hz and side camera 300 Hz

Fig. 3.4 Time sequences of knee joint angles (*left axis*) and anterior tibial translation (*right axis*) in the soccer case. Time 0 (**a**) indicates IC and the *dotted vertical lines* (**b**) and (**c**) indicate the time point 20 and 30 ms after IC, respectively

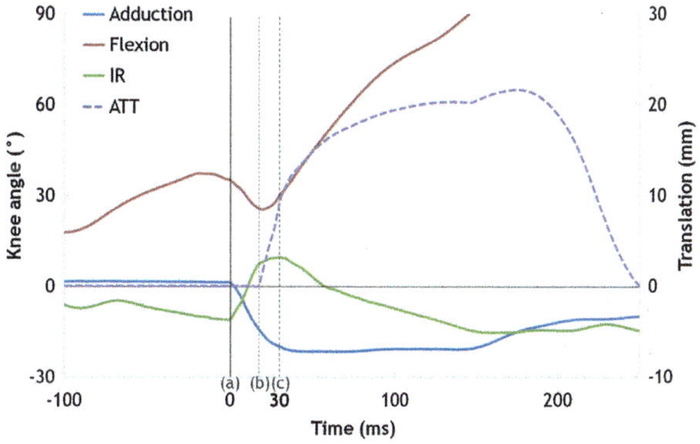

3.2.2 Timing of Noncontact ACL Injuries

Traditionally, it has not been possible to determine the exact timing of ACL injury from video analysis based on simple visual inspection [1–3]. However, using the MBIM technique, abnormal joint configurations, sudden changes in joint angular motion, and the timing of the GRF were assessable. The extracted knee kinematics during ACL injuries using the MBIM technique showed that sudden increases of valgus and internal rotation angles occurred within the first 40 ms after IC. These periods correspond to the average peak vertical GRF in these cases. Moreover, in the case recorded using HD cameras, an abrupt increase in ATT of 9 mm was reached 30 ms after IC. This corresponds to the maximum anterior translation in intact knees [29, 30]. Based on these results, together with the previous studies showing that the ACL was strained shortly (approximately 40 ms) after IC in simulated landings [18, 31], it appears plausible that the injury occurs within 40 ms for the majority of these cases.

3.2.3 Hip Kinematics

We also analyzed hip kinematics in the above ten cases. In contrast to the knee kinematics, hip joint angles remained unchanged at an internally

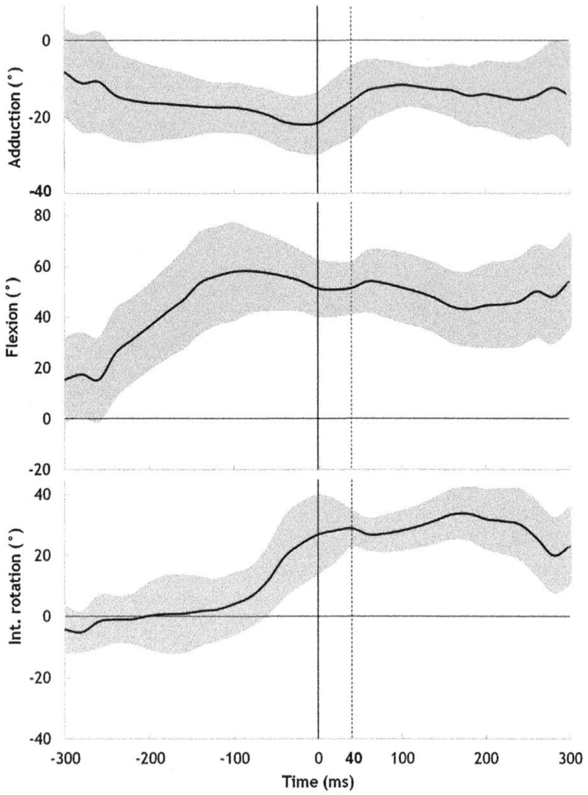

Fig. 3.5 Time sequences of the mean hip angles (°) (*black line*) of the ten cases with 95 % CI (*gray area*). Time 0 indicates IC and the *dotted vertical line* indicates the time point 40 ms after IC

rotated position during the first 40 ms after IC (Fig. 3.5).

Lower extremities act as a kinetic chain during dynamic tasks and the control of hip motion largely affects the knee motion. Decker et al. [32] reported that energy absorption at the hip joint and hip flexion angle at IC were less in females than in males during a drop landing. Schmitz et al. [33] reported that in a single-leg landing, energy absorption at the hip and the total hip flexion displacement were lower in females, even though the peak vertical GRF was larger when compared with males. Furthermore, Hashemi et al. [34] reported in a cadaver study that restricted flexion of the hip at 20° combined with low quadriceps and hamstring force levels in simulated single-leg landing was found to be conductive to ACL injury. A video analysis has shown that ACL-injured subjects' hip flexion and abduction angle was constant during 100 ms after IC, whereas uninjured control subjects' hip flexion increased by 15° in cutting/landing maneuvers [35]. The study using MBIM technique also showed that hip joint angles remained constant during the first 40 ms after IC. Hashemi et al. [36] proposed a mechanism called the "hip extension, knee flexion paradox," i.e., that a mismatch between hip and knee flexion in landing is the cause of ACL injury. In normal conditions, the knee and hip flex together upon landing, whereas in unbalanced landings, the knee is forced to flex while the hip is forced to extend. Under these conditions, the tibia will undergo anterior translation, which will increase the risk of ACL injury.

There are some possible causes of the hip/knee mismatch: (1) In the sagittal plane, an upright or backward-leaning trunk position at IC makes the center of mass posterior to the knee, and increased GRF may encourage more knee flexion than hip flexion and relatively act to extend the hip. (2) In other planes, insufficient hip abductor/external rotator strength or activation can lead to an adducted/internally rotated position of the hip before landing, causing knee valgus after landing. (3) Large hip internal rotation at IC seen in our video analysis could also be an explanation; ACL-injured patients could have limited range of motion in internal rotation [37], and the hip joint may be locked at a large internally rotated position. As a matter of fact, hip dysplasia has also been reported to be a possible risk factor of ACL injury [38]. It has also been reported that decreased range of internal femoral rotation results in greater ACL strain [39].

For these reasons, the fact that there is limited hip joint movement indicates that hip energy absorption may be limited and the knee joint is exposed to larger force, which contribute to ACL injury.

Fact Box 2

- Knee kinematic patterns are consistent, with immediate valgus, internal rotation motion and ATT occurring within 40 ms after initial contact. Peak vertical ground reaction force also occurred at 40 ms after initial contact.
- In the same period, hip kinematics remain constant in an internally rotated position.

3.3 Mechanisms for Noncontact ACL Injury

As previously mentioned, valgus collapse in combination with external rotation (i.e., knee in, toe out) has been frequently identified as an ACL injury mechanism via simple visual inspection of injury video tapes. However, it has been debated whether these kinematics actually represent the cause for ACL injuries or simply are a result of the ACL being torn [3, 22]. The results using the MBIM technique showed that immediate valgus motion occurred within 40 ms after IC. The abrupt internal rotation also occurred during the first 40 ms after IC, and then external rotation was observed, which seems to have occurred after the ACL was torn. In addition, ATT started shortly after IC and increased abruptly until when the injury might have occurred. The discrepancy between the previous studies and the present results could be that the abrupt internal rotation and ATT observed using the MBIM technique analysis appeared not easily detectable from visual inspection alone; the external rotation that occurs afterward is more pronounced and therefore easier to observe. The internal-to-external rotation sequence with ATT has also been reported previously. In a recent cadaver study, the application of pure compressive loads led to ATT and internal tibial rotation of up to 8°, followed by a sudden external rotation of 12° [30]. The combination of internal tibial rotation and ATT is probably caused by joint surface geometry. In this regard, the concave geometry of the medial tibial facet, combined with the slightly convex lateral tibia facet, may cause the lateral femoral condyle to slip back. This may also explain why ACL-injured patients tend to have greater posterior lateral tibial plateau slopes than uninjured controls [40–42].

Combining the results obtained using the MBIM technique with previous findings, the following hypothesis for the mechanism of noncontact ACL injury is proposed (Fig. 3.6): (1) When valgus loading is applied, the MCL becomes taut and lateral compression occurs. (2) This compressive load, as well as the anterior force vector caused by quadriceps contraction, causes a displacement of the femur relative to the tibia where the lateral femoral condyle shifts posteriorly due to the posterior slope of lateral tibial plateau, and the tibia translates anteriorly and rotates internally, resulting in an ACL rupture. (3) After the ACL is torn, the primary restraint to anterior translation of the tibia is gone. This causes the medial femoral condyle to also be displaced posteriorly, resulting in external rotation of the tibia. This external rotation may be exacerbated by the typical movement pattern when athlete plants and cuts, where the foot typically rotates externally relative to the trunk.

3.4 ACL Injury Prevention Based on the Proposed Mechanisms

Based on the mechanisms outlined above, the following strategies to prevent ACL injury are proposed: (1) It is important to acquire a cutting and

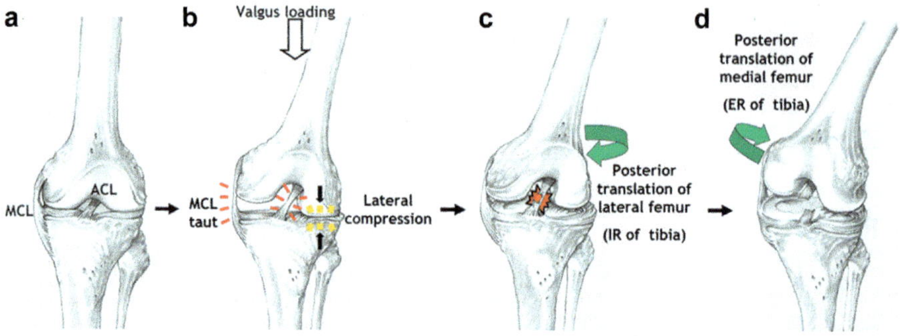

Fig. 3.6 The proposed noncontact ACL injury mechanism. (**a**) An unloaded knee. (**b**) When valgus loading is applied, the MCL becomes taut and lateral compression occurs. (**c**) This compressive load, as well as the anterior force vector caused by quadriceps contraction, causes a lateral femoral posterior displacement, due to the posterior slope of the lateral tibial plateau, and the tibia translates anteriorly and rotates internally, resulting in an ACL rupture. (**d**) After the ACL is torn, the primary restraint to anterior translation of the tibia is gone. This causes the medial femoral condyle to also be displaced posteriorly, resulting in external rotation of the tibia

landing technique avoiding knee valgus and internal rotation during knee flexion and adequate hip flexion to absorb energy from GRF, avoiding excessive hip internal rotation. Preventive efforts should focus not only on the knee joint but also on the hip joint. (2) As ACL injuries occur approximately 40 ms after IC, it is likely that a "feedback" strategy, i.e., an ACL prevention program focusing on correcting joint motion after landing, cannot prevent ACL injury; it takes at least 150–200 ms to react after landing at risk. Prevention efforts should focus on a "feed-forward" strategy that controls knee and hip motion before landing, i.e., training muscular pre-activation and neural control during the pre-landing phase.

Conclusions

1. MBIM technique has enabled detailed video analysis of injury situations that had been limited to simple visual inspection.
2. New mechanisms for noncontact ACL injuries are proposed.
   - ACL injuries are likely to occur within 40 ms after the initial ground contact.
   - Lateral compression caused by valgus loading, as well as the anterior force vector caused by quadriceps contraction, causes a displacement of the femur relative to the tibia where the lateral femoral condyle shifts posteriorly due to the posterior slope of lateral tibial plateau and the tibia translates anteriorly and rotates internally, resulting in an ACL rupture.

   Hip joint angles remain constant at an internally rotated position when ACL injury occurs. This fact indicates that hip energy absorption may be limited and the knee is exposed to larger force, which contributes to the ACL injury.
3. Prevention programs should focus on acquiring a cutting and landing technique that avoids knee valgus and internal rotation during knee flexion and with adequate hip flexion and avoiding excessive hip internal rotation. Moreover, the fact that the ACL injury occurs 40 ms after IC suggests that "feed-forward" strategies, controlling knee and hip motion before landing, may be critical, as "feedback" strategies to correct inappropriate hip and knee motion after landing cannot prevent ACL injuries.

References

1. Boden BP, Dean GS, Feagin JA Jr, Garrett WE Jr (2000) Mechanisms of anterior cruciate ligament injury. Orthopedics 23(6):573–578
2. Krosshaug T, Nakamae A, Boden BP, Engebretsen L, Smith G, Slauterbeck JR, Hewett TE, Bahr R (2007) Mechanisms of anterior cruciate ligament injury in

basketball: video analysis of 39 cases. Am J Sports Med 35(3):359–367
3. Olsen OE, Myklebust G, Engebretsen L, Bahr R (2004) Injury mechanisms for anterior cruciate ligament injuries in team handball: a systematic video analysis. Am J Sports Med 32(4):1002–1012
4. Caraffa A, Cerulli G, Projetti M, Aisa G, Rizzo A (1996) Prevention of anterior cruciate ligament injuries in soccer. A prospective controlled study of proprioceptive training. Knee Surg Sports Traumatol Arthrosc 4(1):19–21
5. Gilchrist J, Mandelbaum BR, Melancon H, Ryan GW, Silvers HJ, Griffin LY, Watanabe DS, Dick RW, Dvorak J (2008) A randomized controlled trial to prevent noncontact anterior cruciate ligament injury in female collegiate soccer players. Am J Sports Med 36(8):1476–1483
6. Mandelbaum BR, Silvers HJ, Watanabe DS, Knarr JF, Thomas SD, Griffin LY, Kirkendall DT, Garrett W Jr (2005) Effectiveness of a neuromuscular and proprioceptive training program in preventing anterior cruciate ligament injuries in female athletes: 2-year follow-up. Am J Sports Med 33(7):1003–1010
7. Myklebust G, Engebretsen L, Braekken IH, Skjolberg A, Olsen OE, Bahr R (2003) Prevention of anterior cruciate ligament injuries in female team handball players: a prospective intervention study over three seasons. Clin J Sport Med 13(2):71–78
8. Olsen OE, Myklebust G, Engebretsen L, Holme I, Bahr R (2005) Exercises to prevent lower limb injuries in youth sports: cluster randomised controlled trial. BMJ 330(7489):449
9. Krosshaug T, Andersen TE, Olsen OE, Myklebust G, Bahr R (2005) Research approaches to describe the mechanisms of injuries in sport: limitations and possibilities. Br J Sports Med 39(6):330–339
10. DeMorat G, Weinhold P, Blackburn T, Chudik S, Garrett W (2004) Aggressive quadriceps loading can induce noncontact anterior cruciate ligament injury. Am J Sports Med 32(2):477–483
11. Yu B, Garrett WE (2007) Mechanisms of non-contact ACL injuries. Br J Sports Med 41(Suppl 1):i47–i51
12. McLean SG, Andrish JT, van den Bogert AJ (2005) Aggressive quadriceps loading can induce noncontact anterior cruciate ligament injury. Am J Sports Med 33(7):1106; author reply 1106–1107
13. McLean SG, Huang X, Su A, Van Den Bogert AJ (2004) Sagittal plane biomechanics cannot injure the ACL during sidestep cutting. Clin Biomech (Bristol, Avon) 19(8):828–838
14. Hewett TE, Myer GD, Ford KR, Heidt RS Jr, Colosimo AJ, McLean SG, van den Bogert AJ, Paterno MV, Succop P (2005) Biomechanical measures of neuromuscular control and valgus loading of the knee predict anterior cruciate ligament injury risk in female athletes: a prospective study. Am J Sports Med 33(4):492–501
15. Quatman CE, Hewett TE (2009) The anterior cruciate ligament injury controversy: is "valgus collapse" a sex-specific mechanism? Br J Sports Med 43(5):328–335
16. Mazzocca AD, Nissen CW, Geary M, Adams DJ (2003) Valgus medial collateral ligament rupture causes concomitant loading and damage of the anterior cruciate ligament. J Knee Surg 16(3):148–151
17. Shin CS, Chaudhari AM, Andriacchi TP (2009) The effect of isolated valgus moments on ACL strain during single-leg landing: a simulation study. J Biomech 42(3):280–285
18. Withrow TJ, Huston LJ, Wojtys EM, Ashton-Miller JA (2006) The effect of an impulsive knee valgus moment on in vitro relative ACL strain during a simulated jump landing. Clin Biomech (Bristol, Avon) 21(9):977–983
19. Speer KP, Spritzer CE, Bassett FH 3rd, Feagin JA Jr, Garrett WE Jr (1992) Osseous injury associated with acute tears of the anterior cruciate ligament. Am J Sports Med 20(4):382–389
20. Matsumoto H (1990) Mechanism of the pivot shift. J Bone Joint Surg Br 72(5):816–821
21. Matsumoto H, Suda Y, Otani T, Niki Y, Seedhom BB, Fujikawa K (2001) Roles of the anterior cruciate ligament and the medial collateral ligament in preventing valgus instability. J Orthop Sci 6(1):28–32
22. Ebstrup JF, Bojsen-Moller F (2000) Anterior cruciate ligament injury in indoor ball games. Scand J Med Sci Sports 10(2):114–116
23. Cochrane JL, Lloyd DG, Buttfield A, Seward H, McGivern J (2007) Characteristics of anterior cruciate ligament injuries in Australian football. J Sci Med Sport 10(2):96–104
24. Krosshaug T, Nakamae A, Boden B, Engebretsen L, Smith G, Slauterbeck J, Hewett TE, Bahr R (2007) Estimating 3D joint kinematics from video sequences of running and cutting maneuvers--assessing the accuracy of simple visual inspection. Gait Posture 26(3):378–385
25. Krosshaug T, Bahr R (2005) A model-based image-matching technique for three-dimensional reconstruction of human motion from uncalibrated video sequences. J Biomech 38(4):919–929
26. Koga H, Nakamae A, Shima Y, Iwasa J, Myklebust G, Engebretsen L, Bahr R, Krosshaug T (2010) Mechanisms for noncontact anterior cruciate ligament injuries: knee joint kinematics in 10 injury situations from female team handball and basketball. Am J Sports Med 38(11):2218–2225
27. Koga H, Bahr R, Myklebust G, Engebretsen L, Grund T, Krosshaug T (2011) Estimating anterior tibial translation from model-based image-matching of a noncontact anterior cruciate ligament injury in professional football: a case report. Clin J Sport Med 21(3):271–274
28. Krosshaug T, Slauterbeck JR, Engebretsen L, Bahr R (2007) Biomechanical analysis of anterior cruciate ligament injury mechanisms: three-dimensional motion reconstruction from video sequences. Scand J Med Sci Sports 17(5):508–519
29. Jakob RP, Staubli HU, Deland JT (1987) Grading the pivot shift. Objective tests with implications for treatment. J Bone Joint Surg Br 69(2):294–299

30. Meyer EG, Haut RC (2008) Anterior cruciate ligament injury induced by internal tibial torsion or tibiofemoral compression. J Biomech 41(16):3377–3383
31. Shin CS, Chaudhari AM, Andriacchi TP (2007) The influence of deceleration forces on ACL strain during single-leg landing: a simulation study. J Biomech 40(5):1145–1152
32. Decker MJ, Torry MR, Wyland DJ, Sterett WI, Richard Steadman J (2003) Gender differences in lower extremity kinematics, kinetics and energy absorption during landing. Clin Biomech (Bristol, Avon) 18(7):662–669
33. Schmitz RJ, Kulas AS, Perrin DH, Riemann BL, Shultz SJ (2007) Sex differences in lower extremity biomechanics during single leg landings. Clin Biomech (Bristol, Avon) 22(6):681–688
34. Hashemi J, Chandrashekar N, Jang T, Karpat F, Oseto M, Ekwaro-Osire S (2007) An alternative mechanism of non-contact anterior cruciate ligament injury during jump-landing: in-vitro simulation. Exp Mech 47:347–354
35. Boden BP, Torg JS, Knowles SB, Hewett TE (2009) Video analysis of anterior cruciate ligament injury: abnormalities in hip and ankle kinematics. Am J Sports Med 37(2):252–259
36. Hashemi J, Breighner R, Chandrashekar N, Hardy DM, Chaudhari AM, Shultz SJ, Slauterbeck JR, Beynnon BD (2011) Hip extension, knee flexion paradox: a new mechanism for non-contact ACL injury. J Biomech 44(4):577–585
37. Gomes JL, de Castro JV, Becker R (2008) Decreased hip range of motion and noncontact injuries of the anterior cruciate ligament. Arthroscopy 24(9):1034–1037
38. Yamazaki J, Muneta T, Ju YJ, Morito T, Okuwaki T, Sekiya I (2011) Hip acetabular dysplasia and joint laxity of female anterior cruciate ligament-injured patients. Am J Sports Med 39(2):410–414
39. Beaulieu ML, Oh YK, Bedi A, Ashton-Miller JA, Wojtys EM (2014) Does limited internal femoral rotation increase peak anterior cruciate ligament strain during a simulated pivot landing? Am J Sports Med 42(12):2955–2963
40. Brandon ML, Haynes PT, Bonamo JR, Flynn MI, Barrett GR, Sherman MF (2006) The association between posterior-inferior tibial slope and anterior cruciate ligament insufficiency. Arthroscopy 22(8):894–899
41. Stijak L, Herzog RF, Schai P (2008) Is there an influence of the tibial slope of the lateral condyle on the ACL lesion? A case–control study. Knee Surg Sports Traumatol Arthrosc 16(2):112–117
42. Hashemi J, Chandrashekar N, Mansouri H, Gill B, Slauterbeck JR, Schutt RC Jr, Dabezies E, Beynnon BD (2010) Shallow medial tibial plateau and steep medial and lateral tibial slopes: new risk factors for anterior cruciate ligament injuries. Am J Sports Med 38(1):54–62

4 In Vivo Biomechanics: Laxity Versus Dynamic Stability

Yuichiro Nishizawa and Scott Tashman

Contents

Y. Nishizawa
Department of Orthopaedic Surgery, University of Pittsburgh, Pittsburgh, PA, USA

Kobe University, Kobe, Japan

S. Tashman, PhD (✉)
Biodynamics Laboratory, Department of Orthopaedic Surgery, University of Pittsburgh, 3820 S. Water St, Pittsburgh, PA 15203, USA
e-mail: tashman@pitt.edu

4.1 Laxity Assessment

Musahl et al. described laxity as the passive response of a joint to an externally applied force or torque in biomechanical terms [60]. Thus, laxity tests for evaluating knee injury assess the passive limits of motion in a particular direction or plane. Through comprehensive laxity testing, it is possible to describe the range of a passive envelope of motion that the joint can achieve within the limits of the low forces typically employed for such testing.

4.1.1 Determining the Passive Envelope of Joint Function

The knee joint consists of multiple hard and soft tissues, including the ACL, medial and lateral collateral ligaments, capsule, menisci, posterolateral complex, and bone/cartilage [20, 33, 37, 43, 51, 55, 57, 59, 80]. In a healthy knee, these structures work synergistically with active muscle forces to control joint motion and maintain knee stability during functional movements. During typical movements, the joint stays well within the limits of its passive motion envelope, to avoid placing tissues at risk of injury. As a result, there are several possible motion paths, and the patterns of joint motion and articular contact vary considerably with loading and activity (even during similar ranges of knee flexion) [5, 56].

V. Musahl et al. (eds.), *Rotatory Knee Instability*, DOI 10.1007/978-3-319-32070-0_4

While laxity tests on cadavers or anesthetized patients can characterize the true passive motion envelope, assessment of laxity in awake subjects may not always reveal the true envelope of motion, since forces are low and there may be influences from neuromuscular activity (conscious or reflexive). After injury, patients often guard during laxity tests, due to pain or fear of subluxation [76]. This may further confound interpretation of laxity assessments.

4.1.2 Assessing Laxity In Vivo: Motion in Response to an Applied Load

Anterior-posterior (A-P) knee laxity after ACL injury or reconstruction is assessed by measuring anterior tibial translation relative to the femur in response to an anterior tibial force applied to the tibia. This assessment can be performed qualitatively (e.g., the widely used anterior drawer and Lachman tests) or using a variety of instrumented devices such as the KT 1000 arthrometer (MEDmetric, San Diego, CA, USA), the Genucom Knee Analysis System (FARO Technologies Inc., Lake Mary, FL, USA), and the Rolimeter (Aircast Europe, Neubeuern, Germany) [9, 14, 15, 22, 52, 63, 73, 75]. Regardless of the method or device used, these assessments consider only a single degree of freedom of motion in response to simplistic, sub-physiological forces with the joint in a non-weight-bearing state and therefore cannot predict the response of the joint to the complex combination of externally applied forces and muscle forces generated during functional movement. Thus, it is not surprising that static A-P laxity tests are poorly correlated with all measures of patient symptoms or functional outcome for ACL-injured subjects, before or after reconstruction [10, 13, 27, 39, 67].

4.1.3 Pivot-Shift Test

The pivot-shift test is commonly used for assessing the combined translational and rotatory knee laxity in ACL-injured and ACL-reconstructed knees [21, 46, 61]. As described by Galway and MacIntosh [21], the test is performed by adducting the hip and passively flexing the knee from full extension while internal tibial torque and valgus stress are applied manually to the knee. A positive pivot shift consists of a palpable anterior tibial subluxation and a subsequent reduction in the tibial plateau from the femoral condyle [21]. Thus, the pivot-shift test assesses the passive response of the knee to multidirectional, dynamic loading. While widely employed for clinical assessment, the classic pivot-shift test is qualitative, and there is considerable variability in the specific technique utilized, with limb position and applied forces differing widely across examiners [40]. However, despite this variability in technique, pivot-shift test measures correlate moderately with knee function, patient satisfaction [39, 41], and the risk for long-term osteoarthritis (OA) [38]. There have been numerous recent efforts to quantify and better standardize the pivot-shift test, employing noninvasive measurement devices, such as electromagnetic tracking [31, 32], accelerometers [44, 45], and video-motion analysis using a handheld tablet [30], which should further improve the validity and clinical applications of the pivot shift.

However, while the pivot-shift test is a dynamic, multiaxial test, it still assesses only the passive envelope of knee motion in response to a specific set of sub-physiological loads in a non-weight-bearing state. It is also subject to guarding by the patients, perhaps to a greater extent than the A-P laxity tests (since the resulting instability can be quite uncomfortable, especially in the acute post-injury period). Two recent studies of patients with acute ACL injury have reported significant differences between quantitative parameters during instrumented pivot-shift tests performed while awake vs. under anesthesia [50, 62]. Therefore, while the pivot-shift exam is clearly superior to simple A-P laxity tests for predicting outcomes, its relationship to functional, dynamic knee behavior remains uncertain.

Fact Box 1
Knee laxity tests assess the envelope of passive knee joint motion, typically in a single direction in response to simple, sub-physiological loading. The pivot-shift examination is a more complex laxity test that assesses joint motion in response to a specific combination of multiaxial loading.

4.2 Laxity vs. Instability

In the orthopedic world, the terms "laxity" and "instability" are often used interchangeably. These terms, however, have significantly different implications with regard to knee function.

4.2.1 Clinical and Functional Interpretations of Stability

As discussed above, knee laxity tests are commonly used to diagnose ACL injury and evaluate knee condition after ACL reconstruction. Clinically, a knee is diagnosed as "unstable" if excessive laxity (as in a positive pivot shift and/or large side-to-side differences in A-P laxity) is found. This laxity-based definition of instability, however, is inconsistent with both the technical definition and the patient's perceptions of stability. Engineers define instability as a dynamic response to a perturbation, resulting in large, unpredictable displacements. Patients are only likely to perceive their knee as unstable if it "gives way" during functional activities [60]. ACL-deficient individuals may experience giving-way symptoms during activities of daily living, but they are more likely to occur during sport activities [8, 19], when forces are higher and neuromuscular demands are greater. Even patients considered "stable" by laxity assessment after ACL reconstruction (i.e., anterior drawer test, Lachman test, and the pivot-shift test are within normal limits) sometimes experience "giving-way" episodes during sport activities. Conversely, not all individuals with clinically unstable knees (failed laxity examinations) experience giving-way episodes, even during high-demand sport activities. Laxity tests are typically performed without the compressive joint forces required to properly engage the conforming condylar surfaces, which play an important role in joint stabilization. Laxity tests (including the pivot shift) also cannot account for the ability of the individual to dynamically stabilize their knee via active muscle forces. While laxity tests may be effective for identifying structural deficits, the results cannot predict joint behavior during dynamic, functional activities. Thus, it is not surprising that clinical and functional outcomes, including the occurrence of patient-reported instability, are poorly or weakly correlated with laxity measures [10, 13, 27, 39, 65, 67]. It is therefore fundamentally incorrect to use the terms laxity and stability interchangeably: laxity is a measure of static response to sub-physiological loads, while true stability can only be assessed during dynamic, functional joint motion and loading.

4.2.2 Proposed Definitions for *Functional* Stability: Terminal and Midrange Instability

Healthy joints rarely operate near the limits of their passive motion envelope. While large and unpredictable loads (such as those that may occur during impact or unpredictable events, i.e., collisions, off-balance jump landings, etc.) may force the joint into positions that exceed its functional envelope, these events are rare and generally cause damage or structural failure. During routine movements, the neuromuscular system is tuned to protect the joint from damage, and sensory elements in tendons, ligaments, muscles, and joint capsule initiate protective inhibitory reflexes as joints approach the limits of their soft tissue constraints. A joint that operates near the limits of its passive envelope during routine, functional loading, due to insufficient soft tissue constraints and/or compromised neuromuscular function, is at high risk of damage. One could refer to such a joint as *terminally* unstable, as it refers to abnormal behavior of the joint at or near its end range of motion.

The literature suggests that there are more subtle forms of joint abnormalities that can alter knee function without pushing the joint to its passive limits or any perception of instability by the patient. Altered rotational and translational knee motion and shifted regions of articular joint contact have been reported during functional activities after ACL reconstruction as well as PCL injury in asymptomatic individuals [26, 70–72]. Such abnormal motions, while not associated with the classic concept of instability, may still place the joint at risk for damage. It has been suggested that healthy cartilage develops in response to loading, resulting in thicker regions where loads are routinely greatest [11, 54, 66]. Since mature cartilage has a very limited capacity to adapt and remodel, any alteration in the load distribution might be detrimental to the articular cartilage [4, 7, 12]. Therefore, if a condition such as ACL injury alters knee kinematics and shifts repetitive loading during routine activities to different regions of cartilage, a degenerative pathway may be initiated [4, 6]. Increased contact point motion during walking has also been associated with knee osteoarthritis, suggesting that "micro-instabilities" below an individual detection threshold may also place a joint at risk [18]. Thus, there appear to be multiple mechanisms by which abnormal functional knee kinematics may be detrimental to joint health, even if the overall excursions remain well within the passive envelope of motion [6]. Since it does not involve motion near the joint's passive limits, this *midrange* instability is most likely unrelated to joint laxity and is probably only be detectable with high-accuracy assessment of joint kinematics during functional movements.

Fact Box 2
Laxity is the passive response of a joint to applied forces. It does not account for the effects of weight-bearing, neuromuscular function, or viscoelasticity of joint tissues. Instability is an abnormal dynamic joint motion that can occur in response to the complex, high-magnitude loads encountered during activities of daily living and sport activities. Laxity does not predict dynamic knee instability. The two concepts are fundamentally distinct and should not be used interchangeably.

4.3 Assessment of Functional Biomechanics

In vitro studies have contributed a wealth of information on the basic biomechanics and passive structural properties of the knee [49, 58, 78]. However, these studies cannot reproduce the complex combination of gravitational, inertial, and active muscular forces that influence knee mechanics during functional activities. Cadaver studies also represent only "time zero" conditions and cannot account for biological responses (such as healing, remodeling, tunnel enlargement, etc.) that can have a significant influence on knee and ligament function [70].

In vivo studies incorporating body-weight loading and active muscular control provide a much more comprehensive and realistic picture of the natural function of the knee joint as a complex neuromusculoskeletal system. However, the studies should incorporate tasks of similar intensity and joint loading as are routine encountered by the individuals being evaluated. The behavior of the knee under low-demand conditions cannot be simply "scaled up" to predict behavior during functional activities, since knee tissues are highly viscoelastic and respond nonlinearly to load magnitude and loading rate [16, 74]. Therefore, studies incorporating body-weight loading during quasi-static activities (e.g., sequential fixed knee angles [34]) or low-effort movements (e.g., half-speed gait [77]) may not predict knee behavior during more complex, demanding tasks. The cartilage is also highly sensitive to shear motion, and increased joint contact velocity has been linked to knee osteoarthritis in both animal models and humans [3, 18]. Thus, well-designed studies, using state-of-the art tools to assess knee kinematics under in vivo, dynamic, high-loading, functionally relevant conditions, are necessary to evaluate the true dynamic function and stability of the knee [70].

4.3.1 Measurement Methods for Dynamic, In Vivo Studies

Several methods for the objective assessment of in vivo motion have been developed. The most common methods utilize high-speed cameras or skin marker-based video-motion capture systems [25, 64]. This method is noninvasive, widely available, and reliable and has been effective for identifying differences in knee kinematics after injury. But conventional motion analysis cannot achieve the submillimeter accuracy required for tissue-relevant measurements (such as changes in cartilage contact), because of the large displacements of skin-mounted markers relative to the underlying bone [23, 24, 28, 48]. Magnetic resonance imaging (MRI) can achieve submillimeter accuracy and enables direct visualization of soft tissue [17], but sample rates are too slow and the imaging environment is too restrictive for most functional movement tasks.

Dynamic radiographic imaging enables direct visualization and three-dimensional tracking of bone motion and has been gaining in popularity over the last decade. Biplane or stereoradiographic imaging systems can generally obtain submillimeter resolution in all three movement planes. Many systems are now in use, with capabilities that vary based on the specific equipment and analysis techniques employed. Conventional "C-arm" fluoroscopy systems are limited by low frame rates (30 Hz or less) and long exposure times (8ms or longer), but are adequate for quasi-static and low-speed activities [42, 69]. Custom-built systems (Fig. 4.1) can achieve much higher sample rates and have validated submillimeter accuracy for more physically demanding tasks, such as running [2, 53]. While dynamic radiographic imaging is more complex, expensive, and invasive due to radiation exposure, it is the only currently available technology that can provide reliable assessment of tibiofemoral kinematics during a variety of functional activities with submillimeter accuracy [2]. As the applications of radiographic methods continue to increase, a more comprehensive understanding of the nature and impact of various degrees and types of instabilities should emerge, leading to definitive answers in terms of the relative merits of different surgical procedures for restoring dynamic joint function and stability.

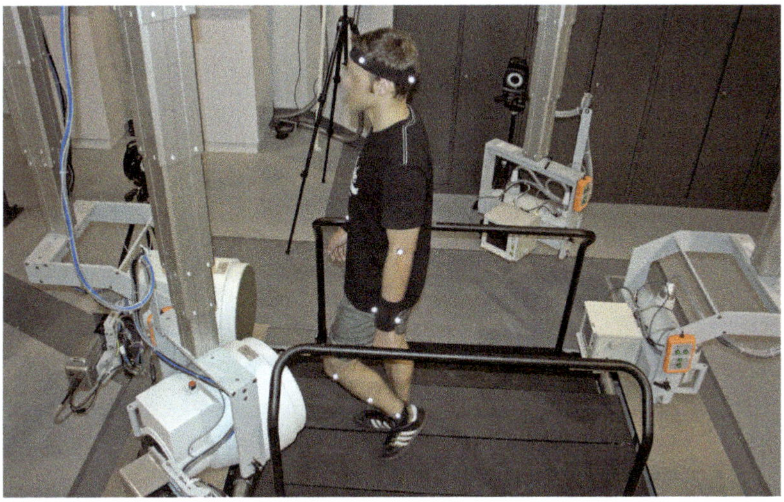

Fig. 4.1 High-speed stereoradiographic imaging system with instrumented treadmill, University of Pittsburgh. Biplane images are acquired simultaneously at up to 180 frame/s

4.3.2 Dynamic Instability After ACL Injury

Satisfactory subjective function can be achieved after ACL reconstruction, even with residual anterior static laxity [29, 36, 79]. Thus, the dynamic behavior of the reconstructed knee during functional activities may be more important for patient outcomes and quality of life than static laxity. Little is known, however, about the relationships between static laxity and dynamic stability. Traditional static laxity assessment (using a KT-1000 arthrometer) was compared to high-accuracy three-dimensional knee kinematics during downhill running using a 250 frame/s dynamic stereo x-ray system [47]. In ACL-reconstructed knees, anterior static knee laxity (absolute KT value for the reconstructed limb) was not significantly correlated with maximum dynamic anterior tibial translation (Spearman's rho = 0.26; $p = 0.23$) (Fig. 4.2). Another recent study comparing instrumented Lachman test (static laxity) to tibial translation during gait (dynamic stability) also found no significant relationship [68]. These studies raise significant doubts about the use of static laxity testing as a surrogate measure for dynamic joint stability.

4.3.3 Factors Affecting Dynamic Stability After ACL Reconstruction

While most methods for ACL reconstruction are similarly effective for restoring laxity (anterior drawer, Lachman, pivot shift) to normal or near-normal levels, dynamic studies have shown that the procedures may fail to restore normal function. Tashman et al. used a 250 frame/s dynamic stereo x-ray (DSX) system to evaluate in vivo knee kinematics during s stressful task (downhill running) for patients who underwent traditional, nonanatomic single-bundle reconstruction by

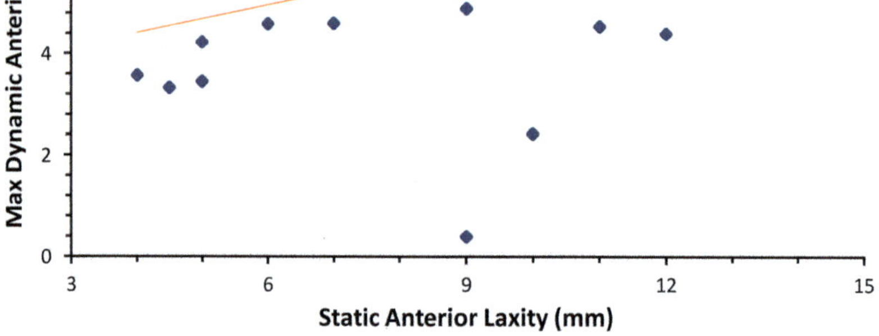

Fig. 4.2 Relationship between dynamic anterior translation during running and static anterior knee laxity in ACL-reconstructed knees. *Vertical axis* is the maximum increase (in mm) of anterior translation of the tibia relative to the femur from foot-strike through mid-stance. *Horizontal axis* is the absolute static laxity of the same knee (also in mm), assessed using KT-1000 arthrometer with manual maximum force. There was no significant correlation between static laxity and dynamic translation

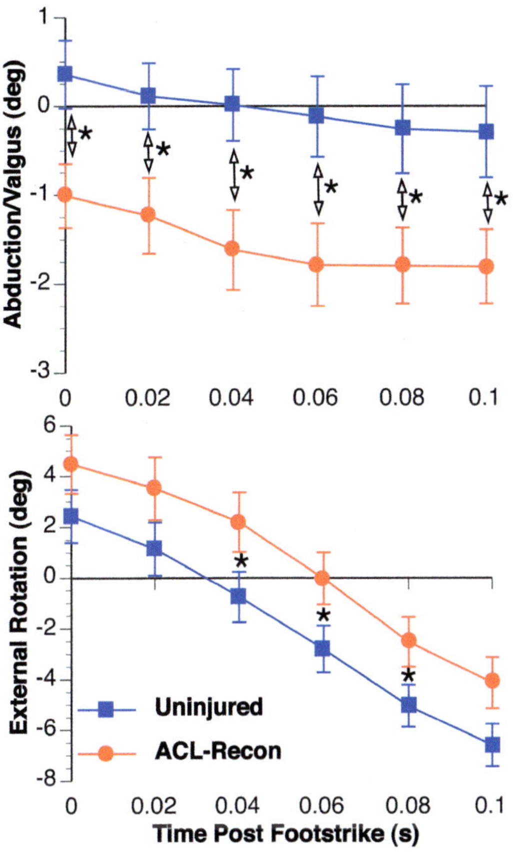

Fig. 4.3 Knee rotational kinematics during the early to mid-stance phase of downhill running, ACL-reconstructed (*red*) vs. contralateral; uninjured (*blue*). *Top*: internal/external rotation. *Bottom*: abduction/adduction. *Vertical lines* are ±1 SE; * $p<0.05$ (Reproduced from Refs. [71, 72])

means of transtibial drilling technique [71, 72]. While the reconstruction restored normal AP translation, reconstructed knees exhibited greater external tibial rotation (3.8±2.3°) and increased adduction (2.8±1.6°) relative to the contralateral, uninjured knees (Fig. 4.3). These rotational changes were associated with shifts in the areas of joint contact (Fig. 4.4) as well as a reduction in medial-compartment joint space under dynamic loading, demonstrating clear "midrange" instability (as defined above) that may place the joint at risk for degenerative changes. Studies such as this contributed to the growing interest in "anatomical" ACL reconstruction techniques, which attempt to place the graft tunnels closer to the native ACL insertion sites. While results of clinical studies on the benefits of anatomic ACL reconstruction for restoring laxity have been mixed, dynamic studies show improved joint stability. Abebe et al., using biplanar fluoroscopy and MR imaging, reported that anatomical femoral placement of the graft in single-bundle reconstruction resulted in a more stable knee during a lunge (Fig. 4.5) [1]. Patients with nonanatomic antero-proximal graft placement had up to 3.4 mm more anterior tibial translation, 1.1 mm more medial tibial translation, and 3.7° more internal tibial translation compared with the contralateral side. Patients with anatomical graft placement had motion that more closely replicated that of the intact knee, with anterior tibial translation within 0.8 mm, medial tibial translation within 0.5 mm, and internal tibial rotation within 1°.

While there is general (but not unanimous) consensus about the benefits of more anatomic graft placement, the merits of double-bundle reconstruction for further improving knee function have yet to be firmly established. Rotational instability has been discussed as a potentially important indicator of surgical outcome, but most studies have primarily relied upon the qualitative pivot-shift examination to evaluate rotational laxity, with inconclusive results and unclear relationships to dynamic function. Studies incorporating high-accuracy measurement methods are currently underway to assess knee kinematics under in vivo, dynamic, high-loading conditions (e.g., [35]). Results of these studies should provide significant insight into the relative performance of anatomic/double-bundle procedures for restoring normal joint motion.

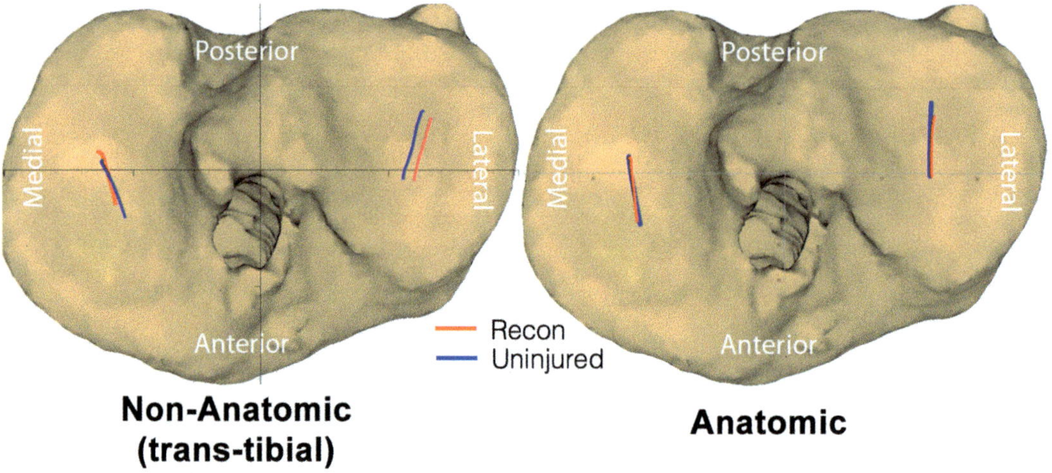

Fig. 4.4 Tibiofemoral contact paths during downhill running, ACL-reconstructed (*red*) vs. contralateral, uninjured knees (*blue*). *Left*: After nonanatomic reconstruction (with femoral tunnels drilled using a transtibial technique), significant differences were found in both the medial and lateral compartments (ANOVA; $p < 0.05$). After anatomic reconstruction (with femoral tunnels drilled using a medial portal technique), no significant differences were found

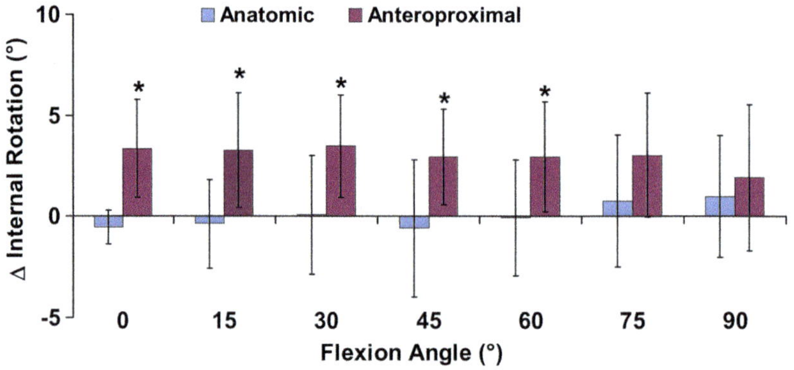

Fig. 4.5 The increase in internal tibial rotation of the reconstructed knee relative to the contralateral intact knee, plotted as a function of flexion (mean and 95 % confidence intervals). Internal tibial rotation was increased (relative to the contralateral, uninjured knees) with anteroproximally placed grafts, while anatomically placed grafts more closely restored normal rotational knee motion. (*$p < 0.05$) (Reproduced from Abebe et al. [1])

Fact Box 3

In vivo studies incorporating body-weight loading and active muscular control provide a much more comprehensive and realistic picture of the natural function of the knee joint as a complex neuromusculoskeletal system. Well-designed studies to assess knee kinematics under in vivo, dynamic, high-loading conditions are necessary to evaluate the relative performance of different procedures for restoring normal joint motion and preventing osteoarthritis after knee injury

Conclusions

Laxity tests are useful for the diagnosis of joint damage, but they have limited value for predicting dynamic joint stability and should not be used as surrogates for dynamic knee function. The pivot-shift test may have some merit for predicting dynamic instability, but remains limited by qualitative assessment and sub-physiological applied loads. Further development of consistent, instrumented methods for standardizing pivot-shift measurements may improve their predictive value, but comparisons with dynamic studies are necessary to establish their validity.

Studies incorporating high-accuracy kinematic assessment during functional activities have shown significant dynamic instabilities in ACL-reconstructed knees, even when normal laxity and pivot shift have been restored. Long-term studies are required to establish the extent to which these dynamic instabilities can adversely affect clinical outcomes and contribute to the development of osteoarthritis after ACL reconstruction.

References

1. Abebe ES, Utturkar GM, Taylor DC, Spritzer CE, Kim JP, Moorman CT, Garrett WE, DeFrate LE (2011) The effects of femoral graft placement on in vivo knee kinematics after anterior cruciate ligament reconstruction. J Biomech 44(5):924–929. doi:10.1016/j.jbiomech.2010.11.028, S0021-9290(10)00654-8
2. Anderst W, Zauel R, Bishop J, Demps E, Tashman S (2009) Validation of three-dimensional model-based tibio-femoral tracking during running. Med Eng Phys 31(1):10–16. doi:10.1016/j.medengphy.2008.03.003, S1350-4533(08)00044-1
3. Anderst WJ, Tashman S (2009) The association between velocity of the center of closest proximity on subchondral bones and osteoarthritis progression. J Orthop Res 27(1):71–77. doi:10.1002/jor.20702
4. Andriacchi TP, Briant PL, Bevill SL, Koo S (2006) Rotational changes at the knee after ACL injury cause cartilage thinning. Clin Orthop Relat Res 442:39–44
5. Andriacchi TP, Dyrby CO (2005) Interactions between kinematics and loading during walking for the normal and ACL deficient knee. J Biomech 38(2):293–298. doi:10.1016/j.jbiomech.2004.02.010
6. Andriacchi TP, Koo S, Scanlan SF (2009) Gait mechanics influence healthy cartilage morphology and osteoarthritis of the knee. J Bone Joint Surg Am 91(Suppl 1):95–101. doi:10.2106/jbjs.h.01408
7. Andriacchi TP, Mundermann A, Smith RL, Alexander EJ, Dyrby CO, Koo S (2004) A framework for the in vivo pathomechanics of osteoarthritis at the knee. Ann Biomed Eng 32(3):447–457
8. Arnold JA, Coker TP, Heaton LM, Park JP, Harris WD (1979) Natural history of anterior cruciate tears. Am J Sports Med 7(6):305–313
9. Balasch H, Schiller M, Friebel H, Hoffmann F (1999) Evaluation of anterior knee joint instability with the Rolimeter. A test in comparison with manual assessment and measuring with the KT-1000 arthrometer. Knee Surg Sports Traumatol Arthrosc 7(4):204–208
10. Barber SD, Noyes FR, Mangine RE, McCloskey JW, Hartman W (1990) Quantitative assessment of functional limitations in normal and anterior cruciate ligament-deficient knees. Clin Orthop Relat Res 255:204–214
11. Carter DR, Beaupre GS, Wong M, Smith RL, Andriacchi TP, Schurman DJ (2004) The mechanobiology of articular cartilage development and degeneration. Clin Orthop Relat Res (427 Suppl):S69–S77. doi:00003086-200410001-00014 [pii]
12. Chaudhari AM, Briant PL, Bevill SL, Koo S, Andriacchi TP (2008) Knee kinematics, cartilage morphology, and osteoarthritis after ACL injury. Med Sci Sports Exerc 40(2):215–222. doi:10.1249/mss.0b013e31815cbb0e
13. Cross MJ, Wootton JR, Bokor DJ, Sorrenti SJ (1993) Acute repair of injury to the anterior cruciate ligament. A long-term followup. Am J Sports Med 21(1):128–131
14. Daniel DM, Malcom LL, Losse G, Stone ML, Sachs R, Burks R (1985) Instrumented measurement of anterior laxity of the knee. J Bone Joint Surg Am 67(5):720–726
15. Daniel DM, Stone ML, Sachs R, Malcom L (1985) Instrumented measurement of anterior knee laxity in patients with acute anterior cruciate ligament disruption. Am J Sports Med 13(6):401–407
16. Dortmans L, Jans H, Sauren A, Huson A (1991) Nonlinear dynamic behavior of the human knee joint--Part II: Time-domain analyses: effects of structural damage in postmortem experiments. J Biomech Eng 113(4):392–396
17. Espregueira-Mendes J, Pereira H, Sevivas N, Passos C, Vasconcelos JC, Monteiro A, Oliveira JM, Reis RL (2012) Assessment of rotatory laxity in anterior cruciate ligament-deficient knees using magnetic resonance imaging with Porto-knee testing device. Knee Surg Sports Traumatol Arthrosc 20(4):671–678. doi:10.1007/s00167-012-1914-9
18. Farrokhi S, Voycheck CA, Klatt BA, Gustafson JA, Tashman S, Fitzgerald GK (2014) Altered tibiofemoral joint contact mechanics and kinematics in patients with knee osteoarthritis and episodic complaints of joint instability. Clin Biomech (Bristol, Avon) 29(6):629–635. doi:10.1016/j.clinbiomech.2014.04.014
19. Feagin JA Jr, Curl WW (1976) Isolated tear of the anterior cruciate ligament: 5-year follow-up study. Am J Sports Med 4(3):95–100
20. Fetto JF, Marshall JL (1979) Injury to the anterior cruciate ligament producing the pivot-shift sign. J Bone Joint Surg Am 61(5):710–714
21. Galway HR, MacIntosh DL (1980) The lateral pivot shift: a symptom and sign of anterior cruciate ligament insufficiency. Clin Orthop Relat Res 147:45–50
22. Ganko A, Engebretsen L, Ozer H (2000) The rolimeter: a new arthrometer compared with the KT-1000. Knee Surg Sports Traumatol Arthrosc 8(1):36–39. doi:10.1007/s001670050008
23. Gao B, Zheng NN (2008) Investigation of soft tissue movement during level walking: translations and rotations of skin markers. J Biomech 41(15):-3189–3195. doi:10.1016/j.jbiomech.2008.08.028, S0021-9290(08)00437-5 [pii]

24. Garling EH, Kaptein BL, Mertens B, Barendregt W, Veeger HE, Nelissen RG, Valstar ER (2007) Soft-tissue artefact assessment during step-up using fluoroscopy and skin-mounted markers. J Biomech 40(Suppl 1):S18–S24. doi:S0021-9290(07)00108-X [pii]
25. Georgoulis AD, Papadonikolakis A, Papageorgiou CD, Mitsou A, Stergiou N (2003) Three-dimensional tibiofemoral kinematics of the anterior cruciate ligament-deficient and reconstructed knee during walking. Am J Sports Med 31(1):75–79
26. Goyal K, Tashman S, Wang JH, Li K, Zhang X, Harner C (2012) In vivo analysis of the isolated posterior cruciate ligament-deficient knee during functional activities. Am J Sports Med 40(4):777–785. doi:10.1177/0363546511435783
27. Harter RA, Osternig LR, Singer KM, James SL, Larson RL, Jones DC (1988) Long-term evaluation of knee stability and function following surgical reconstruction for anterior cruciate ligament insufficiency. Am J Sports Med 16(5):434–443
28. Holden JP, Chou G, Stanhope SJ (1997) Changes in knee joint function over a wide range of walking speeds. Clin Biomech (Bristol, Avon) 12(6):375–382
29. Hong L, Li X, Zhang H, Liu X, Zhang J, Shen JW, Feng H (2012) Anterior cruciate ligament reconstruction with remnant preservation: a prospective, randomized controlled study. Am J Sports Med 40(12):2747–2755. doi:10.1177/0363546512461481
30. Hoshino Y, Araujo P, Ahlden M, Samuelsson K, Muller B, Hofbauer M, Wolf MR, Irrgang JJ, Fu FH, Musahl V (2013) Quantitative evaluation of the pivot shift by image analysis using the iPad. Knee Surg Sports Traumatol Arthrosc 21(4):975–980. doi:10.1007/s00167-013-2396-0
31. Hoshino Y, Kuroda R, Nagamune K, Araki D, Kubo S, Yamaguchi M, Kurosaka M (2012) Optimal measurement of clinical rotational test for evaluating anterior cruciate ligament insufficiency. Knee Surg Sports Traumatol Arthrosc 20(7):1323–1330. doi:10.1007/s00167-011-1643-5
32. Hoshino Y, Kuroda R, Nagamune K, Yagi M, Mizuno K, Yamaguchi M, Muratsu H, Yoshiya S, Kurosaka M (2007) In vivo measurement of the pivot-shift test in the anterior cruciate ligament-deficient knee using an electromagnetic device. Am J Sports Med 35(7):1098–1104, 0363546507299447
33. Hoshino Y, Wang JH, Lorenz S, Fu FH, Tashman S (2012) The effect of distal femur bony morphology on in vivo knee translational and rotational kinematics. Knee Surg Sports Traumatol Arthrosc 20(7):1331–1338. doi:10.1007/s00167-011-1661-3
34. Hosseini A, Gill TJ, Li G (2009) In vivo anterior cruciate ligament elongation in response to axial tibial loads. J Orthop Sci 14(3):298–306. doi:10.1007/s00776-009-1325-z
35. Irrgang JJ, Tashman S, Moore C, Fu FH (2012) Challenge accepted: description of an ongoing NIH-funded randomized clinical trial to compare anatomic single-bundle versus anatomic double-bundle ACL reconstruction. Arthroscopy 28(6):745–747. doi:10.1016/j.arthro.2012.04.003; author reply 747–748
36. Janssen RP, du Mee AW, van Valkenburg J, Sala HA, Tseng CM (2013) Anterior cruciate ligament reconstruction with 4-strand hamstring autograft and accelerated rehabilitation: a 10-year prospective study on clinical results, knee osteoarthritis and its predictors. Knee Surg Sports Traumatol Arthrosc 21(9):1977–1988. doi:10.1007/s00167-012-2234-9
37. Johnson DL, Urban WP Jr, Caborn DN, Vanarthos WJ, Carlson CS (1998) Articular cartilage changes seen with magnetic resonance imaging-detected bone bruises associated with acute anterior cruciate ligament rupture. Am J Sports Med 26(3):409–414
38. Jonsson H, Riklund-Ahlstrom K, Lind J (2004) Positive pivot shift after ACL reconstruction predicts later osteoarthrosis: 63 patients followed 5-9 years after surgery. Acta Orthop Scand 75(5):594–599. doi:10.1080/00016470410001484
39. Kocher MS, Steadman JR, Briggs KK, Sterett WI, Hawkins RJ (2004) Relationships between objective assessment of ligament stability and subjective assessment of symptoms and function after anterior cruciate ligament reconstruction. Am J Sports Med 32(3):629–634
40. Kuroda R, Hoshino Y, Kubo S, Araki D, Oka S, Nagamune K, Kurosaka M (2012) Similarities and differences of diagnostic manual tests for anterior cruciate ligament insufficiency: a global survey and kinematics assessment. Am J Sports Med 40(1):91–99. doi:10.1177/0363546511423634, 0363546511423634
41. Leitze Z, Losee RE, Jokl P, Johnson TR, Feagin JA (2005) Implications of the pivot shift in the ACL-deficient knee. Clin Orthop Relat Res 436:229–236
42. Li G, Van de Velde SK, Bingham JT (2008) Validation of a non-invasive fluoroscopic imaging technique for the measurement of dynamic knee joint motion. J Biomech 41(7):1616–1622. doi:10.1016/j.jbiomech.2008.01.034, S0021-9290(08)00083-3
43. Lipke JM, Janecki CJ, Nelson CL, McLeod P, Thompson C, Thompson J, Haynes DW (1981) The role of incompetence of the anterior cruciate and lateral ligaments in anterolateral and anteromedial instability. A biomechanical study of cadaver knees. J Bone Joint Surg Am 63(6):954–960
44. Lopomo N, Signorelli C, Bonanzinga T, Marcheggiani Muccioli GM, Visani A, Zaffagnini S (2012) Quantitative assessment of pivot-shift using inertial sensors. Knee Surg Sports Traumatol Arthrosc 20(4):713–717. doi:10.1007/s00167-011-1865-6
45. Lopomo N, Zaffagnini S, Signorelli C, Bignozzi S, Giordano G, Marcheggiani Muccioli GM, Visani A (2012) An original clinical methodology for non-invasive assessment of pivot-shift test. Comput Methods Biomech Biomed Engin 15(12):1323–1328. doi:10.1080/10255842.2011.591788
46. Losee RE, Johnson TR, Southwick WO (1978) Anterior subluxation of the lateral tibial plateau. A

diagnostic test and operative repair. J Bone Joint Surg Am 60(8):1015–1030
47. Ma Y, Thorhauer E, Tashman S (2014) Relationships between static laxity and dynamic knee function after ACL reconstruction. Paper presented at the 60th Orthopaedic Research Society Annual Meeting, New Orleans, 15–18 Mar 2014
48. Manal K, McClay Davis I, Galinat B, Stanhope S (2003) The accuracy of estimating proximal tibial translation during natural cadence walking: bone vs. skin mounted targets. Clin Biomech (Bristol, Avon) 18(2):126–131
49. Markolf KL, Park S, Jackson SR, McAllister DR (2008) Simulated pivot-shift testing with single and double-bundle anterior cruciate ligament reconstructions. J Bone Joint Surg Am 90(8):1681–1689. doi:10.2106/jbjs.g.01272
50. Matsushita T, Oka S, Nagamune K, Matsumoto T, Nishizawa Y, Hoshino Y, Kubo S, Kurosaka M, Kuroda R (2013) Differences in Knee Kinematics Between Awake and Anesthetized Patients During the Lachman and Pivot-Shift Tests for Anterior Cruciate Ligament Deficiency. Orthop J Sports Med 1(1):1–6
51. McLean SG, Oh YK, Palmer ML, Lucey SM, Lucarelli DG, Ashton-Miller JA, Wojtys EM (2011) The relationship between anterior tibial acceleration, tibial slope, and ACL strain during a simulated jump landing task. J Bone Joint Surg Am 93(14):1310–1317. doi:10.2106/jbjs.j.00259
52. McQuade KJ, Sidles JA, Larson RV (1989) Reliability of the Genucom Knee Analysis System. A pilot study. Clin Orthop Relat Res 245:216–219
53. Miranda DL, Schwartz JB, Loomis AC, Brainerd EL, Fleming BC, Crisco JJ (2011) Static and dynamic error of a biplanar videoradiography system using marker-based and markerless tracking techniques. J Biomech Eng 133(12):121002. doi:10.1115/1.4005471
54. Miyazaki T, Wada M, Kawahara H, Sato M, Baba H, Shimada S (2002) Dynamic load at baseline can predict radiographic disease progression in medial compartment knee osteoarthritis. Ann Rheum Dis 61(7):617–622
55. Monaco E, Labianca L, Conteduca F, De Carli A, Ferretti A (2007) Double bundle or single bundle plus extraarticular tenodesis in ACL reconstruction? A CAOS study. Knee Surg Sports Traumatol Arthrosc 15(10):1168–1174. doi:10.1007/s00167-007-0368-y
56. Moro-oka TA, Hamai S, Miura H, Shimoto T, Higaki H, Fregly BJ, Iwamoto Y, Banks SA (2008) Dynamic activity dependence of in vivo normal knee kinematics. J Orthop Res 26(4):428–434. doi:10.1002/jor.20488
57. Musahl V, Ayeni OR, Citak M, Irrgang JJ, Pearle AD, Wickiewicz TL (2010) The influence of bony morphology on the magnitude of the pivot shift. Knee Surg Sports Traumatol Arthrosc 18(9):1232–1238. doi:10.1007/s00167-010-1129-x
58. Musahl V, Burkart A, Debski RE, Van Scyoc A, Fu FH, Woo SL (2002) Accuracy of anterior cruciate ligament tunnel placement with an active robotic system: a cadaveric study. Arthroscopy 18(9):968–973. doi:a0180968 [pii]
59. Musahl V, Citak M, O'Loughlin PF, Choi D, Bedi A, Pearle AD (2010) The effect of medial versus lateral meniscectomy on the stability of the anterior cruciate ligament-deficient knee. Am J Sports Med 38(8):1591–1597. doi:10.1177/0363546510364402
60. Musahl V, Hoshino Y, Becker R, Karlsson J (2012) Rotatory knee laxity and the pivot shift. Knee Surg Sports Traumatol Arthrosc 20(4):601–602. doi:10.1007/s00167-011-1844-y
61. Noyes FR, Bassett RW, Grood ES, Butler DL (1980) Arthroscopy in acute traumatic hemarthrosis of the knee. Incidence of anterior cruciate tears and other injuries. J Bone Joint Surg Am 62(5):687–695, 757
62. Ohashi B, Lopomo N, Zaffagnini S, Hoshino Y, Kuroda R, Samuelsson K, Irrgang J, Musahl V (2014) Quantitative measurement of a standardized Pivot-shift: comparison between the awake and the examination under anesthesia in patients with acute ACL injury. Proc Orthop Res Soc 60:1671
63. Oliver JH, Coughlin LP (1987) Objective knee evaluation using the Genucom Knee Analysis System. Clinical implications. Am J Sports Med 15(6):571–578
64. Pappas E, Zampeli F, Xergia SA, Georgoulis AD (2013) Lessons learned from the last 20 years of ACL-related in vivo-biomechanics research of the knee joint. Knee Surg Sports Traumatol Arthrosc 21(4):755–766. doi:10.1007/s00167-012-1955-0
65. Seto JL, Orofino AS, Morrissey MC, Medeiros JM, Mason WJ (1988) Assessment of quadriceps/hamstring strength, knee ligament stability, functional and sports activity levels five years after anterior cruciate ligament reconstruction. Am J Sports Med 16(2):170–180
66. Smith RL, Donlon BS, Gupta MK, Mohtai M, Das P, Carter DR, Cooke J, Gibbons G, Hutchinson N, Schurman DJ (1995) Effects of fluid-induced shear on articular chondrocyte morphology and metabolism in vitro. J Orthop Res 13(6):824–831. doi:10.1002/jor.1100130604
67. Snyder-Mackler L, Fitzgerald GK, Bartolozzi AR 3rd, Ciccotti MG (1997) The relationship between passive joint laxity and functional outcome after anterior cruciate ligament injury. Am J Sports Med 25(2):191–195
68. Sonesson S, Kvist J (2015) Dynamic and static tibial translation in patients with anterior cruciate ligament deficiency initially treated with a structured rehabilitation protocol. Knee Surg Sports Traumatol Arthrosc. doi:10.1007/s00167-015-3714-5
69. Tashman S (2008) Comments on "validation of a non-invasive fluoroscopic imaging technique for the measurement of dynamic knee joint motion". J Biomech 41(15):3290–3291. doi:10.1016/j.jbiomech.2008.07.038; author reply 3292–3293
70. Tashman S, Araki D (2013) Effects of anterior cruciate ligament reconstruction on in vivo, dynamic knee function. Clin Sports Med 32(1):47–59. doi:10.1016/j.csm.2012.08.006

71. Tashman S, Collon D, Anderson K, Kolowich P, Anderst W (2004) Abnormal rotational knee motion during running after anterior cruciate ligament reconstruction. Am J Sports Med 32(4):975–983
72. Tashman S, Kolowich P, Collon D, Anderson K, Anderst W (2007) Dynamic function of the ACL-reconstructed knee during running. Clin Orthop Relat Res 454:66–73. doi:10.1097/BLO.0b013e31802bab3e
73. Torg JS, Conrad W, Kalen V (1976) Clinical diagnosis of anterior cruciate ligament instability in the athlete. Am J Sports Med 4(2):84–93
74. van Dommelen JA, Jolandan MM, Ivarsson BJ, Millington SA, Raut M, Kerrigan JR, Crandall JR, Diduch DR (2006) Nonlinear viscoelastic behavior of human knee ligaments subjected to complex loading histories. Ann Biomed Eng 34(6):1008–1018. doi:10.1007/s10439-006-9100-1
75. van Eck CF, Loopik M, van den Bekerom MP, Fu FH, Kerkhoffs GM (2013) Methods to diagnose acute anterior cruciate ligament rupture: a meta-analysis of instrumented knee laxity tests. Knee Surg Sports Traumatol Arthrosc 21(9):1989–1997. doi:10.1007/s00167-012-2246-5
76. van Eck CF, van den Bekerom MP, Fu FH, Poolman RW, Kerkhoffs GM (2013) Methods to diagnose acute anterior cruciate ligament rupture: a meta-analysis of physical examinations with and without anaesthesia. Knee Surg Sports Traumatol Arthrosc 21(8):1895–1903. doi:10.1007/s00167-012-2250-9
77. Wu JL, Hosseini A, Kozanek M, Gadikota HR, Gill TJ, Li G (2010) Kinematics of the anterior cruciate ligament during gait. Am J Sports Med 38(7):1475–1482. doi:10.1177/0363546510364240, 0363546510364240
78. Yagi M, Wong EK, Kanamori A, Debski RE, Fu FH, Woo SL (2002) Biomechanical analysis of an anatomic anterior cruciate ligament reconstruction. Am J Sports Med 30(5):660–666
79. Yang JH, Yoon JR, Jeong HI, Hwang DH, Woo SJ, Kwon JH, Nha KW (2012) Second-look arthroscopic assessment of arthroscopic single-bundle posterior cruciate ligament reconstruction: comparison of mixed graft versus achilles tendon allograft. Am J Sports Med 40(9):2052–2060. doi:10.1177/0363546512454532
80. Zantop T, Schumacher T, Diermann N, Schanz S, Raschke MJ, Petersen W (2007) Anterolateral rotational knee instability: role of posterolateral structures. Winner of the AGA-DonJoy Award 2006. Arch Orthop Trauma Surg 127(9):743–752. doi:10.1007/s00402-006-0241-3

MRI Laxity Assessment

5

Hélder Pereira, Sérgio Gomes, José Carlos Vasconcelos, Laura Soares, Rogério Pereira, Joaquim Miguel Oliveira, Rui L. Reis, and Joao Espregueira-Mendes

Contents

5.1 Introduction

The algorithms for treatment of anterior cruciate ligament (ACL) injuries have continued to evolve in recent years [42]. These changes have been supported by an improved understanding of joint kinematics and biomechanics as well as from the technical developments introduced for ACL repair techniques [5, 42]. The "double-bundle concept," including the recognition of partial tears of the ACL, has motivated new techniques for reconstruction or augmentation of ACL injuries [38–40, 50]. Individualized ACL repair is now recommended by several authors depending on patient's characteristics, specific demands, and surgeons' experience [1, 42].

H. Pereira (✉)
3B's Research Group – Biomaterials, Biodegradables and Biomimetics, University of Minho, Braga, Portugal

European Institute of Excellence on Tissue Engineering and Regenerative Medicine, Avepark – Parque de Ciência e Tecnologia, Zona Industrial da Gandra, Barco Guimarães 4805-017, Portugal

ICVS/3B's – PT Government Associated Laboratory, Barco Guimarães, Portugal

Ripoll y De Prado Sports Clinic – FIFA Medical Centre of Excellence, Murcia-Madrid, Spain

Orthopedic Department, Centro Hospitalar Póvoa de Varzim, Póvoa do Varzim - Vila do Conde, Portugal
e-mail: helderduartepereira@gmail.com

S. Gomes • J.C. Vasconcelos • L. Soares • R. Pereira
Clínica do Dragão Espregueira-Mendes Sports Centre – FIFA Medical Centre of Excellence, Porto, Portugal

J.M. Oliveira • R.L. Reis • J. Espregueira-Mendes
3B's Research Group – Biomaterials, Biodegradables and Biomimetics, University of Minho, Braga, Portugal

European Institute of Excellence on Tissue Engineering and Regenerative Medicine, Avepark – Parque de Ciência e Tecnologia, Zona Industrial da Gandra, Barco Guimarães 4805-017, Portugal

ICVS/3B's – PT Government Associated Laboratory, Barco Guimarães, Portugal

Clínica do Dragão Espregueira-Mendes Sports Centre – FIFA Medical Centre of Excellence, Porto, Portugal

V. Musahl et al. (eds.), *Rotatory Knee Instability*, DOI 10.1007/978-3-319-32070-0_5

Suboptimal outcomes following ACL repair can be related to an inexact diagnosis and inaccurate preoperative planning. Improved diagnostic capacities are in great need in order to assist in the choice for the best course of treatment for each patient. Several attempts have been made and are currently under development to enhance the capacity of imaging assessment. One of the recent trends is the possibility for dynamic evaluation either using radiographs [20, 51], ultrasound [17], or MRI [12, 25] in order to test simultaneously the functional capacity of the ligaments. Robotics [10, 64] and electronic devices [34] have also been proposed.

This work aims to describe the traditional features of MRI evaluation of ACL tears but also the evolving possibility for dynamic and objective quantification of knee laxity. This concept proposes to enhance the clinical evaluation tests by combining simultaneous MRI imaging assessment.

5.2 The Concept of Rotatory Instability of the Knee

Clinical examination is still one of the most important steps when evaluating the injured knee [41]. Laxity evaluation and grading is considered a key point to success [2, 19]. The most frequently used clinical tests are the Lachman (considered the most sensitive) and the Pivot shift test (considered the most specific) [44]. However, manual clinical examination is difficult to quantify, as it is examiner dependent and lacks intra-tester reliability [2, 26, 27, 36, 53]. Several methods to achieve objective instrumented assessment of the Lachman test [24] have been used [41]. However, some concerns about poor correlation with clinical outcome have been reported [24].

However, the pivot shift has been considered more specific than the Lachman test [4], and it might also be useful in the clinical diagnosis of partial ACL tears [11]. Nevertheless, in a recent study, the clinical grading of the pivot shift has been considered as subjective and inconsistent [19]. In this study, weak correlations were found between the quantitative measurements and the clinical pivot shift grade [19]. Based on that results, the authors suggested to use a simple positive/negative grading and add a quantitative value to register the pivot shift [19]. Many descriptions of the maneuver have been proposed, and many devices have been developed in an attempt to objectively quantify the pivot shift test [36, 40, 41].

If the pivot shift test remains positive after ACL repair, this has been correlated with poor subjective and objective outcome. In such cases, lower rates of return to sports and higher development of degenerative changes have also been reported [21, 31]. One major limitation of the pivot shift test is that it is a non-weight-bearing examination and cannot mimic the true effect of rotatory knee laxity in dynamic weight-bearing conditions [39].

Bony morphology is another aspect, which is known to influence knee stability and the pivot shift phenomenon. Smaller lateral tibial plateau has been reported to be related to higher grade pivot shift test [36]. It has also been suggested that an increased degree of posterior–inferior tibial slope is related to higher pivot shift grade [6]. Moreover, it has also been reported that the distal femoral geometry can influence dynamic rotatory laxity [18].

Besides the bony morphology, features of the ligament itself are also involved in this pivot shift phenomenon. The posterolateral (PL) bundle of the ACL ligament was believed to be the primary responsible for controlling rotational stability; however, the anteromedial (AM) also plays a relevant role [23, 62]. The relative contributions of each bundle are dependent on the knee flexion angle [62].

In terms of all the abovementioned, it is necessary to combine anatomical and functional assessment. The eradication of a positive pivot shift test is considered the most important goal of the ACL repair surgery. Therefore, the first step should be to improve the objective quantification of the pivot shift phenomenon.

MRI has proved its value in anatomic study of the knee. If the "power" of this imaging technology can be combined with the dynamic evaluation of the joint, this will surely provide improvements of pre- and postoperative assessment. Moreover, this dynamic evaluation using the MRI device should enable joint assessment in different degrees of flexion and combine anterior–posterior and rotational forces.

5.3 Comprehensive Evaluation of ACL Tear on MRI

Previous studies have reported a general 78–100 % sensitivity and 68–100 % specificity of MRI for the diagnosis of ACL tears [16, 47, 56, 61]. In recent studies an accuracy of approximately 95 % has been reported [3]. The diagnosis of proximal, partial, or chronic tears has been considered as more challenging and accounts for most of the persistent errors in interpretation [3]. Sensitivity is also significantly decreased in cases of multi-ligament injury [3, 49]. Recently, 3-tesla imaging has improved the distinction of the AM and PL bundles; however, it has not significantly increased the MRI accuracy for detection of ACL injuries [60]. Concerning MRI analysis, about 70 % of ACL tears occur in the middle part of the ligament, 7–20 % occur near its femoral origin, and only 3–10 % are identified at the tibial insertion [45, 46].

MRI protocols for the knee joint are designed to yield diagnostic images of the ACL as well as the menisci, bones, articular cartilage, and other ligamentous structures of the knee. The requirements for optimal meniscus and cartilage imaging are more demanding than what is needed for diagnostic ACL imaging. In general, a protocol that enables proper imaging of the menisci and cartilage will also satisfactorily demonstrate the ACL. For that reason, several centers image patients in full knee extension, although the ACL is better evaluated with the knee in approximately 30° of flexion [30].

T2 sequences are most relevant for the diagnosis of acute ACL ruptures [33]. However, in most centers, the regular protocol for knee MRI evaluation includes T2-weighted sequences (or proton-weighted fat-suppressed) in 2–3 orthogonal planes and one T1-weighted sequence in either the sagittal or coronal plane [14, 33]. Lately, fast spin echo fat saturation sequences have proven to be quicker and more sensitive to injury than conventional T2-weighted spin echo images and have been increasingly replacing these sequences [16].

When evaluating an MRI examination, the observer must be familiar with the "normal" and "abnormal" features and routinely inspect the ACL in all planes [16]. The method of acquisition of sagittal images for ACL study has varied over time. A frequent recommendation, in order to achieve images closer to the long axis of the ACL, is to perform sagittal oblique slices at 10–15° perpendicular to a bicondylar line tangent to the posterior margins of the medial and lateral femoral condyles [16]. However, several centers now advise that the true sagittal plane (perpendicular to the bicondylar line) is superior for evaluation of the ACL and meniscus as well (Unpublished data, Mayo Clinic, Jacksonville, Fla. Presented at Society of Skeletal Radiology, March 2009).

5.3.1 Acute ACL Tear

The changes of the ACL tissue itself, which permit a high accuracy in the diagnosis of an acute tear, are considered the primary signs of ACL tear (Fact Box 1) [13, 29]. The axis of the ACL is abnormal if it is clearly more horizontal than a line projected along the intercondylar roof (Blumensaat line) on sagittal images (Fig. 5.1) [13]. An angle of less than 45° of the long axis of the ACL relative to a line parallel to the tibial plateau, also known as "the ACL angle," is reported to be sensitive and specific for an ACL rupture [32].

Fact Box 1. Summary of Primary and Secondary MRI Signs of Acute ACL Tear

Primary signs (enable the diagnostic per se)	*Secondary signs* (its absence does not exclude the diagnosis of ACL tear)
Non-visualization of the ACL	Pivot shift bone bruises/osteochondral fractures
Rupture of the substance of the ACL noticed by abnormal increased signal intensity	Anterior translocation of the tibia
ACL abrupt angulation or wavy appearance	Segond fracture: high association with ACL injury
Abnormal axis of the ACL	Fracture of the tibial spine: less reliably associated with ACL tear

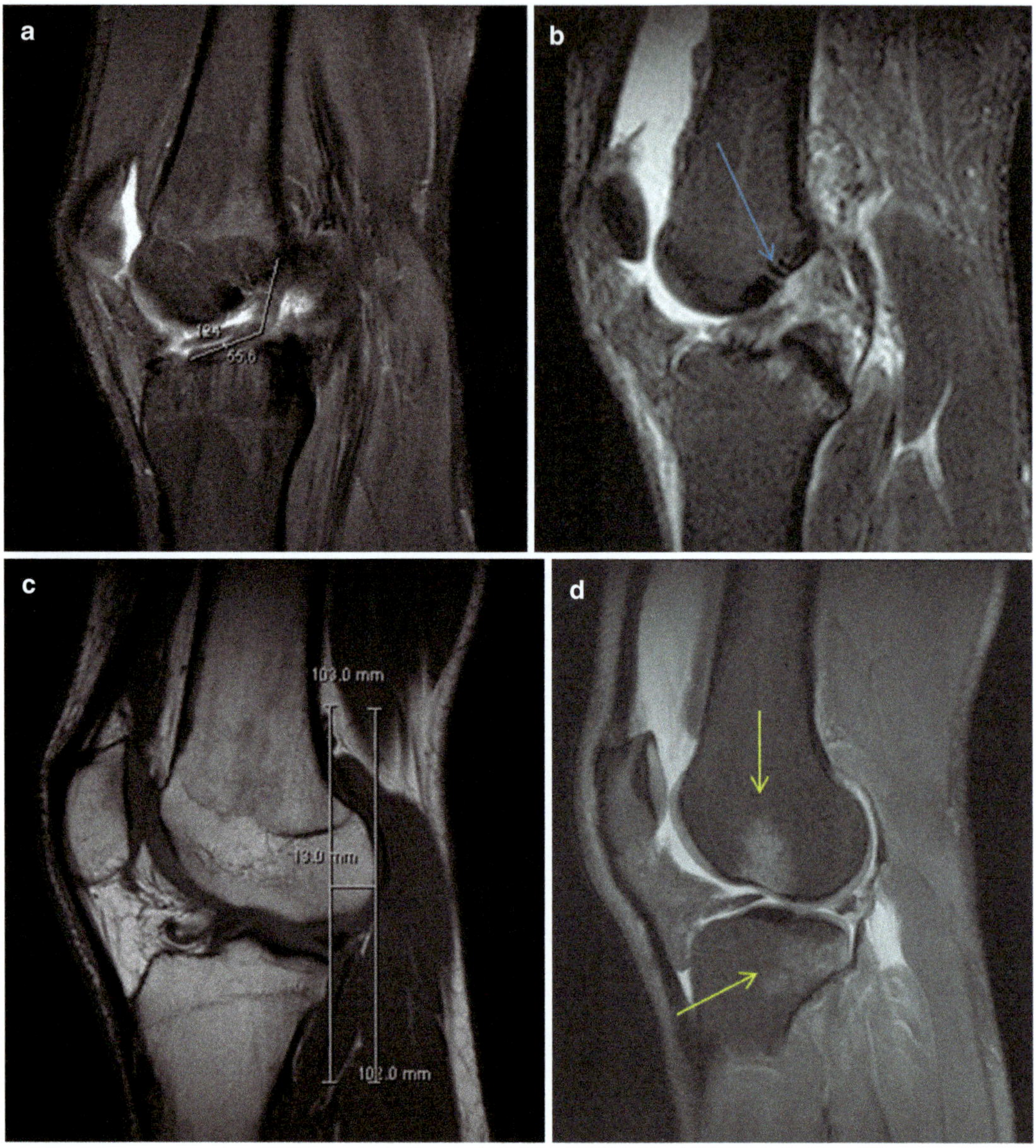

Fig. 5.1 Examples of primary signs of acute ACL tear: ACL abrupt angulation (**a**) and rupture of the substance of the ACL noticed by abnormal increased signal intensity (*blue arrow*) (**b**). Examples of secondary signs of acute ACL tear: anterior translocation of the tibia (10 mm in this example) (**c**) and bone femoral and tibial bruises (*yellow arrows*) (**d**)

A common finding of an acute ACL rupture is non-visualization of the ligament. Focal edema and/or hemorrhage are seen where the "normal" ACL is expected to be found. Enlargement and increased internal signal intensity, while preserving intact fascicles have been described as interstitial tear (or delaminated tear). This type of tear must be differentiated from mucoid degeneration of the intact ACL [13, 16].

Axial images should also be carefully reviewed to assess the proximal ACL close to the lateral wall of the intercondylar notch [48]. The secondary signs of acute ACL rupture are MRI findings that do not correspond to the ACL proper but are correlated to the injury mechanism (Fact Box 1). The absence of such signs does not exclude the diagnosis of ACL rupture [7, 16]. However, they are useful when primary signs are found to be ambiguous [7].

When a rotatory injury of the ACL occurs, there is a movement of external rotation of the lateral femoral condyle (LFC) relative to the fixed tibia. This way, the LFC causes an impact to the posterolateral tibial plateau, which might give origin to bone bruises and/or fractures of one or both bones [35]. The LFC bone bruise is usually found close to the anterior horn lateral meniscus. However, if such injuries occur at higher degrees of flexion, these bruises will be found more posteriorly. The tibial bone bruise/fracture usually occurs at the posterolateral corner of the tibia [35].

Anterior translocation of the tibia indirectly suggests ACL insufficiency [9]. If this anterior translocation exceeds 5 mm, an acute or chronic ACL tear is probable to be found [9]. A Segond fracture (Fig. 5.2) has a 75–100 % association with ACL tear [46]. The Segond fracture is described as an elliptical, vertical, 3 × 10-mm bone fragment parallel to the lateral tibial cortex about 4 mm distal to the plateau [8]. These types of fractures have historically been attributed to traction avulsion of the middle third of the meniscotibial capsular ligament [8]. The iliotibial band and lateral collateral ligament complex might also play a role [8].

Tibial spine fractures occur in approximately 5 % of adults with traumatic ACL insufficiency. The ACL insertion usually takes place immediately lateral and anterior to the tibial spine. For this reason, tibial spine fractures can be seen in patients with a normally functioning ACL. Tibial spine avulsion resulting in ACL insufficiency is usually related to a hyperextension injury mechanism. In children, tibial spine fractures are often isolated, while in adults the injury is frequently associated to high-energy injuries [55].

In addition, there are five specific fractures that are statistically associated with ACL injuries and should also be taken into account (table 5.1) [7, 16].

One study reported that kissing bone bruises on the anterior femur and tibia suggest a hyperextension mechanism and were found in association with ACL tears in approximately 50 % [54]. Avulsion fractures of the proximal fibula,

Table 5.1 Fractures commonly associated with ACL injury

Segond fracture (high probability of ACL injury)
Deep-lateral femoral-notch sign fracture (high probability of ACL injury)
Tibial spine avulsion fracture (intermediate probability of ACL injury)
Fracture of the posterolateral corner of the tibia (intermediate probability of ACL injury)
Arcuate fibular head fracture (intermediate probability of ACL injury)

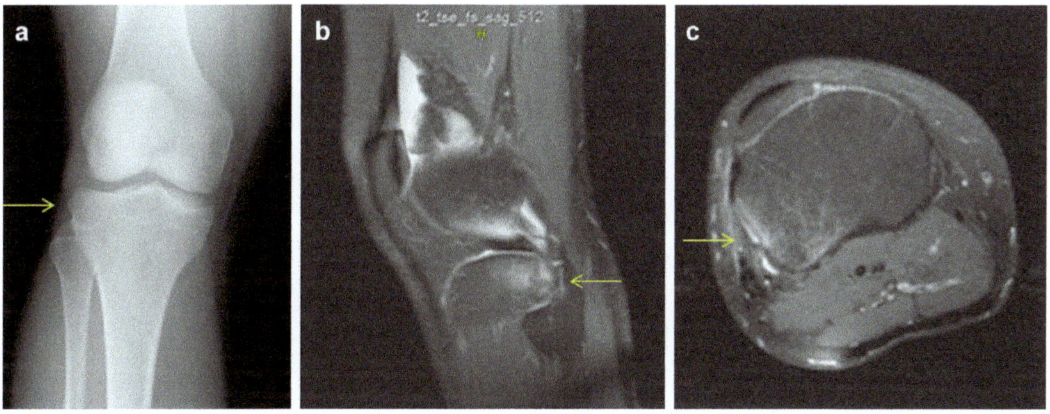

Fig. 5.2 Example of Segond fracture is difficult to identify on radiographs (*yellow arrows*) (**a**) but better clarified on MRI T2 sagittal view (**b**) and axial view (**c**)

also known as the arcuate sign, can indicate a hyperextension/varus knee injury which usually may affect the lateral collateral ligament complex, and the ACL might also be injured [22]. In severe hyperextension injuries, the posterior cruciate ligament might be damaged, and even popliteal neurovascular injuries can occur [63].

5.3.2 Chronic ACL Tear

Chronic ACL ruptures are often associated to meniscal injuries and secondary osteoarthritis. The signs of ACL injury are basically the same as in the acute setting except that bone bruises and edema are usually no longer visible and T1-weighted sequences are of greater importance [57].

A fragmented ACL is the most common MRI finding in the case of a chronic injury [57]. Complete non-visualization of the ACL may also occur and include the "empty notch" sign [45].

The chronically torn ACL may attach to the posterior cruciate ligament (the so-called ACL on PCL) [52]. This phenomenon is more often noticed during arthroscopic observation and is less frequently visible on MRI [52]. The chronic non-displaced ruptured ACL might have a normal appearance once mature collagenous scarring is difficult to distinguish from the normal collagenous hypointense ligament [57].

In the presence of a positive clinical assessment (positive Lachman or pivot shift test result), a negative MRI should be interpreted as a possible false negative.

5.3.3 Partial ACL Tear

Partial ruptures of the ACL account for 10–43 % of all ACL injuries [15, 29, 37, 48] and have reported an even higher percentage in the pediatric population [43]. While MRI is effective in differentiating the normal from abnormal ACL, it is less reliable in terms of the diagnosis of partial ruptures [28]. Even 3-tesla MRI devices have failed to overcome this limitation [58, 59].

5.4 Dynamic and Objective MRI Assessment of the Knee: Porto-Knee Testing Device (PKTD)

The PKTD (Fig. 5.3) is a knee laxity-testing device designed for the measurement of anterior–posterior tibial translation and rotational laxity of the knee during an MRI examination [12]. This way it combines the assessment of "anatomy" and "function" during the same examination [40].

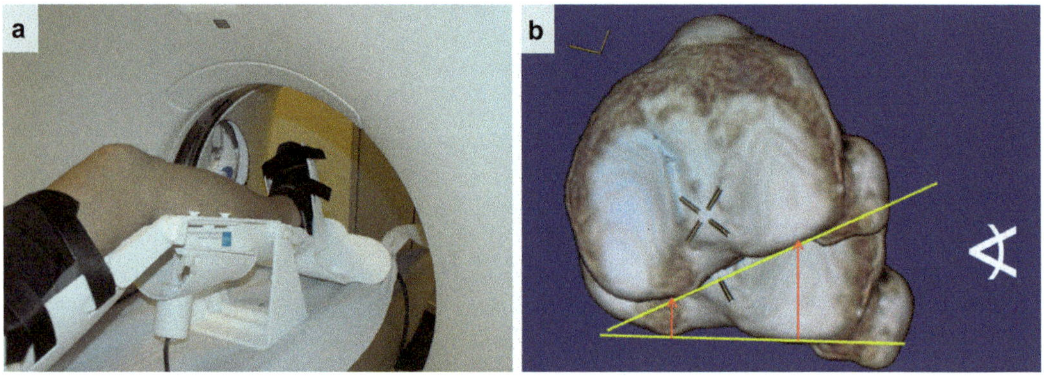

Fig. 5.3 Porto-knee testing device (PKTD®) inside MRI equipment (**a**); CT 3D axial view representation of tibial internal rotation and anterior translation after load application by the PKTD (**b**)

PKTD is built on polyurethane which permits it to be used during MRI scans. The knee is placed under stress caused by the inflation of pneumatic cuffs permitting the examiner to control the magnitude of load transmission up to 46.7×10^3 N/m^2 applied in the posterior proximal calf region.

The PKTD enables the examiner to study at different degrees of knee flexion and different degrees of external/internal rotation as decided by the footplate. When required, it can also be used for evaluation of PCL injuries (Fig. 5.4). This is done by changing the position of the cuff, thus transmitting force to be applied to the anterior aspect of the tibia in a posterior direction. The study of rotational laxity is possible once the MRI images are acquired with 1-mm spacing and 3D reconstruction.

The measurement (in mm) is performed using a line that is perpendicular to the tibial slope crossing the most posterior point of the tibial plateau and its distance to a parallel line crossing the most posterior point of the femoral condyle. This process is repeated with or without pressure for medial and lateral compartments, with or without rotation, identifying the same points as the bony landmarks (Fig. 5.5).

The amount of anterior translation, in millimeters, of the medial and lateral tibial plateaus with different combination of rotation is calculated by the difference of each of the two points (without and with pressure) (Fig. 5.6). The method can include the assessment of ACL-deficient knees alone or side-to-side comparison. Axial images can quantify the angles relative to the posterior intercondylar line and the posterior tibial line in degrees (Figs. 5.4 and 5.6). This is another aspect of assessment of rotational laxity in MRI evaluation currently under intense research.

It has been clinically demonstrated that PKTD–MRI method is reliable in the assessment of anterior–posterior translation (comparing to KT-1000) and rotatory laxity (compared with lateral pivot shift under anesthesia) of the ACL-deficient knee.

It has also shown capacity to identify partial ruptures (confirmed later by arthroscopic

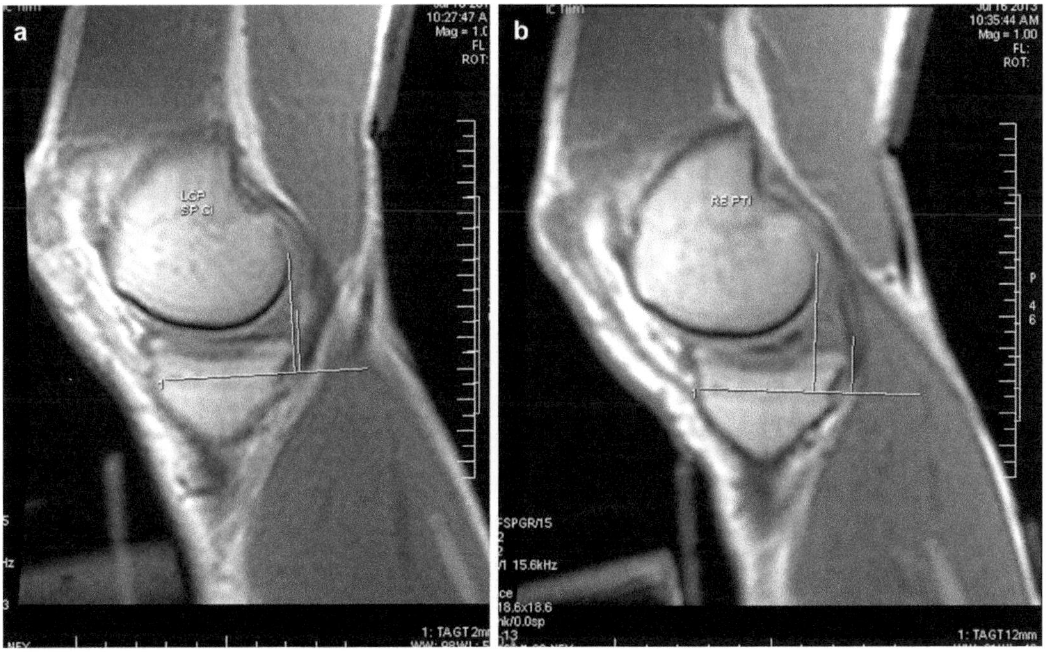

Fig. 5.4 MRI–PKTD® evaluation of a patient with posterior cruciate ligament rupture: (**a**) sagittal view without load, distance between medial posterior condyle and medial tibial plateau; (**b**) sagittal view with the load directed posteriorly and with external rotation, distance between medial posterior condyle and medial tibial plateau

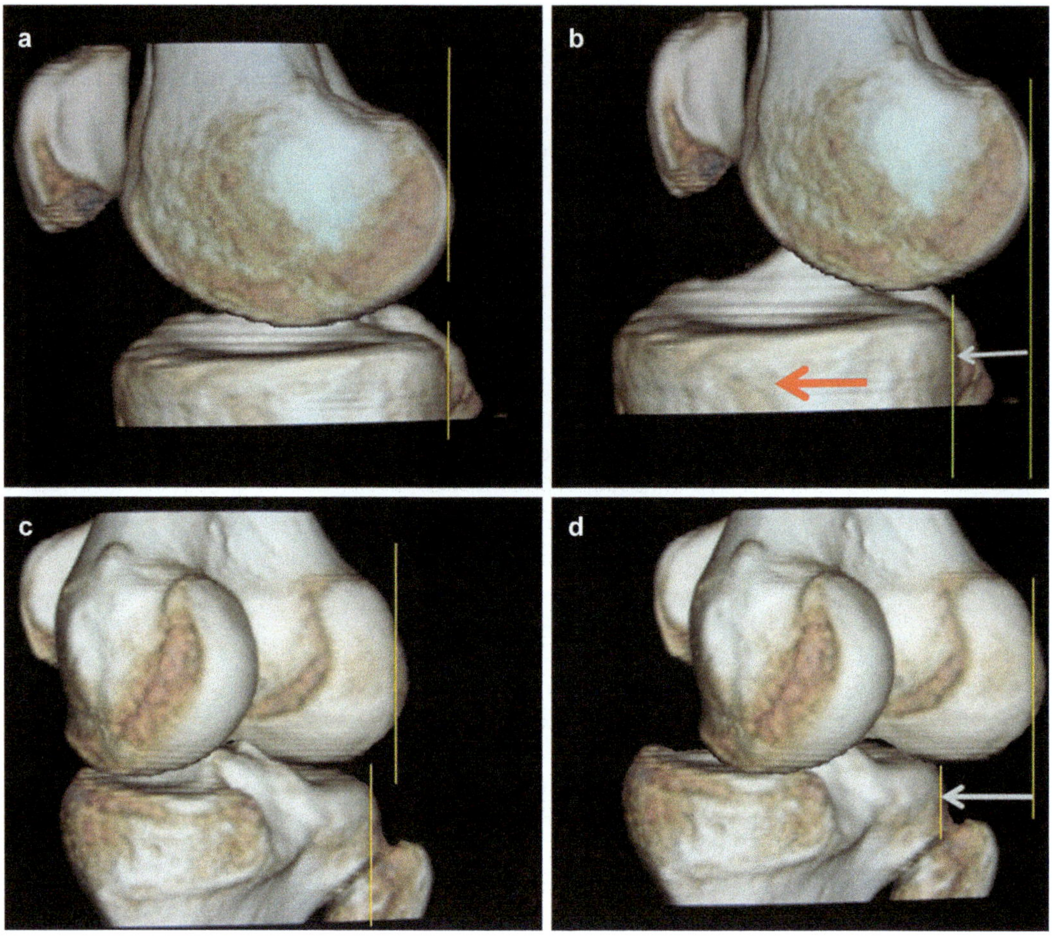

Fig. 5.5 CT 3D representation of the effect of PKTD® effect on anterior translation for medial compartment (**a**, **b**) and lateral compartment (**c**, **d**)

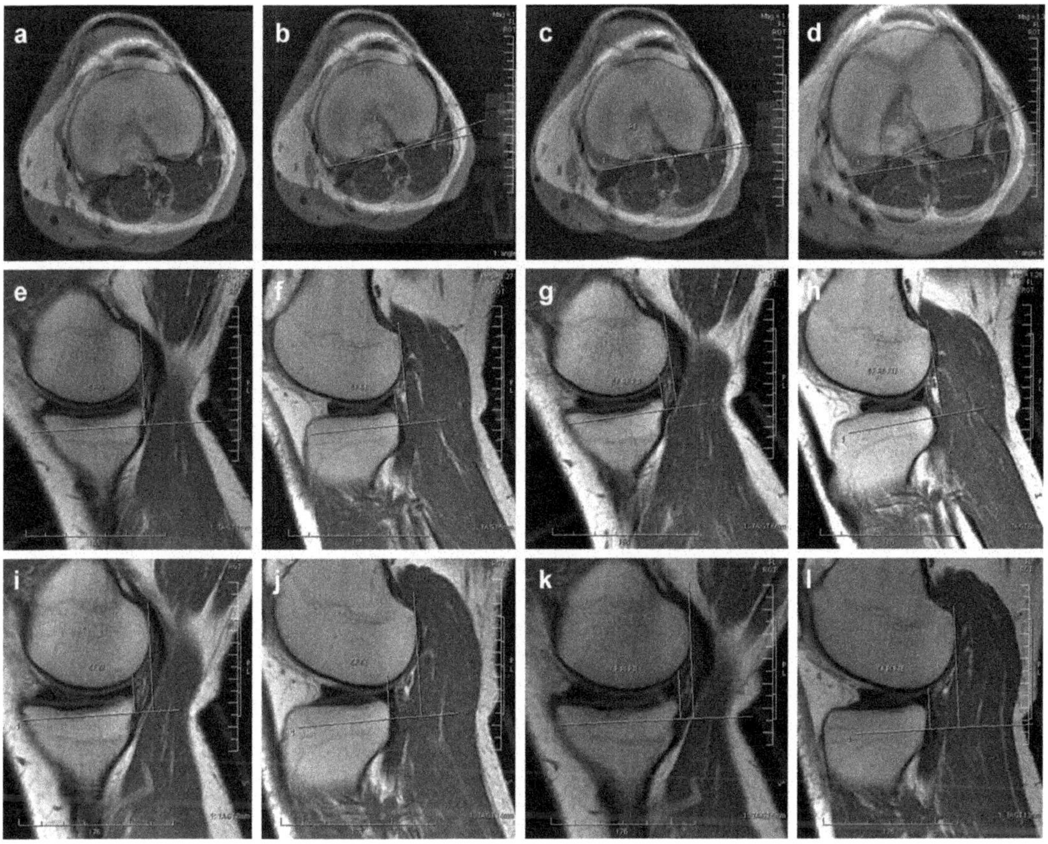

Fig. 5.6 MRI–PKTD® evaluation of a patient with ACL rupture: (**a**) choice of the adequate image for bony landmarks; (**b**) posterior intercondylar line and posterior tibial line without pressure (5°); (**c**) angle with load application in anterior direction and external rotation (3°); (**d**) angle with load application in anterior direction and internal rotation (12°); (**e**) sagittal view without load, distance between medial posterior condyle and medial tibial plateau (1 mm); (**f**) sagittal view without pressure, distance between lateral posterior condyle and lateral tibial plateau (5 mm); (**g**) sagittal view without anterior pressure but with external rotation, distance between medial posterior condyle and medial tibial plateau (6 mm); (**h**) sagittal view without anterior pressure but with external rotation, distance between lateral posterior condyle and lateral tibial plateau (6 mm); (**i**) sagittal view with anterior pressure, distance between medial posterior condyle and medial tibial plateau (8 mm); (**j**) sagittal view with anterior load, distance between lateral posterior condyle and lateral tibial plateau (14 mm); (**k**) sagittal view with anterior load and internal rotation, distance between medial posterior condyle and medial tibial plateau (5 mm); (**l**) sagittal view with anterior load and internal rotation, distance between lateral posterior condyle and lateral tibial plateau (13 mm)

findings). However, by putting stress on the ACL during the examination, the method permits to simultaneously evaluate the mechanical behavior of partial ruptures and improve the visualization of "biologic"/signal features of the ruptured and the remaining bundle (Fact Box 2).

Fact Box 2. Advantages of PKTD: MRI Evaluation Protocol

- Preserves all anatomical possibilities of MRI
- Enables knee assessment at several degrees of flexion
- Enables anterior–posterior and rotational forces during the exam
- Uses bony landmarks to measure translation
- Enables objective quantification of the amount of produced translation for medial and lateral compartments
- Dynamic evaluation assists in evaluation of partial tears
- Enables assessment of posterior instability (posterior cruciate ligament or combined injuries).

Ongoing research is now focused to improve the possibilities of this method to identify populations with increased risk factors for ACL rupture [40].

Conclusion

MRI protocols for knee study should include spin echo or fat-saturated fast spin echo images in all three planes, including T1- and T2-weighted sagittal images. Currently, sagittal images are more frequently obtained in the true orthogonal plane. The examiner must be familiar with normal and abnormal appearances of the ACL in all planes. Primary and secondary signs of ACL rupture should be scrutinized. Frequently associated fractures/patterns should also be checked. One should be aware of the lower accuracy of MRI for partial tears and chronic tears. There is much room for progress in MRI investigations of the ACL. Continued technological advances in imaging instrumentation, software, and contrast agents will probably result in faster and more informative MRI examinations in the near future. New types of sequences are emerging every year. Moreover, dynamic MRI evaluation is under development in order to become easier, faster, and more useful compared with the current static imaging.

References

1. Araujo PH, Kfuri Junior M, Ohashi B, Hoshino Y, Zaffagnini S, Samuelsson K, Karlsson J, Fu F, Musahl V (2014) Individualized ACL reconstruction. Knee Surg Sports Traumatol Arthrosc 22(9):1966–1975. doi:10.1007/s00167-014-2928-2
2. Arilla FV, Yeung M, Bell K, Rahnemai-Azar AA, Rothrauff BB, Fu FH, Debski RE, Ayeni OR, Musahl V (2015) Experimental execution of the simulated Pivot-Shift Test: a systematic review of techniques. Arthrosc 31:2445–2454. doi:10.1016/j.arthro.2015.06.027
3. Behairy NH, Dorgham MA, Khaled SA (2009) Accuracy of routine magnetic resonance imaging in meniscal and ligamentous injuries of the knee: comparison with arthroscopy. Int Orthop 33(4):961–967. doi:10.1007/s00264-008-0580-5
4. Benjaminse A, Gokeler A, van der Schans CP (2006) Clinical diagnosis of an anterior cruciate ligament rupture: a meta-analysis. J Orthop Sports Phys Ther 36(5):267–288. doi:10.2519/jospt.2006.2011
5. Bjornsson H, Desai N, Musahl V, Alentorn-Geli E, Bhandari M, Fu F, Samuelsson K (2015) Is double-bundle anterior cruciate ligament reconstruction superior to single-bundle? a comprehensive systematic review. Knee Surg Sports Traumatol Arthrosc 23(3):696–739. doi:10.1007/s00167-013-2666-x
6. Brandon ML, Haynes PT, Bonamo JR, Flynn MI, Barrett GR, Sherman MF (2006) The association between posterior-inferior tibial slope and anterior cruciate ligament insufficiency. Arthrosc 22(8):894–899. doi:10.1016/j.arthro.2006.04.098
7. Brandser EA, Riley MA, Berbaum KS, el-Khoury GY, Bennett DL (1996) MR imaging of anterior cruciate ligament injury: independent value of primary and secondary signs. AJR Am J Roentgenol 167((1):121–126. doi:10.2214/ajr.167.1.8659355
8. Campos JC, Chung CB, Lektrakul N, Pedowitz R, Trudell D, Yu J, Resnick D (2001) Pathogenesis of the segond fracture: anatomic and MR imaging evidence

of an iliotibial tract or anterior oblique band avulsion. Radiology 219(2):381–386. doi:10.1148/radiology.219.2.r01ma23381
9. Chan WP, Peterfy C, Fritz RC, Genant HK (1994) MR diagnosis of complete tears of the anterior cruciate ligament of the knee: importance of anterior subluxation of the tibia. AJR Am J Roentgenol 162(2):355–360. doi:10.2214/ajr.162.2.8310927
10. Citak M, Suero EM, Rozell JC, Bosscher MR, Kuestermeyer J, Pearle AD (2011) A mechanized and standardized pivot shifter: technical description and first evaluation. Knee Surg Sports Traumatol Arthrosc 19(5):707–711. doi:10.1007/s00167-010-1289-8
11. DeFranco MJ, Bach BR Jr (2009) A comprehensive review of partial anterior cruciate ligament tears. J Bone Joint Surg Am 91(1):198–208. doi:10.2106/JBJS.H.00819
12. Espregueira-Mendes J, Pereira H, Sevivas N, Passos C, Vasconcelos JC, Monteiro A, Oliveira JM, Reis RL (2012) Assessment of rotatory laxity in anterior cruciate ligament-deficient knees using magnetic resonance imaging with Porto-knee testing device. Knee Surg Sports Traumatol Arthrosc 20(4):671–678. doi:10.1007/s00167-012-1914-9
13. Falchook FS, Tigges S, Carpenter WA, Branch TP, Stiles RG (1996) Accuracy of direct signs of tears of the anterior cruciate ligament. Can Assoc Radiol J (Journal l'Association canadienne des radiologistes) 47(2):114–120
14. Fitzgerald SW, Remer EM, Friedman H, Rogers LF, Hendrix RW, Schafer MF (1993) MR evaluation of the anterior cruciate ligament: value of supplementing sagittal images with coronal and axial images. AJR Am J Roentgenol 160(6):1233–1237. doi:10.2214/ajr.160.6.8498224
15. Fruensgaard S, Johannsen HV (1989) Incomplete ruptures of the anterior cruciate ligament. J Bone Joint Surg 71(3):526–530
16. Giaconi JC, Allen CR, Steinbach LS (2009) Anterior cruciate ligament graft reconstruction: clinical, technical, and imaging overview. Top Magn Reson Imaging : TMRI 20(3):129–150. doi:10.1097/RMR.0b013e3181d657a7
17. Grzelak P, Podgorski MT, Stefanczyk L, Domzalski M (2015) Ultrasonographic test for complete anterior cruciate ligament injury. Indian J Orthop 49(2):143–149. doi:10.4103/0019-5413.152432
18. Hoshino Y, Kuroda R, Nagamune K, Araki D, Kubo S, Yamaguchi M, Kurosaka M (2012) Optimal measurement of clinical rotational test for evaluating anterior cruciate ligament insufficiency. Knee Surg Sports Traumatol Arthrosc 20(7):1323–1330. doi:10.1007/s00167-011-1643-5
19. Hoshino Y, Musahl V, Irrgang JJ, Lopomo N, Zaffagnini S, Karlsson J, Kuroda R, Fu FH (2015) Quantitative evaluation of the Pivot Shift - relationship to clinical Pivot Shift Grade: a prospective international multicenter study. Orthop J Sports Med 3(2 suppl):56–72. doi:10.1177/2325967115s00108
20. Isberg J, Faxen E, Brandsson S, Eriksson BI, Karrholm J, Karlsson J (2006) KT-1000 records smaller side-to-side differences than radiostereometric analysis before and after an ACL reconstruction. Knee Surg Sports Traumatol Arthrosc 14(6):529–535. doi:10.1007/s00167-006-0061-6
21. Jonsson H, Riklund-Ahlstrom K, Lind J (2004) Positive pivot shift after ACL reconstruction predicts later osteoarthrosis: 63 patients followed 5–9 years after surgery. Acta Orthop Scand 75(5):594–599. doi:10.1080/00016470410001484
22. Juhng SK, Lee JK, Choi SS, Yoon KH, Roh BS, Won JJ (2002) MR evaluation of the "arcuate" sign of posterolateral knee instability. AJR Am J Roentgenol 178(3):583–588. doi:10.2214/ajr.178.3.1780583
23. Kato Y, Maeyama A, Lertwanich P, Wang JH, Ingham SJ, Kramer S, Martins CQ, Smolinski P, Fu FH (2013) Biomechanical comparison of different graft positions for single-bundle anterior cruciate ligament reconstruction. Knee Surg Sports Traumatol Arthrosc 21(4):816–823. doi:10.1007/s00167-012-1951-4
24. Kocher MS, Steadman JR, Briggs KK, Sterett WI, Hawkins RJ (2004) Relationships between objective assessment of ligament stability and subjective assessment of symptoms and function after anterior cruciate ligament reconstruction. Am J Sports Med 32(3):629–634
25. Kothari A, Haughom B, Subburaj K, Feeley B, Li X, Ma CB (2012) Evaluating rotational kinematics of the knee in ACL reconstructed patients using 3.0 Tesla magnetic resonance imaging. Knee 19(5):648–651. doi:10.1016/j.knee.2011.12.001
26. Kuroda R, Hoshino Y, Kubo S, Araki D, Oka S, Nagamune K, Kurosaka M (2011) Similarities and Differences of Diagnostic Manual Tests for Anterior Cruciate Ligament Insufficiency: A Global Survey and Kinematics Assessment. Am J Sports Med. doi:10.1177/0363546511423634, 0363546511423634 [pii]
27. Lane CG, Warren R, Pearle AD (2008) The pivot shift. J Am Acad Orthop Surg 16(12):679–688, doi: 16/12/679 [pii]
28. Lawrance JA, Ostlere SJ, Dodd CA (1996) MRI diagnosis of partial tears of the anterior cruciate ligament. Injury 27(3):153–155
29. Lee K, Siegel MJ, Lau DM, Hildebolt CF, Matava MJ (1999) Anterior cruciate ligament tears: MR imaging-based diagnosis in a pediatric population. Radiology 213(3):697–704. doi:10.1148/radiology.213.3.r99dc26697
30. Lee SY, Matsui N, Yoshida K, Doi R, Matsushima S, Wakami T, Fujii M, Yoshiya S, Kurosaka M, Yamamoto T (2005) Magnetic resonance delineation of the anterior cruciate ligament of the knee: flexed knee position within a surface coil. Clin Imaging 29(2):117–122. doi:10.1016/j.clinimag.2004.04.024
31. Leitze Z, Losee RE, Jokl P, Johnson TR, Feagin JA (2005) Implications of the pivot shift in the ACL-deficient knee. Clin Orthop Relat Res 436:229–236

32. Mellado JM, Calmet J, Olona M, Gine J, Sauri A (2004) Magnetic resonance imaging of anterior cruciate ligament tears: reevaluation of quantitative parameters and imaging findings including a simplified method for measuring the anterior cruciate ligament angle. Knee Surg Sports Traumatol Arthrosc 12(3):217–224. doi:10.1007/s00167-003-0431-2
33. Mink JH, Levy T, Crues JV 3rd (1988) Tears of the anterior cruciate ligament and menisci of the knee: MR imaging evaluation. Radiology 167(3):769–774. doi:10.1148/radiology.167.3.3363138
34. Muller B, Hofbauer M, Rahnemai-Azar AA, Wolf M, Araki D, Hoshino Y, Araujo P, Debski RE, Irrgang JJ, Fu FH, Musahl V (2015) Development of computer tablet software for clinical quantification of lateral knee compartment translation during the pivot shift test. Comput Methods Biomech Biomed Engin 19:1–12. doi:10.1080/10255842.2015.1006210
35. Murphy BJ, Smith RL, Uribe JW, Janecki CJ, Hechtman KS, Mangasarian RA (1992) Bone signal abnormalities in the posterolateral tibia and lateral femoral condyle in complete tears of the anterior cruciate ligament: a specific sign? Radiology 182(1):221–224. doi:10.1148/radiology.182.1.1727286
36. Musahl V, Voos J, O'Loughlin PF, Stueber V, Kendoff D, Pearle AD (2010) Mechanized pivot shift test achieves greater accuracy than manual pivot shift test. Knee Surg Sports Traumatol Arthrosc 18(9):1208–1213. doi:10.1007/s00167-009-1004-9
37. Noyes FR, Mooar LA, Moorman CT 3rd, McGinniss GH (1989) Partial tears of the anterior cruciate ligament. progression to complete ligament deficiency. J Bone Joint Surg 71(5):825–833
38. Ochi M, Adachi N, Deie M, Kanaya A (2006) Anterior cruciate ligament augmentation procedure with a 1-incision technique: anteromedial bundle or posterolateral bundle reconstruction. Arthroscopy 22(4):463 e461–465. doi:10.1016/j.arthro.2005.06.034, S0749-8063(05)01560-4 [pii]
39. Ohashi B, Ward J, Araujo P, Kfuri M, Pereira H, Espregueira-Mendes J, Musahl V (2014) Partial ACL Ruptures: knee laxity measurements and Pivot Shift. In: Doral MN, Karlsson J (eds) Sports injuries. Springer, Berlin/Heidelberg, pp 1–16. doi:10.1007/978-3-642-36801-1_85-1
40. Pereira H, Fernandes M, Pereira R, Jones H, Vasconcelos JC, Oliveira JM, Reis RL, Musahl V, Espregueira-Mendes J (2014) ACL injuries identifiable for Pre-participation imagiological analysis: risk factors. In: Doral MN, Karlsson J (eds) Sports injuries. Springer, Berlin/Heidelberg, pp 1–15. doi:10.1007/978-3-642-36801-1_80-1
41. Pereira H, Sevivas N, Pereira R, Monteiro A, Oliveira JM, Reis RL, Espregueira-Mendes J (2012) New tools for diagnosis, assessment of surgical outcome and follow-up. In: Hernández JA, Monllau JC (eds) Lesiones ligamentosas de la rodilla. Marge Médica Books Barcelona, Spain, pp 185–198
42. Pereira H, Sevivas N, Pereira R, Monteiro A, Sampaio R, Oliveira J, Reis R, Espregueira-Mendes J (2014) Systematic approach from Porto School. In: Siebold R, Dejour D, Zaffagnini S (eds) Anterior cruciate ligament reconstruction. Springer, Berlin/Heidelberg, pp 367–386. doi:10.1007/978-3-642-45349-6_34
43. Prince JS, Laor T, Bean JA (2005) MRI of anterior cruciate ligament injuries and associated findings in the pediatric knee: changes with skeletal maturation. AJR Am J Roentgenol 185(3):756–762. doi:10.2214/ajr.185.3.01850756
44. Prins M (2006) The Lachman test is the most sensitive and the pivot shift the most specific test for the diagnosis of ACL rupture. Aust J Physiother 52(1):66. doi:http://dx.doi.org/10.1016/S0004-9514(06)70069-1
45. Remer EM, Fitzgerald SW, Friedman H, Rogers LF, Hendrix RW, Schafer MF (1992) Anterior cruciate ligament injury: MR imaging diagnosis and patterns of injury. Radiogr Rev Publ Radiol Soc N Am, Inc 12(5):901–915. doi:10.1148/radiographics.12.5.1529133
46. Resnick D (1995) Diagnosis of bone and joint disorders. 3rd edn. WB Saunders Co, Philadelphia
47. Robertson PL, Schweitzer ME, Bartolozzi AR, Ugoni A (1994) Anterior cruciate ligament tears: evaluation of multiple signs with MR imaging. Radiology 193(3):829–834. doi:10.1148/radiology.193.3.7972833
48. Roychowdhury S, Fitzgerald SW, Sonin AH, Peduto AJ, Miller FH, Hoff FL (1997) Using MR imaging to diagnose partial tears of the anterior cruciate ligament: value of axial images. AJR Am J Roentgenol 168(6):1487–1491. doi:10.2214/ajr.168.6.9168712
49. Rubin DA, Kettering JM, Towers JD, Britton CA (1998) MR imaging of knees having isolated and combined ligament injuries. AJR Am J Roentgenol 170(5):1207–1213. doi:10.2214/ajr.170.5.9574586
50. Sonnery-Cottet B, Lavoie F, Ogassawara R, Scussiato RG, Kidder JF, Chambat P (2010) Selective anteromedial bundle reconstruction in partial ACL tears: a series of 36 patients with mean 24 months follow-up. Knee Surg Sports Traumatol Arthrosc 18(1):47–51. doi:10.1007/s00167-009-0855-4
51. Staubli HU, Noesberger B, Jakob RP (1992) Stress radiography of the knee. Cruciate ligament function studied in 138 patients. Acta Orthop Scand Suppl 249:1–27
52. Stoller D (1997) Magnetic resonance imaging in orthopaedics and sports medicine. 2nd edn. Lippincott-Raven, Philadelphia
53. Swain MS, Henschke N, Kamper SJ, Downie AS, Koes BW, Maher CG (2014) Accuracy of clinical tests in the diagnosis of anterior cruciate ligament injury: a systematic review. Chiropr Man Therap 22:25. doi:10.1186/s12998-014-0025-8
54. Terzidis IP, Christodoulou AG, Ploumis AL, Metsovitis SR, Koimtzis M, Givissis P (2004) The appearance of kissing contusion in the acutely injured knee in the athletes. Br J Sports Med 38(5):592–596. doi:10.1136/bjsm.2003.006718
55. Toye LR, Cummings DP, Armendariz G (2002) Adult tibial intercondylar eminence fracture: evaluation with MR imaging. Skeletal Radiol 31(1):46–48. doi:10.1007/s00256-001-0440-5
56. Tung GA, Davis LM, Wiggins ME, Fadale PD (1993) Tears of the anterior cruciate ligament: primary and sec-

ondary signs at MR imaging. Radiology 188(3):661–667. doi:10.1148/radiology.188.3.8351329
57. Vahey TN, Broome DR, Kayes KJ, Shelbourne KD (1991) Acute and chronic tears of the anterior cruciate ligament: differential features at MR imaging. Radiology 181(1):251–253. doi:10.1148/radiology.181.1.1887042
58. Van Dyck P, De Smet E, Veryser J, Lambrecht V, Gielen JL, Vanhoenacker FM, Dossche L, Parizel PM (2012) Partial tear of the anterior cruciate ligament of the knee: injury patterns on MR imaging. Knee Surg Sports Traumatol Arthrosc 20(2):256–261. doi:10.1007/s00167-011-1617-7
59. Van Dyck P, Vanhoenacker FM, Gielen JL, Dossche L, Van Gestel J, Wouters K, Parizel PM (2011) Three tesla magnetic resonance imaging of the anterior cruciate ligament of the knee: can we differentiate complete from partial tears? Skeletal Radiol 40(6):701–707. doi:10.1007/s00256-010-1044-8
60. Van Dyck P, Vanhoenacker FM, Lambrecht V, Wouters K, Gielen JL, Dossche L, Parizel PM (2013) Prospective comparison of 1.5 and 3.0-T MRI for evaluating the knee menisci and ACL. J Bone Joint Surg Am 95(10):916–924. doi:10.2106/JBJS.L.01195
61. Winters K, Tregonning R (2005) Reliability of magnetic resonance imaging of the traumatic knee as determined by arthroscopy. N Z Med J 118(1209):U1301
62. Yasuda K, van Eck CF, Hoshino Y, Fu FH, Tashman S (2011) Anatomic single- and double-bundle anterior cruciate ligament reconstruction, part 1: basic science. Am J Sports Med 39(8):1789–1799. doi:10.1177/0363546511402659
63. Yu JS, Goodwin D, Salonen D, Pathria MN, Resnick D, Dardani M, Schweitzer M (1995) Complete dislocation of the knee: spectrum of associated soft-tissue injuries depicted by MR imaging. AJR Am J Roentgenol 164(1):135–139. doi:10.2214/ajr.164.1.7998526
64. Zaffagnini S, Bignozzi S, Martelli S, Imakiire N, Lopomo N, Marcacci M (2006) New intraoperative protocol for kinematic evaluation of ACL reconstruction: preliminary results. Knee Surg Sports Traumatol Arthrosc 14(9):811–816. doi:10.1007/s00167-006-0057-2

Software Applications

6

Amir Ata Rahnemai-Azar, Justin W. Arner, Jan-Hendrik Naendrup, and Volker Musahl

Contents

A.A. Rahnemai-Azar • J.W. Arner
J.-H. Naendrup
Department of Orthopaedic Surgery, University of Pittsburgh, Pittsburgh, PA, USA

V. Musahl (✉)
Department of Orthopaedic Surgery, UPMC Center for Sports Medicine, Pittsburgh, PA, USA
e-mail: vmusahl@gmail.com

6.1 Software Application for Quantification of Rotatory Laxity

The pivot shift is a dynamic test that evaluates rotatory laxity by applying complex axial and rotational loads. In contrast to other physical examinations, the pivot shift test has been shown to be associated with patient-reported outcome and osteoarthritis after anterior cruciate ligament (ACL) reconstruction surgery [25, 27]. However the interpretation of this test is difficult as it can be highly variable among examiners and is subjective [17].

Several methods, such as surgical navigation systems [28] and electromagnetic tracking system [21], have been proposed to objectively quantify joint laxity during the pivot shift test in patients. However, their application in clinical settings is limited due to expense, their invasiveness, and/or cumbersome use. These issues limit the practical assessment of contralateral limb for comparison. Recently two software products named “PIVOT” and “KiRA” have been introduced that attempt to quantify this test by measuring lateral tibial compartment translation and acceleration of the tibial dislocation during pivot shift testing.

6.1.1 PIVOT Software

Tibial translation has been suggested as a more realistic kinematic determinant of grading of the

V. Musahl et al. (eds.), *Rotatory Knee Instability*, DOI 10.1007/978-3-319-32070-0_6

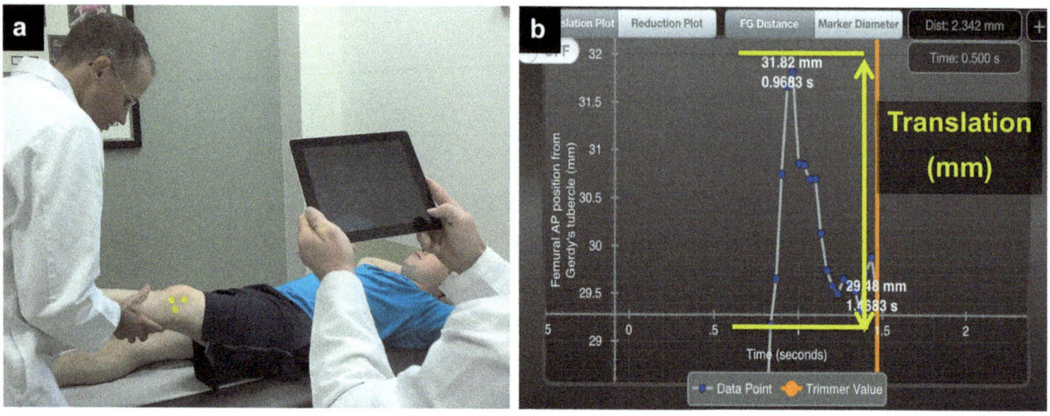

Fig. 6.1 (**a**) Testing setup for the PIVOT software. (**b**) The software interface demonstrating the reduction curve. The difference between the maximum and minimum points of the reduction curve determines the lateral compartment translation

pivot shift test, rather than rotation [8]. This is highlighted in a study by Bedi et al. [3] using a computer navigation system, which demonstrated that anterior translation of the lateral compartment of the knee correlates with the grade of the pivot shift test. This translation is visualized during the pivot shift test, which is the principle of this specific software. Utilizing a digital camera to record the video of examination, it then must be analyzed. One way to analyze this information is by using ImageJ software (National Institutes of Health, Bethesda, MD, USA) (ImageJ software is explained in Sect. 6.2.2 of the current chapter). However, this method is time-consuming and is not applicable in routine clinical practice.

The PIVOT software, which can be installed on a computer tablet, records video of the pivot shift test and using custom software to calculate the translation in less than 30 s [37]. To improve visualization of the image analysis technique, circular markers are attached to the skin over three bony landmarks on the lateral side of the knee. The following landmarks were selected as they are easily identifiable: (1) lateral epicondyle of the knee, (2) Gerdy's tubercle, and (3) fibular head. The color of the circular markers should contrast with the patient's skin, and a solid colored background should be used to reduce the noise from the surroundings.

To obtain a quantitative pivot shift, the assistant utilizes the software, which incorporates a tablet's camera to record the movement of the markers while the examiner performs the examination (Fig. 6.1a). The software scans the images in real time and utilizes custom algorithms that shade the entire image except the markers by adjusting the brightness and contrast. The software then automatically tracks the movement of the markers and calculates the translation of the pivot point defined by the intersection of the line between markers on the fibular head and Gerdy's tubercle with a perpendicular line crossing the femoral condyle marker (Fig. 6.2). After tracking the markers, the software provides a reduction plot that represents backward reduction of the tibia during pivot shift testing. From this plot the amount of translation can be determined by selecting the maximum and minimum points of the plot at the time of the reduction (Fig. 6.1b). Further, the pivot shift test can be quantified in the contralateral knee for comparison or the injured knee after reconstruction surgery and during follow-up period. In addition, by using application of sterilized markers, the quantification of pivot shift test can be performed intraoperatively.

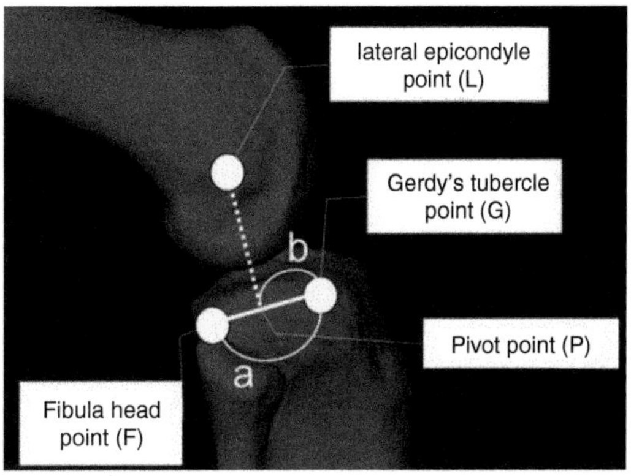

Fig. 6.2 The pivot point is defined of by intersection of the line between markers on the fibular head and Gerdy's tubercle with the perpendicular line crossing the femoral condyle marker. The translation of the pivot point during examination presents the lateral compartment translation

The validity of the software and its application has been investigated in controlled laboratory settings. The maximum error of the software in quantifying the movement of the markers was determined to be less than 6 % at distances of tablet and the patient between 75 and 126 cm and a deviation angle of less than 45° [37]. Moreover, the reliability of the pivot software in predicting the 3D bony motion during the pivot shift test has been evaluated in a cadaveric study utilizing an electromagnetic tracking system. It has been demonstrated that lateral compartment translation measured by PIVOT software has strong correlation with 3D bony motion with about three times higher translation in bony motion (Pearson correlation, 0.75–0.79, $p < 0.05$). Moreover, the intra-examiner reliability of the methodology was also demonstrated to be strong (intra-class correlation coefficient = 0.70–0.82).

In a group of ACL-injured patients, it was demonstrated that the PIVOT software can consistently detect and quantify lateral compartment translation [20]. The quantitative results from PIVOT software have also been validated by clinical grade of pivot shift test where the incremental increase in lateral compartment translation measured by software was associated with increase in clinical grade of the pivot shift test [22].

The software has been recently utilized to investigate the role of different knee structures on rotatory laxity of the knee during the pivot shift test. Using quantitative pivot shift results from the PIVOT software, it has been demonstrated that in ACL-injured patients, concomitant injury to the medial meniscus, lateral meniscus, or lateral capsule, as well as an increased lateral tibial plateau slope, results in higher rotatory laxity. Overall PIVOT software provides an easy, noninvasive, and reliable tool to quantify the pivot shift test.

Fact Box 1
PIVOT software is able to measure lateral compartment translation during the pivot shift test with an acceptable accuracy. The actual 3D bony motion is approximately three times higher than the measured value by software.

6.1.2 Inertial Sensors

Acceleration of the tibial reduction during the pivot shift test has been suggested for objective measurement of the pivot shift test. This parameter has been positively correlated with clinical grading of the pivot shift test [21]. The acceleration of the pivot shift test can be quantified by invasive and noninvasive methods such as electromagnetic tracking systems [21], surgical navigation systems [28], and triaxial inertial accelerometers [6, 10, 29, 32]. Inertial sensors track the position and orientation of an object relative to a known starting point without a need for external references.

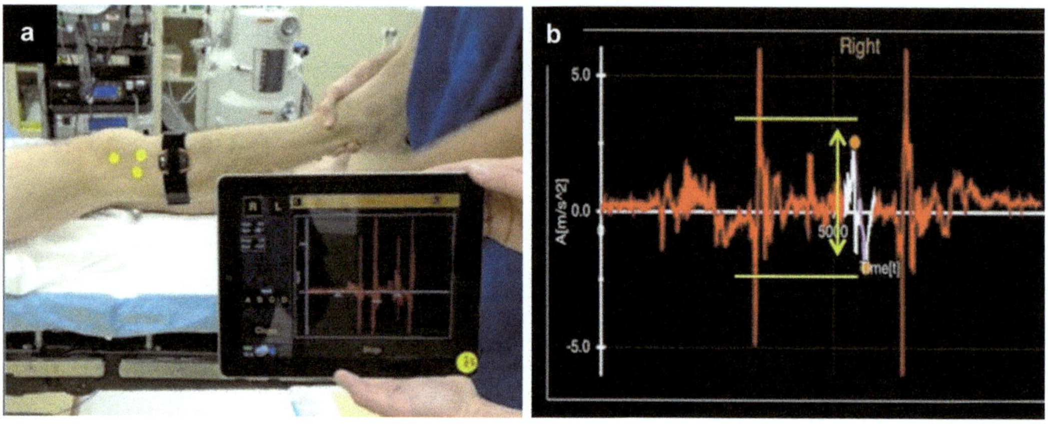

Fig. 6.3 (**a**) Up Setup for the KiRA software and the inertial sensors: the sensor is tightly secured in the anterolateral side of the tibia between anterior tuberosity and Gerdy's tubercle. The axis of the sensor is aligned with the mechanical axis of the tibia. (**b**) The acceleration curve obtained from KiRA software. The *yellow arrow* demonstrates the acceleration range

Lopomo et al. described a noninvasive methodology of acquiring acceleration during the pivot shift test using a single commercial triaxial accelerometer sensor strapped to the skin and custom software referred to as KiRA (KiRA, Orthokey LLC, Lewes, DE, USA) [30]. The sensor is mounted noninvasively on the lateral side of the tibia between the lateral aspect of anterior tuberosity and Gerdy's tubercle by means of a strap, while the main axis is aligned with the mechanical axis of the tibia. This position is chosen to ensure the optimal stability and to minimize skin artifact. Moreover, in this position, the lateral compartment acceleration can be most easily acquired (Fig. 6.3a).

The 3D acceleration during the pivot shift test is sent wirelessly via standard Bluetooth 2.0 to a computer tablet equipped with KiRA software. The software is developed in order to manage the receiving of the data from the sensor and analyze the acceleration data to a patient database [48]. The software adjusts the acceleration modulus for the gravitational component and provides an acceleration curve in the software interface in a live mode. The software automatically identifies the appropriate curve relating to the pivot shift phenomenon and calculates a series of acceleration components by analyzing the curve (Fig. 6.3b):

a_{max}: the maximum value of the limb acceleration

a_{min}: the minimum value of the limb acceleration

a_{range}: range of acceleration determined by the difference of a_{max} and a_{min}

Slope: mean slope of the corresponding curve, which is indicative of smoothness

The KiRA system has been validated by an electromagnetic tracking system and surgical navigation system and has been determined to be a feasible method of the measurement of knee kinematics. Using a cadaveric specimen, Araujo et al. demonstrated good correlation between acceleration measured by the KiRA system and the electromagnetic tracking system (Pearson's correlation coefficient = 0.75) [2]. Similarly, the absolute 3D acceleration range obtained from the KiRA system demonstrated a good positive correlation (Pearson's correlation coefficient = 0.72, $p < 0.05$) and moderate predictability ($R^2 = 0.51$) when compared with anteroposterior acceleration simultaneously measured by surgical navigation during in vivo studies. The acceleration obtained from the KiRA system also correlates with clinical grading of the pivot shift test by in vitro and in vivo studies [1]. The

KiRA system has also demonstrated fair/good intra-tester reliability (ICC: 0.76–0.90).

In a cohort of 66 patients, knees with an ACL injury demonstrate greater a_{max}, lower a_{min}, greater a_{range} (with mean difference of 1.6 ± 1.5 m/s^2, $p < 0.05$), and greater acceleration slope (with mean difference of 8.6 ± 13.7 m/s^3, $p < 0.05$) compared with intact knees [30]. Of the abovementioned parameters, a_{range} most clearly distinguished intact and ACL-injured knees. The probability of a correct diagnosis of ACL injury was 70 % using only the slope of the curve and 80 % using only the a_{range}. Although the diagnosis of an ACL injury by only results of a pivot shift examination is not common in clinical practice, the currently reported accuracy for this methodology indicates necessity of improvement.

This methodology of quantifying of acceleration with the KiRA software is user-friendly as it involves the use of a small sensor and uses a wireless connection and does not require any anatomic registration. In a group of 100 patients with ACL injuries, Berruto et al. [4] demonstrated that the use of KiRA is promising and reliable. They also found that the efficacy of the system has a learning curve, as the specificity of diagnosis of ACL injury increased significantly with further use and experience with the device. Moreover, it needs to be considered that the acceleration during the examination is dependent on the load applied and technique of the pivot shift test, which underlines the necessity of performing a standardized maneuver to reduce variability [19, 38].

Some studies suggest developing algorithms to establish the diagnosis of ACL insufficiency by in-depth analysis of data from pivot shift testing. With regression analysis of the data obtained from inertial sensors during examination of both limbs under general anesthesia, ACL insufficiency can be diagnosed with 97 % accuracy [6]. The accuracy of the algorithm increased by using training data from more subjects. For instance, to reach a 97 % accuracy, the algorithm needed to use data from 61 subjects, whereas with data of less than 20 subjects, diagnostic accuracy was poor. Once again, it is of note that any diagnostic device with accuracy of less than 100 % needs to be complemented with other modalities to eliminate potential misdiagnosis and achieve optimal outcome.

> **Fact Box 2**
> Acceleration of the tibial reduction is a determinant of pivot shift test. The acceleration measured using KiRA has been validated and shown to have strong correlation with acceleration of the bones.

6.1.3 Future Direction of Quantification of Rotatory Laxity

By measuring six degrees of freedom of motion, Bull et al. demonstrated that every patient with an ACL injury has a different "envelope of motion" during the pivot shift test [8]. Kinematics of rotatory laxity during the pivot shift test consists of different aspects.

Objective quantification of the pivot shift test warrants methods that are able to easily and reliably measure different aspects of rotatory laxity during the pivot shift test in a routine clinical setting. The preliminary results from a cohort of ACL-injured patients using the PIVOT and KiRA systems support findings from Bull et al., where rotatory knee laxity is widely distributed in these patients (Fig. 6.4). This further emphasizes the need for individualized treatment of ACL-injured patients rather than the traditional "one fits all" treatment approach.

The abovementioned software products do not represent the "gold standard" method for measurement of rotatory laxity, nor do other devices used to measure kinematics of the pivot shift test. These software products, however, allow clinicians who desire to obtain objective quantification of the pivot shift exam by providing the opportunity to do so portably, accurately, and with data recording capabilities. The ultimate goal of performing a quantitative pivot shift would be to classify patients' rotatory laxity

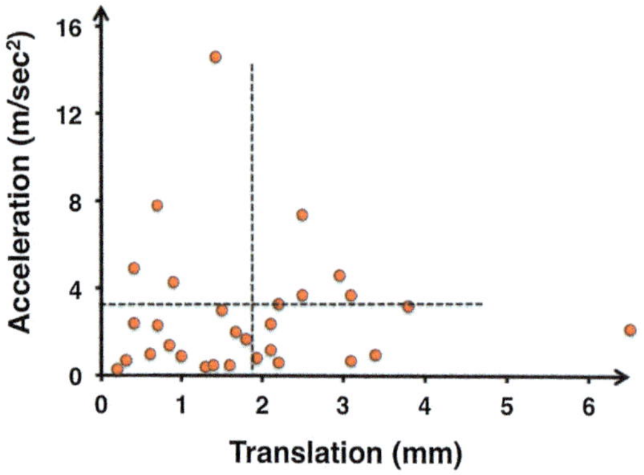

Fig. 6.4 Results from a group of anterior cruciate ligament-injured patients. Each *red dot* represents side to side difference of kinematics of pivot shift kinematics in one patient. The translation and acceleration were acquired by PIVOT and KiRA system, respectively. *Dashed line* represents the median number for translation and acceleration

patterns and accordingly assist in decision-making with respect to improving functional outcome.

6.2 Software Products with General Application

Apart from the abovementioned software products with specific application in the assessment of rotatory laxity, other more generalized technologies exist that are designed to perform more daily tasks that are useful in orthopedic practice. These range from simple user interfaces to more complex research tools.

6.2.1 Smart Phone Application Programs (Apps)

A wide range of apps designed to be used by smartphones and computer tablets have been developed in recent years due to their convenience and ease of use and profit potential [11, 12]. Many are general medical apps and are not specific to orthopedics like drug references and BMI calculator apps. Examples of apps with specific utilization in orthopedics include examination evaluation apps [46] (Goniometer, Knee Goniometer, Forearm Goniometer), outcome tools (OrthoScore, JointScore), radiographic measurement aids (iGonio, Hallux Angles), and apps for reference books. Some of these apps are free, while some require payments by users and others are supported by academic centers or industry. Few websites provide reviews of the apps dedicated to the field of orthopedics [44].

Surveys have demonstrated that medical trainees and faculty rely on their mobile devices to meet their clinical needs [7]. However, it should be noted that some of these resources are of varying quality without any standardization or peer review, which raises concerns in terms of their accuracy and application. Users must check the accuracy and validity of the software products before their application in clinical practice.

6.2.2 Medical Image Processing Programs

Image processing programs began to grow substantially since digital imaging equipment was introduced to the medical field in mid-1980s. Several processing programs have been developed in recent years that are applicable in the field of orthopedics. Commonly used processing programs include ImageJ (National Institutes of Health, Bethesda, MD, USA) and OsiriX (OsiriX Foundation, Geneva, Switzerland). These software products are easily accessible to scientific community free of charge and allow users to display, edit, and analyze images from radiological modalities (e.g., plain radiographs, magnetic resonance imaging) or other medical images (e.g., histology, photography) [13, 23]. ImageJ is a public domain, Java-based program and can process many image formats including TIFF, GIF, PNG, JPEG, BMP, and DICOM.

OsiriX, runs under Mac OS X (Apple Inc.) and has comparable abilities with ImageJ in terms of opening different file formats and processing the images. The goal is to obtain quantitative knowledge from medical imaging such as alignment of the bones and measurement of area and volume of different anatomical structures. For instance, by utilizing this software, researchers were able to measure area of ACL insertion site or demonstrate shifting of the graft inside the bone tunnel by comparing the distance between centroid of the graft and tunnel [13, 23, 45]. Moreover, the open source nature of these software programs allows the freedom to create additions or plug-ins to the main software with the ability to perform specific tasks.

Some programs such as Mimics (Materialise, Leuven, Belgium) and Geomagic (Research Triangle Park, NC, USA) are used for segmentation of clinical images and development of three-dimensional (3D) designs and models. The 3D models can be made from a series of two-dimensional medical image data or by scanning the physical object. These programs have a significant role in investigation of anatomy and relation of the structures as well as simulation of realistic geometries by finite element modeling [26, 47]. These programs, however, require a relatively costly licensure from the company to use and are associated with a considerable learning curve.

6.2.3 Telemedicine

Telemedicine is the use of information technologies to provide clinical healthcare while there is a distance between the patient and provider. Telecommunication is performed by means of free public communication software products [15] (e.g., Skype) or specific communication platforms designed for healthcare [9]. These technologies are applied to different areas of telemedicine such as teleradiology [16, 43], teleconsultation [5, 34], and tele-rehabilitation [36].

Although telemedicine is touted to improve healthcare by, for example, providing healthcare to remote areas and reducing cost, it also limits the physical examination and creates opportunities for privacy violation and data breach. It is thus necessary that clinicians avoid any activities that are noncompliant with safety and privacy regulations under the Health Information Portability and Accountability Act (HIPAA). Further, some programs require substantial bandwidths, which limit their use.

6.2.4 Educational Tools

New technologies have made a large impact on medical and orthopedic education and training. Many educational software products allow self-learning with benefits of including multimedia content and interactive communications. Further, technology has allowed large searchable complied databases and textbooks, which many times are faster and more convenient for learning and research. The ease of access of bullet style references such as Wheeless Orthopaedics and Orthobullets have become very popular, but many question their simplicity.

One developing sector in the field of orthopedic education is training by virtual learning environments or so called "virtual reality." These systems were first developed in the early 1940s to generate onboard flight simulation for aviators' trainings. However their application is now expanded to different branches of science including medicine. These systems are generally composed of hardware equipped with the training software [31].

In the field of orthopedics, these systems have been used in simulation training of different joints such as hip [39], shoulder [18, 33], and knee [24, 35]. The simulator programs allow trainees to repeat and rehearse in order to build a required surgical skill and usually provide feedback during the training session (Fig. 6.5). It is proposed in several studies that orthopedic surgery simulation will result in a decrease in surgical time, associated costs, and improve patient safety [14, 40–42]. However, further validation studies as well as research prospective studies must be performed to provide sound recommendations.

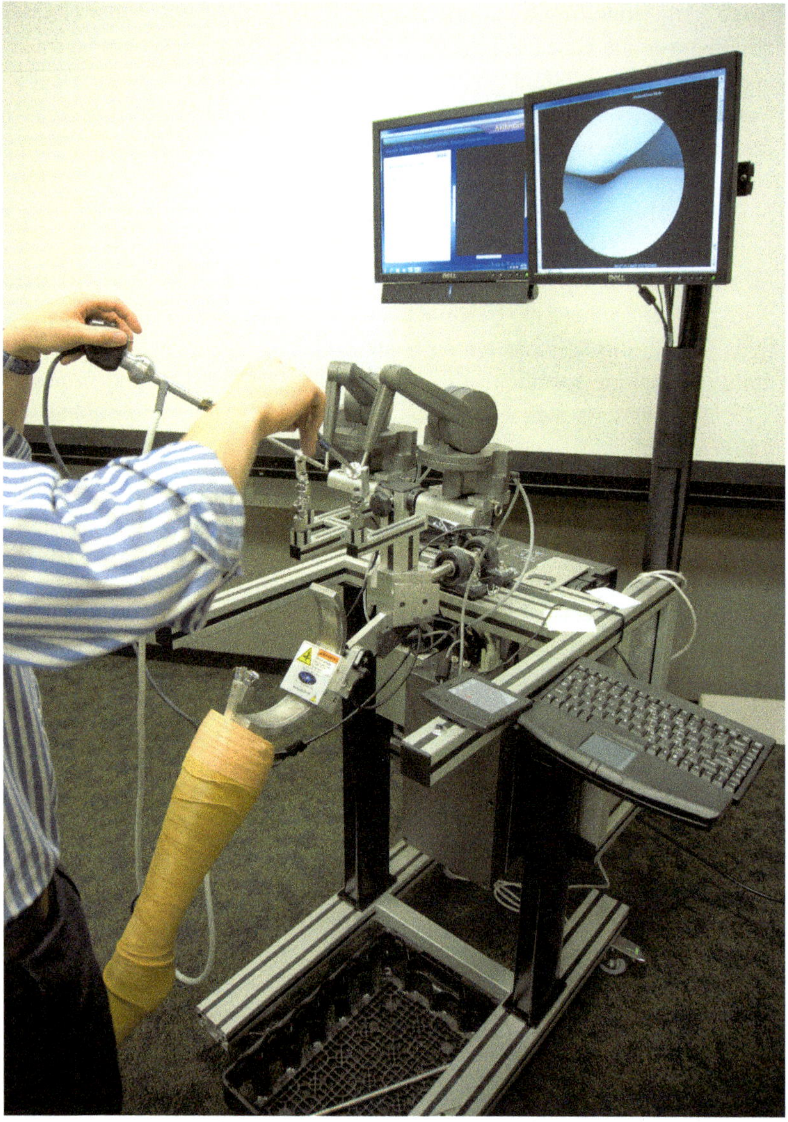

Fig. 6.5 Knee arthroscopy simulator. The "virtual reality" replicates both visualization and feeling of the knee arthroscopy. Examiner observes performing surgery by surgical tools (arthroscope and probe) in the right screen and a series of haptic devices provide instant tactile response. A "mentor" program that runs along the simulation software (left screen) guides the examiner through the joint arthroscopy and provides feedback

Conclusion

Objective measurement of complex aspects of the pivot shift test has become more feasible by new technologies that provide clinicians with the ability to perform quantitative testing in an office setting as well as an operation room. Portability, being noninvasive, inexpensive, and the possibility of its use on the contralateral knee make it possible that these technologies will soon play significant roles in the care of patients with knee ligamentous injuries.

References

1. Ahlden M, Araujo P, Hoshino Y, Samuelsson K, Middleton KK, Nagamune K, Karlsson J, Musahl V (2012) Clinical grading of the pivot shift test correlates best with tibial acceleration. Knee Surg Sports Traumatol Arthrosc Off J ESSKA 20(4):708–712
2. Araujo PH, Ahlden M, Hoshino Y, Muller B, Moloney G, Fu FH, Musahl V (2012) Comparison of three non-invasive quantitative measurement systems for the pivot shift test. Knee Surg Sports Traumatol Arthrosc Off J ESSKA 20(4):692–697

3. Bedi A, Musahl V, Lane C, Citak M, Warren RF, Pearle AD (2010) Lateral compartment translation predicts the grade of pivot shift: a cadaveric and clinical analysis. Knee Surg Sports Traumatol Arthrosc Off J ESSKA 18(9):1269–1276
4. Berruto M, Uboldi F, Gala L, Marelli B, Albisetti W (2013) Is triaxial accelerometer reliable in the evaluation and grading of knee pivot-shift phenomenon? Knee Surg Sports Traumatol Arthrosc Off J ESSKA 21(4):981–985
5. Blank E, Lappan C, Belmont PJ Jr, Machen MS, Ficke J, Pope R, Owens BD (2011) Early analysis of the United States Army's telemedicine orthopaedic consultation program. J Surg Orthop Adv 20(1):50–55
6. Borgstrom PH, Markolf KL, Wang Y, Xu X, Yang PR, Joshi NB, Yeranosian MG, Petrigliano FA, Hame SL, Kaiser WJ, McAllister DR (2015) Use of inertial sensors to predict pivot-shift grade and diagnose an ACL injury during preoperative testing. Am J Sports Med 43(4):857–864
7. Boruff JT, Storie D (2014) Mobile devices in medicine: a survey of how medical students, residents, and faculty use smartphones and other mobile devices to find information. J Med Libr Assoc 102(1):22–30
8. Bull AM, Earnshaw PH, Smith A, Katchburian MV, Hassan AN, Amis AA (2002) Intraoperative measurement of knee kinematics in reconstruction of the anterior cruciate ligament. J Bone Joint Surg 84(7): 1075–1081
9. Daruwalla ZJ, Wong KL, Thambiah J (2014) The application of telemedicine in orthopedic surgery in Singapore: a pilot study on a secure, mobile telehealth application and messaging platform. JMIR Mhealth Uhealth 2(2):e28
10. Debandi A, Maeyama A, Hoshino Y, Asai S, Goto B, Smolinski P, Fu FH (2013) The effect of tunnel placement on rotational stability after ACL reconstruction: evaluation with use of triaxial accelerometry in a porcine model. Knee Surg Sports Traumatol Arthrosc Off J ESSKA 21(3):589–595
11. Duncan SF, Hendawi TK, Sperling J, Kakinoki R, Hartsock L (2015) iPhone and iPad use in orthopedic surgery. Ochsner J 15(1):52–57
12. Franko OI (2011) Smartphone apps for orthopaedic surgeons. Clin Orthop Relat Res 469(7):2042–2048
13. Fujii M, Sasaki Y, Araki D, Furumatsu T, Miyazawa S, Ozaki T, Linde-Rosen M, Smolinski P, Fu FH (2014) Evaluation of the semitendinosus tendon graft shift in the bone tunnel: an experimental study. Knee Surg Sports Traumatol Arthrosc. 2014 Dec 4. pp.1–5. [Epub ahead of print] PubMed PMID: 25472684
14. Gomoll AH, O'Toole RV, Czarnecki J, Warner JJ (2007) Surgical experience correlates with performance on a virtual reality simulator for shoulder arthroscopy. Am J Sports Med 35(6):883–888
15. Good DW, Lui DF, Leonard M, Morris S, McElwain JP (2012) Skype: a tool for functional assessment in orthopaedic research. J Telemed Telecare 18(2):94–98
16. Hammel R, Kovalski N, Zimmerman DR (2010) Mobile telephone-based remote orthopedic consultation. AJR Am J Roentgenol 195(4):W307
17. Hefti F, Muller W, Jakob RP, Staubli HU (1993) Evaluation of knee ligament injuries with the IKDC form. Knee Surg Sports Traumatol Arthrosc Off J ESSKA 1(3–4):226–234
18. Henn RF 3rd, Shah N, Warner JJ, Gomoll AH (2013) Shoulder arthroscopy simulator training improves shoulder arthroscopy performance in a cadaveric model. Arthrosc J Arthroscopic Relat Surg Off Publ Arthrosc Assoc N Am Int Arthrosc Assoc 29(6):982–985
19. Hoshino Y, Araujo P, Ahlden M, Moore CG, Kuroda R, Zaffagnini S, Karlsson J, Fu FH, Musahl V (2012) Standardized pivot shift test improves measurement accuracy. Knee Surg Sports Traumatol Arthrosc Off J ESSKA 20(4):732–736
20. Hoshino Y, Araujo P, Ahlden M, Samuelsson K, Muller B, Hofbauer M, Wolf MR, Irrgang JJ, Fu FH, Musahl V (2013) Quantitative evaluation of the pivot shift by image analysis using the iPad. Knee Surg Sports Traumatol Arthrosc Off J ESSKA 21(4):975–980
21. Hoshino Y, Kuroda R, Nagamune K, Yagi M, Mizuno K, Yamaguchi M, Muratsu H, Yoshiya S, Kurosaka M (2007) In vivo measurement of the pivot-shift test in the anterior cruciate ligament-deficient knee using an electromagnetic device. Am J Sports Med 35(7): 1098–1104
22. Hoshino Y, Musahl V, Irrgang JJ, Lopomo N, Zaffagnini S, Karlsson J, Kuroda R, Fu F (2015) Quantitative evaluation of the Pivot shift test, relationship to clinical pivot shift grade. Paper presented at the American Orthopaedic Society for Sports Medicine, Orlando
23. Iriuchishima T, Ryu K, Aizawa S, Fu FH (2016) The difference in centre position in the ACL femoral footprint inclusive and exclusive of the fan-like extension fibres. Knee Surg Sports Traumatol Arthrosc Off J ESSKA 24:254–259
24. Jackson WF, Khan T, Alvand A, Al-Ali S, Gill HS, Price AJ, Rees JL (2012) Learning and retaining simulated arthroscopic meniscal repair skills. J Bone Joint Surg Am 94(17):e132
25. Jonsson H, Riklund-Ahlstrom K, Lind J (2004) Positive pivot shift after ACL reconstruction predicts later osteoarthrosis: 63 patients followed 5–9 years after surgery. Acta Orthop Scand 75(5):594–599
26. Kim JG, Chang MH, Lim HC, Bae JH, Lee SY, Ahn JH, Wang JH (2015) An in vivo 3D computed tomographic analysis of femoral tunnel geometry and aperture morphology between rigid and flexible systems in double-bundle anterior cruciate ligament reconstruction using the transportal technique. Arthrosc J Arthroscopic Relat Surg Off Publ Arthrosc Assoc N Am Int Arthrosc Assoc 31(7):1318–1329
27. Kocher MS, Steadman JR, Briggs KK, Sterett WI, Hawkins RJ (2004) Relationships between objective assessment of ligament stability and subjective assessment of symptoms and function after anterior cruciate

ligament reconstruction. Am J Sports Med 32(3): 629–634

28. Lane CG, Warren RF, Stanford FC, Kendoff D, Pearle AD (2008) In vivo analysis of the pivot shift phenomenon during computer navigated ACL reconstruction. Knee Surg Sports Traumatol Arthrosc Off J ESSKA 16(5):487–492
29. Lopomo N, Signorelli C, Bonanzinga T, Marcheggiani Muccioli GM, Visani A, Zaffagnini S (2012) Quantitative assessment of pivot-shift using inertial sensors. Knee Surg Sports Traumatol Arthrosc Off J ESSKA 20(4):713–717
30. Lopomo N, Zaffagnini S, Signorelli C, Bignozzi S, Giordano G, Marcheggiani Muccioli GM, Visani A (2012) An original clinical methodology for non-invasive assessment of pivot-shift test. Comput Methods Biomech Biomed Engin 15(12):1323–1328
31. Mabrey JD, Reinig KD, Cannon WD (2010) Virtual reality in orthopaedics: is it a reality? Clin Orthop Relat Res 468(10):2586–2591
32. Maeyama A, Hoshino Y, Debandi A, Kato Y, Saeki K, Asai S, Goto B, Smolinski P, Fu FH (2011) Evaluation of rotational instability in the anterior cruciate ligament deficient knee using triaxial accelerometer: a biomechanical model in porcine knees. Knee Surg Sports Traumatol Arthrosc Off J ESSKA 19(8): 1233–1238
33. Martin KD, Cameron K, Belmont PJ, Schoenfeld A, Owens BD (2012) Shoulder arthroscopy simulator performance correlates with resident and shoulder arthroscopy experience. J Bone Joint Surg Am 94(21): e160
34. Mauer UM, Kunz U (2010) Management of neurotrauma by surgeons and orthopedists in a military operational setting. Neurosurg Focus 28(5):E10
35. McCarthy AD, Moody L, Waterworth AR, Bickerstaff DR (2006) Passive haptics in a knee arthroscopy simulator: is it valid for core skills training? Clin Orthop Relat Res 442:13–20
36. Moffet H, Tousignant M, Nadeau S, Merette C, Boissy P, Corriveau H, Marquis F, Cabana F, Ranger P, Belzile EL, Dimentberg R (2015) In-home telerehabilitation compared with face-to-face rehabilitation after total knee arthroplasty: a noninferiority randomized controlled trial. J Bone Joint Surg Am 97(14):1129–1141
37. Muller B, Hofbauer M, Rahnemai-Azar AA, Wolf M, Araki D, Hoshino Y, Araujo P, Debski RE, Irrgang JJ, Fu FH, Musahl V (2016) Development of computer tablet software for clinical quantification of lateral knee compartment translation during the pivot shift test. Comput Methods Biomech Biomed Engin 19: 217–228
38. Musahl V, Hoshino Y, Ahlden M, Araujo P, Irrgang JJ, Zaffagnini S, Karlsson J, Fu FH (2012) The pivot shift: a global user guide. Knee Surg Sports Traumatol Arthrosc Off J ESSKA 20(4):724–731
39. Pollard TC, Khan T, Price AJ, Gill HS, Glyn-Jones S, Rees JL (2012) Simulated hip arthroscopy skills: learning curves with the lateral and supine patient positions: a randomized trial. J Bone Joint Surg Am 94(10):e68
40. Srivastava S, Youngblood PL, Rawn C, Hariri S, Heinrichs WL, Ladd AL (2004) Initial evaluation of a shoulder arthroscopy simulator: establishing construct validity. J Shoulder Elbow Surg Am Shoulder Elbow Surg [et al]) 13(2):196–205
41. Tay C, Khajuria A, Gupte C (2014) Simulation training: a systematic review of simulation in arthroscopy and proposal of a new competency-based training framework. Int J Surg 12(6):626–633
42. Thomas GW, Johns BD, Marsh JL, Anderson DD (2014) A review of the role of simulation in developing and assessing orthopaedic surgical skills. Iowa Orthop J 34:181–189
43. Toomey RJ, Ryan JT, McEntee MF, Evanoff MG, Chakraborty DP, McNulty JP, Manning DJ, Thomas EM, Brennan PC (2010) Diagnostic efficacy of handheld devices for emergency radiologic consultation. AJR Am J Roentgenol 194(2):469–474
44. Top ortho apps. http://toporthoapps.com. Accessed 29 July 2015
45. Wang JH, Kim JG, Ahn JH, Lim HC, Hoshino Y, Fu FH (2012) Is femoral tunnel length correlated with the intercondylar notch and femoral condyle geometry after double-bundle anterior cruciate ligament reconstruction using the transportal technique? An in vivo computed tomography analysis. Arthrosc J Arthrosc Relat Surg Off Publ Arthrosc Assoc N Am Int Arthrosc Assoc 28(8):1094–1103
46. Wellmon RH, Gulick DT, Paterson ML, Gulick CN (2015) VValidity and Reliability of Two Goniometric Mobile Apps: Device, Application and Examiner Factors. J Sport Rehabil. [Epub ahead of print] PubMed PMID: 25945601
47. Yang JH, Chang M, Kwak DS, Wang JH (2014) Volume and contact surface area analysis of bony tunnels in single and double bundle anterior cruciate ligament reconstruction using autograft tendons: in vivo three-dimensional imaging analysis. Clin Orthop Surg 6(3):290–297
48. Zaffagnini S, Lopomo N, Signorelli C, Marcheggiani Muccioli GM, Bonanzinga T, Grassi A, Raggi F, Visani A, Marcacci M (2014) Inertial sensors to quantify the pivot shift test in the treatment of anterior cruciate ligament injury. Joints 2(3):124–129

Part II

Historical Perspective

7 Knee Rotation: The Swiss School

Michael T. Hirschmann and Werner Müller

Contents

7.1 Introduction

Rotation of the knee is a result of a complex teamwork between various active and passive structures [2, 3, 13]. Specific injuries to one or multiple of the involved structures may cause some form of rotatory laxity [2, 3, 13]. In this regard, there are only few anatomical structures that are solely responsible for one specific function [2, 3, 11, 13]. Generally, each function of the knee is the result of a complex interplay of several anatomical structures [2, 3, 11–13].

The knee joint offers six degrees-of-freedom (DOF) range of motion. Rotational movement consists of flexion-extension, internal-external, and varus-valgus [2, 3, 13]. Translational movement is possible in the anterior-posterior and medial-lateral directions, as well as by compression and distraction of the knee joint (Fig. 7.1) [2, 3, 13]. Each of these six DOF of motion results in complex function within the envelope of motion [2, 3, 13, 14].

This chapter aims to give a historical review and perspective as to how knee rotation is accomplished by a complex interplay of active structures, such as muscles and tendons, and passive structures, such as ligaments and joint capsule. In addition, the different types of rotatory injuries and instabilities are systematically classified and highlighted.

7.2 Screw Home Mechanism (Automatic Rotation)

As early as 1853, Meyer described an automatic external rotation during the last 20° of extension [8]. The terminal sulcus of the lateral femoral condyle is an anatomic consequence of the automatic rotation [11]. In case of a chronic laxity of

M.T. Hirschmann (✉) • W. Müller
Department of Orthopaedic Surgery and Traumatology, Kantonsspital Baselland (Bruderholz, Liestal, Laufen), Bruderholz CH-4101, Switzerland
e-mail: michael.hirschmann@ksbl.ch; Michael.Hirschmann@unibas.ch; http://www.kneedoctor.ch

V. Musahl et al. (eds.), *Rotatory Knee Instability*, DOI 10.1007/978-3-319-32070-0_7

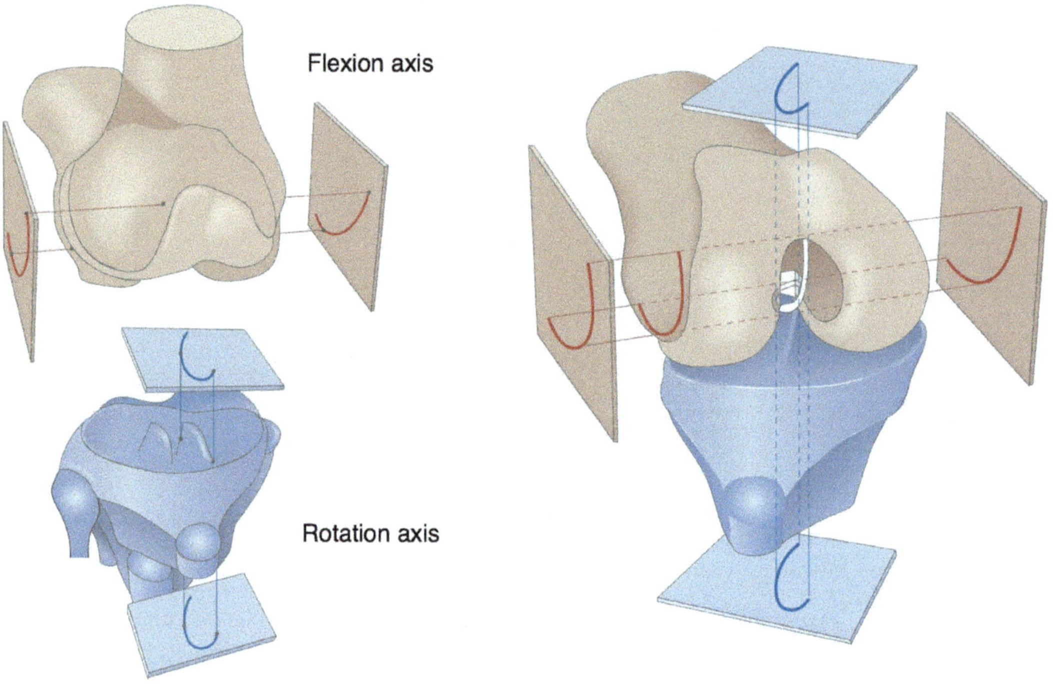

Fig. 7.1 The knee joint has six degrees of freedom for rotation and translation

the knee, a posttraumatic genu recurvatum can be observed, whereby the forces acting on the knee are not sufficiently controlled when the knee moves from flexion to extension. This may lead to hammering of the lateral femoral condyle into the anterior tibial plateau, which is a finding that also been described by Morscher [10].

The screw home mechanism (automatic rotation), which happens at end of extension, is only possible if the medial and lateral femoral condyle have different lengths [11]. In addition, the rotational axes of active knee rotation (medial of PCL and eminence in posterior tibial half) and automatic rotation (near center of lateral tibial condyle) are different [11].

Fact Box 1
The screw home mechanism represents an automatic external rotation in the last 20° of extension. It is passively controlled by the length of the medial and lateral femoral condyles and actively by the popliteal tendon.

7.3 Active Rotation

Active rotation can be performed through activation of extensor and flexor muscles, which depends on the rotation axis and "punctum fixum" and "punctum mobile" [11]. Clearly, active rotation represents a complex interplay of several muscles and tendons [11].

7.3.1 Active Rotation (Extensor Muscles)

Active rotation through extensor muscles is mainly enabled by the function of the quadriceps muscle [11].

The quadriceps muscle consists of four muscle bellies, including the rectus femoris, the vastus medialis, the vastus lateral, and the vastus intermedius muscles [11]. The course of the rectus femoris tendon and the vastus intermedius muscle over the patella and patellar tendon is angled by approximately 10–15° [11]. This orientation leads to an internal rotation of the tibia in relation to the femur [11]. Depending on the "punctum fixum," the tibia is internally rotated (e.g., when tibia is hanging freely) or the femur is externally rotated (e.g., when the tibia is fixed) [11].

The vastus medialis and lateralis muscles are important structures in active knee rotation [11]. The vastus medialis muscle acts as an internal rotator of the tibia but also plays a role in deloading the lateral patellofemoral joint [11]. The vastus lateralis muscle limits further internal rotation of the tibia and deloads the lateral patellofemoral joint [11]. Interestingly, the function of both muscles is dependent on the rotation of the knee [11]. In the externally rotated knee, the vastus medialis muscle is highly active, whereas in the internally rotated knee the vastus lateralis is more active [11].

Fact Box 2
Active knee rotation via extensor muscles is mainly enabled by the quadriceps muscle and controlled by its different arms.

7.3.2 Active Rotation (Flexor Muscles)

The most important internal rotator of the knee, which only acts at the knee, is the popliteus muscle [3, 11, 12]. Other active internal rotators all act on two joints (hip and knee) [3, 11, 12], which includes the sartorius, gracilis, semitendinosus, and semimembranosus muscles [11].

Fact Box 3
Active knee rotation via the flexor muscles is enabled by the popliteus muscle, the sartorius, the gracilis, the semitendinosus, and the semimembranosus muscles.

The popliteus muscle and tendon system consist of three main tendon arms [11]. The first tendon arm, which consists of synovial reflections above and below the meniscus, also known as popliteo-meniscal fascicles, is directed toward the posterior wall of the lateral meniscus [11]. The second one represents the popliteofibular ligament, which connects the fibular head and the popliteus tendon [11]. It is the thickest part of the popliteus system [11]. The third tendon arm runs underneath the LCL to its insertion, which is slightly ventral and distal to the femoral LCL insertion [11].

The popliteus muscle belly is located on the medial backside of the proximal tibia [11].

A torn popliteofibular ligament leads to increased rotational freedom of the popliteus tendon [11]. In such an injury, the popliteus tendon is unconstrained from the popliteofibular ligament restraints and approximately 1 cm longer, thereby allowing more tibial rotation [3, 11].

The popliteus tendon has several functions:

1. Internal rotator of the tibia (when the femur is fixed)
2. External rotator of the femur (when the foot is fixed)
3. Near extension as a lateral stabilizer, together with the biceps muscle and tractus iliotibialis
4. Flexor of knee due to its location posterior to flexion axis

Fact Box 4
The popliteus muscle and tendon system has three tendon arms, including the popliteo-meniscal fascicles, the popliteofibular ligament, and a third tendon arm which runs underneath the LCL to its insertion. The most important functions of the popliteus system are internal rotation of the tibia (when the femur is fixed), external rotation of the femur (when the foot is fixed), and lateral stabilization and flexion of the knee.

The most important external rotator of the knee, which only acts on one joint, is the biceps muscle. Other active external rotators are running over two joints, the hip and knee.

The biceps muscle, in particular the short head, acts as an external rotator and is an antagonist of the popliteal muscle [3, 11]. The flexor function of the biceps muscle is much greater than the popliteal muscle [3, 11].

Other important groups of external rotators are the tensor fasciae latae and gluteus maximus muscles, which act indirectly through a band-like structure, the tractus iliotibialis (ITT) [3, 11].

Fact Box 5

The most important external rotator acting on only one joint is the biceps muscle. The flexor function of the biceps muscle is greater than the popliteal muscle. Other external rotators are the tensor fasciae latae and gluteus maximus muscles, which act indirectly through a band-like structure, the tractus iliotibialis (ITT).

The ITT attaches at Gerdy's tubercle and functions as an anterolateral stabilizer of the knee joint [3, 11]. The Kaplan fibers, which connect the ITT with the distal lateral femoral condyle, represent a dynamic ligamentous junction [11]. It diverts the strong forces of the tensor fasciae latae and gluteus maximus muscles [11]. Due to the relation of the ITT to the flexion axis of the knee, it has the extraordinary function as being both a flexor and extender [11]. During the last 30° of extension, the ITT acts as an extensor, in a knee flexed more than 30° as flexor and external rotator [11].

Fact Box 6

The tractus iliotibialis (ITT) attaches at Gerdy's tubercle and functions as anterolateral stabilizer of the knee joint. The Kaplan fibers, which connect the ITT with the distal lateral femoral condyle, divert the strong forces of the tensor fasciae latae and gluteus maximus muscle. During the last 30° of extension, the ITT acts as an extender, whereas in a knee flexed more than 30°, it acts as a flexor and external rotator.

7.4 Passive Rotational Stabilizers

Active rotation by the aforementioned structures is only possible when passive stabilizers guide and limit these rotational activities [3, 11]. The most important passive stabilizer of knee rotation includes the cruciate ligaments, the menisci, and the capsule-ligamentous structures, including the posterior capsule [3, 11].

The ACL is considered to have two or even three primary functional bundles: the anteromedial (AM), posterolateral (PL), and intermediate (IM) bundles [2, 3]. These bundles are named with regard to their tibial insertions [2, 3]. During passive motion, the AM portion of the ACL lengthens with knee flexion, while the PL portion of the ACL shortens [2, 3]. The PL bundle is dominant at 20° of knee flexion [2, 3] (Figs. 7.2 and 7.3).

Fact Box 7

The most important passive stabilizers of knee rotation include the cruciate ligaments, the menisci, and the capsule-ligamentous structures, including the posterior capsule.

The PCL is the strongest ligament of the knee and consists of multiple bundles. Most researchers describe two to three bundles, including the anterolateral (ALB), the posteromedial (PMB), and the intermediate bundles [3, 11, 12]. However, Mommersteeg et al. found six to ten bundles and multiple fascicles [9]. Both the lengths and the widths of the PCL are larger than those of the ACL.

The PCL is the primary restraint to posterior tibial translation and a secondary restraint to external tibial rotation [7, 16].

The menisci form a mobile containment on the tibial plateau adapting to the rolling gliding and rotating movement of the femoral condyles [3, 11, 12]. The incongruity of femoral condyle and tibial plateau is compensated by the medial and lateral menisci [6]. In addition, the medial meniscus is connected to the medial collateral ligament. The medial posterior horn is fixed to

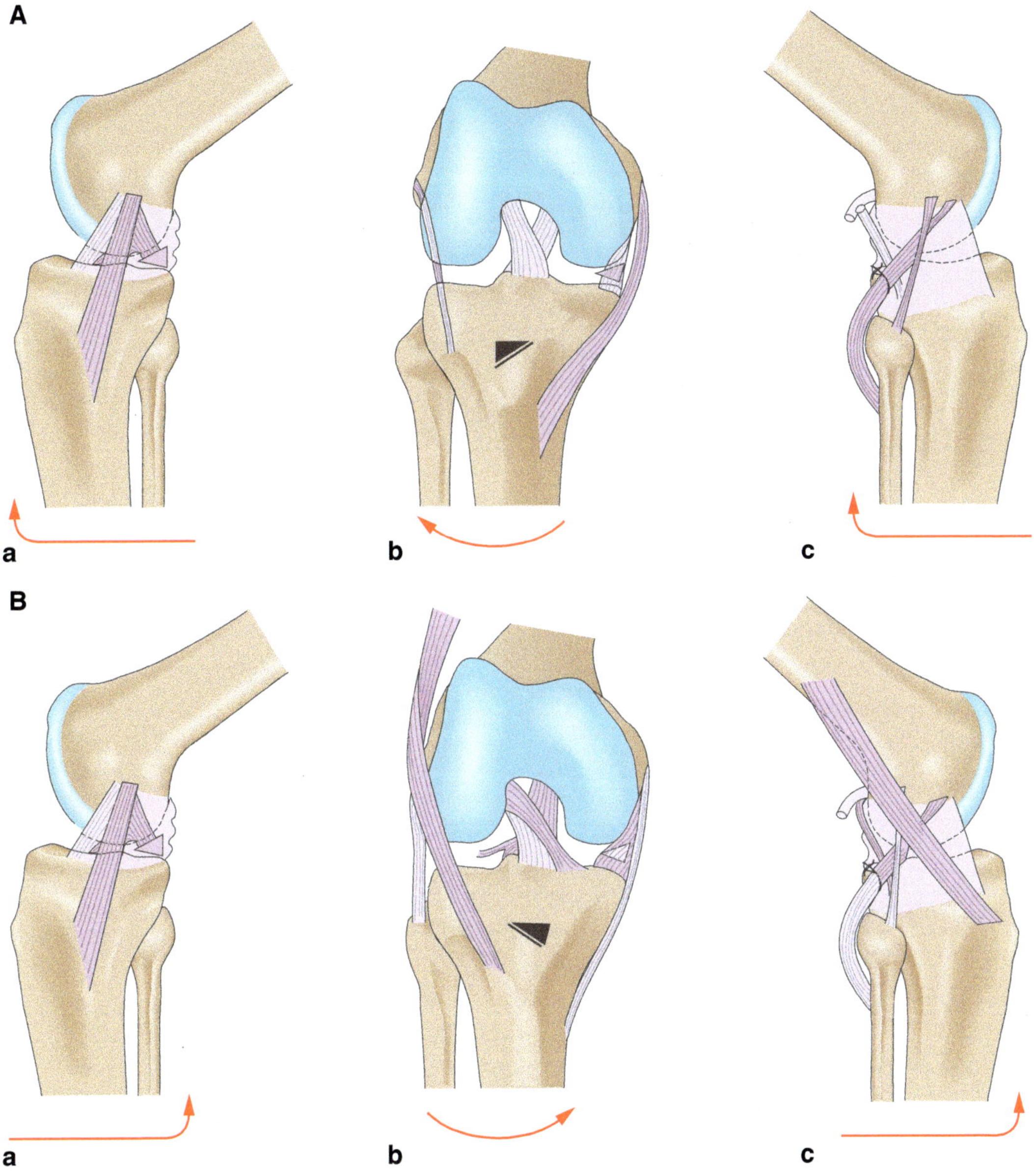

Fig. 7.2 Laxity in 30° flexion and ER (first row. 2A) and IR (second row, 2B). (**a**) Medial view, (**b**) frontal view, (**c**) lateral view. *In 30° flexion and ER***:** Tight: medial collateral ligament, semimembranosus corner, lateral collateral ligament, popliteal corner. Loose: ACL, less loose PCL. *In 30° flexion and IR***:** Tight: semimembranosus corner, ACL, PCL, LFTLA, arcuate ligament. Loose: MCL and LCL

the posterior oblique ligament (POL) and functions as an important secondary co-restraint to the ACL and with its parallel orientation to the PCL also a co-restraint for the PCL [3, 6, 11, 12].

The fibers of the posterior capsule are orientated in a V-shaped manner [11]. Medially, it is

Fact Box 8
The incongruity of the femoral condyle and the tibial plateau is compensated for by the medial and lateral menisci.

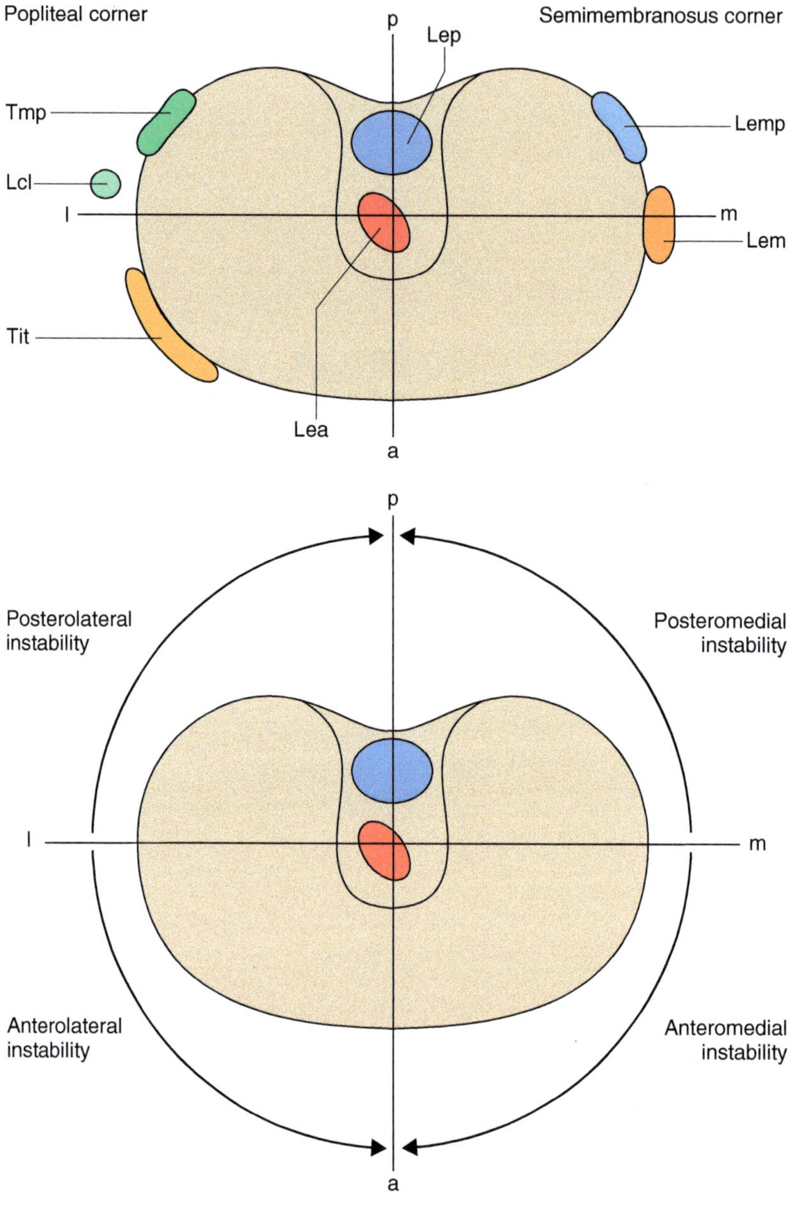

Fig. 7.3 Schematic illustration of the right tibial plateau divided in four quadrants. Seven major passive stabilizers of the knee are shown. These are ACL, PCL as central pivot, MCL, posterior oblique ligament, iliotibial tract, LCL, popliteal tendon. *a* anterior, *p* posterior, *m* medial, *l* lateral, *PCL* posterior cruciate ligament, *MCL* medial collateral ligament, *POL* posterior oblique ligament, *ITT* iliotibial tract, *ACL* anterior cruciate ligament, *LCL* lateral collateral ligament, *Popl.T* popliteal tendon

the popliteal oblique ligament, which builds a triangle with the semimembranosus muscle, whereas laterally it is the arcuate ligament [11]. Another important passive structure stabilizing the posterior capsule is the fabella and the structures attaching to it [11]. The most prominent structures are the popliteal oblique ligament, the fabellofibular ligament, and the lateral gastrocnemius tendon [11]. A fabella is found in only 20% of all knee joints, however [11].

In addition, in early textbooks and publications, a capsule-ligamentous thickening of the anterolateral capsule has been mentioned and named as the anterolateral ligament (ALL). Others have named it as mid-third lateral capsular ligament, anterior oblique band, capsule-osseous layer of the ITT, or lateral capsular ligament [1, 4, 5, 11]. However, its clear function and anatomic description has been vague and inconsistent.

The origin of the ALL is on the lateral femoral epicondyle proximally and posterior to the popliteus tendon insertion [15]. It inserts on the lateral meniscus and tibia 5 mm distal to the tibiofemoral joint and posterior to Gerdy's tubercle [15]. However, still considerable variation exists in the description of the ALL.

The ALL is most tight during combined flexion and internal tibial rotation. Hence, it serves as stabilizer for internal rotation in flexion >35° [15]. It has no function against anterior tibial translation [15].

Fact Box 9
Posterior stabilizers are the thick posterior capsule, the popliteal oblique ligament, the arcuate ligament, the fabella, and the structures attaching to it such as the popliteal oblique ligament, the fabellofibular ligament, and the lateral gastrocnemius tendon.

The ALL represents a thickening of the anterolateral capsule. It originates at the lateral femoral epicondyle proximally and posterior to the popliteus tendon insertion and inserts on the lateral meniscus and tibia 5 mm distal to the tibiofemoral joint and posterior to Gerdy's tubercle. It serves as a stabilizer for internal rotation in >35° knee flexion.

7.5 Classification of Rotatory Laxity

Typical examples of rotatory laxities are presented and illustrated in Figs. 7.4, 7.5, 7.6, 7.7, 7.8, 7.9, and 7.10. Also, combined rotatory laxities are seen in clinical practice [4, 5, 11–13].

7.5.1 Anteromedial Rotatory Laxity

A typical finding of this type of rotatory laxity is that the medial tibia excessively rotates anteriorly, and the medial joint gap is opening. Injured structures are typically (ordered by injury severity) the semimembranosus tendon complex, the medial collateral ligament complex, and the ACL [11, 12].

7.5.2 Anterolateral Rotatory Laxity

A typical finding of this type of rotatory laxity is that the lateral tibia excessively rotates anteriorly, and the lateral joint gap is opening. Injured structures are typically (ordered by injury severity) the lateral anterior femorotibial ligament (LFTLA), which is part of the ITT, the ACL, and the popliteal corner [11, 12].

7.5.3 Posterolateral Rotatory Laxity

A typical finding of this type of rotatory laxity is that the lateral tibia rotates excessively posteriorly, and the lateral joint gap opens. Injured structures are typically (ordered by injury severity) the popliteal corner, LCL, and PCL [11, 12].

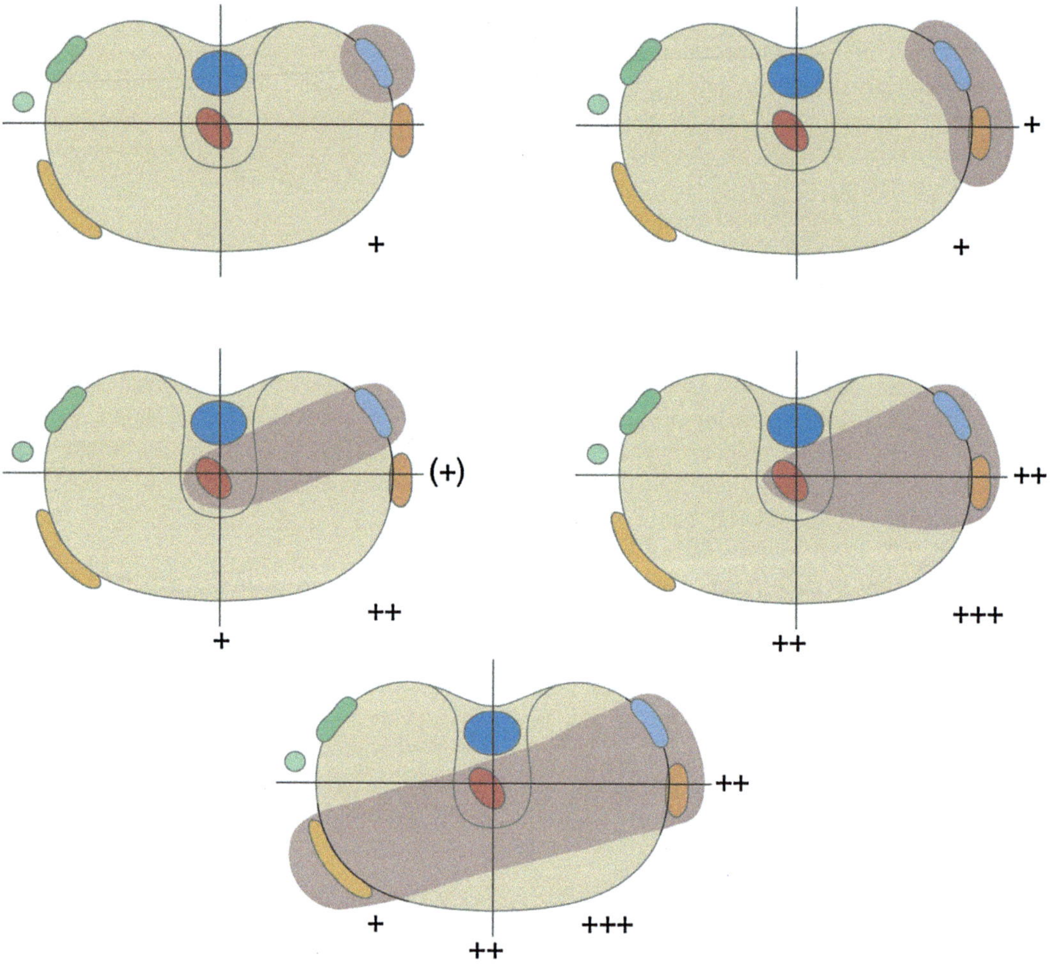

Fig. 7.4 Several types of anteromedial laxity are shown here: (**a**) Lesion of posterior oblique ligament presenting as anteromedial laxity (+). (**b**) Combined lesion of posterior oblique ligament and MCL presenting as anteromedial instability (+) and valgus laxity (+). (**c**) Combined lesion of posterior oblique ligament and ACL presenting as anteromedial laxity (++), anterior drawer in neutral rotation (+), and valgus laxity (+). (**d**) Combined lesion of posterior oblique ligament, MCL and ACL presenting as anteromedial instability (+++), anterior drawer in neutral rotation (++), and valgus laxity (++). (**e**) Combined lesion of posterior oblique ligament, MCL, ACL, and LFTLA presenting as anteromedial laxity (+++), anterior drawer in neutral rotation (++), anterolateral laxity (+), valgus instability (++), lateral pivot shift (+). Genu recurvatum (+)

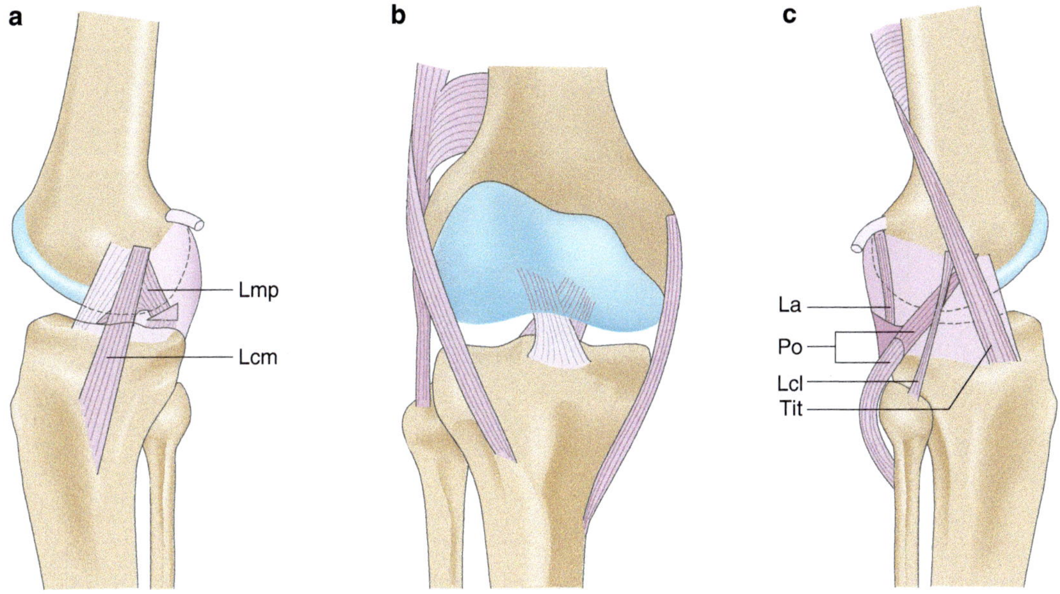

Fig. 7.5 Laxity in extension. Tight: MCL (*Lcm*), posterior oblique ligament (*Lcmp*), LFTLA, LCL, popliteal corner, posterior capsule, ACL, and PCL. *Po* popliteal tendon

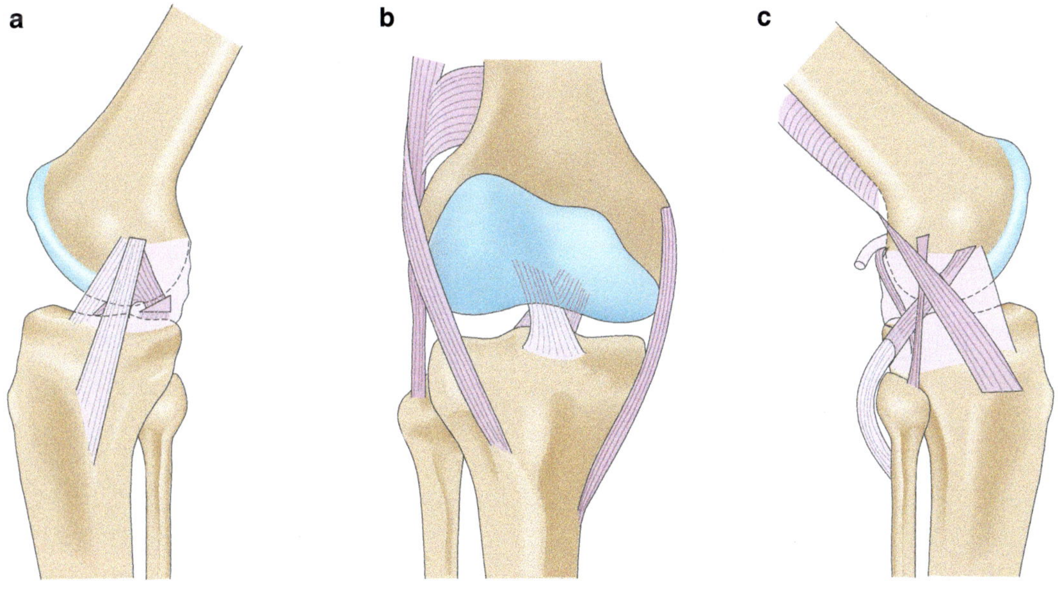

Fig. 7.6 Laxity in 30° flexion and normal rotation. Less tight than in extension: MCL, semimembranosus corner, LFTLA, LCL, and PCL. Loose: ACL

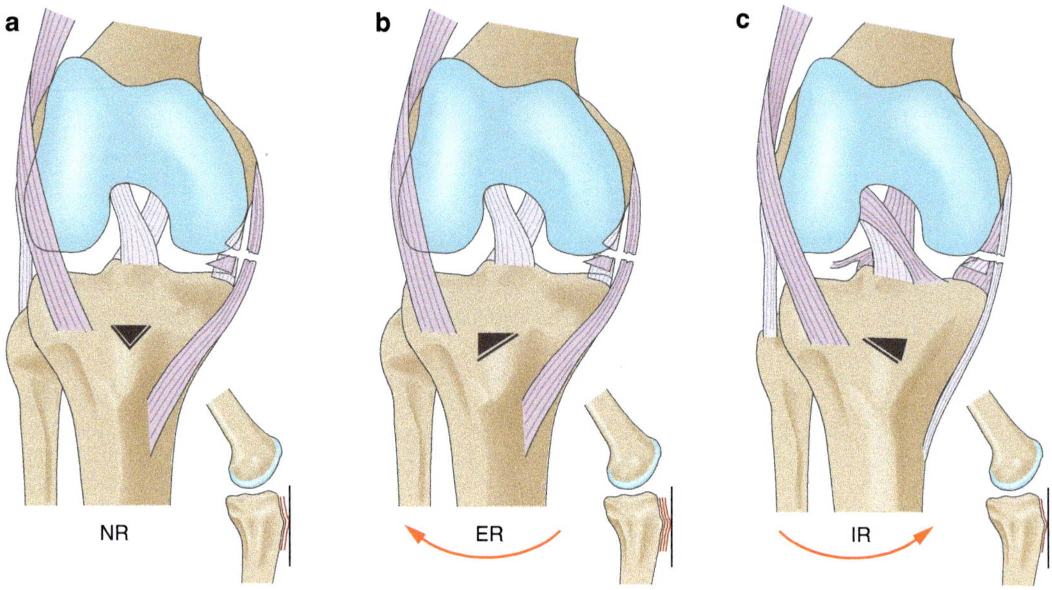

Fig. 7.7 Laxity in 30° flexion and anterior tibial translation. (**a**) In neutral rotation (*NR*). Tight: ACL. Slightly tight: semimembranosus corner, LFTLA. (**b**) In external rotation (*AR*). Tight: MCL, semimembranosus corner, LCL. Loose: ACL, PCL, LFTLA. (**c**) In internal rotation (*IR*). Tight: ACL, PCL, LFTLA. Slightly tight: semimembranosus corner

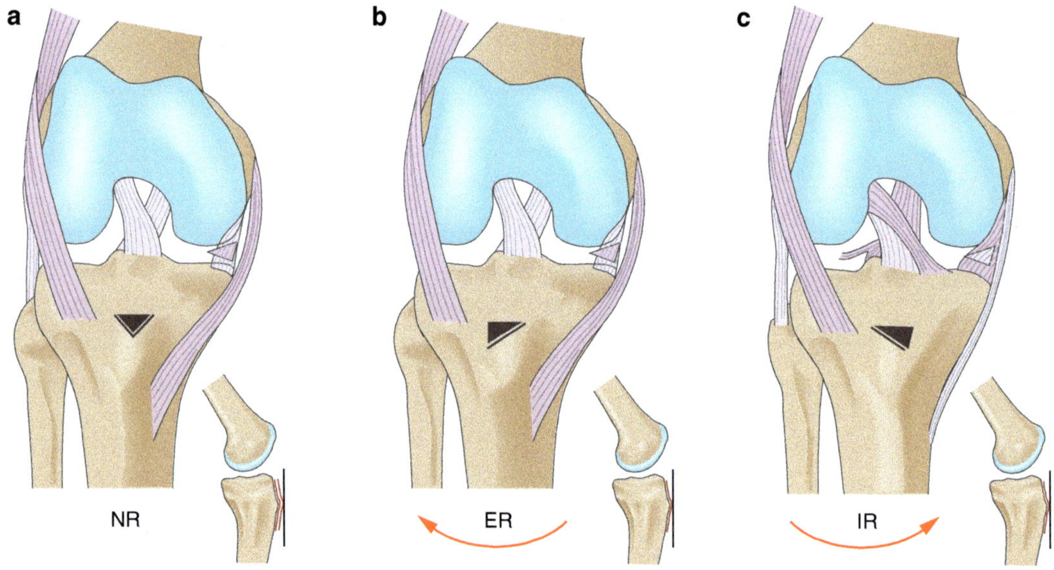

Fig. 7.8 Laxity in 30° flexion and anterior tibial translation with torn MCL. After tear of MCL, anterior tibial translation is (**a**) in neutral rotation (*NR*): Same as in uninjured knee. (**b**) In external rotation (*AR*). Increased, more than in NR. (**c**) In internal rotation (*IR*). Same as in uninjured knee – both cruciates and LFTLA are tight

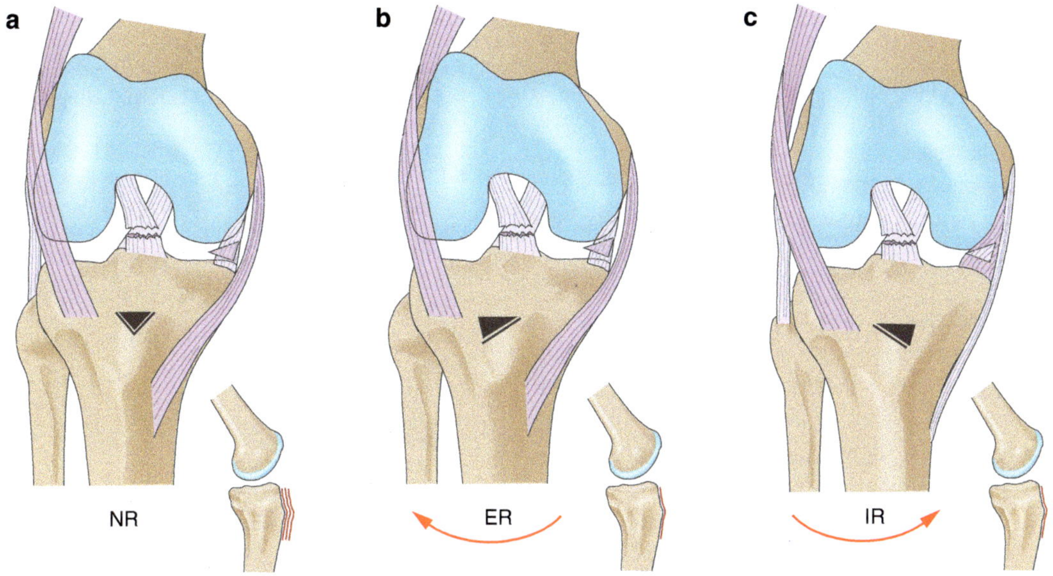

Fig. 7.9 Laxity in 30° flexion and anterior tibial translation with torn ACL. After tear of ACL, anterior tibial translation is (**a**) in neutral rotation (*NR*): Increased, more than in uninjured knee. (**b**) in external rotation (*AR*). Normal, not increased as ACL is loose in this position. (**c**) In internal rotation (*IR*). Normal, not increased as LFTLA and semimembranosus corner act as stabilizer

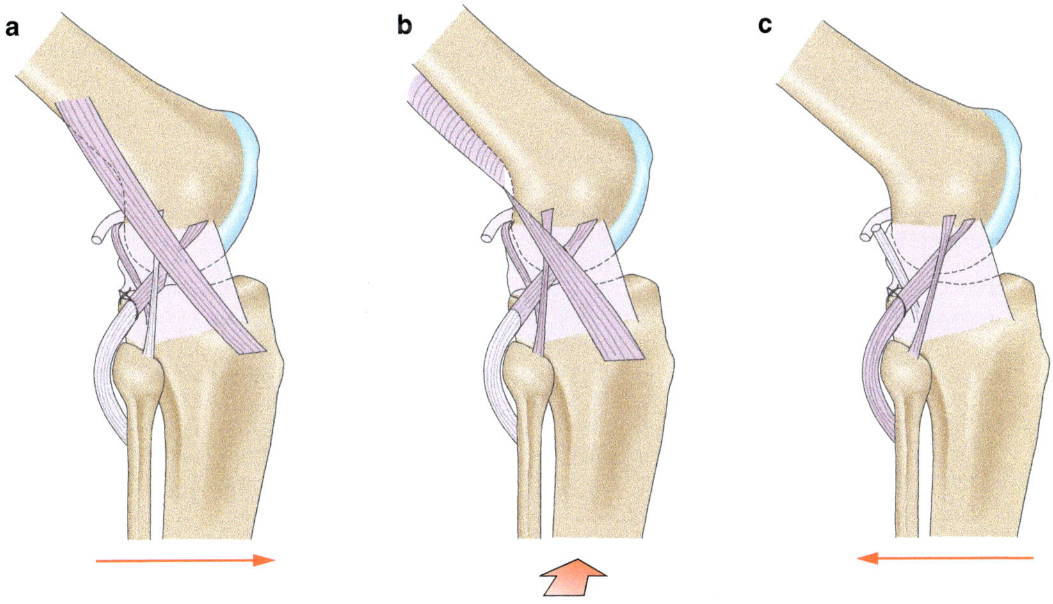

Fig. 7.10 Lateral ligamentous structures in 30° flexion. (**a**) In anterior tibial translation. Tight: LFTLA, part of arcuate ligament. (**b**) In varus stress. Tight: LFTLA, LCL, part of arcuate ligament, popliteal tendon. (**c**) In posterior tibial translation. Tight: LCL, popliteal tendon, and part of arcuate ligament

7.5.4 Posteromedial Rotatory Laxity

A typical finding of this type of rotatory laxity is that the medial tibia excessively rotates anteriorly and the lateral joint gap opens. Injured structures are typically (ordered by injury severity) semimembranosus corner, MCL, ACL partially, and PCL [11, 12].

Conclusion

A historical review and perspective are presented about how knee rotation is accomplished by a complex interplay of active structures, such as muscles and tendons, and passive structures, such as ligaments and joint capsule. The different types of rotatory injuries are systematically classified and highlighted.

References

1. Dodds AL, Halewood C, Gupte CM, Williams A, Amis AA (2014) The anterolateral ligament: anatomy, length changes and association with the segond fracture. J Bone Joint Surg Br 96(3):325–331. doi:10.1302/0301-620X.96B3.33033
2. Feagin J, Hirschmann MT, Muller W (2015) Understand, respect and restore anatomy as close as possible! Knee Surg Sports Traumatol Arthrosc. doi:10.1007/s00167-015-3635-3
3. Hirschmann MT, Muller W (2015) Complex function of the knee joint: the current understanding of the knee. Knee Surg Sports Traumatol Arthrosc. doi:10.1007/s00167-015-3619-3
4. Hughston JC, Andrews JR, Cross MJ, Moschi A (1976) Classification of knee ligament instabilities. Part I: the medial compartment and cruciate ligaments. J Bone Joint Surg Am 58(2):159–172
5. Hughston JC, Andrews JR, Cross MJ, Moschi A (1976) Classification of knee ligament instabilities. Part II: the lateral compartment. J Bone Joint Surg Am 58(2):173–179
6. Kapandji IA (1999) Funktionelle Anatomie der Gelenke. Band 2 Untere Extremität. Hippokrates Verlag GmbH, Stuttgart
7. Kennedy NI, Wijdicks CA, Goldsmith MT, Michalski MP, Devitt BM, Aroen A, Engebretsen L, LaPrade RF (2013) Kinematic analysis of the posterior cruciate ligament, part 1: the individual and collective function of the anterolateral and posteromedial bundles. Am J Sports Med 41(12):2828–2838. doi:10.1177/0363546513504287
8. Meyer H (1853) Die Mechanik des Kniegelenkes. Arch Anat Physiol Wiss Med:497–547
9. Mommersteeg TJ, Kooloos JG, Blankevoort L, Kauer JM, Huiskes R, Roeling FQ (1995) The fibre bundle anatomy of human cruciate ligaments. J Anat 187(Pt 2):461–471
10. Morscher E (1976) Traumatische Knorpelimpression an den Femurkondylen. Hefte Unfallheilkd 127: 71–78
11. Mueller W (1982) The knee: form, function, and ligament reconstruction. Springer, Berlin/Heidelberg/New York
12. Muller W (1977) Current aspects of functional anatomy of the knee joint. Hefte Unfallheilkd (129):131–137
13. Musahl V, Zaffagnini S, LaPrade R, Hirschmann MT, Karlsson J (2015) The challenge of treating complex knee instability. Knee Surg Sports Traumatol Arthrosc. doi:10.1007/s00167-015-3665-x
14. Noyes FR, Cummings JF, Grood ES, Walz-Hasselfeld KA, Wroble RR (1991) The diagnosis of knee motion limits, subluxations, and ligament injury. Am J Sports Med 19(2):163–171
15. Vincent JP, Magnussen RA, Gezmez F, Uguen A, Jacobi M, Weppe F, Al-Saati MF, Lustig S, Demey G, Servien E, Neyret P (2012) The anterolateral ligament of the human knee: an anatomic and histologic study. Knee Surg Sports Traumatol Arthrosc 20(1):147–152. doi:10.1007/s00167-011-1580-3
16. Wijdicks CA, Kennedy NI, Goldsmith MT, Devitt BM, Michalski MP, Aroen A, Engebretsen L, LaPrade RF (2013) Kinematic analysis of the posterior cruciate ligament, part 2: a comparison of anatomic single- versus double-bundle reconstruction. Am J Sports Med 41(12):2839–2848. doi:10.1177/0363546513504384

Knee Rotation: The Lyon School

8

Sébastien Lustig, Timothy Lording, Dan Washer, Olivier Reynaud, and Philippe Neyret

Contents

S. Lustig (✉) • D. Washer • O. Reynaud • P. Neyret
Department of Orthopaedic, Albert Trillat Center, Lyon North University Hospital, Lyon, France
e-mail: sebastien.lustig@gmail.com

T. Lording
Department of Orthopaedic, Melbourne Orthopaedic Group, Melbourne, VIC, Australia

8.1 Introduction

Modern reconstruction techniques for anterior cruciate ligament (ACL) injury have achieved good results for the majority of patients; however, there remains a group for whom rotational instability is still an issue [3]. Lateral extra-articular reconstruction procedures were described to address anterolateral rotational laxity. Widely used during the 1970s and 1980s, today, lateral extra-articular reinforcement has again been proposed as a possible solution to failure in ACL reconstruction. In the past 5 years, there has been an improvement in the understanding of the complex anatomy of the lateral capsule, leading to a better recognition of reasons why reconstruction of the ALL, in combination with an intra-articular ACL reconstruction, may improve rotational stability in ACL-deficient knees.

8.2 Knee Rotation Control: The Rationale for Early Lateral Extra-Articular Procedures

ACL injury generally produces both translational and rotational abnormalities. Early attempts at surgical intervention, both intra- and extra-articular, attempted to address only anterior tibial translation [14]. In 1979, Slocum and Larson, recognizing the importance of rotational instability in the ACL-deficient knee, introduced

V. Musahl et al. (eds.), *Rotatory Knee Instability*, DOI 10.1007/978-3-319-32070-0_8

the concept of rotational laxity and described a "rotational stability test" [16]. Their work focused on anteromedial rotation associated with medial-sided injury, and they went on to develop a pes anserinus transfer to hold the tibia in internal rotation [17].

Evidence for damage to the lateral structures of the knee in ACL injury was described as early as 1879. Prior to the invention of radiographs, Ségond described an avulsion fracture of the proximal tibia during cadaveric experiments to reproduce ACL injury. He hypothesized that this avulsion, from just posterior to the iliotibial tract insertion, was the insertion site of the middle third of the lateral capsular ligament [15]. Studies have shown the incidence of ligamentous injuries associated with acute anterolateral rotatory instability. In 36 knees, the authors found only four with isolated ACL injury, 26 with ACL and additional lateral injury (to the lateral capsular ligament, the iliotibial tract, or both), and six knees with lateral capsular ligament injury alone [11].

Lateral extra-articular procedures were promoted as having a biomechanical advantage over intra-articular reconstruction in terms of rotational control. This was due to the longer lever arm of a laterally based reconstruction to resist torque. Ellison described the ACL as, "the hub of the wheel" and noted, "it is easier to control rotation of a wheel at its rim than at its hub" [5].

Fact Box 1

1. Evidence for damage to the lateral structures of the knee in ACL injury was described as early as 1879.
2. Lateral extra-articular procedures were promoted as having a biomechanical advantage over intra-articular reconstruction in terms of rotational control.
3. This is due to the longer lever arm of a laterally based reconstruction to resist torque.

8.3 Recent Advances

8.3.1 Anatomy

The anatomy of the knee remains incompletely understood, particularly in regard to the functional anatomy of the lateral side. Numerous authors have described a structure connecting the lateral femoral condyle, lateral meniscus, and lateral tibial plateau [8, 18, 20]. This structure has been described as part of the iliotibial tract, a capsular thickening, or a ligament in its own right and has been variously referred to as the "capsulo-osseous layer" of the iliotibial tract, the "mid-third lateral capsular ligament," the "lateral capsular ligament" [1], and most recently the "anterolateral ligament" [20].

Vincent and colleagues identified a structure, which they termed the anterolateral ligament, in 30 consecutive total knee arthroplasties, as well as 10 cadaver knees [21]. At cadaveric dissection, the structure was found to arise from just anterior to the popliteus tendon insertion in nine knees or from the popliteus tendon itself in one. It was closely associated with the lateral meniscus at the junction of its anterior and middle thirds. Its insertion was onto the anterolateral proximal tibia, 5 mm from the articular cartilage and always posterior to the most posterior border of Gerdy's tubercle. Histological analysis demonstrated a distinct fibrous structure, with some fibers inserting onto the meniscus. Recent published work by Claes and colleagues has identified this structure in 40 of 41 cadaveric knees [2]. They found the structure to originate posterior and proximal to the popliteus tendon insertion, on the lateral femoral epicondyle, and noted no connections between this structure and the iliotibial band.

Terry suggested that injury to the capsulo-osseous layer of the iliotibial band may be responsible for the variety of clinical findings in the ACL-injured knee [19], and failure to address associated injuries is a recognized cause of failed ACL reconstruction [22]. Future research should help to standardize nomenclature and clarify the biomechanics of this ligament. Should this confirm a role in the restraint of rotatory laxity, lateral extra-articular techniques may be shown to be more anatomical than once thought and may be able to be modified to be truly anatomical reconstructive procedures.

8.3.2 Combined Procedures

Isolated extra-articular procedures are no longer recommended [13]. Their role in combined procedures with modern intra-articular techniques, however, is less clear.

Engebretsen showed that an iliotibial tenodesis reduced the force in an ACL graft by an average of 43 % [6]. Load sharing between an intra- and extra-articular reconstruction has been demonstrated, and it has been suggested that the extra-articular procedure may have a role in protecting the intra-articular reconstruction during the healing phase [4]. While these studies did not use anatomical intra-articular reconstructions, they suggest a role for extra-articular procedures in combined operations in some cases.

Monaco and colleagues compared ten anatomical single-bundle reconstructions with lateral extra-articular reinforcement with ten double-bundle ACL reconstructions using a navigation system [9]. They found no difference in anteroposterior translation between the two groups but a significant reduction in internal rotation at 30° of knee flexion in the extra-articular reinforcement group.

Early lateral procedures tended to use iliotibial band as graft material. The strength of this material depends on the width harvested; however, it is generally weaker than hamstring tendons and able to withstand significantly lower maximum stresses [12]. More recently, techniques have been described using hamstring tendon for lateral reinforcement.

Marcacci has described a technique of intra- and extra-articular reconstruction using hamstring tendons [7]. The gracilis and semitendinosus tendons are stripped, but their tibial insertions maintained. The sutured graft is then passed through a tibial tunnel and over the top of the lateral femoral condyle. A groove is formed in the lateral femur for stability and bone healing, and the tendons fixed with two bone staples. The remaining graft is passed deep to the iliotibial band and secured at Gerdy's tubercle.

At 11 years follow-up of 54 knees in high level athletes, Marcacci reported 90.7 % excellent or good results using the International Knee Documentation Committee (IKDC) score [8]. Three knees (5.5 %) showed a slight pivot shift.

Neyret has described a technique using a bone-patella tendon-bone intra-articular graft and a gracilis tendon graft for the extra-articular reinforcement [10]. The gracilis is threaded through a drill hole in one of the bone blocks, to create a continuous graft. The patella tendon graft is passed anterograde through a femoral and tibial tunnel, locking the gracilis tendon in the femoral tunnel with the press fit of the bony block. The two free limbs are then passed deep to the LCL and through either end of a bony tunnel through Gerdy's tubercle and sutured to one another.

Fact Box 2

1. The role of extra-articular procedures in combined procedures with modern intra-articular techniques is still unclear.
2. Advances in understanding the complex lateral anatomy and biomechanics of the knee are crucial for the development of more anatomical procedures.
3. Some authors report excellent or good results at midterm follow-up after combined intra- and extra-articular ACL reconstruction.

8.4 Current Technique in Albert Trillat Center (Lyon)

8.4.1 Surgical Indications

We have several indications for adding an extra-articular tenodesis to an intra-articular ACL reconstruction. In general, our philosophy is to perform the procedure in cases where the expected failure rate is increased. Our primary indication for an extra-articular tenodesis is a 3+ pivot shift on physical examination. In these patients, an intra-articular graft alone may not completely control excessive anterior tibial translation and internal rotation in the lateral compartment. These are generally patients with chronic ACL deficiency. It is unusual for us to perform an extra-articular reconstruction in the acute setting. Similarly, patients with generalized hyper laxity are treated with the combined procedure. We also consider extra-articular augmentation in patients who plan to return to collision sports. The additional constraint may help protect these knees from the high loads seen in these sports and may decrease the re-rupture rate. We also consider an extra-articular tenodesis in patients less than 20 years of age. It has been shown that these patients are at an increased risk of re-rupture of an isolated intra-articular graft. Finally, we perform this procedure in cases of revision ACL surgery. Objective laxity is greater in patients with failed ACL reconstructions, especially those that have undergone concomitant medial meniscectomies (because of the role of the posterior horn of the medial meniscus in anteroposterior laxity, especially in ACL-deficient knees), and the addition of an extra-articular tenodesis has improved the results of revision ACL surgery in some studies.

Fact Box 3

Indications for adding extra-articular tenodesis to intra-articular ACL reconstruction:

- 3+ pivot shift
- Generalized hyper laxity
- Plan to return to collision sports
- Age less than 20 years
- Revision ACL surgery (especially for patients that have undergone concomitant medial meniscectomies)

8.4.2 Surgical Contraindications

The addition of an extra-articular reconstruction is contraindicated in ACL-deficient patients that have an associated posterolateral corner injury. In this situation, the lateral augmentation may fix the tibia in a posterolaterally subluxed position. We also do not perform an extra-articular reconstruction in skeletally immature patients because of the risk of injury to the femoral physis. Older studies have shown increased risk of lateral tibiofemoral degeneration after an isolated extra-articular reconstruction. This may have been a result of overtensioning of the graft leading to overconstraint of the lateral compartment or may have been related to the 4–6 weeks of postoperative immobilization that was standard at that time. We have not seen lateral tibiofemoral arthritis in our extra-articular patients where the lateral meniscus was intact.

8.4.3 Preoperative Planning

Physical examination remains the most important factor in deciding when to add an extra-articular procedure to an intra-articular ACL reconstruction. The examiner must be skilled in performing both the Lachman test to assess anterior translation and the pivot shift test to assess rotatory laxity. KT-1000 measurements and anterior tibial stress radiographs can help quantify global anterior laxity, but a measurement of the translation of the individual tibiofemoral compartments would be more useful to identify patients who would benefit from an extra-articular procedure. Several research techniques, including computer-assisted measurements, are being developed to quantitate the rotatory laxity of the knee, but these are not yet widely available. Radiographs should be obtained in all patients with suspected knee injuries. The presence of a Segond fracture confirms that there has been injury to the ALL. In our experience, MRI does not help the surgeon in the decision of when to add an extra-articular procedure. In cases of revision ACL surgery, old operative reports should be obtained to know what grafts will be available and what instrumentation might be required to remove previously placed hardware.

8.4.4 Surgical Technique

Two different surgical approaches can be utilized. One option is to use an extended anterior incision that will allow access to both the patellar tendon and the iliotibial band. Alternatively, two incisions can be used: an anteromedial one for harvesting the patellar tendon and a lateral incision for the extra-articular procedure. Subcutaneous skin flaps are raised and a central 10 mm strip of patellar tendon is harvested. The patellar bone block is 9 × 25 mm to allow for easy graft passage, while the 25 mm long tibial bone block is harvested as a trapezoid being 10 mm wide at the tendon insertion and fanning out to 12 mm distally. A passing stitch of #2 reinforced nonabsorbable suture is placed through a small drill hole in each bone block. The patella tendon graft is then placed in a moist saline sponge until ready for passage.

Next, the lateral skin flap is dissected subcutaneously to expose the iliotibial band and Gerdy's tubercle. A distally based strip of iliotibial band 10 mm wide and 70–100 mm long is harvested using a scalpel and scissors (Fig. 8.1). A whip stitch of #2 suture is placed in the proximal end of the graft. Next, the surgeon should identify the fibular collateral ligament and its attachment on the femur. Dissection is carried out so that a clamp can be passed underneath the ligament.

An arthroscopic evaluation of the knee joint is then undertaken and any associated intra-articular pathology is addressed. The ACL remnant is debrided. A femoral tunnel guide pin is drilled with an outside-in guide starting just 5 mm posterior and proximal to the FCL femoral insertion (Fig. 8.2) and exiting inside the knee joint at the center of the ACL femoral attachment. The guide pin is then reamed up to a 10 mm diameter tunnel. Finally, a 9 mm tibial tunnel is created in the center of the ACL tibial footprint using standard technique.

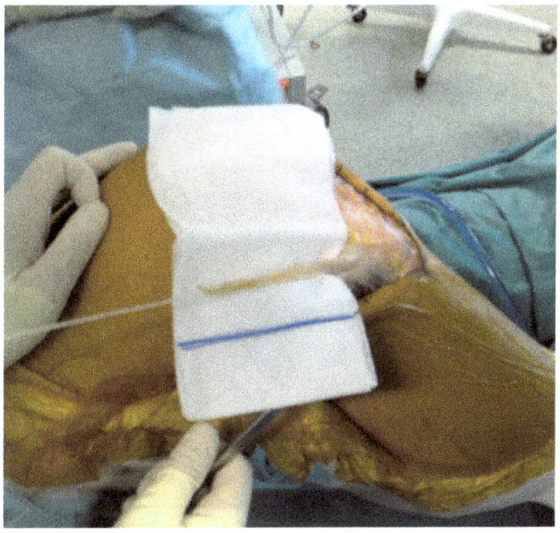

Fig. 8.1 A distally based strip of iliotibial band 10 mm wide and 70–100 mm long is harvested using a scalpel and scissors

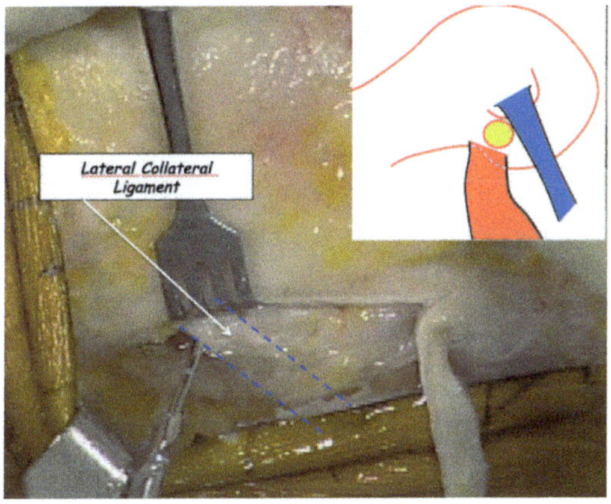

Fig. 8.2 A femoral tunnel guide pin is drilled with an outside-in guide starting just 5 mm posterior and proximal to the FCL femoral insertion

A passing suture is then placed through both tunnels and a second passing stitch placed through the femoral tunnel and exiting out the anteromedial portal. With the patellar bone block leading, the graft is then passed proximal to distal until the tibial bone block is just about to enter the femoral tunnel. The strip of iliotibial band is then passed underneath the FCL (Fig. 8.3) and then pulled into the femoral tunnel (Fig. 8.4). With the leg held in 30° of flexion and neutral

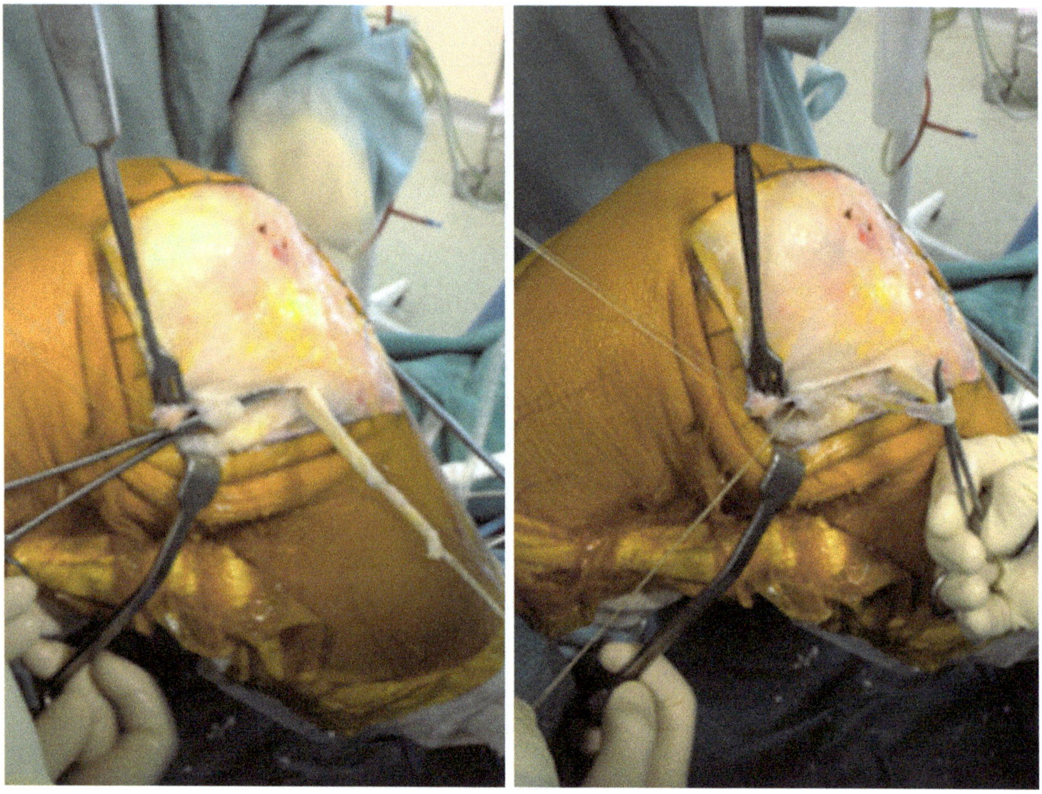

Fig. 8.3 The strip of iliotibial band is passed underneath the FCL

rotation, tension is applied through the iliotibial band sutures. The tibial bone plug is then press fit into the femoral tunnel with the aid of a bone tamp. This provides secure fixation for both the patellar tendon graft and the extra-articular reconstruction. The leg is then brought out into full extension, and the patellar bone plug is tensioned and secured with a 9 mm tibial interference screw. The split in the iliotibial band is closed with #1 absorbable suture, and if necessary, a limited lateral retinacular release is performed to avoid increased pressure on the lateral facet of the patella.

8.4.5 Postoperative Management

Patients who have undergone the combined intra- and extra-articular ACL reconstruction undergo the same rehabilitation protocol at isolated intra-articular ACL reconstruction patients. The knee is immobilized in a hinged brace at 0° for the first 2 weeks while the patient is at rest. The patient is allowed range of motion as tolerated. Weight bearing is progressed as pain, swelling, and quadriceps strength allows. Full range of motion is expected by 6 weeks. After the first 6 weeks, no brace is required. Closed-chain exercises are emphasized the first 3 months. In patients with isolated ACL reconstructions, assuming normal motion, no effusion and sufficient strength, running, and sports-specific conditioning is allowed at 3 months. In patients with no severe laxity, return to play can be allowed at 6 months because the extra-articular augmentation protects the ACL graft during pivoting activities.

8.4.6 Complications to Avoid

All complications that can occur with an isolated intra-articular ACL reconstruction can

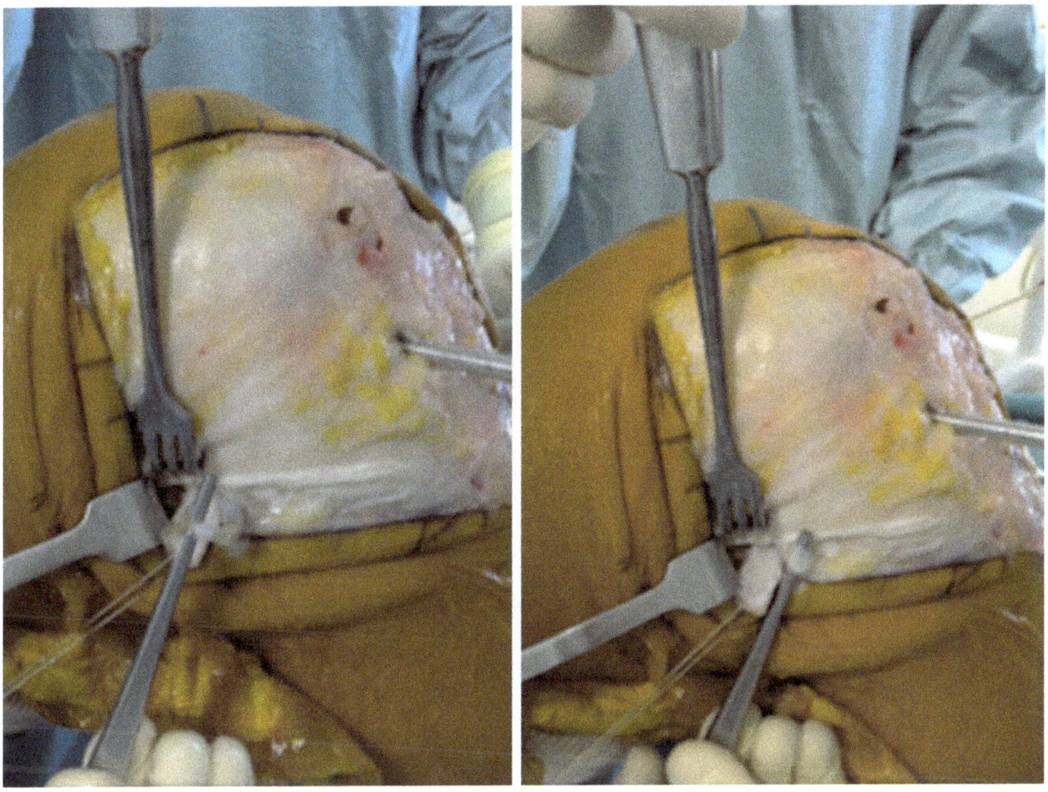

Fig. 8.4 The strip of iliotibial band is then pulled into the femoral tunnel

happen with this combined procedure. These include infection, stiffness, errors in tunnel placement, and residual laxity. The extra-articular ACL reconstruction described above should not be performed as an isolated procedure as it will not adequately control anterior tibial translation nor completely restore normal knee kinematics in young, active patients. Care must be taken to avoid over-constraining rotational laxity. We believe that appropriately tensioning the graft and maintaining the knee in neutral rotation during fixation can avoid this complication. Graft placement is also critical. The starting point for the outside-in femoral tunnel is extremely important to reproduce the femoral attachment point of the ALL. The surgeon must also insure that the tibial bone block achieves excellent fixation in the femoral tunnel while being fully seated. Appropriately trimming the graft and trialing with tunnel sizers prior to graft passage can minimize these problems. The closure of the IT band split can over-tension the lateral retinaculum, causing lateral patellar facet overload. Performing a lateral retinacular release can help avoid this complication. Finally, pain and lateral tenderness can occur if the extra-articular reconstruction is passed superficial to the FCL. Making sure the graft passes beneath the FCL will avoid this complication.

Conclusions

Lateral extra-articular reinforcement in conjunction with intra-articular reconstruction may be an important option in the control of rotational laxity of the knee. Advances in understanding the complex lateral anatomy and biomechanics of the knee may allow the development of more anatomical procedures. Improved diagnostic techniques should help to identify patients most likely to benefit. Further research is needed to clarify the indications for this procedure in high-risk and revision cases.

1. Lateral extra-articular reinforcement in conjunction with intra-articular reconstruction may be an important option in the control of rotational laxity of the knee.
2. Advances in understanding the complex lateral anatomy and biomechanics of the knee is crucial for the development of more anatomical procedures.
3. We describe a personal technique combining BTB ACL reconstruction with extra-articular reinforcement using iliotibial band graft.
4. Improved diagnostic techniques should help to identify patients most likely to benefit.

References

1. Campos J, Chung C, Lektrakul N, Pedowitz R, Trudell D, Yu J et al (2001) Pathogenesis of the segond fracture: anatomic and MR imaging evidence of an iliotibial tract or anterior oblique band avulsion1. Radiology 219:381–386
2. Claes S, Vereecke E, Maes M, Victor J, Verdonk P, Bellemans J (2013) Anatomy of the anterolateral ligament of the knee. J Anat 223:321–328
3. Dejour H, Walch G, Neyret P, Adeleine P (1988) Results of surgically treated chronic anterior laxities: apropos of 251 cases reviewed with a minimum follow-up of 3 years. Rev Chir Orthop Reparatrice Appar Mot 74:622–636. (In French)
4. Draganich L, Reider B, Ling M, Samuelson M (1990) An in vitro study of an intraarticular and extraarticular reconstruction in the anterior cruciate ligament deficient knee. Am J Sports Med 18:262–266
5. Ellison A (1978) Anterolateral rotatory instability. In: Funk FJ Jr (ed) Symposium on the athlete's knee, surgical repair and reconstruction, American Academy of Orthopaedic Surgeons. Mosby, St. Louis, pp 178–193
6. Engebretsen L, Lew W, Lewis J, Hunter R (1990) The effect of an iliotibial tenodesis on intraarticular graft forces and knee joint motion. Am J Sports Med 18:169–176
7. Marcacci M, Zaffagnini S, Iacono F, Neri M, Loreti I, Petitto A (1998) Arthroscopic intra- and extra-articular anterior cruciate ligament reconstruction with gracilis and semitendinosus tendons. Knee Surg Sports Traumatol Arthrosc 6:68–75
8. Marcacci M, Zaffagnini S, Giordano G, Iacono F, Presti M (2009) Anterior cruciate ligament reconstruction associated with extra-articular tenodesis: a prospective clinical and radiographic evaluation with 10- to 13-year follow-up. Am J Sports Med 37:707–714
9. Monaco E, Labianca L, Conteduca F, De Carli A, Ferretti A (2007) Double bundle or single bundle plus extraarticular tenodesis in ACL reconstruction? Knee Surg Sports Traumatol Arthrosc 15:1168–1174
10. Neyret P, Demey G, Servien E, Lustig S (2012) Traité de chirurgie de genou. Elsevier Masson, Issy-les-Moulineaux. (In French)
11. Norwood L, Andrews J, Meisterling R, Glancy G (1979) Acute anterolateral rotatory instability of the knee. J Bone Joint Surg Am 61:704–709
12. Noyes F, Butler D, Grood E, Zernicke R, Hefzy M (1984) Biomechanical analysis of human ligament grafts used in knee-ligament repairs and reconstructions. J Bone Joint Surg Am 66:344–352
13. Pearl A, Bergfeld J, American Orthopaedic Society for Sports Medicine (1992) Extraarticular reconstruction in the anterior cruciate ligament deficient knee. Human Kinetics Publishers, Champaign
14. Schindler O (2011) Surgery for anterior cruciate ligament deficiency: a historical perspective. Knee Surg Sports Traumatol Arthrosc 20:5–47
15. Ségond P (1879) Recherches cliniques et expérimentales sur les épanchements sanguins du genou par entorse. Progès Médicale, Paris. (In French)
16. Slocum D, Larson R (1968) Rotatory instability of the knee. Its pathogenesis and a clinical test to demonstrate its presence. J Bone Joint Surg Am 50:211–225
17. Slocum D, Larson R (1968) Pes anserinus transplantation. A surgical procedure for control of rotatory instability of the knee. J Bone Joint Surg Am 50:226–242
18. Terry G, Hughston J, Norwood L (1986) The anatomy of the iliopatellar band and iliotibial tract. Am J Sports Med 14:39–45
19. Terry G, Norwood L, Hughston J, Caldwell K (1993) How iliotibial tract injuries of the knee combine with acute anterior cruciate ligament tears to influence abnormal anterior tibial displacement. Am J Sports Med 21:55–60
20. Vieira E, Teixeira da Silva R, dos Santos Berlfein P, Abdalla R, Cohen M (2007) An anatomic study of the iliotibial tract. Arthroscopy 23:269–274
21. Vincent JP, Magnussen RA, Gezmez F, Uguen A, Jacobi M, Weppe F et al (2011) The anterolateral ligament of the human knee: an anatomic and histologic study. Knee Surg Sports Traumatol Arthrosc 20:147–152
22. Wright R, Huston L, Spindler K, Dunn W, Haas A et al., The MARS Group (2010) Descriptive epidemiology of the Multicenter ACL Revision Study (MARS) cohort. Am J Sports Med 38:1979–1986

Knee Rotation: The Torg School

9

Eric J. Kropf, Jared W. Colón, and Joseph S. Torg

Contents

E.J. Kropf (✉) • J.W. Colón • J.S. Torg
Department of Orthopaedic Surgery and Sports Medicine, Lewis Katz School of Medicine at Temple University, Philadelphia, PA, USA
e-mail: Eric.Kropf@tuhs.temple.edu; jared.colon@temple.edu; joseph.torg@temple.edu

9.1 Historical Perspective

The 1970s brought about a drastic shift in the clinical treatment of anterior cruciate ligament (ACL) injuries. Previously, the diagnosis of ACL insufficiency was difficult and not obvious or reproducible during conventional physical examination. During this period, the main technique used to make the clinical diagnosis of an ACL tear was the anterior drawer sign. The anterior drawer test was performed by applying an anterior stress to the tibia with the knee flexed to 90° and the foot placed in internal, external, and neutral rotation. However, this test was often insufficient with a high false-negative rate for isolated ACL injury. The anterior drawer test was often only "positive" when associated with significant meniscal or capsular injury [2].

When a positive anterior drawer sign was demonstrated, conventional treatment of this era was to reduce the drawer at 90° of flexion and attempt to restore tension in the joint capsule [6, 11, 12]. This required a long phase of immobilization and rigorous rehabilitation. At the time, the ACL itself was rarely repaired or reconstructed. Instead, the procedure would render the joint stable through capsular contracture or fibrosis, while the ACL itself remained nonfunctional or absent. As a result, patient function did not typically return to the level of the uninjured knee with an intact ACL [2].

In 1976, Joseph Torg authored "Clinical diagnosis of anterior cruciate instability in the ath-

V. Musahl et al. (eds.), *Rotatory Knee Instability*, DOI 10.1007/978-3-319-32070-0_9

lete," which was published in the American Journal of Sports Medicine. This landmark paper provided the first clearly defined description of the Lachman test, a knee examination technique used to determine the status of the ACL in an attempt to improve clinical diagnosis and understanding of ACL instability. In many ways, the theories and perspectives outlined here drove the early phases of developing our current understanding of knee laxity and instability [14].

It is important to put Torg's work into historical perspective, realizing that his purported view on the importance of proper diagnosis of ACL insufficiency went against mainstream thought at the time. However, it was also clearly acknowledged the "enigma" presented by the ACL. Great diversity of opinion surrounded ACL injury, such as injury mechanisms, efficacy of diagnostic techniques, and treatment and management protocols. This is evident in observations published by Helfet [5] who stated that "occasionally, when operating for a torn medial cartilage, one finds that the anterior cruciate ligament has been torn from its insertions in the tibia... but this knee does not demonstrate anterior-posterior instability preoperatively or postoperatively, and removal of the cartilage cures all symptoms. It is not possible to diagnose the coincidental rupture of the cruciate ligament before operations." Elsewhere in the publication, Helfet stated that "isolated ruptures of the cruciate ligament are rare and of little clinical significance."

Furthermore, in 1970, Smillie [13] published on various issues surrounding the use of the drawer sign in clinical examination. He stated, "the drawer sign is 'minimal' in isolated ruptures of the anterior cruciate ligament," and went on to say that "if the sign is 'maximal,'" it is likely that "the medial ligament has been involved," therefore defining limitation at the time in diagnosing isolated ACL ruptures on clinical examination. Smillie also recognized that it is difficult to perform the drawer sign following acute injury because of factors such as pain, hemarthrosis, and muscle spasms. Finally, he stated that when an isolated rupture of the ACL occurred, "the anterior cruciate ligament alone is not the factor controlling instability, and a repair does not necessarily improve function. When rupture is associated with a tear of the medial meniscus, treatment is meniscectomy, the ruptured ligament being ignored."

Helfet and Smillie summarized the thought process at the time, which was a lack of understanding of isolated ruptures of the ACL and their clinical significance due to limitations in diagnosing an isolated ACL tear with intact menisci, capsule, and collateral ligaments. On the other hand, supporters of the Lachman test and its theories challenged this concept and looked further. They believed that the ultimate key to advancing the understanding of ACL injury and subsequent treatment was to improve clinical diagnostic techniques.

Supporters of the Lachman test also rejected the thought process of the previously mentioned authors, believing that the authors' statements regarding the ACL were a gross oversimplification of the problem. The supporters believed that ACL deficiency posed a greater long-term problem than was understood at the time and pointed to several publications in support of their ideas.

In 1955, O'Donoghue reported on the end results of patients with major ligamentous knee injuries and their progression to medial compartment disease [12]. The study found that 50 out of 69 patients (72 %) had tears of the ACL and based on the analysis of these cases, O'Donoghue concluded that ACL instability ultimately caused significant disability. Surgical repair of the ligament was therefore warranted and recommended.

In addition to O'Donoghue's study, supporting evidence was found in a study by Kennedy et al. [9] around the same time. Kennedy had recently studied 50 patients with ACL tears and concluded that isolated tears of the ligament do occur. He found that there is a high incidence of associated medial meniscal damage in knees with ACL tears (40 % of patients in his study). However, he still concluded that an acceptable result could be seen in a high percentage of patients with or without ACL repair.

Thirdly, Allman in 1971 [3] was quoted as saying that, in some individuals with ACL tears that are not surgically repaired, the injury begins a cascade of events that causes progressive disability and disruption of integral structures within the knee, leading to "the beginning of the end." The author goes on to describe the deficit in indications for surgical versus nonsurgical cases that was characteristic of the time, but most importantly the author stressed the functional importance of the ACL.

In turn, Torg clearly believed that a deeper understanding of the ACL was required and would undoubtedly lead to improved management of athletes with traumatic knee injuries. In his paper, he begins with a description of the anterior drawer test, which at that time was the classic clinical examination used to diagnose ACL ruptures. He then describes the Lachman test, the focus of his paper, and the paradigm-shifting clinical test for orthopedic surgeons everywhere.

At the time of Torg's publication, it differed from other reports in two ways. First, it was understood that the ACL was of great clinical significance, and, second, the necessity of improving clinical diagnostic methods to more accurately and fully understand the entire spectrum of the injury was advocated. In pushing the understanding of the day, Torg was able to emphasize that a better diagnosis and treatment plan was possible by improving one of the most important tools available to physicians everywhere: the clinical examination.

9.2 The Anterior Drawer Test

In 1976, classic orthopedic teaching relied on the anterior drawer test to make a clinical diagnosis of ACL deficiency. The test was performed with that patient supine and the affected knee at 90° of flexion. The examiner would then attempt to translate the tibia anteriorly with respect to the femur by pulling on the posterior surface of the proximal end of the tibia (Fig. 9.1). A positive anterior drawer sign resulted when anterior translation of the tibia with respect to the femur was observed. This test was unquestionably relied upon, despite the fact that its origins were "obscure." In "Clinical diagnosis of anterior cruciate instability in the athlete," clinical experience with 172 ACL ruptures was described. Through that experience, it is concluded that the anterior drawer test was unreliable [14].

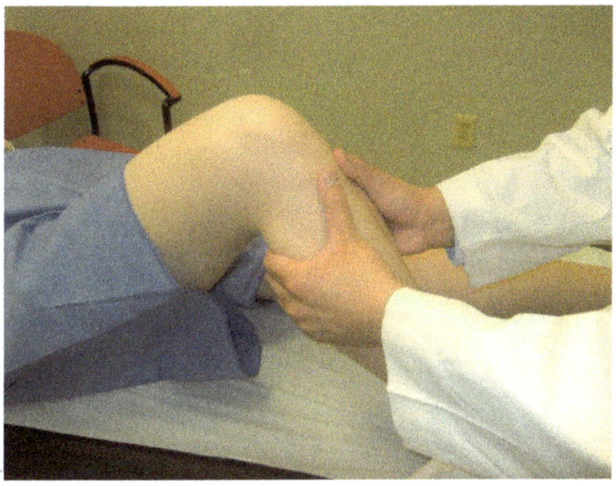

Fig. 9.1 The Anterior Drawer Test

Torg believed there to be three main causes for false-negative anterior drawer tests or scenarios where ACL injury was either unrecognized or underappreciated (Fact Box 1). First, in the setting of acute ACL injury, there are typically an accompanying tense hemarthrosis and reactive synovitis in the joint space. These conditions preclude knee flexion to 90°, thus making it difficult to perform the drawer test with accuracy. Second, acutely following injury, the body experiences protective muscle spasms, such that in "the well-muscled, well-conditioned athlete" this would "generate considerable force" [14]. The resultant problem would be extreme difficulty in attempt to anteriorly translate the tibia against the opposed hamstring spasm. The vector analysis clearly demonstrates this issue. Third, the anatomy of the medial compartment of the knee when flexed to 90° versus relatively extended presents the main barrier to effective anterior translation of the tibia when performing the drawer test. The convex posterior surface of the medial femoral condyle is more congruent with the more concave medial tibial plateau in flexion. In addition, the presence of the posterior horn of the medial meniscus further prevents anterior translation of the tibia due to the supporting effect it produces against the posterior aspect of the medial femoral condyle (Fig. 9.2).

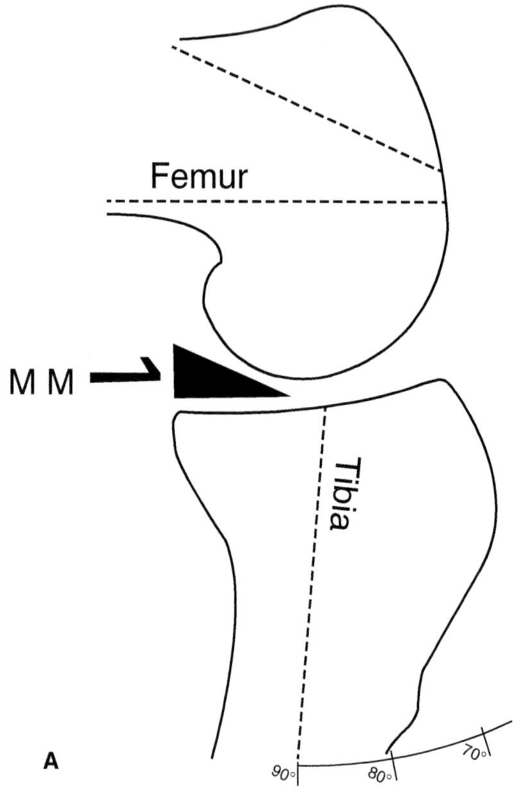

Fig. 9.2 Diagram displaying the relationship between the medial femoral condyle, medial meniscus, and the tibia with the knee in 90° of flexion and viewed in a sagittal plane. Medial meniscus causes a "door stopper" effect preventing efficient anterior translation of the tibia during the anterior drawer test. *MM* medial meniscus (Reproduced with permission from Torg et al. [14])

Fact Box 1: Causes of False-Negative Anterior Drawer Tests [14]

1. Acute hemarthrosis precluding knee flexion to 90°
2. Protective muscle spasms preventing anterior tibial translation
3. Anatomical configuration of knee in flexion preventing effective anterior tibial translation

Based on these observations, the study by Torg concluded that "significant 'anterior drawering' occurred only after peripheral separation of the posterior horn of the medial meniscus or disruption of the medial capsular and/or posterior oblique ligaments" [14]. This observation that combined injury to the ACL and medial meniscus resulted in greater joint instability was novel and began to advance our understanding of the effects produced by combined knee ligament injuries.

9.3 The Lachman Test

In response to the problems with the anterior drawer test presented above, "Clinical diagnosis of anterior cruciate instability in the athlete" proposed a new method for diagnosing ACL ruptures known as the Lachman test. The test received its name from John W. Lachman, MD, who was chairman and professor of Orthopaedic Surgery at Temple University at the time of the publication. For several years prior to the publication of "Clinical diagnosis of anterior cruciate instability in the athlete," Lachman had been teaching this "simple, reliable, and reproducible clinical test to demonstrate anterior cruciate ligament instability" [14].

The Lachman test is performed with the patient supine and "the knee held between full extension and 15° of flexion." The examiner would stabilize the femur with one hand and with the other hand apply firm pressure to the posterior aspect of the proximal tibia, attempting to translate it anteriorly relative to the femur

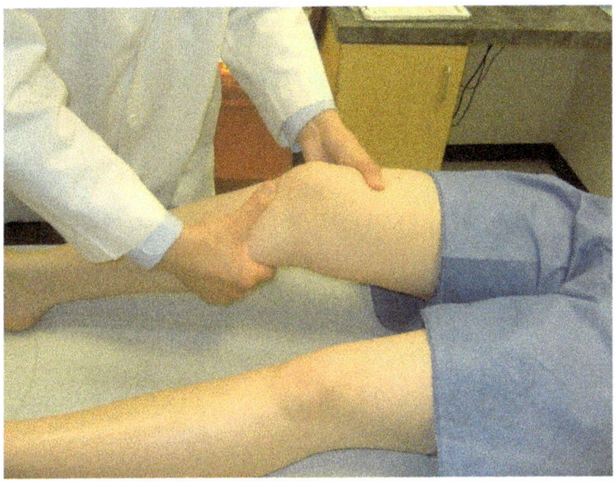

Fig. 9.3 The Lachman test

(Fig. 9.3). A positive test, correlating with an anterior cruciate ligament tear, was described as the feeling of a "proprioceptive and/or visual anterior translation of the tibia in relation to the femur with a characteristic "mushy" or "soft" end point." This is in stark contrast to the "hard" end point characteristic of a negative Lachman test, indicating that the ACL is intact [14].

Furthermore, visual assessment is a valuable diagnostic indicator of ACL insufficiency. When viewed from the lateral aspect of the knee, anterior translation occurring in the presence of a positive test would eliminate the normal slope of the infrapatellar tendon between the patella and its insertion on the anterior aspect of the proximal tibia [14].

The Lachman test was developed to avert the previously mentioned issues that were associated with anterior drawer test (Fact Box 2). First, the reduced degree of flexion allowed the knee to assume a comfortable position even in the presence of hemarthrosis or reactive synovitis and decreased the likelihood of guarding, which precludes the execution of a proper test. Second, the effect of hamstring spasm is virtually negated as the force required to translate the tibia anteriorly is applied in a vector perpendicular to the pull of the hamstring muscle complex. Third, with the knee in relative extension, the contact area is between the tibial plateau, the medial meniscus, and the distal weight-bearing surface of the femur. Because this surface is relatively flat compared to the posterior femoral condyle, obstruction of anterior tibial translation is greatly reduced (Fig. 9.4). The Lachman test is able to overcome the difficulties associated with performing the anterior drawer test, giving the clinician greater acuity for diagnosing isolated ACL injury [14].

Fact Box 2: Benefits of Lachman Test [14]

1. Eliminates effect of acute hemarthrosis on successfully performing exam
2. Negates force generated by hamstring spasms
3. Produces optimal anatomical configuration for anterior tibial translation

9.3.1 The Grading System

Nearly a decade after initial publication detailing the Lachman exam, Torg and colleagues established a grading system to assess the degree of joint instability for ACL disruption based on the extent of anterior tibial translation. The grading system ranges from I (least severe) to grade IV (most extensive injury and instability). The degree of anterior translation corresponding to each level was quantified using a knee arthrometer [4].

A grade I tear is defined as a positive Lachman test with the proprioceptive detection of a "soft" or "mushy" end point upon anterior tibial translation. Further appreciation of the positive test could be seen when placing the thumb on the joint line during the examination and comparing the difference between the injured leg and the contralateral side. In Torg's study, grade I tears were associated with an anterior displacement of between 1 and 6 mm. A grade II tear was determined based on detection of the soft end point described above as well as visible anterior tibial translation. A distinguishing characteristic of a grade II tear was the disappearance of the normal slope of the infrapatellar tendon between the patella and its insertion on the anterior aspect of the proximal

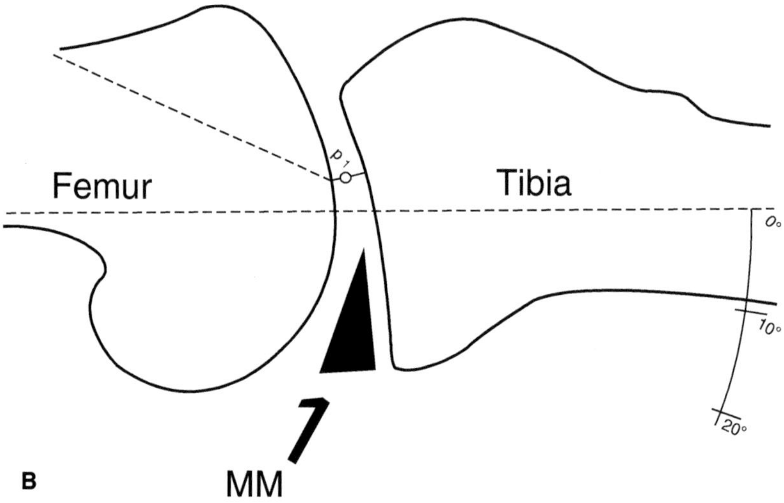

Fig. 9.4 When the knee is in extension, the configuration of the joint components are changed such that the "door stopper" effect caused by the medial meniscus is relieved, allowing anterior tibial translation to occur unobstructed. *MM* medial meniscus (Reproduced with permission from Torg et al. [14]) (Figures reproduced with permission from: Torg JS, Conrad W, Kalen V. *Am J Sports Med* Volume 4, Issue 2. Pp. 84–93, ©1976 by SAGE Publications. Reprinted by Permission of SAGE Publications)

tibia. Grade II tears involved a displacement between 3 and 9 mm. A grade III tear was seen when the tibia displays passive anterior subluxation without a need for the examiner to provide a force. Placing a 4×4×6 in. block underneath the tibia just distal to the joint reproduces the same degree of subluxation. Similar to a grade II tear, the slope of the infrapatellar tendon will disappear as well. Grade III tears were associated with tibial translation ranging from 6 to 16 mm. A grade IV injury is defined in patients who were able to actively displace the tibia anteriorly by contracting the quadriceps muscle while either sitting or standing with the knee in flexion. The force produced through the muscle contraction alone is sufficient to translate the tibia anteriorly. Grade IV tears demonstrate anterior displacement ranging from 10 to 20 mm [4].

This grading system was to serve as a basis to guide treatment and management of patients with varying degrees of knee instability. In a proposed algorithm, grade I tears could be treated with a conservative course of bracing and rehabilitation. Grade II tests were generally indicative of injury to a combination of structures, usually one or both menisci in addition to the ACL. In such cases, arthroscopy was suggested as the proper course of treatment, along with bracing and subsequent rehabilitation. In some cases, an extra-articular cruciate substitution procedure was performed. Grade III tears required ACL repair or reconstruction as well as meniscal repair in the young active patient. Finally, a grade IV tear necessitated ACL repair or reconstruction and possibly medial capsular repair or reefing due to the extreme degree of instability [4].

9.3.2 External Verification

Following the publication of "Clinical diagnosis of anterior cruciate instability in the athlete" in 1976, multiple other authors have validated the Lachman test in clinical application. In 1983, DeHaven [3] found that the Lachman test is "much more reliable" than the anterior drawer test in diagnosing isolated anterior cruciate tears, being positive in 85 % of patients without anesthesia and nearly 100 % in patients with anesthesia. In the same year, Larson [10] also noted that the Lachman test is "one of the most accurate and sensitive tests" used to diagnose ACL injury. Johnson [7] notes that the Lachman test can "greatly increase the accuracy of the clinical examination."

In 1982 Jonsson et al. [8] reported findings comparing the accuracy of the anterior drawer and Lachman tests performed on unanesthetized patients following acute ACL rupture. Their results showed that the Lachman test had a much higher diagnostic accuracy, with 39 out of 45 patients having a positive Lachman test whereas only 15 out of 45 had a positive anterior drawer test. Jonsson et al. concluded that the Lachman test is a "valuable diagnostic tool" and should be regularly utilized to evaluate the status of the ACL.

More recently, Benjaminse et al. [1] in 2006 concluded that the Lachman test has a high diagnostic accuracy from a meta-analysis of over 2,000 patients. This study pooled results from varied publications between 1980 and 1995. The Lachman test has had great longevity in the accurate clinical diagnosis of ACL injuries worldwide.

Conclusions

Four decades ago, "Clinical diagnosis of anterior cruciate instability in the athlete" emphasized the importance of complete and accurate clinical diagnosis, sought to improve exam skills, and opened the door to a greater understanding of combined knee injury patterns. This publication clearly noted differences in knee laxity patterns with various combined knee ligament injuries. The Lachman test has become a key component of the physical examination to effectively and efficiently diagnose varied degrees of knee instability. Treatment algorithms have been developed and advanced throughout the subsequent decades based on the clinical information afforded by the Lachman test.

The "Torg School of Thought" was integral to the advancement of the field of ACL management and surgery. The limitations of conventional wisdom and physical exam testing were challenged. This drove forward our understanding of knee instability, clinical diagnostic testing, and the appreciation for combined knee ligament injuries. Torg's contributions serve as a strong foundation to our current day understanding of knee laxity and instability.

The Lachman test, originally described in 1976 by Dr. Joseph Torg, has become a key method to diagnose ACL insufficiency. The Lachman test still drives treatment algorithms today. The widespread clinical application of this simple and reproducible test has improved our ability to diagnose and quantify ACL injury. These works represent key advances in the early understanding of knee laxity and rotational instability.

References

1. Benjaminse A, Gokeler A, van der Schans CP (2006) Clinical diagnosis of an anterior cruciate ligament rupture: a meta-analysis. J Orthop Sports Phys Ther 36(5):267–288
2. Chambat P, Guier C, Sonnery-Cottet B et al (2013) The evolution of ACL reconstruction over the last fifty years. Int Orthop 37(2):181–186
3. DeHaven KE (1983) Arthroscopy in the diagnosis and management of the anterior cruciate ligament deficient knee. Clin Orthop Relat Res 172:52–56
4. Gurtler RA, Stine R, Torg JS (1987) Lachman test evaluated. quantification of a clinical observation. Clin Orthop Relat Res 216:141–150
5. Helfet A (1974) Disorders of the knee. Lippincott Co, Philadelphia, pp 92–93
6. Hughston JC, Eilers AF (1973) The role of the posterior oblique ligament in repairs of acute medial (collateral) ligament tears of the knee. J Bone Joint Surg Am 55(5):923–940
7. Johnson RJ (1983) The anterior cruciate ligament problem. Clin Orthop Relat Res 172:14–18
8. Jonsson T, Althoff B, Peterson L et al (1982) Clinical diagnosis of ruptures of the anterior cruciate ligament: a comparative study of the lachman test and the anterior drawer sign. Am J Sports Med 10(2):100–102
9. Kennedy JC, Weinberg HW, Wilson AS (1974) The anatomy and function of the anterior cruciate ligament. As determined by clinical and morphological studies. J Bone Joint Surg Am 56(2):223–235

10. Larson RL (1983) Physical examination in the diagnosis of rotatory instability. Clin Orthop Relat Res 172:38–44
11. Nicholas JA (1973) The five-one reconstruction for anteromedial instability of the knee. indications, technique, and the results in fifty-two patients. J Bone Joint Surg Am 55(5): 899–922
12. O'Donoghue DH (1955) An analysis of end results of surgical treatment of major injuries to the ligaments of the knee. J Bone Joint Surg Am 37-A(1):1–13
13. Smillie I (1970) Injuries of the knee joint. The Williams and Wilkins Co, Baltimore, p 152
14. Torg JS, Conrad W, Kalen V (1976) Clinical diagnosis of anterior cruciate ligament instability in the athlete. Am J Sports Med 4(2):84–93

Knee Rotation: The HSS School

10

Ryan M. Degen, Thomas L. Wickiewicz, Russell F. Warren, Andrew D. Pearle, and Anil S. Ranawat

Contents

R.M. Degen (✉) • T.L. Wickiewicz • R.F. Warren
A.D. Pearle • A.S. Ranawat
Sports Medicine and Shoulder Service,
Hospital for Special Surgery, 535 East 70th Street,
New York, NY 10021, USA
e-mail: degenr@hss.edu; ranawatanil@hss.edu

10.1 Introduction

While anterior cruciate ligament (ACL) reconstruction is one of the most commonly performed procedures in sports medicine, it has taken centuries to achieve the level of understanding required to perform these procedures in their current fashion [16, 38, 48]. In fact, the ACL has garnered significant interest from scientists and clinicians since the early 1800s. Early descriptions of its function and subsequent case reports of injury began to appear in the literature in the late 1830s [48]. However, it was not until the early 1900s that the first ACL repair was performed. At the time, concerns existed about the ability to perform a suture repair of remnant ACL fibers, and various reconstruction techniques were proposed by Hey Groves and O'Donoghue in subsequent years [24, 38, 45]. However, these early surgical descriptions received little attention as they were followed by a controversial debate over the role of operative versus nonoperative treatment of ACL injuries, with many surgeons concluding that operative intervention was unwarranted. It was not until the late 1960s that a renewed interest for ACL repair was seen after poor outcomes were noted following nonoperative treatment.

V. Musahl et al. (eds.), *Rotatory Knee Instability*, DOI 10.1007/978-3-319-32070-0_10

10.2 ACL Repair

In the early 1970s, John Marshall (Fig. 10.1) began his surgical career at Hospital for Special Surgery (HSS) as chief of the sports medicine service. Based on prior interests stemming from his time as a veterinarian studying the ACL in dogs, he began similar research, closely studying the functional role and significance of the ACL in humans. Through this early research, Marshall taught us much of what is known about the ACL today. His early cadaveric studies contributed to the identification of two distinct bundles of the ligament, while subsequent sectioning studies helped determine its role in resisting anterior tibial translation and tibial rotation [19, 21].

Dr. Marshall was also intrigued by the work of his colleagues, including John Feagin, who published some of the earliest results following ACL repair, and Anders Alm, who investigated the use of the medial third of the patellar tendon for ACL reconstruction [1, 17]. In combination with their early treatment successes, Dr. Marshall also noted associations with further intra-articular injuries in patients treated conservatively, with poor functional outcomes, and began attempting primary surgical repair of these injuries [54]. This was a technically challenging procedure that involved passing multiple sutures through the remnant fibers of the ACL, with the sutures then passed through bone tunnels in the femur and tibia and tied to tension the repair and approximate the torn ends (Fig. 10.2) [37]. The authors noted that this was much simpler for femoral peel-off injuries rather than mid-substance tears. Although early results reported by Marshall et al. identified good outcomes in a series of 70 primary repairs, with high rates of return to sport (93 %), residual laxity was identified on anterior drawer testing in all patients [36]. Around the same time, MacIntosh also described good success with suture repair of the femoral origin behind the lateral condyle, the so-called over-the-top repair [35]. Unfortunately, further follow-up studies of both Marshall and MacIntosh's series of patients revealed relatively poor and unpredictable outcomes following primary suture repair in isolation, with high rates of residual laxity and reinjury [28]. Consequently, it was felt that repair alone was insufficient and further research into alternative reconstruction strategies began.

Marshall went on to describe a modification of the "over-the-top" procedure, whereby a central strip of the iliotibial band was harvested and left attached to Gerdy's tubercle distally, with the proximal end of the IT band passed

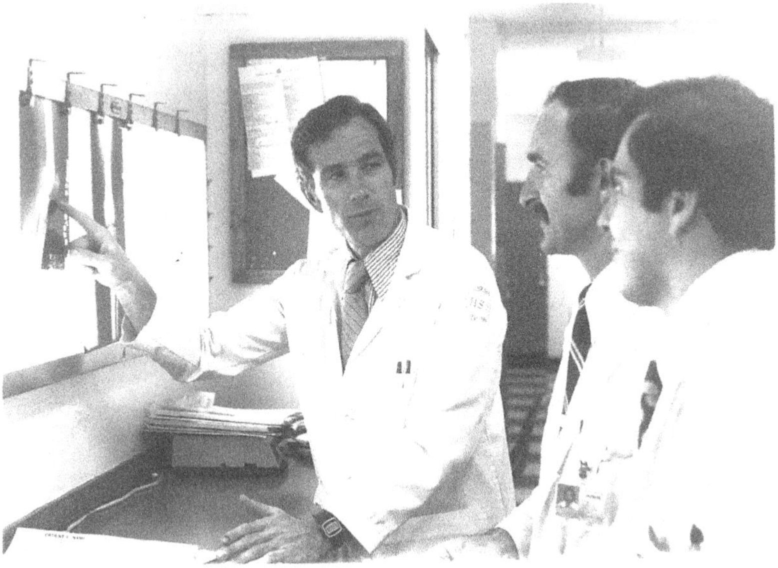

Fig. 10.1 Dr. John Marshall (*left*) and Dr. Russell Warren (*right*)

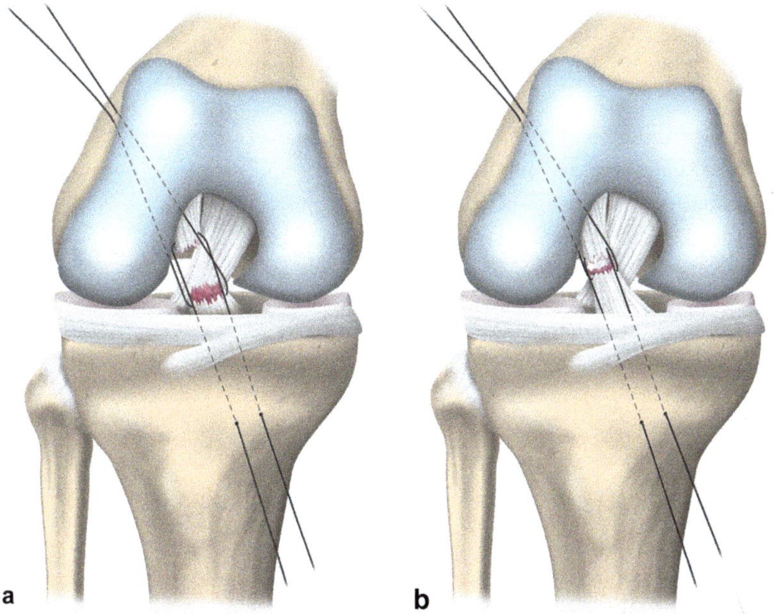

Fig. 10.2 ACL suture repair with sutures passed through remnant fibers (**a**) and subsequently passed through bone tunnels and tied to re-approximate the torn ends (**b**) (Reprinted with permission from Kaplan et al. [28])

behind the lateral femoral condyle through the joint, exiting anteriorly through a drill hole in the tibia [37]. This resulted in an extra-articular-based augmentation of their repair, which quickly became common practice at the time. While this augmentation was initially performed in the minority of patients undergoing primary repair in the initial surgical series (<10 %), high rates of recurrent instability or failure lead to increased use of augmentation as isolated repair was felt to be insufficient [18]. Similarly encouraged by the potential for achieving some degree of healing of the native ACL, Warren and Wickiewicz continued a series of primary suture repair cases that were augmented with a semitendinosus tendon reconstruction, much like the IT band augmentation, fixed in the over-the-top position [49]. This also involved a period of 6 weeks postoperative cast immobilization. Both of these augmented repairs produced improved results compared with repair in isolation. Additionally, the added benefit of the actual repair of the native ACL remnant was felt to add little compared to the IT band or semitendinosus augmentation. Consequently, primary repair was largely abandoned in favor of reconstructive techniques.

10.3 Extra-articular Procedures

Around the same time as the transition to augmented repair, concern existed that perhaps rotatory instability, attributable to capsular injury, may be a more significant contributing factor to residual knee instability. Helfet remarked that, while the cruciate ligaments may act as checkreins to anterior-posterior translation, it is possible that they may simply act as “guide ropes” that ultimately rely on capsular structures to limit translation [23]. If true, this would allow restoration of stability with extra-articular reconstruction or tenodesis alone. As such, several other extra-articular procedures were described around that time to restrict rotation and restore knee laxity. Nicholas described the “Five-One” procedure in 1972, which involved a pes anserinus transfer, medial meniscectomy, posteromedial capsular reefing, posterior MCL advancement, and vastus medialis advancement [41]. In addition, this procedure was followed by a period of casting for 6 weeks. While certainly limiting rotation, this procedure failed to address the increased anterior tibial translation and also resulted in significant motion loss and was eventually abandoned. Similarly, both Lemaire and MacIntosh described lateral extra-articular tenodeses, using a strip of fascia lata laterally to limit tibial translation or subluxation attributed to anterolateral rotation [8, 27, 31]. While these extra-articular tenodeses were successful in the describing surgeons' hands, both Kennedy and subsequently Warren and Marshall reported inferior results when relying solely on these procedures, recommending reconstruction of the ACL itself [29, 55]. Moving forward, these extra-articular procedures were instead recommended as augments to intra-articular reconstruction in patients where instability could be attributed to more complex rotatory instability [48].

Thereafter, MacIntosh described an extra-articular-based reconstruction using a continuous strip of the extensor mechanism, including quadriceps tendon, prepatellar fascia, and patellar tendon [38]. Similar to the modified "over-the-top" procedure, the tibial insertion of the patellar tendon was left intact and the graft passed retrograde through the joint, exiting posterior to the lateral femoral condyle where it was sutured to a periosteal window or stapled to the distal femur for fixation. Marshall suggested a modification for this quadriceps tendon substitution (QTS) graft, as the region or prepatellar fascia was frequently quite thin [37]. They suggested incorporating a folded-down strip of quadriceps tendon or synthetic material to augment this region, with the resultant procedure commonly referred to as the "Marshall MacIntosh" procedure, popularized in the late 1970s [14, 38, 48].

Kornblatt et al. reviewed the experience following the "Marshall MacIntosh" procedure, or quadriceps tendon substitution procedure, at HSS [30]. They noted that 20 % of patients were classified as failures at an average of 4 years of follow-up, with 40 % of patients demonstrating some form of a residual positive pivot shift test. In a similar study, the authors investigated the addition of a lateral sling procedure in conjunction with reconstruction using this quadriceps tendon substitution graft. They reported that clinical failure rates dropped to 4 %, with a residual pivot shift detectable in only 11.5 % of patients, leading them to recommend the routine use of a lateral sling procedure when this type of ACL reconstruction was performed [30]. However, the results of this first study led to a change in clinical practice, with adoption of intra-articular reconstructions in subsequent years.

Fact Box 1: ACL repair

(a) Primary ACL repair using primitive suturing techniques resulted in high failure rates with residual laxity.
(b) Augmentation with IT band tenodesis did improve clinical success rates.
(c) The role of ACL repair with all-arthroscopic, modern-day repair techniques remains to be determined.

10.4 Intra-articular Reconstruction

While first described in Germany [1], and subsequently in North America [15], the central third bone-patellar tendon-bone autograft was adopted as the primary graft choice at HSS after review of the Marshall MacIntosh outcomes. This decision was based on previous literature that had demonstrated excellent tensile stress of this graft [13, 42] and positive early clinical results [15]. Following adoption of this graft for primary ACL reconstruction, an ensuing review of clinical outcomes demonstrated improved failure rates of only 5 %, with residual pivot shift tests noted in 16 % of patients, both of which were significant improvements when compared with the outcomes following the Marshall MacIntosh procedure [43]. An additional follow-up study reviewed the role of the lateral sling procedure in patients who had undergone ACL reconstruction with bone-patellar tendon-bone autograft. They found that there was no conferred benefit by adding this procedure, with the added risk of approximately 40 % of patients experiencing lateral-sided knee pain postoperatively [44]. Consequently, the authors recommended reconstruction with autogenous patellar tendon-bone autograft without a lateral sling tenodesis unless clinically indicated. These clinical results lead to the popularization and widespread use of this graft as a primary choice for many surgeons across the United States.

10.5 Arthroscopic or Arthroscopically Assisted Reconstruction

Technologic advances allowed for the development of arthroscopic equipment in the early 1980s. This was roughly around the time that intra-articular reconstructions were accepted as the primary method of treatment for ACL ruptures. As arthroscopic equipment became readily available and surgeon's experience with this technology improved, efforts were made to incorporate this technology to improve surgical accuracy of tunnel placement during ACL reconstruction while also reducing the degree of invasiveness of the procedure. The arthroscope was first used as part of a two-incision technique to reconstruct the ACL in 1985. It was used to visualize the tibial tunnel as it was being drilled, while the femoral tunnel was created in an outside-in fashion with a rear-entry guide ensuring a high, posterior femoral tunnel [14].

Results of the first cases of arthroscopically assisted reconstructions combined with early range of motion performed at HSS revealed excellent outcomes with 93 % of knees having less than 4 mm of translation and 84 % having less than 3 mm of translation on arthrometric measurements using the KT-1000 [12]. Good to excellent outcome scores were achieved in 87 % of patients utilizing the HSS rating system. More importantly, the rates of postoperative patellofemoral pain and the need for manipulation for postoperative stiffness were reduced by 42 % and 33 %, respectively, when compared with open reconstructions with postoperative immobilization performed at the same hospital. The researchers concluded that arthroscopically assisted reconstructions were beneficial as they conferred a similar stabilizing effect to open reconstruction, with a reduction in postoperative stiffness with the morbidity of the arthrotomy obviated, as well as improved visualization of the anatomic placement of the bone tunnels.

With time, all-arthroscopic reconstructions became the standard of care in subsequent years as training improved and technologic advances made it feasible. This was first made feasible by rear-entry femoral drill guides that allowed outside-in drilling of the femoral tunnel under arthroscopic visualization in the mid- to late 1980s. In the early 1990s, the transition was made to a single-incision transtibial reconstruction [25]. By the mid- to late 1990s, a single-incision, arthroscopic ACL reconstruction was considered the standard of care. This was subsequently improved with the invention of arthroscopic drills and offset guides allowing for inside-out drilling in a more anatomic position [14].

10.6 Hamstring Reconstruction

While excellent results have been demonstrated following arthroscopic ACL reconstruction with patellar tendon autograft, the procedure is not without risks. Patellofemoral pain, patellar fractures, and patella baja are all potential complications that have resulted in ongoing study into alternative graft sources to reduce associated complications. Lipscomb is credited with the first report of using both the semitendinosus and gracilis hamstring tendons for reconstruction of the ACL [34]. While cyclic loading studies demonstrated equivalent mechanical properties to patellar tendon autograft, limited clinical data was available when this graft was first adopted. At HSS, Williams et al. reported on the 2-year outcomes of patients who underwent ACL reconstruction using quadrupled hamstring autograft [56]. They identified a reduction in tibial translation on the Lachman and pivot shift tests in 89 % of patients, with a 7 % re-rupture rate. Factoring in clinical outcome scores, a total of 11 % of patients were considered failures. Objective arthrometric data revealed higher rates of increased translation compared with patients reconstructed with patellar tendon autograft; however, these measures did not correlate with subjective outcome scores. While successful outcomes were achieved using hamstring autograft, they were slightly inferior to those with patellar tendon autograft with minimally higher rates of re-rupture. This may relate to poor fixation devices for hamstring autografts at the time, nonspecific rehabilitation protocols extrapolated to hamstring reconstruction, or may relate to the nonanatomic positioning of reconstruction grafts. A retrospective analysis of the effect of graft choice on postoperative infection rates was also performed at our institution. Interestingly, hamstring autografts were associated with higher rates of postoperative infection (1.4 %) compared with patellar tendon autograft (0.49 %) and allograft reconstructions (0.44 %), although the exact reasons for this are unclear [3].

Fact Box 2: ACL reconstruction

(a) Central third patellar tendon autograft provided improved stability and lower failure rates compared with extra-articular-based reconstructions.
(b) Early results with patellar tendon autograft suggest lateral IT band tenodesis may be unnecessary.
(c) Tunnel placement is key to restore ACL isometry and prevent early failures or residual instability.
(d) Caution should be employed with transtibial femoral tunnels as they contribute to vertical, nonanatomic reconstructions with poor rotational control.

10.7 Secondary Stabilizers

In addition to the importance of anatomic ACL reconstruction to restoring knee stability, there are several secondary stabilizers that also restrict translation that must be considered at the time of surgical reconstruction. Injuries to these structures, or variations in local anatomy, can potentially expose the reconstruction to undue stress that may result in early failure [4, 43].

Previous cadaveric studies performed at HSS have demonstrated the importance of meniscal preservation. Sectioning of the medial meniscus in an ACL-deficient knee resulted in a further significant increase in anterior tibial translation compared with isolated ACL transection [33]. Consequently, it was theorized that meniscal preservation can be protective of the reconstruction and prevent excessive translation [33]. The lateral meniscus did not appear to have the same effect on anterior tibial translation when sectioned in an ACL-deficient knee [32]. However, a more recent follow-up study in our lab performed with the assistance of computer navigation to track translation identified that the lateral meniscus does play an important role in resisting lateral compartment translation in response to combined translation and rotatory forces [39]. Additional work in a cadaveric model following single-bundle ACL reconstruction has demonstrated that both medial and lateral meniscectomies alone, or in combination, can limit the ability of the ACL reconstruction to resist the pivot shift [47].

The collateral ligaments have also been shown to play an integral role in resisting both translation and rotational moments about the knee. Sectioning studies of both the medial collateral ligament and lateral collateral ligament (as part of the posterolateral ligament complex) in conjunction with ACL transection lead to significantly greater anterior tibial translation [51, 52]. Recognizing these injuries and either performing delayed reconstruction to allow collateral ligament healing or combined repair or reconstruction of these ligaments will reduce loads placed on the ACL reconstruction.

In conjunction with the recognized effect of LCL and posterolateral corner injuries, the iliotibial (IT) band has been shown to contribute to tibial translation and rotation. This was initially demonstrated by Bach et al., where they demonstrated that hip abduction, which reduces the tension in the IT band, resulted in a greater degree of pivot shift in ACL-deficient knees [2]. More recently, a cadaveric study with sequential release of the IT band following ACL transection resulted in significantly greater anterior tibial translation in both the medial and lateral compartments and a correspondingly higher grade of pivot shift test [50]. Combined with injury to the anterolateral capsule, these results may provide support for anterolateral ligament reconstruction.

Finally, variations in bony morphology can also contribute to both anterior tibial translation and the magnitude of the pivot shift. Increased slope changes the resting position of the tibia, shifting this anteriorly, although cadaveric testing did not identify an associated increase in the magnitude of anterior tibial translation [53]. However, increased tibial slope was shown to increase anterior translation during a simulated pivot shift examination, although the exact mechanism is unclear [53]. A follow-up study to quantify the magnitude of this effect demonstrated poor correlation between slope and kinematic testing [20]. However, this follow-up study did identify that increased lateral femoral condyle width and length are associated with increased translation and pivot shift grade following ACL injury. These patients are considered "lateral compartment dominant" and should be considered as high risk for clinical instability following ACL injury and potentially even following reconstruction. These patients may potentially represent a population that would benefit from additive extra-articular tenodesis.

Fact Box 3: Secondary stabilizers

(a) Menisci and collateral ligaments are important secondary stabilizers.
(b) Meniscal preservation and collateral ligament repair should be considered to protect ACL reconstruction.
(c) Increased tibial slope may also contribute to instability and reconstruction failure.

10.8 ACL Isometry

As arthroscopic equipment and skill improved in the mid- to late 1990s, the use of a posterior incision became superfluous, and reconstructions were largely completed with all-inside techniques. However, failure rates were higher than anticipated, with as few as 40 % of patients reporting that their reconstructed knee felt "normal" [9]. Subsequently, increased attention has been placed on the accuracy of surgical reconstruction. As our knowledge has improved in terms of the complexity of the anatomical origin and insertion of the ACL, as well as the function of its two individual bundles, there has been improved recognition that single-bundle transtibial reconstructions often place the graft in a vertical, nonanatomic position [10, 22]. A comparative study performed at our institution investigated the effect of drilling technique on both tunnel placement and accuracy. While both the transtibial and anteromedial (AM) portal drilling techniques were capable of accurately restoring femoral footprint anatomy, this came at the expense of tibial footprint restoration for the transtibial group [10]. Tibial tunnel placement was significantly more posterior in the transtibial group in order to gain access to the femoral footprint for drilling of the femoral tunnel, thereby leaving the graft much more vertical compared with the AM portal group. This has been shown to reduce the ability to resist rotational forces, often associated with a residual pivot shift after reconstruction.

Follow-up studies have identified similar findings. One study utilized computer navigation software (Fig. 10.3) to track postoperative motion following both a conventional, transtibial single-bundle reconstruction and a horizontal single-bundle reconstruction, more consistent with an AM portal reconstruction technique [11]. This study identified an improved ability to resist both translational and rotational forces with a horizontal graft, suggesting that AM portal techniques aimed at more anatomic reconstruction may confer improved joint stability in single-bundle reconstruction. Similar findings were noted in a cadaveric study comparing tibial translation following ACL reconstruction with a fixed femoral tunnel and three different tibial tunnels. The more anterior tibial tunnel reconstructions better resisted translation and rotation [5]. The only caveat to this point is that increasingly anterior tibial tunnels must be observed for the risk of potential graft impingement in extension and increased risk of re-rupture. Finally, an additional study assessed the

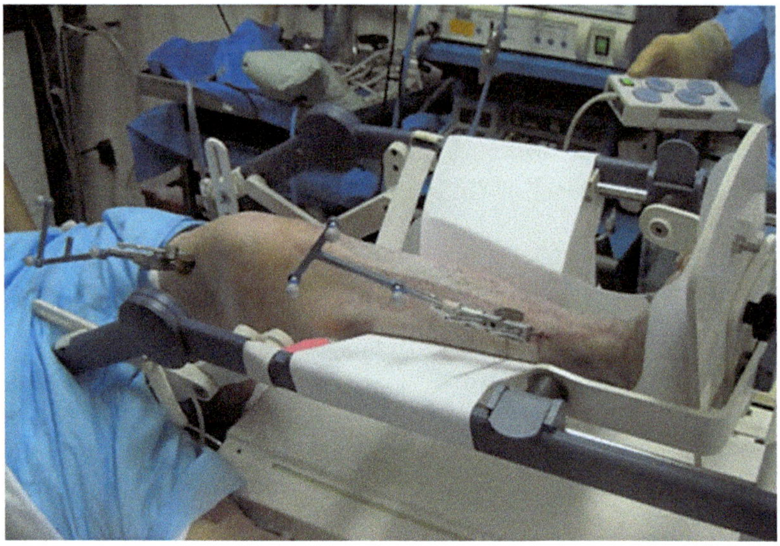

Fig. 10.3 Computer navigation tracking devices used to assess in vitro translational kinematics following surgical reconstruction

effect of both tunnel position and graft size on time-zero knee kinematics [5]. This study identified that restoration of native footprint anatomy with the reconstruction was most important and that a larger graft could not overcome the deleterious effect of a malpositioned tunnel during single-bundle ACL reconstruction [6].

Surgical navigation software has also been utilized to assess the isometry of different ACL reconstructions, simulating reconstruction of the anteromedial (AM) bundle and the posterolateral (PL) bundle, a central reconstruction, and the conventional transtibial reconstruction (PL tibia to AM femur). In this study, Pearle et al. identified that all reconstructions are anisometric; however, a reconstruction that replicates the AM bundle position demonstrates the most favorable isometric profile. While achieving an AM tunnel position on both the tibia and femur is often challenging via transtibial drilling, these data suggest that mirroring the orientation of the AM bundle may be advantageous in a single-bundle reconstruction [46].

10.9 Double-Bundle Reconstruction

Improved restoration of native ligament orientation, with either an AM bundle reconstruction or central single-bundle reconstruction, has been shown to provide improved time-zero knee kinematics and laxity [6]. With the recognized differences in the behavior of the different bundles, double-bundle reconstruction has been theorized to offer the advantage of a more dynamic reconstruction, with improved ability to resist both rotational and translational loads in all positions of knee flexion. Unfortunately, most clinical comparisons have been made between this technique and the conventional transtibial, nonanatomic reconstruction. A study in the HSS biomechanics laboratorium was subsequently performed utilizing a matched-pair cadaveric model to compare the effect of a double-bundle reconstruction with an anatomical, AM portal single-bundle reconstruction on translation and pivot shift kinematics [7]. Both the double-bundle and center-center single-bundle reconstructions adequately reduced anterior translation with Lachman testing [7]. However, the double-bundle reconstruction was significantly better at reducing the time-zero pivot shift by reducing the anterior translation of the lateral tibial plateau more than the single-bundle reconstruction. This difference was magnified in the presence of concomitant meniscal pathology, leading authors to conclude that double-bundle reconstruction may be indicated in patients with "at-risk" knees, with either concomitant meniscal pathology or a high-grade pivot shift preoperatively [7]. However, these results should be interpreted with caution, as there is limited clinical data to support the use of double-bundle reconstructions. The only randomized study comparing single- and double-bundle reconstruction was unable to detect clinically significant differences in outcome measures or translation testing postoperatively [26]. Additionally, similar studies in the HSS biomechanics laboratorium have suggested the possibility that double-bundle reconstructions may over-constrain the kinematics of the knee compared with single-bundle reconstructions [40].

10.10 Future Directions

Interestingly, we have come full circle, with much of the current research focusing on renewed methods of performing historic procedures. This includes a renewed interest in studying the potential role and outcomes with ACL repair using modern surgical techniques, as well as further study of anterolateral ligament reconstruction, mirroring the concepts of Lemaire and MacIntosh's lateral extra-articular tenodeses. Additionally, further cadaveric work with computer-assisted navigation will continue to provide useful information regarding optimal reconstruction techniques. Together, the information gained from these areas will provide exciting information in years to come, which will undoubtedly continue to improve the surgical reconstructive techniques.

Conclusion

ACL injuries and the techniques of associated surgical management continue to evolve. While methods of repair and reconstruction have improved over the past few decades, the ideal reconstruction method remains elusive and continual study is required to improve on existing techniques in order to provide our patients with the best possible clinical outcome.

References

1. Alm A, Gillquist J, Strömberg B (1974) The medial third of the patellar ligament in reconstruction of the anterior cruciate ligament. A clinical and histologic study by means of arthroscopy or arthrotomy. Acta Chir Scand Suppl 445:5–14
2. Bach BR, Warren RF, Wickiewicz TL (1988) The pivot shift phenomenon: results and description of a modified clinical test for anterior cruciate ligament insufficiency. Am J Sports Med 16:571–576
3. Barker JU, Drakos MC, Maak TG, Warren RF, Williams RJ, Allen AA (2010) Effect of graft selection on the incidence of postoperative infection in anterior cruciate ligament reconstruction. Am J Sports Med 38:281–286
4. Battaglia MJ, Cordasco FA, Hannafin JA, Rodeo SA, O'Brien SJ, Altchek DW, Cavanaugh J, Wickiewicz TL, Warren RF (2007) Results of revision anterior cruciate ligament surgery. Am J Sports Med 35:2057–2066
5. Bedi A, Maak T, Musahl V, Citak M, O'Loughlin PF, Choi D, Pearle AD (2011) Effect of tibial tunnel position on stability of the knee after anterior cruciate ligament reconstruction: is the tibial tunnel position most important? Am J Sports Med 39:366–373
6. Bedi A, Maak T, Musahl V, O'Loughlin P, Choi D, Citak M, Pearle AD (2011) Effect of tunnel position and graft size in single-bundle anterior cruciate ligament reconstruction: an evaluation of time-zero knee stability. Arthrosc J Arthrosc Relat Surg Elsevier Inc 27:1543–1551
7. Bedi A, Musahl V, O'Loughlin P, Maak T, Citak M, Dixon P, Pearle AD (2010) A comparison of the effect of central anatomical single-bundle anterior cruciate ligament reconstruction and double-bundle anterior cruciate ligament reconstruction on pivot-shift kinematics. Am J Sports Med 38:1788–1794
8. Bertoia JT, Urovitz EP, Richards RR, Gross AE (1985) Anterior cruciate reconstruction using the MacIntosh lateral-substitution over-the-top repair. J Bone Joint Surg Am 67:1183–1188
9. Biau DJ, Tournoux C, Katsahian S, Schranz P, Nizard R (2007) ACL reconstruction: a meta-analysis of functional scores. Clin Orthop Relat Res 458: 180–187
10. Bowers AL, Bedi A, Lipman JD, Potter HG, Rodeo SA, Pearle AD, Warren RF, Altchek DW (2011) Comparison of anterior cruciate ligament tunnel position and graft obliquity with transtibial and anteromedial portal femoral tunnel reaming techniques using high-resolution magnetic resonance imaging. Arthrosc J Arthrosc Relat Surg Elsevier Inc 27:1511–1522
11. Brophy RH, Pearle AD (2009) Single-bundle anterior cruciate ligament reconstruction: a comparison of conventional, central, and horizontal single-bundle virtual graft positions. Am J Sports Med 37: 1317–1323
12. Buss DD, Warren RF, Wickiewicz TL, Galinat BJ, Panariello R (1993) Arthroscopically assisted reconstruction of the anterior cruciate ligament with use of autogenous patellar-ligament grafts. Results after twenty-four to forty-two months. J Bone Joint Surg Am 75:1346–1355

13. Butler D, Noyes F, Grood E, Miller E, Malek M (1979) Mechanical properties of transplants for the anterior cruciate ligament. Orthop Trans 3:180–181
14. Chambat P, Guier C, Sonnery-Cottet B, Fayard JM, Thaunat M (2013) The evolution of ACL reconstruction over the last fifty years. Int Orthop 37:181–186
15. Clancy WG, Nelson DA, Reider B, Narechania RG (1982) Anterior cruciate ligament reconstruction using one-third of the patellar ligament, augmented by extra-articular tendon transfers. J Bone Joint Surg Am 64:352–359
16. Davarinos N, O'Neill BJ, Curtin W (2014) A brief history of anterior cruciate ligament reconstruction. Adv Orthop Surg 2014:1–6
17. Feagin J (1972) Experience with isolated tears of the anterior cruciate ligaments. A report of 36 cases. Am Acad Orthop Surg Annu Meet Washington, DC
18. Feagin JA, Curl WW (1976) Isolated tear of the anterior cruciate ligament: 5-year followup study. J Sports Med Am 3:95–100
19. Furman W, Marshall JL, Girgis FG (1976) The anterior cruciate ligament. A functional analysis based on postmortem studies. J Bone Joint Surg Am 58:179–185
20. Galano GJ, Suero EM, Citak M, Wickiewicz T, Pearle AD (2012) Relationship of native tibial plateau anatomy with stability testing in the anterior cruciate ligament-deficient knee. Knee surgery. Sport Traumatol Arthrosc 20:2220–2224
21. Girgis FG, Marshall JL, Monajem A (1975) The cruciate ligaments of the knee joint. Anatomical, functional and experimental analysis. Clin Orthop Relat Res 106:216–231
22. Harner CD, Honkamp NJ, Ranawat AS (2008) Anteromedial portal technique for creating the anterior cruciate ligament femoral tunnel. Arthroscopy 24:113–115
23. Helfet A (1963) The management of internal derangements of the knee. Lippincott Williams & Wilkins, Philadelphia
24. Hey-Groves EW (1917) Operation for the repair of the crucial ligaments. Lancet 2:274
25. Howell SM, Wallace MP, Hull ML, Deutsch ML (1999) Evaluation of the single-incision arthroscopic technique for anterior cruciate ligament replacement. A study of tibial tunnel placement, intraoperative graft tension, and stability. Am J Sports Med 27:284–293
26. Hussein M, van Eck CF, Cretnik A, Dinevski D, Fu FH (2012) Prospective randomized clinical evaluation of conventional single-bundle, anatomic single-bundle, and anatomic double-bundle anterior cruciate ligament reconstruction: 281 cases with 3- to 5-year follow-up. Am J Sports Med 40:512–520
27. Ireland J, Trickey EL (1980) Macintosh tenodesis for anterolateral instability of the knee. J Bone Joint Surg Br 62:340–345
28. Kaplan N, Wickiewicz TL, Warren RF (1990) Primary surgical treatment of anterior cruciate ligament ruptures. A long-term follow-up study. Am J Sports Med 18(4):354–358
29. Kennedy JC, Stewart R, Walker DM (1978) Anterolateral rotatory instability of the knee joint. An early analysis of the Ellison procedure. J Bone Joint Surg Am 60:1031–1039
30. Kornblatt I, Warren RF, Wickiewicz TL (1988) Long-term followup of anterior cruciate ligament reconstruction using the quadriceps tendon substitution for chronic anterior cruciate ligament insufficiency. Am J Sports Med 16:444–448
31. Lemaire M (1975) Chronic knee instability. Technics and results of ligament plasty in sports injuries. J Chir (Paris) 110:281–294
32. Levy IM, Torzilli PA, Gould JD, Warren RF (1989) The effect of lateral meniscectomy on motion of the knee. J Bone Joint Surg Am 71:401–406
33. Levy IM, Torzilli PA, Warren RF (1982) The effect of medial meniscectomy on anterior-posterior motion of the knee. J Bone Joint Surg Am 64:883–888
34. Lipscomb AB, Johnston RK, Snyder RB (1981) The technique of cruciate ligament reconstruction. Am J Sports Med 9:77–81
35. MacIntosh DL (1974) Acute tears of the anterior cruciate ligament. Over-the-top repair. Am Acad Orthop Surg Annu Meet Dallas, Texas
36. Marshall JL, Warren RF, Wickiewicz TL (1982) Primary surgical treatment of anterior cruciate ligament lesions. Am J Sports Med 10:103–107
37. Marshall JL, Warren RF, Wickiewicz TL, Reider B (1979) The anterior cruciate ligament: a technique of repair and reconstruction. Clin Orthop Relat Res 143:97–106
38. McCulloch PC, Lattermann C, Boland AL, Bach BR (2007) An illustrated history of anterior cruciate ligament surgery. J Knee Surg 20:95–104
39. Musahl V, Citak M, O'Loughlin PF, Choi D, Bedi A, Pearle AD (2010) The effect of medial versus lateral meniscectomy on the stability of the anterior cruciate ligament-deficient knee. Am J Sports Med 38: 1591–1597
40. Musahl V, Voos JE, O'Loughlin PF, Choi D, Stueber V, Kendoff D, Pearle AD (2010) Comparing stability of different single- and double-bundle anterior cruciate ligament reconstruction techniques: a cadaveric study using navigation. Arthroscopy 26:S41–S48
41. Nicholas JA (1973) The five-one reconstruction for anteromedial instability of the knee. Indications, technique, and the results in fifty-two patients. J Bone Joint Surg Am 55:899–922
42. Noyes FR, Butler DL, Grood ES, Zernicke RF, Hefzy MS (1984) Biomechanical analysis of human ligament grafts used in knee-ligament repairs and reconstructions. J Bone Joint Surg Am 66:344–352
43. O'Brien SJ, Warren RF, Pavlov H, Panariello R, Wickiewicz TL (1991) Reconstruction of the chronically insufficient anterior cruciate ligament with the central third of the patellar ligament. J Bone Joint Surg Am 73:278–286
44. O'Brien SJ, Warren RF, Wickiewicz TL, Rawlins BA, Allen AA, Panariello R, Kelly AM (1991) The iliotibial band lateral sling procedure and its effect on the

results of anterior cruciate ligament reconstruction. Am J Sports Med 19:21–24; discussion 24–25
45. O'Donoghue DH (1955) Analysis of end results of surgical treatment of major injuries to ligaments of the knee. J Bone Joint Surg 37A:1–13
46. Pearle AD, Shannon FJ, Granchi C, Wickiewicz TL, Warren RF (2008) Comparison of 3-dimensional obliquity and anisometric characteristics of anterior cruciate ligament graft positions using surgical navigation. Am J Sports Med 36:1534–1541
47. Petrigliano FA, Musahl V, Suero EM, Citak M, Pearle AD (2011) Effect of meniscal loss on knee stability after single-bundle anterior cruciate ligament reconstruction. Knee Surgery. Sport Traumatol Arthrosc 19:86–93
48. Schindler OS (2012) Surgery for anterior cruciate ligament deficiency: a historical perspective. Knee Surg Sport Traumatol Arthrosc 20:5–47
49. Sgaglione NA, Warren RF, Wickiewicz TL, Gold DA, Panariello RA (1990) Primary repair with semitendinosus tendon augmentation of acute anterior cruciate ligament injuries. Am J Sports Med 18:64–73
50. Suero EM, Njoku IU, Voigt MR, Lin J, Koenig D, Pearle AD (2013) The role of the iliotibial band during the pivot shift test. Knee Surg Sport Traumatol Arthrosc 21:2096–2100
51. Sullivan D, Levy IM, Sheskier S, Torzilli PA, Warren RF (1984) Medial restraints to anterior-posterior motion of thc knee. J Bone Joint Surg Am 66:930–936
52. Veltri DM, Deng XH, Torzilli PA, Warren RF, Maynard MJ (1995) The role of the cruciate and posterolateral ligaments in stability of the knee. A biomechanical study. Am J Sports Med 23:436–443
53. Voos JE, Suero EM, Citak M, Petrigliano FP, Bosscher MRF, Citak M, Wickiewicz TL, Pearle AD (2012) Effect of tibial slope on the stability of the anterior cruciate ligament-deficient knee. Knee Surg Sport Traumatol Arthrosc 20:1626–1631
54. Warren RF, Marshall JL (1978) Injuries of the anterior cruciate and medial collateral ligaments of the knee. A retrospective analysis of clinical records – part I. Clin Orthop Relat Res 136:191–197
55. Warren RF, Marshall JL (1978) Injuries of the anterior cruciate and medial collateral ligaments of the knee. A long-term follow-up of 86 cases – part II. Clin Orthop Relat Res 136:198–211
56. Williams RJ, Hyman J, Petrigliano F, Rozental T, Wickiewicz TL (2004) Anterior cruciate ligament reconstruction with a four-strand hamstring tendon autograft. J Bone Joint Surg Am 86-A:225–232

Development of Arthrometry 11

Najeeb Khan, Eric Dockter, Donald Fithian, Ronald Navarro, and William Luetzow

Contents

N. Khan, MD
Kaiser Permanente, San Marcos Outpatient Medical Center, 400 Craven Rd, San Marcos, CA 92078, USA

E. Dockter, MD • D. Fithian, MD
Kaiser Permanente, El Cajon Medical Offices, 250 S Travelodge Dr, El Cajon, CA 92020, USA

R. Navarro, MD (✉)
Kaiser Permanente, South Bay Medical Center, Coastline MOB, 25821 S. Vermont Ave, Harbor City, CA 90710 USA
e-mail: Ronald.A.Navarro@kp.org

W. Luetzow, MD
Kaiser Permanente, Garfield Specialty Center, 5893 Copley Dr, San Diego, CA 92111 USA

11.1 Introduction

In the evaluation of ligamentous injury, orthopedists estimate the amount of displacement, endpoint feel, and rotation when performing the Lachman and pivot shift examinations. These exams and the reported results depend on experience, training, and ability [51]. The subjective nature of physical examination makes the need for objective and standardized clinical measures of knee laxity obvious.

Researchers in the late 1970s developed arthrometry to quantify their physical examination findings in order to better study knee kinematics. Instrumented measurement of knee motion can assist the surgeon to diagnose and document pathologic laxity in the injured knee compared with the normal side. Postoperative measurements can grade knee laxity with respect to the contralateral and presumed normal knee. Objective quantitative ligament testing devices provide the opportunity to compare populations of patients more accurately.

The first quarter century of knee ligament arthrometry was dominated by the first generation

V. Musahl et al. (eds.), *Rotatory Knee Instability*, DOI 10.1007/978-3-319-32070-0_11

of devices and methods which focused on measuring single-plane AP translation due to the technological limitations of the time. The second generation of arthrometry includes robotics, multiple-plane measurements, and smartphone applications and may bring about a more sophisticated and nuanced understanding of knee joint kinematics. This chapter gives specific details and comparisons about each of these first- and second-generation devices.

11.2 Assessing Knee Laxity

There are many techniques for assessing knee laxity [71]:

- Manual clinical testing/physical examination: This is the oldest known technique for assessing knee laxity and will remain a critical component of evaluating ligament function. There are no associated costs or side effects, and results are immediate. However, there is limited ability to compare results between surgeons. Measurements are inexact, idiosyncratic, and patient factors (cooperation, muscle guarding) can compromise results. Arthrometry devices provide a more objective and reliable measurement of displacement in response to a specified load. The portable devices can be used in the clinic and operating room. Results from different devices cannot be generalized or compared with each other, and each device has shortcomings. The next generation of arthrometry may obviate some of these deficiencies.
- Intraoperative navigation: An examination under anesthesia eliminates issues related to guarding and cooperation. Data derived from computer navigation can be accurate and precise but require invasive techniques. An important flaw is that data are garnered only from the limb undergoing operation.
- Stress radiography: This is also an excellent technique which provides reproducible results but requires additional equipment, personnel, radiation exposure, and associated costs.
- Computerized systems with mechanical load application: This represents at least one branch of the next generation of ligament arthrometry. These systems are not yet generally available for clinical use and remain in development.

11.3 First-Generation Knee Ligament Arthrometry

11.3.1 UCLA Instrumented Clinical Testing Apparatus

The first arthrometer device was designed and tested by a researcher and mechanical engineer at UCLA named Keith Markolf in 1978 [47]. This device, and later a similar portable device [46], measured tibial translation in both anteroposterior (AP) and varus/valgus planes and provided a response curve over tibial displacement. The response curve to displacement was an important feature to this device and provided the examiner with stiffness data (Fig. 11.1).

To use this device, the reclining patient's knee was flexed to 20° and the distal femur (encompassing the condyles and patella) was clamped to a weighted base. The foot was secured in a plate that controls rotation, thus allowing measurements in internal and external tibial rotation. A spring-loaded plunger was applied to the tibial tubercle and force is applied to the tibia via an instrumented load cell. Continuous force vs. displacement data was garnered on a graph plotter. Sagittal motion was measured at 200 N of applied anterior force, and anterior stiffness (slope of the anterior loading curve) was calculated at 100 N. The inclusion of stiffness as a measurement did not yield data that was clinically useful.

As with all arthrometric devices, an accurate test requires (a) patient cooperation to relax muscles and remove guarding as a confounding factor and (b) multiple preliminary trials to center the device at the resting state of the knee.

An in vitro study, in which selective supporting structures were released and then put through biomechanical testing, showed a mean translation of 6.6 mm (±2.5 mm) with a force of 100 N before ACL failure. Maximal anterior displacement occurred in all cadaver knees at 30° of flexion [48]. This result was duplicated and verified 14 years later by Bach et al. using the KT-1000 arthrometer [5].

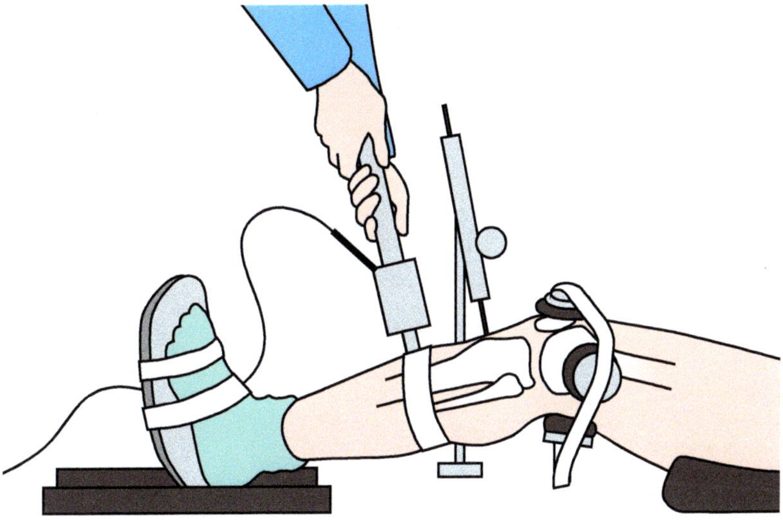

Fig. 11.1 UCLA Instrumented clinical testing apparatus is the first knee ligament arthrometer. This device provides a continuous force vs. displacement response curve. Sagittal plane tibial motion and the firmness of the end point both anteriorly and posteriorly can be assessed

The UCLA device was able to correctly diagnose ACL deficiency with up to 95 % accuracy and compared favorably to other arthrometers [65] but was not manufactured and thus not available outside of the UCLA research laboratories. Although it was used primarily as a research device at UCLA, Markolf's design established several principles which many other subsequent arthrometers have incorporated.

11.3.2 Genucom Knee Analysis System

The Genucom knee analysis system was developed by the FARO Medical Technologies Company in the early 1980s. It contained an electrical goniometer and a computer which provided digital measurements of knee motion in 6 degrees of freedom. Using this device, the patient was placed in a seated position with the tibia secured. An electronic goniometer measured knee joint displacement in the AP plane and a dynamometer measured forces and moments on the knee joint in six planes. Numerical and graphical data was displayed on a digital screen.

Early studies validated the Genucom device with respect to physical examination [52] and provided evidence of reliability [33, 49]. However, other researchers reported issues with intra-observer consistency and variability due to the application of the device [79]. The attempt to measure knee motion accurately and reliably in six planes was laudable, but this was an ambitious undertaking that ultimately became a victim in an era of computational and design limitations. A series of studies which compared different arthrometer designs ultimately showed the Genucom device to have less reliability and clinical utility than other similar arthrometers [1, 59, 69, 72]. Clinicians have largely abandoned this device and it is no longer available.

11.3.3 Stryker

The Stryker Knee Laxity Tester was introduced in the mid-1980s. This was a simple analog device which measures anterior and posterior displacement of the tibial tubercle with respect to the patella. While some clinicians championed its clinical use [9], others reported that the Stryker device had issues with sensitivity and interobserver reliability [36]. The Stryker device is no longer manufactured and has long been abandoned for clinical use.

11.3.4 Shino Knee Testing Apparatus [66]

Introduced in 1987, this apparatus was a heavy steel frame which contains a chair and linked measurement device that captures the thigh and leg

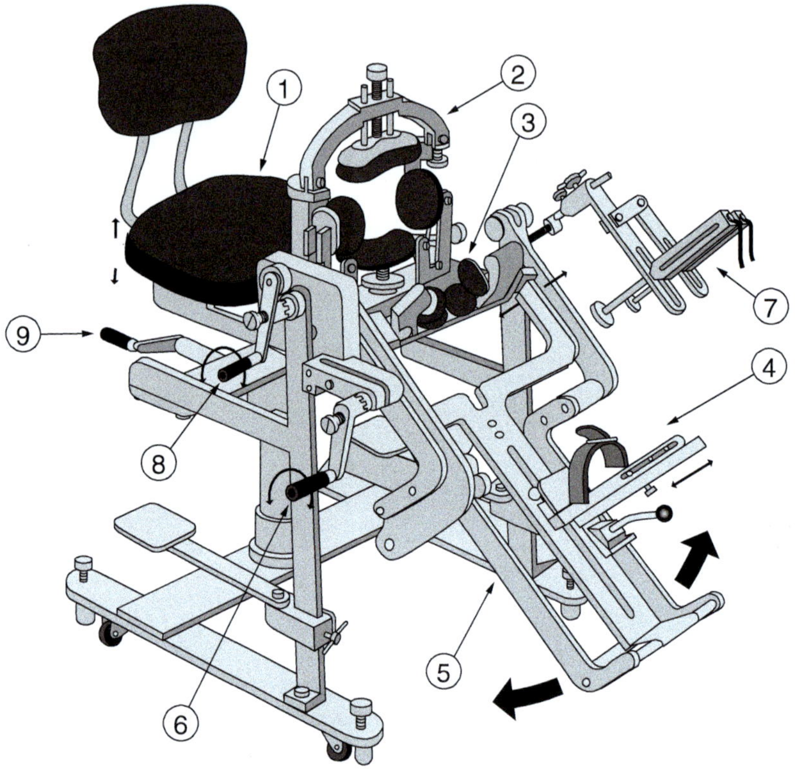

Fig. 11.2 Shino knee testing apparatus. *1* Chair, *2* Four adjustable metal shells with sand filled pads to clamp distal thigh, *3* Four sand filled pads to clamp proximal tibia, *4* Hinged foot holder to allow full rotation of tibia, *5* Legrest, *6* Lever that allows adjustment of the angle of flexion of the knee, *7* Two displacement transducers, *8* Lever to adjust anteroposterior force, *9* Lever to adjust height and angle of chair

independently. Knee flexion angle was adjustable, though recommended at 20°. The patient reclined to allow muscular relaxation. The tibia was controlled by a clamp just below the tibial tubercle, and anterior and posterior forces were applied to the tibia manually by a lever connected to a gear system. Displacement was amplified by a gear system, quantified by a strain gauge load cell, and then fed into a computer to produce a graph.

The gear system was a unique feature, which allowed the examiner to apply forces exceeding 200 N without significant effort. Shino et al. reported an average ACL injured-to-normal difference in anterior displacement of 6.7 mm ± 3.3. Edixhoven et al. developed a comparable apparatus, with similar limitations stemming from the stationary nature of the device [23]. Neither is currently available on the market (Fig. 11.2).

11.3.5 KT-1000

Dale Daniel and colleagues established a weekly acute knee clinic in 1981 that was populated by patients who presented to any of the San Diego facilities with an acute knee injury. This clinic captured most, if not all of acutely injured knees with hemarthrosis. The KT-2000 and the subsequent KT-1000 models were developed in partnership by Dale Daniel and engineer Lawrence Malcolm with the goals of (a) assisting the clinician in diagnosing ligament disruption by detecting pathologic laxity, (b) documenting the amount of pathologic laxity, and (c) measuring the ability of ligament surgery to reestablish normal knee motion [18]. The KT-1000 calculates the amount of displacement occurring at the joint line. The initial intention was to build a measuring device that would capture translation of the tibia in the AP plane, translation of the tibia in the medial/lateral plane, and rotation of the tibia about the proximal/distal axis [55, 56]. Technical design and computational limitations of that time forced the developers to limit their aims to measuring AP tibial translation only.

Dale Daniel provided the clinical setting for bench-to-bedside research, methodology, and scientific vision. Lawrence Malcolm was an engineering professor at the University of California in San Diego who built prototypes and ultimately the KT-1000. He formed the Medmetric Company and devoted his time and energy on knee ligament arthrometry.

Physical therapist Mary Lou Stone was a key player in the research and development of knee ligament arthrometry. In order to minimize bias in the study, she gathered all arthrometry data independently apart from the primary investigators (pre- and postoperatively).

The KT-2000 preceded the KT-1000 and is similar in all ways except the addition of a graph plotter that records force displacement relationships on an x-y plotter. The KT-1000 had a simple analog dial, which made this device even more portable and easy to use.

11.3.5.1 Examination Technique

Obtaining precise, accurate, and reproducible data from the KT-1000 requires that the examiner uses and positions the device in a reliable and standardized fashion. It also requires a cooperative patient who is able to relax the quadriceps and core musculature during the examination.

The patient is positioned in a supine position with the knees held supported in a slightly flexed position (between 20° and 40°) so that that patella is well seated in the trochlea. A firm thigh support is placed proximal to the knee joint and a foot rest limits and equalizes tibial external rotation. The KT-1000 is placed on the anterior leg and secured by two Velcro straps (Fig. 11.3). The uninvolved knee is always tested first to establish normal values for the patient, followed by the involved knee. The proximal sensor pad is lined up with the inferior border of the patella and the distal pad lays distal to the joint line at the tibial tubercle (Fig. 11.4). This device measures relative motion in millimeters between these two sensor pads. The examiner then determines the zero point or resting state of the knee by performing multiple anterior and posterior translations of the leg. A consistent resting state is found and the device is calibrated to measure bidirectional laxity from this point.

With the patella stabilized, the handle on the device is pulled to effectively translate the tibia anteriorly. A characteristic audible tone is heard at 15 lb (67 N), 20 lb (89 N), and 30 lb (133 N), respectively. For the musically curious, the tones are G5, Ab4, and C5. To test a manual maximum displacement, the patella is again stabilized manually, while the proximal anteromedial leg is grasped and pulled anteriorly with firm force (Fig. 11.5). This is repeated multiple times until a consistent anterior translation amount is measured. Estimated force generated by this test ranges from 135 to 180 N, depending on the examiner's effort and strength.

The examiner utilized the analog display to record the tibial translation at 15 lb, 20 lb, and 30 lb and at manual maximum for each knee

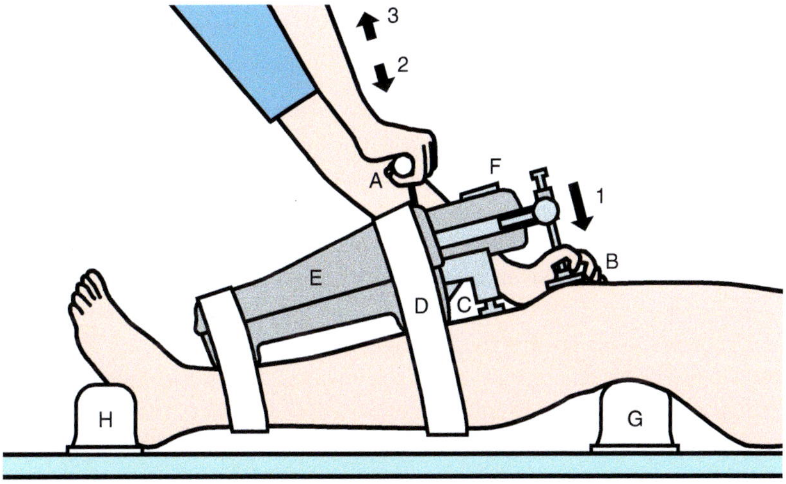

Fig. 11.3 Components of the KT-1000: (*A*) Force handle, (*B*) Patellar sensor pad, (*C*) Tibial tubercle sensor pad, (*D*) Velcro straps, (*E*) Arthrometer body, (*F*) Displacement dial, (*G*) Thigh support, (*H*) Foot support. (*1*) The stabilizing hand rests against the lateral thigh and applies 2–5 lb of pressure on the patellar sensor pad to keep it in contact with the patella. (*2*) and (*3*), Posterior and anterior forces are applied

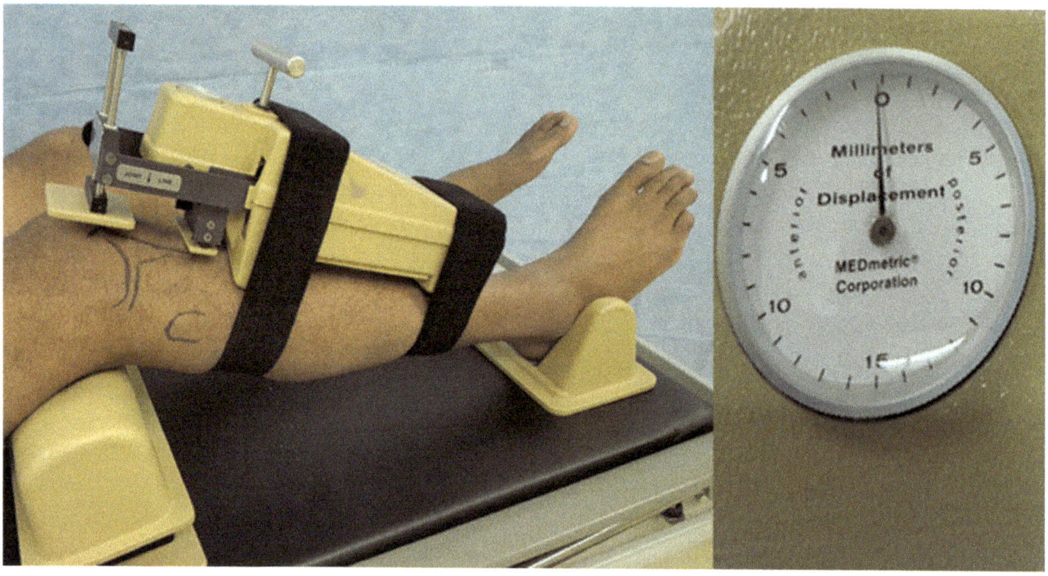

Fig. 11.4 The KT-1000 positioned on knee of patient with drawn anatomical landmarks (*left*). The analog dial displays the amount of displacement in both anterior and posterior directions (*right*)

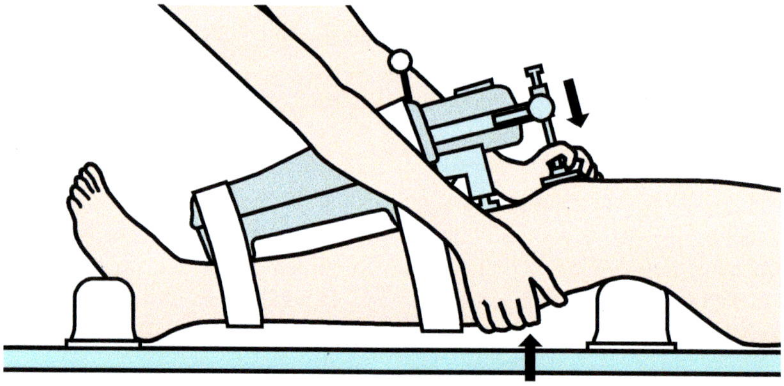

Fig. 11.5 KT-1000, maximum manual measurement. The limbs are positioned with the included thigh and foot supports. While the patellar sensor pad is stabilized with one hand, the other hand applies a strong anterior displacement force directly to the proximal calf. Care is taken to avoid extending the knee

(Fig. 11.4). The side-to-side difference at the manual maximum is calculated and is the most reliable clinical parameter. Compliance index, defined as the difference in tibial displacement between the two displacement forces (15 and 20 lbs), was studied extensively and found to be less useful [60].

It is crucial that the effort and strength used on the uninvolved knee matches that of the involved or injured knee. Consistent arthrometer placement and angle of force vector when displacing the leg is also important, as malpositioning and varying the angle of displacement can yield inconsistent and inaccurate data [38]. Practice and experience with the KT-1000 have been shown to improve the reliability of measurements [7, 8]. The ability of the patient to avoid guarding and quadriceps contraction is critical to obtaining a reliable, precise, and accurate result. The two greatest sources of measurement error with this device are lack of muscle relaxation and inability to stabilize the patellar sensor pad.

Arthrometric examination under anesthesia is often undertaken to obviate the challenges posed by patient guarding and apprehension. Multiple independent studies have shown that arthrometric data taken under anesthesia is improved in all variables, including displacement and side-to-side differences [18, 32, 78].

Fact Box 1

The two greatest sources of measurement error with the KT-1000 are lack of muscle relaxation and inability to stabilize the patellar sensor pad.

11.3.5.2 KT-1000 vs. MRI

Sensitivity rates for MRI detection of a complete ACL tear range from 67 to 97 % [17, 58, 74, 77], with larger magnets tending to be more sensitive. Differentiating a complete from a partial ACL tear on MRI is much less specific. This is a key distinction because complete tears more often result in clinical instability necessitating surgical intervention, in comparison with partial tears.

KT-1000 has a similar sensitivity to MRI and greater specificity in terms of partial vs. complete ACL tears. Using arthroscopy as the standard of measurement, partial tears can be differentiated from complete tears with a sensitivity of 80 % and a specificity of 100 % [62].

Liu et al. [41] reported in 1995 that a 0.5 T magnet is 97 % sensitive in detecting ACL pathology but only 82 % for complete rupture. KT-1000 testing was found to be much more accurate (97 %), with the conclusion that the diagnosis and the decision to reconstruct a complete ACL tear can be reliably made clinically without a preoperative MRI. Most clinicians, however, continue to complete a preoperative MRI to evaluate for concomitant meniscal and chondral injury. MRI is best used as an adjunct to arthrometry, as pathologic knee laxity and dysfunction is more closely tied to patient satisfaction than intra-articular appearance on imaging.

11.3.5.3 KT-1000 and ACL Deficiency

Independent in vitro sectioning studies [13, 20] have shown that the mean difference with 89 N of anterior translation between an ACL intact and deficient state is 6.7 mm with a fairly wide range of increase in anterior displacement (Fig. 11.6). In vivo results are similar. The arthrometric parameters of normal and abnormal

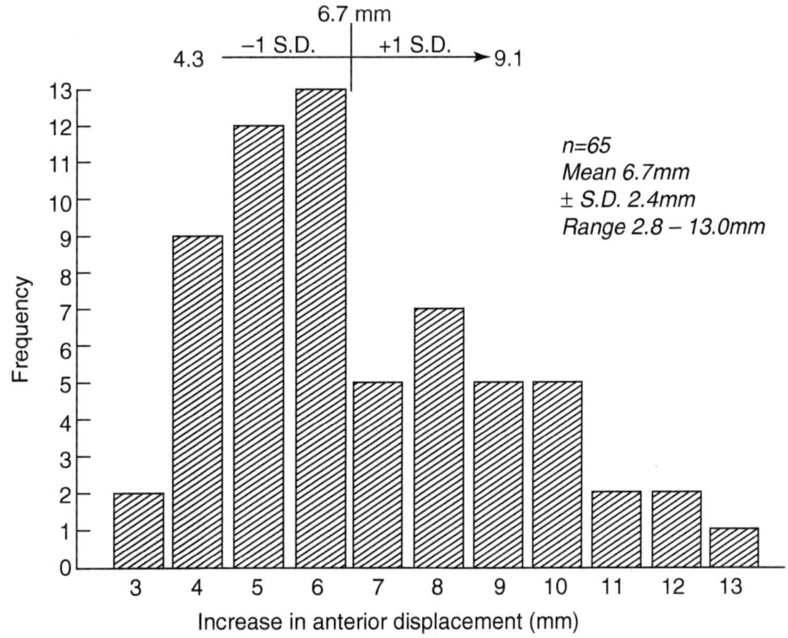

Fig. 11.6 Effect of anterior cruciate ligament (ACL) sectioning on anterior displacement. The difference of anterior displacement between the ACL intact knee followed by transection of ACL on 65 fresh cadaveric specimens

knees were established in a series of classic studies by Daniel et al. and Malcom et al. [20, 45]. Normal subjects can have a side-to-side difference of up to 2 mm [20] and were found to have a wide range of normal laxity and minimal side-to-side differences. The mean difference in a normal subject in the manual maximum test was 0.8 mm, whereas the range of displacement in these normal knees was 5–15.0 mm. Absolute translations were not nearly as helpful as the side-to-side differences due to these wide ranges. A side-to-side difference of 3 mm or greater at 89 N or at manual maximum was considered diagnostic of ACL insufficiency.

The average maximum displacement and manual side-to-side difference for chronic and acute ACL injuries are similar [5, 20, 21]. Daniel et al. reported a side-to-side difference of 5.6 mm for a chronic ACL injury and 5.0 mm for an acute injury.

Absolute displacement can also be helpful; a maximum manual translation of greater than 10 mm is sensitive for ACL injury, whereas the side-to-side difference of greater than 3 mm is both sensitive and specific [5, 21]. The primacy of maximum manual displacement clinical utility has been verified in several studies [5, 60, 70, 80].

11.3.5.4 Surgical Results

Direct primary ACL repair has largely been abandoned in part due to arthrometric data that showed persistent laxity after repair. Higgins and Steadman reported KT-1000 data on 24 skiers who underwent non-augmented ACL repair [31]. Maximum manual side-to-side differences after ACL repair showed a wide range (4.5–13.5 mm ± 2.3), placing a significant portion of these patients above the threshold for a failed surgery. Although some patients reported good outcomes, repair proved to produce unreliable and unpredictable outcome.

Multiple studies have reported preoperative and postoperative arthrometry data [2–4, 24, 29, 30], with Daniel's group being the first to do so [45]. In a classic series of outcome-based studies, Bach et al. reported on 2-year (minimum) and subsequently 5- to 9-year postoperative KT-1000 data [3, 4]. At a mean of 36 months, mean maximum manual side-to-side differences were reduced from 6.5 mm preoperatively to 1.1 mm postoperatively. Mean data for the longer-term study was similar, with only 4 % of postoperative patients having a maximum manual side-to-side difference greater than 5 mm. Bach et al. reported a strong correlation between a postoperative side-to-side difference of greater than 5 mm and a demonstrable pivot shift, representing failure of reconstruction.

Three independent meta-analyses [27, 28, 40] have reported in favor of patellar tendon autograft compared with hamstring autograft in terms of postoperative maximum manual side-to-side difference. Both graft choices improved clinical laxity; however, patellar tendon autografts were more likely to result in reconstructions with normal Lachman, normal pivot shift, KT-1000 manual maximum side-to-side difference <3 mm, and fewer results with significant flexion loss. In contrast, hamstring grafts had a reduced incidence of patellofemoral symptoms, kneeling pain, and extension loss. Improved arthrometric scores correlated with patient satisfaction and patellar tendon autograft. Other studies have also shown greater residual laxity for hamstring grafts but could not show a difference in outcome scores or return-to-play rates [24]. More recent studies have reported equivalent outcomes including KT-1000 arthrometer side-to-side differences between hamstring and patellar tendon groups [14, 34, 35], ostensibly due to updated techniques and fixation devices.

11.3.5.5 Limitations

There are multiple limitations to the KT-1000. Although not steep, there is a learning curve to using the KT-1000. Inter-user reliability can be as high as 95 %, with experience being the most important factor that increases reliability [7, 8].

The direction and rate at which force is applied are uncontrolled and thus affect interobserver reliability. Multiple factors, such as patient size, patient cooperation, clinician experience, and even hand dominance of the examiner [64], can influence the results.

Patient factors can skew KT-1000 data. There is an assumption that the contralateral knee is normal and can serve as a control for the injured knee. If the contralateral knee is reported to be functional and asymptomatic, this is most likely an acceptable control. If there has been previous injury and/or surgery, the validity of side-to-side difference data is limited [62]. The inability of the patient to completely relax the quadriceps and core musculature and avoid guarding precludes the ability to complete a KT-1000 examination. Examination under anesthesia may need to be considered for some. Another patient factor is obesity. Motion of the soft tissue envelope of a very large leg may obfuscate motion at the joint line, thereby invalidating the arthrometry data. Finally, ipsilateral PCL injury renders KT-1000 testing nonspecific, as the resting state of the knee is in posterior subluxation which increases overall sagittal translation.

The clinical relevance of anterior displacement measures has been challenged. Arguably the most important outcome with knee ligament injuries is patient satisfaction. Ligament arthrometry provides objective and numerical data for an outcome that is subjective. This has been studied extensively in the postoperative patient after ACL reconstruction. Kocher et al. reported that instrumented knee laxity and Lachman examination had no significant relationships with any subjective variables of symptoms and function postoperatively. The pivot shift examination, not KT-1000 data, however, had significant associations with satisfaction, giving way sensation, overall knee function, sports participation, and Lysholm score [37]. Other researchers have also reported on the lack of correlation between arthrometric data and functional scores postoperatively [22, 68]. Multiple researchers have reported no correlation between KT-1000 data and restoration of functional kinematic patterns [14, 15, 54], presumed to be due to the purely sagittal plane measurements inherent to KT-1000 testing. There is also no correlation between anterior displacement measures and the development of osteoarthritis after ACL reconstruction [76].

Perhaps the most important limitation of the KT-1000 is that it only measures AP laxity and does not measure rotation. Thus, a normal KT-1000 result can be seen with a malpositioned graft that may restrict AP motion while allowing a pivot shift phenomenon. This is a valid criticism, though it must be tempered by the understanding that the first quarter century of arthrometry by all researchers and developers was dominated by single-plane measurements due to design and computational limitations.

Despite these challenges, arthrometry remains one of the few objective measures that knee surgeons have to evaluate knee motion. The concepts of objective and reliable measurements of knee motion continue to be explored and refined.

The success of the KT-1000 stems from its reliability, portability, affordability, mass production, ease of use, and the simple goal of measuring one plane of motion. The KT-1000 is considered the standard of arthrometric testing devices and was a required component in research manuscripts by most journals for many years. This device has helped shape our understanding of knee motion and has been used in hundreds of articles. A search on MEDLINE in July of 2015 yielded 819 articles reporting the use of the KT-1000. A similar search on PubMed produced 881. While the use of the KT-1000 continues in many clinical settings throughout the world, the Medmetric Corporation is defunct and the KT-1000 device is no longer manufactured.

11.3.6 Kneelax

The Kneelax arthrometer is essentially a modernized version of the KT-1000. Mechanically similar in appearance and technical operations, the data are processed and displayed on a computer screen. Side-to-side differences were not found to be significantly different between the Kneelax and the KT-1000 in a validation study [53]. This device is available on the European market.

11.3.7 Vermont Knee Laxity Device (VKLD)

The VKLD was developed to evaluate AP displacement of the tibia relative to the femur during non-weight bearing, weight bearing, and the transition between these two conditions [75]. The patient is secured to a reclined seat with the feet secured to independent footplates which can be used to simulate weight bearing. Reliability and accuracy data for this device are sparse but support its use [67]. The developers of the VKLD are credited with being the first to broach the relationship between knee laxity measurements and weight bearing. This device is not available on the market.

11.3.8 CA-4000 Electrogoniometer

Previously called the Acufex Knee Signature System, this is an electrogoniometer that measures tibial AP translation, varus/valgus angulation, internal/external rotation, and flexion angle. The device is strapped to the thigh and calf and the subject is seated with the knee at 30° flexion. The examiner then applies external forces with a handheld load cell while an electronic goniometer provides data. This examination can be repeated with the patient performing functional activities on an exercise machine [69].

The CA-4000 was unique in that it measured four degrees of freedom and allowed functional testing. Although most studies have reported good accuracy and reliability compared with other arthrometers [26, 59, 61], this device is no longer available on the market.

11.3.9 Dyonics Dynamic Cruciate Tester

The Dyonics device measured AP displacement and is one of the first computerized arthrometers. Only one study has evaluated this device [1], reporting a higher false-positive result than other arthrometers. The Dyonics arthrometer was available for a brief period in the 1990s and is not currently available on the market.

11.3.10 Rolimeter

The Rolimeter is a compact, lightweight, and relatively simple device that measures sagittal translation. This is a steel device that has two pads which contact the patient connected by a bar (Fig. 11.7). Like the KT-1000, the Rolimeter is secured to the anterior tibia and manually stabilized at the patella. A stylus at the level of the tibial tubercle provides displacement data. Inter- and intra-tester reliability is high in both experienced and inexperienced users, though ultimately some experience optimizes results [50]. It has been shown to be at least as accurate as the KT-1000 in its ability to differentiate an ACL-deficient knee from a normal. Maximum manual side-to-side difference data from the Rolimeter and the KT-1000 correlated strongly to KT-1000 data, which validates the Rolimeter as a method to assess anterior laxity of the knee [6, 57]. The Rolimeter has many advantages. The simple design lends this device to sterilization and can be used intraoperatively. It is also relatively inexpensive and easy to use. Perhaps the biggest advantage of all is that the Rolimeter is currently the only first-generation arthrometer available on the market.

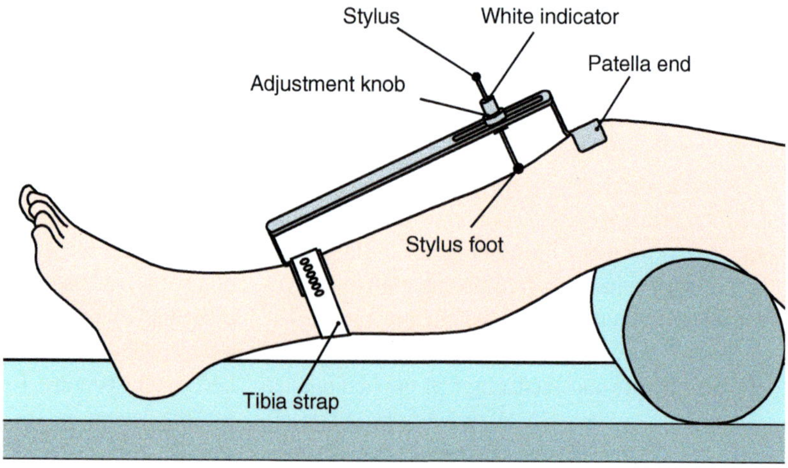

Fig. 11.7 Rolimeter. This device is centered over the patella and secured to the leg. The stylus is placed over the tibial tubercle, allowing a measurement of translation between the patella and the tibial tubercle

Fact Box 2
The success of the KT-1000 stems from its reliability, portability, affordability, mass production, ease of use, and the simple goal of measuring one plane of motion. The KT-1000 is considered the standard of arthrometric testing devices and was a required component in research manuscripts by most journals for many years.

11.4 Second-Generation Knee Ligament Arthrometry

Single-plane arthrometry represents the first generation whereas robotics, multiple-plane measurements, and smartphone applications represent the second generation. Robotic systems have the potential to apply standardized and reproducible magnitude, direction, and rate of force to the leg. The increased complexity and power of modern software combined with the miniaturization of hardware leads to the ability to measure knee motion with much more precision, accuracy, and sophistication than when arthrometry was first described in 1978.

Several methodologies have been identified and developed to quantify pivot shift test. However, clinical professionals are still lacking a "gold standard" method for the quantification of knee joint dynamic laxity.

11.4.1 Quantitative Pivot Shift Application

As the presence of pivot shift postoperatively correlates most closely with a poor patient satisfaction [39], measuring pre- and postoperative pivot shift is an obvious target. Tsai et al. have developed an image analysis technique for quantitatively assessing the pivot shift using universally available handheld computers [73]. This method holds great promise, remains in development, and is discussed in an earlier chapter of this book.

11.4.2 KneeKG

The KneeKG system [44] is a noninvasive navigational technique for assessing three-dimensional (3D) knee kinematics. This technique holds great promise in the clinic and gait lab and will be discussed in a later chapter in this book.

11.4.3 Rotameter

The Rotameter device and method is based on the dial test with the patient lying prone and the knee flexed to 30° [42]. Unique from first-generation arthrometers, the Rotameter only measures rotation in degrees in conjunction with applied torque and does not measure sagittal translation. The patient's leg is secured in a boot, which is fixed to a handlebar that allows transfers of different torques to the knee. The developers have reported high inter- and intra-observer reliability and have compared this device favorably to digital navigation. A clinical trial [43] with postoperative Rotameter data revealed a very small range (1° or less) and no significant rotational differences between the operated and contralateral knees. This device is discussed in a later chapter in this book.

11.4.4 GNRB

The GNRB knee laxity testing device (GeNouRoB, Montenay, France) is a computerized system that applies an anteriorly directed load to the knee to evaluate anterior laxity. A linear jack exerts gradually increasing thrust forces according to the examiner: 67, 89, 134, 150, or 250 N on the upper section of the calf. A displacement transducer (0.1 mm precision) records the relative displacement of the anterior tibial tubercle with respect to the femur. Associated software is able to compare not only side-to-side differences in the absolute amount of anterior tibial translation but also differences in the slope between 100 N and the maximum force applied [12]. This system has compared favorably with the KT-1000 [16], may be able to identify partial ACL tears [63], and even showed greater reproducibility than TELOS stress radiography [10]. This device is available to purchase in Europe.

11.4.5 Robotic Knee Test (RKT)

The RKT system developed by Branch et al. evaluates rotation stability by applying rotational torques to the knee with a computer-driven motor and measures kinematics with an electromagnetic measuring system [11]. Intra-rater correlation was measured at 0.97, making this a very reliable and reproducible instrument. This device is not devised for intraoperative use and is not yet available on the market. The RKT system will be discussed in a subsequent chapter of this book.

11.4.6 SmartJoint

Ferretti et al. have developed a smartphone-based arthrometer which is secured to the leg by way of a dedicated leg support. Maximum manual testing provides tibial translation data much in the same way as the KT-1000, with comparable and reliable data [25]. In the near future, a mobile phone arthrometer application may be a reliable alternative to the KT-1000 for measuring anterior tibial translation.

Conclusions

Instrumented measurements can be used to document knee laxity, establish the diagnosis of cruciate ligament dysfunction, assess post-operative laxity restoration, and provide a means to compare results over a variety of parameters. The first generation of arthrometry focused on measuring single-plane AP translation due to the technological limitations of the time. Because first-generation arthrometry measures AP translation only, it provides static information and can be influenced by both patient (guarding, cooperation) and clinician (experience) factors. The second generation of arthrometry promises to bring greater accuracy, precision, portability, and the ability to measure multiple planes and rotation.

Ligament arthrometry is an important part of a clinical evaluation. Regardless of the device used, arthrometry is not meant to displace the importance of history, physical examination, imaging, and other diagnostics. When used in conjunction with history, physical exam, and imaging, the clinician can better understand the injured knee and formulate an appropriate plan in sync with the patient's goals.

Fact Box 3

- Arthrometry is an important part of the clinical evaluation and provides an objective tool in evaluating knee ligamentous injury.
- Multiple first-generation arthrometers were developed based on principles developed and tested by Markolf, Daniel, and Malcolm.
- KT-1000 is still considered the gold standard in objective AP measurement of knee ligamentous laxity despite the fact it is no longer in production.
- Second-generation arthrometers have the promise of creating greater precision, accuracy, portability, and the ability to measure laxity in multiple planes.

References

1. Anderson AF, Snyder RB, Federspiel CF, Lipscomb AB (1992) Instrumented evaluation of knee laxity: a comparison of five arthrometers. Am J Sports Med 20:135–140
2. Bach BR Jr, Jones GT, Hager CA, Sweet FA, Luergans S (1995) Arthrometric results of arthroscopically assisted anterior cruciate ligament reconstruction using autograft patellar tendon substitution. Am J Sports Med 23:179–185
3. Bach BR Jr, Levy ME, Bojchuk J, Tradonsky S, Bush-Joseph CA, Khan NH (1998) Single-incision endoscopic anterior cruciate ligament reconstruction using patellar tendon autograft. Minimum two year follow-up evaluation. Am J Sports Med 26:30–40
4. Bach BR Jr, Tradonsky S, Bojchuk J, Levy ME, Bush-Joseph CA, Khan NH (1998) Arthroscopically

assisted anterior cruciate ligament reconstruction using patellar tendon autograft. Five- to nine year follow-up evaluation. Am J Sports Med 26:20–29
5. Bach BR Jr, Warren RF, Flynn WM, Kroll M, Wickiewiecz TL (1990) Arthrometric evaluation of knees that have a torn anterior cruciate ligament. J Bone Joint Surg Am 72:1299–1306
6. Balasch H, Schiller M, Friebel H, Hoffmann F (1999) Evaluation of anterior knee joint instability with the Rolimeter: a test in comparison with manual assessment and measuring with the KT-1000 arthrometer. Knee Surg Sports Traumatol Arthrosc 7: 204–208
7. Ballantyne BT, French AK, Heimsoth SL, Kachingwe AF, Lee JB, Soderberg GL (1995) Influence of examiner experience and gender on inter-rater reliability of KT-1000 arthrometer measurements. Phys Ther 75:898–906
8. Berry J, Kramer K, Binkley J et al (1999) Error estimates in novice and expert raters for the KT-1000 arthrometer. J Orthop Sports Phys Ther 29:49–55
9. Boniface RJ, Fu FH, Ilkhanipour K (1986) Objective anterior cruciate ligament testing. Orthopedics 9:391–393
10. Bouguennec N et al (2015) Comparative reproducibility of TELOS and GNRB for instrumental measurement of anterior tibial translation in normal knees. Orthop Traumatol Surg 101:301–305
11. Branch T, Browne J, Campbell J et al (2010) Rotational laxity greater in patients with contralateral anterior cruciate ligament injury than healthy volunteers. Knee Surg Sports Traumatol Arthrosc 18:1379–1384
12. Branch T, Mayr HO, Browne JE, Campbell JC, Stoehr A, Jacobs CA (2010) Instrumented examination of anterior cruciate ligament injuries: minimizing flaws of the manual clinical examination. Arthroscopy 26:997–1004
13. Burks RT, Lelan R (1988) Determination of graft tension before fixation in anterior cruciate ligament reconstruction. Arthroscopy 4:260
14. Chouliaras V, Ristanis S, Moraiti C, Stergiou N, Georgoulis A (2007) Effectiveness of reconstruction of the anterior cruciate ligament with quadrupled hamstrings and bone-patellar tendon- bone autografts. An in vivo study comparing tibial internal-external rotation. Am J Sports Med 35:189–196
15. Chouliaras V, Ristanis S, Moraiti C, Tzimas V, Stergiou N, Georgoulis A (2009) Anterior cruciate ligament reconstruction with a quadrupled hamstrings tendon autograft does not restore tibial rotation to normative levels during landing from a jump and subsequent pivoting. J Sport Med Phys Fitness 49:64–70
16. Collette M, Courville J, Forton M, Gagnière B (2012) Objective evaluation of anterior knee laxity; comparison of the KT-1000 and GNRB arthrometers. Knee Surg Sports Traumatol Arthrosc 20(11):2233–2238
17. Craig JC, Go L, Belchinger J et al (2005) Three-tesla imaging of the knee: initial experience. Skeletal Radiol 34:453–461
18. Dahlstedt LJ, Dalen N (1989) Knee laxity in cruciate ligament injury: value of examination under anesthesia. Acta Orthop Scan 60:181
19. Daniel D, Stone ML (1990) Instrumented measurement of knee motion. In: O'Connor J (ed) Knee ligaments: structure, function, injury, and repair. Raven Press, New York, pp 421–426
20. Daniel DM, Malcom LL, Losse G et al (1985) Instrumented measurement of anterior laxity of the knee. J Bone Joint Surg 67A:720–726
21. Daniel DM, Stone ML, Sachs R, Malcom L (1985) Instrumented measurement of anterior knee laxity in patients with acute anterior cruciate ligament disruption. Am J Sports Med 13:401–407
22. Eastlack M, Axe M, Snyder-Mackler L (1999) Laxity, instability, and functional outcome after ACL injury: copers versus noncopers. Med Sci Sports Exerc 31:210–215
23. Edixhoven P, Huiskes R, De Graaf R, van Rens TJ, Slooff TJ (1987) Accuracy and reproducibility of instrumented knee-drawer tests. J Orthop Res 5:378–387
24. Feller JA, Webster KE (2003) A randomized comparison of patellar tendon and hamstring tendon anterior cruciate ligament reconstruction. Am J Sports Med 31:564–573
25. Ferretti A, Valeo L, Mazza D, Muliere L, Iorio P, Giovannetti G, Conteduca F, Iorio R (2014) Smartphone versus knee ligament arthrometer when size does not matter. Int Orthop 38(10):2197–2199
26. Fleming BC, Johnson RJ, Shapiro E, Fenwick J, Howe JG, Pope MH (1992) Clinical versus instrumented knee testing on autopsy specimens. Clin Orthop Relat Res 282:196–207
27. Freedman KB, D'Amato MF, Nedeff DD et al (2003) Arthroscopic anterior cruciate ligament reconstruction: a meta-analysis comparing patellar tendon and hamstring tendon autografts. Am J Sports Med 32:2
28. Goldblatt JP, Fitzsimmons SE, Balk E, Richmond JC (2005) Reconstruction of the anterior cruciate ligament: meta-analysis of patellar tendon versus hamstring tendon autograft. Arthroscopy 21(7):791–803
29. Harter RA, Osternig LR, Singer KM, James SL, Larson RL, Jones DC (1988) Long-term evaluation of knee stability and function following surgical reconstruction for anterior cruciate ligament insufficiency. Am J Sports Med 16:434–443
30. Harter RA, Osternig LR, Singer KM (1989) Instrumented Lachman tests for the evaluation of anterior laxity after reconstruction of the anterior cruciate ligament. J Bone Joint Surg Am 71:975–983
31. Higgins RW, Steadman JR (1987) Anterior cruciate ligament repairs in world class skiers. Am J Sports Med 15:439
32. Highgenboten CL, Jackson AW, Jansson KA, Meske NB (1992) KT-1000 arthrometer: conscious and unconscious test results using 15, 20, and 30 pounds of force. Am J Sports Med 20:450–454
33. Highgenboten CL, Jackson A, Meske NB (1989) Genucom, KT-1000, and Stryker knee laxity

measuring device comparisons. Device reproducibility and interdevice comparison in asymptomatic subjects. Am J Sports Med 17:743–746
34. Holm I, Oiestad BE, Risberg MA, Aune AK (2010) No difference in knee function or prevalence of osteoarthritis after reconstruction of the anterior cruciate ligament with 4-strand hamstring autograft versus patellar tendon-bone autograft: a randomized study with 10-year follow-up. Am J Sports Med 38(3):448–454
35. Keays SL, Bullock-Saxton JE, Keays AC, Newcombe PA, Bullock MI (2007) A 6-year follow-up of the effect of graft site on strength, stability, range of motion, function, and joint degeneration after anterior cruciate ligament reconstruction: patellar tendon versus semitendinosus and Gracilis tendon graft. Am J Sports Med 35(5):729–739
36. King JB, Kumar SJ (1989) The Stryker knee arthrometer in clinical practice. Am J Sports Med 17:649–650
37. Kocher M, Steadman J, Briggs K, Sterett W, Hawkins R (2004) Relationships between objective assessment of ligament stability and subjective assessment of symptoms and function after anterior cruciate ligament reconstruction. Am J Sports Med 32:629–634
38. Kowalk DL, Wojtys EM, Disher J et al (1993) Quantitative analysis of the measuring capabilities of the KT-1000 knee ligament arthrometer. Am J Sports Med 21:744
39. Leitze Z, Losee RE, Jokl P, Johnson TR, Feagin JA (2005) Implications of the pivot shift in the ACL-deficient knee. Clin Orthop Relat Res 436:229–236
40. Li S, Su W, Zhao J, Xu Y, Bo Z, Ding X, Wei Q (2011) A meta-analysis of hamstring autografts versus bone-patellar tendon-bone autografts for reconstruction of the anterior cruciate ligament. Knee 18(5):287–293
41. Liu SH, Osti L, Henry M, Bocchi L (1995) The diagnosis of acute complete tears of the anterior cruciate ligament. Comparison of MRI, arthrometry and clinical examination. J Bone Joint Surg Br 77:586–588
42. Lorbach O, Brockmeyer M, Kieb M et al (2012) Objective measurement devices to assess static rotational knee laxity: focus on the rotameter. Knee Surg Sports Traumatol Arthrosc 20(4):639–644
43. Lorbach O, Kieb M, Brogard P, Maas S, Pape D, Seil R (2012) Static rotational and sagittal knee laxity measurements after reconstruction of the anterior cruciate ligament. Knee Surg Sports Traumatol Arthrosc 20(5):844–850
44. Lustig S, Magnussen RA, Cheze L, Neyret P (2012) The KneeKG system: a review of the literature. Knee Surg Sports Traumatol Arthrosc 20(4):633–638
45. Malcom LL, Daniel DM, Stone ML, Sachs R (1985) The measurement of anterior knee laxity after ACL reconstructive surgery. Clin Orthop Relat Res 196:35–41
46. Markolf KL, Amstutz HC (1987) The clinical relevance of instrumented testing for ACL insufficiency. Experience with the UCLA clinical knee testing apparatus. Clin Orthop Relat Res 223:198–207
47. Markolf KL, Graff-Radford A, Amstutz HC (1978) In vivo knee stability. A quantitative assessment using an instrumented clinical testing apparatus. J Bone Joint Surg Am 60:664–674
48. Markolf KL, Mensch JS, Amstutz HG (1976) Stiffness and laxity of the knee: the contributions of the supporting structures – a quantitative in vitro study. J Bone Joint Surg Am 58:583
49. McQuade KJ, Sidles JA, Larson RV (1989) Reliability of the genucom knee analysis system. A pilot study. Clin Orthop Relat Res 245:216–219
50. Muellner T, Bugge W, Johansen S, Holtan C, Engebretsen L (2001) Inter- and intra-tester comparison of the rolimeter knee tester: effect of tester's experience and the examination technique. Knee Surg Sports Traumatol Arthrosc 9:302–306
51. Noyes F, Grood E, Cummings J, Wroble R (1991) Analysis of the pivot-shift phenomenon. The knee motion and subluxations induced by different examiners. Am J Sports Med 19:148–155
52. Oliver JH, Coughlin LP (1987) Objective knee evaluation using the Genucom Knee Analysis System. Clinical implications. Am J Sports Med 15:571–578
53. Paine R, Lowe W (2012) Comparison of Kneelax and KT-1000 knee ligament arthrometers. J Knee Surg 25(2):151–154
54. Papannagari R, Gill T, DeFrate L, Moses J, Petruska A, Li G (2006) In vivo kinematics of the knee after anterior cruciate ligament reconstruction. Am J Sports Med 34:2006–2012
55. Patent 4712542. N.d. Print
56. Patent 4969471. N.d. Print
57. Pollet V, Barrat D, Meirhaeghe E, Vaes P, Handelberg F (2005) The role of the Rolimeter in quantifying knee instability compared to the functional outcome of ACL-reconstructed versus conservatively-treated knees. Knee Surg Sports Traumatol Arthrosc 13:12–18
58. Prodromos CC, Han YS, Keller BL et al (2005) Stability of hamstring anterior cruciate ligament reconstruction at two to eight year follow. Arthroscopy 21:138–146
59. Queale WS, Snyder-Mackler L, Handling KA, Richards JG (1994) Instrumented examination of knee laxity in patients with anterior cruciate deficiency: a comparison of the KT-2000, Knee Signature System, and Genucom. J Orthop Sports Phys Ther 19:345–351
60. Rangger C, Daniel DM, Stone ML, Kaufman K (1993) Diagnosis of an ACL disruption with KT-1000 arthrometer measurements. Knee Surg Sports Traumatol Arthrosc 1:60–66
61. Riederman R, Wroble RR, Grood ES, VanGinkel L, Shaffer BL (1991) Reproducibility of the knee signature system. Am J Sports Med 19:660–664
62. Rijke AM, Perrin DH, Goitz HT et al (1994) Instrumented arthrometry for diagnosing partial versus complete anterior cruciate ligament tears. Am J Sports Med 22:294
63. Robert H, Nouveau S, Gageot S, Gagniere B (2009) A new knee arthrometer, the GNRB: experience in ACL complete and partial tears. Orthop Traumatol Surg Res 95:171–176

64. Sernert N, Helmers J, Kartus C, Ejerhed L, Kartus J (2007) Knee laxity measurements examined by a left-handed and a right-hand-dominant physiotherapist, in patients with anterior cruciate ligament injuries and healthy controls. Knee Surg Sports Traumatol Arthrosc 15:1181–1186
65. Sherman OH, Markolf KL, Ferkel RD (1987) Measurements of anterior laxity in normal and anterior cruciate absent knees with two instrumented test devices. Clin Orthop Relat Res 215:156–161
66. Shino K, Inoue M, Horibe S, Nakamura H, Ono K (1987) Measurement of anterior instability of the knee. J Bone Joint Surg 69B:608–613
67. Shultz SJ, Shimokochi Y, Nguyen AD, Schmitz RJ, Beynnon BD, Perrin DH (2007) Measurement of varus-valgus and internal-external rotational knee laxities in vivo, part I: assessment of measurement reliability and bilateral asymmetry. J Orthop Res 25:989–996
68. Snyder-Mackler L, Fitzgerald G, Bartolozzi AI et al (2009) The relationship between passive joint laxity and functional outcome after anterior cruciate ligament injury. Am J Sports Med 25:191–195
69. Steiner ME, Brown C, Zarins B, Brownstein B, Koval PS, Stone P (1990) Measurement of anterior-posterior displacement of the knee. A comparison of the results with instrumented devices and with clinical examination. J Bone Joint Surg Am 72:1307–1315
70. Strand T, Solheim E (1995) Clinical tests versus KT-1000 instrumented laxity test in acute anterior cruciate ligament tears. Int J Sports Med 16:51–53
71. Thomas P et al (2010) Instrumented examination of anterior cruciate ligament injuries: minimizing flaws of the manual clinical examination branch. Arthroscopy 26(7):997–1004
72. Torzilli PA, Panariello RA, Forbes A, Santner TJ, Warren RF (1991) Measurement reproducibility of two commercial knee test devices. J Orthop Res 9:730–737
73. Tsai A, Musahl V, Steckel H et al (2008) Rotational knee laxity: reliability of a simple measurement device in vivo. BMC Musculoskelet Disord 9:35
74. Tsai KJ, Chiang H, Jiang CC (2004) Magnetic resonance imaging of anterior cruciate ligament rupture. BMC Musculoskelet Disord 8:21
75. Uh BS, Beynnon BD, Churchill DL, Haugh LD, Risberg MA, Fleming BC (2001) A new device to measure knee laxity during weightbearing and non-weightbearing conditions. J Orthop Res 19:1185–1191
76. Van Der Hart C, Van Den Bekerom M, Patt T (2008) The occurrence of osteoarthritis at a minimum of ten years after reconstruction of the anterior cruciate ligament. J Orthop Surg 3:24
77. Vellet AD, Lee DH, Munk PL et al (1995) Anterior cruciate ligament tear: prospective evaluation of diagnostic accuracy of middle and high field strength MR imaging at 1.5 and 0.5 T. Radiology 197:826–830
78. Wang CWBB (1990) Clinical diagnosis of ACL-deficient knees. J Orthop Surg 7:139
79. Wroble RR, Grood ES, Noyes FR, Schmitt DJ (1990) Reproducibility of Genucom Knee Analysis system testing. Am J Sports Med 18:387–395
80. Wroble RR, Van Ginkel LA, Grood ES, Noyes FR, Shaffer BL (1990) Repeatability of the KT-1000 arthrometer in a normal population. Am J Sports Med 18:396–399

Development of the IKDC Forms 12

Allen F. Anderson, James J. Irrgang, and Christian N. Anderson

Contents

A.F. Anderson, MD (✉) • C.N. Anderson, MD
Tennessee Orthopaedic Alliance, 4230 Harding Road, Suite 1000, Nashville, TN 37205, USA
e-mail: AndersonAF@toa.com

J.J. Irrgang, PhD, PT, ATC
Department of Orthopedic Surgery, University of Pittsburg, Pittsburg, PA, USA

12.1 Historic Methods

The evolution of knee surgery has been predicated on the development, refinement, and evaluation of new surgical techniques. Historically, empiric assessment was used to document the relative efficacy of treatment. This unscientific approach often resulted in erroneous conclusions by researchers.

The problem lies not in veracity but rather in human nature, subjective interpretation of variables, and the difficulty of evaluating results. Even the most consciousness researcher, especially the surgeon, is subject to bias. The knowledge and perceptual ability of the examiner is an important variable. Experienced examiners frequently produce appreciable differences in translation and rotation when evaluating the limits of knee motion. Even when the examiners produce the same displacement, the correct interpretation depends on accurate perception of the motion.

The complexity of the knee and the number of criteria used to assess results make accurate evaluation even more difficult. Anderson et al. [1] found that the problem was exacerbated by the number of operative procedures and diverse methods of evaluation described in the 1980s. They [1] reported that, during that decade, 52 articles were published in the *American Journal of Sports Medicine* and the *Journal of Bone and Joint Surgery American* on conservative or operative treatment of the ACL-deficient knee. Twenty-eight

V. Musahl et al. (eds.), *Rotatory Knee Instability*, DOI 10.1007/978-3-319-32070-0_12

different operative procedures were described, including primary repair, five extra-articular procedures, 13 intra-articular procedures, and 9 combined intra- and extra-articular reconstructions. The results of these procedures were rated as good or excellent in the majority of cases, although they were evaluated with 38 different rating scales.

The consensus among the researchers who have compared rating scales is that the differences are sufficiently great to preclude predicting results from one scale based on another and that inconsistency among these scales created an impediment to progress in the field.

12.2 Development of the IKDC Standard Knee Evaluation Form

The consensus was that a uniform scale was vital to the evaluation of treatment. Under the leadership of John Feagin from the United States and Werner Mueller from Switzerland, and the auspices of the American Orthopaedic Society for Sports Medicine and the European Society of Knee Surgery and Arthroscopy, the International Knee Documentation Committee (IKDC) was formed in 1987 to develop a standardized, international documentation system.

The initial objectives of the committee were to develop a form that was one page, including only the essential reproducible criteria necessary to evaluate results and to develop a form simple enough to be used by any clinician, both with and without research assistance. Second, the form was developed only for acute ACL injuries, but it was anticipated that this would serve as a foundation for a more comprehensive evaluation system, allowing for a valid scientific analysis of knee function. The first step was to agree on standard terminology to document knee motion and function. Next, the clinical examination of the limits of knee motion was critiqued, and a core of measurements was adopted. Finally, methods for documentation of activity, evaluation of limb function, and assessment of symptoms were evaluated, and a format was designed to record these observations.

12.3 Development of Standard Terminology

The discrepancy in the implied meaning of terms used in the literature has been an impediment to international communication. To improve communication, the IKDC met in New York in August 1987 to discuss standard terminology [6]. Noyes, Grood, and Torzilli [24] submitted definitions of terms for motion, position of the knee, and injuries of the ligaments. The committee critiqued, revised, and adopted a standard set of definitions. The following definitions are among those adopted [24]:

Motion: the act or process of changing position. Motion is described as the rate and direction of change.

Displacement: the net effect of motion; a change in position between two points without regard to the path followed. Displacement may be described by a change in translation or in rotation, each of which has three degrees of freedom.

Translation: motion of a rigid body in which all lines remain parallel to their original orientation. By convention, knee translation is described as motion of the tibia relative to the femur. Translation of the tibia may be mediolateral, anteroposterior, or proximodistal. Translation is measured in millimeters. The reference point normally used to measure translation is midway between the medial and lateral margins of the joint.

Rotation: a type of motion or displacement in which all points move about an axis. Rotations of the knee may be flexion-extension, internal-external, and abduction-adduction.

Range of motion: the displacement occurring between two limits of movement for each degree of freedom. Range of motion does not indicate the extremes of motion. For motion other than flexion-extension, range of motion depends on the angle of knee flexion.

Limits of knee motion: the extreme positions of movement possible for each of the 6 degrees of freedom. The term *limits of knee motion* is more specific than *range of motion*. It indicates where motion begins and ends and includes range of motion. There are 12 limits of motion, two for each 6 degrees of freedom. Ligament injury increases the limits of knee motion. The European system describes the limits of flexion and extension with three numbers: the maximum extension, neutral position, and flexion.

Coupled motions: a displacement or motion in 1 or more degrees of freedom caused by a load applied in another degree of freedom. Coupled motions occur during the clinical examination. An anterior displacement force applied during the Lachman test causes anterior translation and internal rotation of the tibia. A posterior displacement force results in posterior translation and external rotation. The amount of motion depends on the force applied and the constraints of the coupled motion. For example, constraint of rotation during the Lachman test significantly diminishes anterior translation.

Laxity: a lack of tension; looseness, referring to a normal or abnormal range of motion. In the first context, laxity is used to describe a lack of tension in a ligament and, in the second, as a looseness of a joint. This ambiguous term should be used to indicate lack of tension in the ligament. The degree of laxity should be specified as either normal or abnormal. Laxity should not be used in the context of looseness of a joint; the motion should be specified. The term *anterior translation* is preferable to *anterior joint laxity*.

Instability is another ambiguous term that has been used in two ways. First, it is used to describe the symptoms of giving way and, second, as the sign of increased joint motion. Rather than use *instability* to refer to symptoms, it is preferable to describe the event (i.e., giving way with activity). It is incorrect to designate a specific anatomic structure as the cause of ACL instability; rather, instability should only be used in the general sense to indicate excessive motion of the tibia as the result of traumatic injury.

Fact Box 1
The discrepancy in the implied meaning of terms used in the literature has been an impediment to international communication.

12.4 Limits of Knee Motion Evaluation

The methods of examination that have been used to determine the limits of knee motion are qualitative and clinician specific. Even experienced examiners may produce and perceive appreciable differences in displacement. Accurate assessment of translation and rotation is more demanding in ligament injuries, which increase more than one limit of motion. In these circumstances, clinicians have difficulty identifying either the starting or ending positions for the tibia.

The objectives of the second IKDC meeting in Zurich, Switzerland, in 1988 were, first, to agree on the clinical tests essential to evaluation of knee motion limits and, second, to identify the conditions that maximize the accuracy and reproducibility of measurements.

The consensus was that reproducibility depends on specifying the conditions of the tests. Clinical and laboratory studies confirm that the position of the knee at the initiation of testing affects displacement. The site of measurement must be identified, and the magnitude, direction, and point of application of force should be specified. Measurements in translation should be reported in millimeters and rotation in degrees. Changes in any of these conditions will result in different interpretations of the tests.

Subsequently, the IKDC convened in Jackson Hole, Wyoming, in July 1988 for its third meeting. The objective of this meeting was to determine the accuracy of the clinical tests and conditions for testing adopted at the Zurich meeting. Three studies were performed to assess the reproducibility of clinical measurements, differences in test techniques, and clinical accuracy in estimating knee displacement [24–26].

Ten patients were examined by eleven IKDC members to determine the reproducibility of clinical measures [24]. Nine of the ten patients had sustained a ligament injury. The examination technique and recording system were standardized and reviewed by the examiners before testing. The patients also underwent an instrumented knee examination with the KT-1000, KSS, and Genucom.

The examiners estimated anteroposterior translation in millimeters and rotation in degrees, at both 25 and 90° of flexion. A thigh support was used to facilitate relaxation and standardize testing at 25° of flexion. When testing at 90° of flexion, the sole of the foot supported the limb. The sagittal knee profile or quadriceps active drawer test was used to evaluate the normal anatomic position.

Varus-valgus stress tests were measured at 0° and 25° of flexion. The pivot shift and reverse pivot shift tests were performed with the tibia in internal, neutral, and external rotation. These tests were graded in the following manner: 0 = none, 1 = glide, 2 = moderate, and 3 = severe.

The results of this study demonstrated that, even with benefit of standardized test techniques, a significant discrepancy existed in the examiner's estimation of displacement. The greatest differences occurred in the evaluation of anteroposterior translation. One clinician recorded a side-to-side difference of greater than 3 mm in all eight patients, and another examiner only reported one patient with a side-to-side difference of greater than 3 mm. Analysis of the data revealed that the correlation between the examiners was better for total anteroposterior translation than for either anterior or posterior displacement.

The second study was performed to identify the differences in examination techniques contributing to the discrepancy in estimation of displacement. Another objective of this study was to determine the accuracy of the clinicians' estimate of tibiofemoral displacement [25]. In this study, 11 members of the IKDC examined two cadaver knees that were instrumented with a device to measure three-dimensional motion. The examiners' estimation of joint displacement was compared with the actual measurements recorded by the instrumented spatial linkage system. The ACL and MCLs were cut in one knee. The examination included estimation of anteroposterior displacement, mediolateral joint opening, and internal/external rotation.

The examiners were accurate in diagnosing injuries of these ligaments. Nine of the ten examiners correctly diagnosed a complete tear of the ACL and MCL, and the other two diagnosed partial tears of the ACL and MCL.

The examiners were not as accurate with the rotation tests. Seven of the eleven examiners misinterpreted the external tibial rotation associated with MCL injury as injury to the posterolateral ligaments. This error indicated that the examiners were incapable of determining if the medial tibial plateau came forward or the lateral tibial plateau went back. The tests that assess rotation are not accurate, even for experienced examiners.

The actual measurements of anterior tibial translation produced during the Lachman tests range from 7 to 16 mm. The discrepancy in displacement related to differences in the position of the knee at the initiation of testing (range of flexion of 2–25°) and the magnitude of displacement forces. The constraint of coupled motions did not significantly influence the measured displacement. Only three examiners estimated anterior displacement within 2 mm of the measured value, five estimated the displacement between 2 and 4 mm, and the estimates of two examiners were more than 5 mm different from the measured value.

Significant differences in displacement were produced by the examiners for both internal/external rotation and mediolateral joint opening. The knee flexion angle at the initiation of testing varied widely among the examiners. Some examiners started the mediolateral opening test with the femoral condyle in contact with the tibial plateau, and others did not. Even so, the examiners were more accurate in estimating medial joint opening; either of the examiners estimated displacement within 3 mm of the measured displacement.

In summary, only six of the examiners estimated true anteroposterior displacement within a range of 2 mm, tibial rotation within 5 mm, and medial joint opening within 3 mm.

Fact Box 2
The reproducibility of the clinical examination depends on specifying the conditions of the tests, including magnitude and direction of force, site of measurement, and point of application of force. However, even in the best of circumstances, large variations may exist in clinician's estimates of displacement. Consequently, objective estimation of pathologic knee laxity by clinicians is qualitative, at best, and therefore cannot be validated.

These studies demonstrate that limb position, site of measurement, and application of force should be standardized. Even under the best circumstances, large variations may exist in clinicians' estimates of displacement. Consequently, instrumented or stress radiography measurements should be used to report clinical results. The rotation tests are even more difficult to assess than either anterior posterior or mediolateral displacement. Evaluation of rotary subluxation is subject to error and the rotational test cannot be validated.

12.5 Analysis of the Pivot Shift Test

In the third study conducted at the Jackson Hole meeting, each member of the IKDC performed their versions of the pivot shift test on the instrumented cadaveric limbs [25]. Like the anteroposterior displacement tests, the beginning test position varied between examiners, although it was typically close to extension. The difference in maximum anterior translation of the medial tibial plateau recorded during the pivot shift ranged from 6 to 17 mm, and the maximum subluxation of the lateral plateau ranged from 14 to 20 mm among the examiners.

Analysis of the data confirmed that the examiners constrain knee motion when performing the pivot shift test. The coupled knee motions of anterior translation and internal tibial rotation were induced to produce anterior subluxation. The examiners who internally rotated the tibia most in performing the test also limited anterior translation of the medial tibial plateau. One examiner performed the test in internal, neutral, and external rotation. The greatest translation of both the medial and lateral tibial plateaus occurred in neutral and external rotation of the tibia. The committee recommended avoiding internal tibial rotation when performing the pivot shift test.

The variability of measurement indicated the pivot shift could only be considered a qualitative test. At that time, in vivo measurement devices were not available to quantitate displacement in millimeters; consequently, the committee recommended grading the pivot shift: negative; 1+, glide; 2+, clunk; 3+, gross.

After analyzing the data of these three studies, the committee recommended but did not validate instrumented or radiographic measurement of the Lachman test, at 25° of flexion, total anteroposterior translation at 70° of flexion, and medial and lateral joint opening at 20° of flexion, and the qualitative, pivot shift, and reverse pivot shift tests.

12.6 Documentation of Activity

By consensus, the committee agreed that limitation of knee function may be masked by involuntary low-activity levels. The criterion "return to sports" was considered imprecise because different activities place different demands on the knee. The IKDC field tested a comprehensive form evaluating the level of difficulty, intensity, and exposure. Intensity describes the level of activity as occupational, light recreational sports, vigorous recreational sports, or competitive sports. Exposure, the best estimate of the number of hours per year at a given functional level and intensity, was recorded only for participation of more than 50 h/year.

Changes in activity may occur for knee-related or non-knee-related reasons. A decline in athletic activity and participation is inherent with aging, and a question was included to specify the reasons for any changes in activity.

After field testing the comprehensive form, the committee selected the minimum criteria necessary to evaluate activity. The functional tests are as follows: I, strenuous; II, moderate; III, light; and IV, sedentary. These are based on the demands that certain activities place on the knee. Assessment of activity is equally important for patients who do not participate in sports. Heavy manual work was assigned a level II rating, light work a level III rating, and activities of daily living a level IV rating.

The level of activity at which the patient is able to perform, without significant symptoms, is recorded before injury, before treatment, and after treatment. Credit is not given for participation in activities that cause significant symptoms (i.e., "knee abusers"). Two questions were included in the IKDC form to determine how the knee affected activity. One of these questions – "How does your knee affect your activity level?" – was graded 0–3.

12.7 Symptoms and Impairment

The committee recognized that the magnitude of symptoms and impairments is difficult to quantitate, and the collection of data is prone to bias. Even so, this important category has been included in every rating scale.

The symptoms and impairments were evaluated in the field test. The symptoms of pain, swelling, and giving way were universal to earlier knee rating systems. Giving way indicates an event precipitated by a pathologic tibiofemoral shift. It should not be mistaken for the buckling caused by weakness or other conditions. Partial giving way is not associated with falling or swelling, although these events are included in full giving way.

Patients with pathologic conditions frequently decrease activity to avoid symptoms. To detect these patients and prevent an exaggerated symptom score, the committee adopted the philosophy of relating symptoms to activity. Other patients who are capable of performing strenuous activities without symptoms may avoid them by choice. To prevent a reduction of a symptom score in these cases, patients are asked to grade the highest activity at which they can participate without symptoms, even if they are not participating at that level.

In general, the impairments had not been included in the published rating scales, and the IKDC did not consider them among the minimal essential criteria. The subjective assessment questions and evaluation of symptoms in the IKDC form provide an overall assessment of impairment.

12.8 Compartment and Roentgenographic Findings

Restoration of stability and prevention of degenerative changes are long-term goals of knee reconstruction, but evaluation of success in attaining this goal is difficult. Early degenerative changes cannot be accurately evaluated without visual inspection, and roentgenographic changes occur late in the course of osteoarthritis. Assessment of crepitation was included in the IKDC form to detect early compartment changes. Unfortunately, only limited conclusions may be drawn from the evaluation of crepitation. The collection of data is subject to examiner bias, and crepitation may not indicate articular cartilage abnormality. Crepitation associated with pain is a significant finding that is graded more stringently.

Roentgenographic changes are also qualitatively graded. A mild grade indicates flattening of the femoral condyle, subchondral sclerosis, or small osteophytes. The moderate and severe grades had progressive joint narrowing in addition to these changes.

Evaluations of compartment and roentgenographic findings are not included in the final evaluation of the IKDC form. These data are qualitative and influenced by investigator bias.

12.9 Functional Tests

The IKDC critiqued the methods that have been used to evaluate limb function. Gait analysis, instrumented strength testing (i.e., Cybex evaluation), agility tests, and hop tests provide quantitative data that compare the involved knee to the normal knee. Instrumented examination was excluded because it requires expensive equipment that is not universally available.

The single-leg hop is more accurate and easier to perform than the agility tests. Although a normal score does not preclude giving way with activity, an abnormal score is correlated with significant functional limitations. The single-leg hop test is a useful screening test that provides quantitative data [27]. Like the compartment and roentgenographic findings, the results are recorded but not graded.

12.10 Rating Results

Rating results are fundamental to the evaluation and comparison of different methods of treatment. The methods of grading that have been used reflect differences in philosophy, which are as diverse as the rating scales themselves. Most scales have used a numeric system to assign points to each variable. In some scales, points are added to produce a single-digit total score, whereas others categorize the results as excellent, good, fair, or poor. Tegner and Lysholm [34] and Feagin and Blake [7] recommended separate scores for symptoms, subjective function, and clinical findings.

Numeric grading systems are popular because they are easy to understand, although some investigators condemn assigning points to variable, stating that this practice requires an arbitrary judgment of the relative importance of a variable to the knee as a whole. The numbers reflect the values of the author and not necessarily the clinical outcome. Apley once declared that "we should resist the seductive simplicity of numerical scores and we should abandon the practice of adding unrelated scores" [3].

The IKDC adopted the system used by Noyes et al. [23] and the Swiss knee group [21], in which the lowest grade within a group determines the group grade and the worst group grade determines the final evaluation.

Fact Box 3
The original IKDC Knee Ligament Standard Evaluation Form made an important contribution by serving as a rudimentary form that functioned as a foundation for a more advanced evaluation system.

The IKDC Knee Ligament Standard Evaluation Form was published in 1993 [12] but never validated. It made an important contribution by serving as a rudimentary form that functioned as a foundation for more advanced evaluation systems. The future goals of the IKDC were to refine the standard form, identify additional important and reproducible criteria, and develop a comprehensive method of evaluation.

12.11 Evidence-Based Medicine

A new paradigm of assessment, evidence-based medicine, called into question our fundamental basis of learning. An important tenet of evidence-based medicine is the conscientious, explicit, and judicious use of current best evidence in making decisions about the care of individual patients. The best research evidence places emphasis on patient-centered research related to the accuracy of diagnosis, power of prognostic identification, and efficacy and safety of surgical interventions.

Historically, researchers did not have outcome instruments to accurately measure the quality of life impacting complaints (with an ACL tear, those complaints may be subjective, pain, instability, and functional limitations). Therefore, researchers were forced to use surrogate measures (i.e., objective measures such as range of motion, strength, and laxity) for what the surgeon and patient really cared about. Although these impairment measures appear to have accuracy because they can be reduced to a number, they often suffer from poor intra-rater and inter-rater reliability because these measures contain elements of subjective measurements by the examiner as documented by the IKDC studies. In addition, they have poor correlation with important domains of health to the patient. Consequently, the relationship between impairment of body structures and function to activity limitations and participation restrictions is not direct. For example, some authors have demonstrated there is no relationship between anterior displacement measured with KT-1000 and patient-reported activity and participation [17, 32].

Fact Box 4

Although these impairment measures appear to have accuracy because they can be reduced to a number, they often suffer from poor intra-rater and inter-rater reliability because these measures contain elements of subjective measurements by the examiner as documented by the IKDC studies.

In contrast to objective measures, many subjective clinical measures might not appear to be reliable or valid but, when rigorously tested using well-established scientific methods, actually can be shown to be very reliable and valid. Activity and participation are of utmost concern to the patients. Therefore, health-related quality of life should be the primary outcome measure "how is the patient doing?". The secondary outcome should be "how is the knee doing?".

In March 1997, at John Feagin's request, the AOSSM Board of Directors moved to support the revision of the knee ligament evaluation form created by the IKDC. The board's interest in revision stemmed from the success of the initial form, as demonstrated by its widespread use, and the opportunity to integrate advances in the measurement of medical outcomes into the knee ligament form, making it more broadly applicable and credible.

Three members of the committee and Chad Munger from Data Harbor met in Sun Valley in June 1997 and developed the following objectives:

- To update the current objective portion of the IKDC form, enhance assessment of injuries and develop new modules for the objective evaluation of the PCL and patellofemoral components of the knee.
- Develop a new subjective evaluation form to assess patient-reported outcomes for measurement of function and symptoms.
- Evaluation of the psychometric properties of each module of the knee ligament evaluation form.
- Publish and disseminate results of testing.

Thereafter, between July and October 1997, the committee developed a work plan, budget, and list of additional individuals needed to ensure complete international representation and clinical expertise. The committee's preliminary work plan estimated development and testing for approximately 2.5 years, including psychometric evaluation and publication. In the fall of 1997, work on the revision process began. Members of the AOSSM included Allen Anderson (Chairman), John Bergfield, Art Boland, Mininder Kocher, John Feagin, Christopher Harner, Nick Motahi, John Richmond, Don Shelbourne, and Glenn Terry. ESSKA members included Hans Uli Staeubli, Roland Jakob, Philippe Neyret, Jorgen Hoeher, and Werner Mueller. APOSSM members included K. M. Chan, Masahiro Kurosaka, James Irrgang, M.S., P.T. psychometrician/consultant; Chad Munger, Data Harbor consultant; and John Fulkerson, ex officio. Committee members were assigned one of three work groups related to the ACL, PCL, or patellofemoral joint. Each member was charged with reviewing background material for the purposes of identifying new items or revisions to existing items that could be included in the objective portion of the form.

The other major objective included the development of a valid, reliable, and responsive IKDC Subjective Knee Form that would serve as an appropriate means by which to evaluate a variety of knee impairments, including ligament and meniscal injury, articular cartilage lesions, and patellofemoral pain. In this regard, the development of a single instrument that is valid for a variety of conditions affecting the knee could simplify data collection and also provide an opportunity to compare the impact of different knee conditions on the individual's level of symptoms, function, and sports activity. This objective influenced all phases of the IKDC development.

Finally, the committee felt that it was critical to develop a worldwide consensus of opinion to create a standard outcome form that would provide a uniform method of evaluation and facilitate the sharing of results and solving clinical problems.

The committee devised a demographic module primarily from the current health assessment module of modems. This module includes age, sex, race, and education items, as well as a fully tested comorbidity index. The general health questionnaire, SF36, was included because patients with knee conditions may have other health-related problems which would be reflected in lower scores on outcome assessment.

Between October 1997 and March 1998, three revisions of each form were completed, involving the addition, deletion, and modification of hundreds of items. By March 1998, the committee agreed to a testable version of the form, consisting of 42 questions.

At that time, James Irrgang Ph.D., P.T., A.T.C., a psychometrician who worked closely with the orthopedic community, was recruited by the committee to assist in the design and implementation of a study to evaluate the validity, reliability, and sensitivity of the revised form.

Field testing of the demographic, subjective, and objective assessment modules began in April 1998. Over an 8–10-week period, 144 patients completed the demographic and subjective modules. During this same period of time, the objective module was completed by 31 patients. The results were summarized and presented to the committee in Vancouver, British Columbia. Key findings were as follows:

- There were very few missing data for all of the items on the demographic module.
- There were substantial missing data for many of the items on the subjective module. This was particularly problematic for the items that were related to symptoms (i.e., pain, swelling, giving way, and locking). Additionally, the proportion of missing data was greater for items located at the end of the instrument, indicating the need to shorten the instrument to lessen the burden on patients.
- There were substantial missing data for many of the items included on the objective module. Items that were related to prior surgery, procedure, and diagnosis codes, status of the menisci, range of motion, and KT-1000 and hop tests had the greatest proportion of missing data.

Fact Box 5
The IKDC Subjective Knee Form was pilot tested on 144 patients. The results were used to modify the objective and subjective models. Field testing was performed by having 222 patients complete the subjective model and 211 the objective model. The results of analysis were used to modify the modules.

With the input of the committee, the results were used to modify the subjective and objective modules. Further testing of the revised subjective and objective modules was undertaken in August 1998. Two hundred twenty-two (222) patients completed the subjective module, and the objective module was completed for 211 patients. The results were summarized and reported to the committee in Boston, MA, in November 1998.

A summary of the results presented to the committee follows:

Subjective Module

- Problems with missing data for items on the subjective module were resolved. Most items had less than 10 % missing responses, and items with the highest proportion of missing responses continued to be those related to symptoms.
- An exploratory factor analysis indicated there was a single dominant trait underlying responses to the subjective module. Most of the items had a high loading on this dominant trait (i.e., there were high correlations between the item and the dominant trait). Broadly, this dominant trait reflected a combination of symptoms, function, and sports activity, which implies that it is reasonable to combine the item scores into a single total score to reflect an individual's level of function. Items with a low loading on the dominant factor were considered by the committee for elimination.
- A Rasch analysis was also performed to evaluate the subjective module. Overall, the results indicated that the Rasch model adequately fit the data. Collectively, the items measured a broad range of function. Several misfitting items (i.e., those items that did not conform to Rasch model) were identified and considered for elimination by the committee.
- A stepwise regression analysis was performed using the individual items to predict the total score (i.e., the sum of the item scores). The results indicated that 99.9 % of the variance of the total score could be predicted by 24 of the 42 items included on the scale. The committee used these results during the item reduction process.

Objective Module

- Problems with missing data on this version of the objective module were reduced. Most of the missing data were related to information that was not routinely measured or recorded during the history and physical examination, such as diagnosis and procedure codes, as well as the status of the menisci. Portions of the physical examination that continued to have a high proportion of missing data included crepitus, harvest site pathology, and one-legged hop and KT-1000 tests. A high proportion of the data for documentation of knee extension could not be interpreted as recorded on the form.
- An exploratory factor analysis was performed to determine the structure of the objective module. The results indicated that there were four or five factors underlying the objective module, and as a result, an orthogonal rotation was performed to clarify the meaning of the factors. Components of the objective module that loaded on the first factor included most of the laxity tests (Lachman, A-P translation, varus and valgus rotation, and pivot shift). The second factor represented crepitus and radiographic narrowing of the joint. The third factor represented loss of motion. The fourth and fifth factors represented the posterior drawer and reverse pivot shift tests, respectively. Given that the correlation between each of these factors was zero. These results question the validity of combining the results of the objective module into a single score.

Fact Box 6

Factor analysis demonstrated that it was reasonable to combine all the questions in the IKDC Subjective Knee Form into a single score.

The above results were used to modify the subjective and objective modules. By considering the statistical properties and content of the individual items, the committee reduced the subjective module from 42 items to 19 items. To modify the objective module, findings from the physical examination were separated from the historical data.

At the conclusion of the meeting in Boston, the committee requested additional information concerning the reduced version of the subjective module. This included a comparison of an individual's rating of function on an 11-point scale (i.e., 0–10) to a rating of function using the 4-point scale included in the original IKDC guidelines (i.e., normal to severely abnormal). Evidence that the items performed the same for those with and without a ligament injury was also requested. The data that were analyzed above were used to address these questions. To better describe the sample, the centers that submitted the original data were asked to provide demographic information including the subjects' age, sex, and diagnosis. The results were provided to the committee at its meeting in Anaheim, CA.

A summary of the findings is as follows:

- The rating of function on an 11-point scale was similar to the rating of function on the 4-point scale. The correlation between the two items was .71.
- An exploratory analysis of the reduced item set demonstrated a single dominant trait underlying the item responses. All of the items, except for the item related to locking, loaded highly on this trait.
- The Rasch model fit the data well. The items continued to measure a broad range of ability.
- To compare performance of the items for those with a ligament injury to those without a ligament injury, the diagnosis code was used to split the sample into two subsamples (i.e., those with a ligament injury and those without a ligament injury). A Rasch analysis was performed separately on each subsample. If the items performed the same for each group, one would expect the item statistics (i.e., the item difficulty parameters) to be the same for each sample. The results supported this premise. Thus, it appears that the items performed the same for those with a ligament injury compared to those without a ligament injury. Similar findings were found when the sample was split by age (i.e., the items performed the same for young and old individuals).
- Three scoring methods were compared. This included summing the item scores, summing the item scores using the results of the factor analysis to weight the items, and using the Rasch model to score the instrument. All three scoring methods yielded similar results. The distributions of the scores for each method were also similar. Additionally, the correlation between the three scoring methods ranged from .993 to .998. Thus, for simplicity sake, summing the scores was a satisfactory method to score the subjective module.

Several changes were made to some items in the subjective module during the committee meeting in 1999 in Anaheim, CA. To assess the effects of these changes and to describe the psychometric properties of the final version of the subjective module, additional data was gathered with the revised subjective module.

In 2001, the final version of the IKDC Subjective Knee Form (SKF), consisting of 18 questions, was administered to 590 patients with ligament injuries, meniscal injuries, patellofemoral pain, and osteoarthritis, to provide additional evidence that performance of the instrument was not dependent on diagnosis [13]. The average age of the patients was 37.5 years old and 52.6 % were males. In the sample, 76 % participated in sports activity; 19 % were competitive athletes, and 57 % were recreational athletes.

Fact Box 7

In 2001, the final version of the IKDC (SKF), consisting of 18 questions, was administered to 590 patients with ligament injuries, meniscal injuries, patellofemoral pain, and osteoarthritis.

The factor analysis demonstrated that it is reasonable to combine all of the questions in the IKDC Subjective Knee Score into a single score. Other patient-reported measures of symptoms and function have applied differential scoring based on the author's perception of what is important and how it should be scored rather than on statistical evidence.

Three different methods of scoring were evaluated. These included adding unweighted scores for the questions, a weighted sum of the questions that used the factor loadings from the factor analysis, and a method based on item response theory. The correlations among the three methods of scoring were all high. Additionally, the method of adding unweighted scores and the method based on item response theory identified the same five highest and lowest scoring subjects. Given these results and the simplicity of adding the unweighted scores was recommended over the other two methods of scoring.

The IKDC SKF has acceptable levels of internal consistency. A high value of coefficient alpha (0.92) indicated that the questions consistently measure the underlying construct of symptoms, function, and sports activity in patients with a variety of knee problems. The underlying concept for internal consistency is that the consistency with which a patient responds from one question to the next can be used to provide an estimate of reliability for the total test score [22].

Test-retest reliability and responsiveness are important characteristics of a rating scale designed to measure change over time [16]. Test-retest reliability reflects measurement error associated with repeated measurement when the patient's status remains the same. Thus, high levels of test-retest reliability imply that repeated measurements yield consistent scores when a patient's symptoms, function, and sports activity have remained constant. The IKDC SKF had high (0.94) levels of test-retest reliability.

Fact Box 8
Psychometric analysis demonstrated that the IKDC SKF functions similarly, regardless of age, sex, or diagnosis.

A major objective in the development of the IKDC SKF was to create a form that would be appropriate for patients with a variety of knee impairments, including ligament and meniscal injuries, articular cartilage lesions, and patellofemoral conditions. Item response theory was used to determine if the IKDC SKF would perform the same for young versus old, for men versus women, or for patients with different knee problems. The results indicated that, with few exceptions, the questions and therefore the entire form functioned similarly regardless of age, sex, or diagnosis.

12.12 Responsiveness

The next step in testing was to determine responsiveness of the IKDC SKF. Responsiveness is the ability of a form to detect minimal clinically important differences when the patient's status has changed [9]. Demonstration of responsiveness requires administration of the instrument on two or more occasions to patients who are expected to undergo change. To provide evidence for responsiveness, the IKDC SKF was administered longitudinally to 207 patients who had a variety of knee problems [14].

In summary, the IKDC SKF, a well-standardized outcome instrument, has been proven to be reliable, valid, and responsive for any measure of change in symptoms, function, and sports activity over time in patients with a variety of knee impairments.

Fact Box 9
The minimal detectable change, the change in score necessary to be certain that the change is greater than the measurement error of the outcome instrument, was 12.5. The minimal clinically important difference, the change in score necessary for the patient to perceive change that is clinically relevant, was 11.5.

12.13 Normative Data

The next step in standardization of the IKDC SKF was the collection of normative data. The primary purpose of this study was to provide clinicians and researchers with normative data that would place scores, changes in scores, and scores from male or female patients of different ages within the context of normal population values. Normative comparison facilitates the interpretation of results on the IKDC form for patient management decisions and for comparison between groups of patients by demonstrating how close patients come to the normal range of functioning.

The Subjective Knee Evaluation Form was mailed to 600 people in each of 8 age/gender categories (18–24 years, 25–34 years, 35–50 years, and 51–65 years for both male subjects and female subjects) [2]. Participants were drawn from a panel of 550,000 households (1,300,000 subjects) representative of noninstitutionalized persons in the United States and were matched to data from the United States Census Bureau on geographical region, market size, income, and household size.

Fact Box 10
Normative data were determined in each of 8 age/gender categories by testing 5,246 subjects.

Results Complete data were available for 5,246 knees. Twenty-eight percent of respondents reported an injury, weakness, or other problem with one or both knees. Normative data were determined for respondents as a whole and for the subset of respondents with no history of knee problems. Scores on the IKDC Subjective Knee Evaluation Form vary by age, gender, and history of knee problems. The normative data published in 2006 allow clinicians to interpret how patients with knee injuries are functioning relative to their age- and gender-matched peers and will enable researchers to determine the clinical outcome of treatment [2].

12.14 Pedi-IKDC

Fact Box 11
The pediatric IKDC was developed and psychometric characteristics were determined on 589 patients, ages 6–18, with a variety of knee disorders.

A crucial feature of evaluating the psychometric properties of the IKDC SKF is demonstration of validity for the target population. The use of a validated outcome measure is not necessarily appropriate for pediatric patients. Patient-reported outcome measures rely on literacy and comprehension of questions that children may not understand. Consequently, cognitive interviews were conducted to determine how well children understood the components of the IKDC SKF [15]. This study revealed that children had difficulty comprehending and answering certain questions. Based on the specific areas of misunderstanding, a modified IKDC SKF (pedi-IKDC) was developed, and psychometric characteristics were determined on 589 patients, ages 6–18, with a variety of knee disorders [18]. The pedi-IKDC SKF demonstrated overall acceptable psychometric performance for outcome assessment of children and adolescents with various knee disorders [4].

12.15 Future Directions

In October 2014, the AOSSM Board voted to update the IKDC SKF by developing a computerized adapted test and integrating it with Patient-Reported Outcomes Measurement Information System (PROMIS) physical and functional computer-adaptive tests (CAT). The rationale for converting the existing IKDC SKF to a CAT is that it would enable the IKDC SKF to continue to be used as a measure of physical function and other dimensions of health overall more efficiently without increasing the total number of items

2000
IKDC KNEE EXAMINATION FORM

Patient Name:________________________ **Date of Birth:** __/__/__
Day Month Year

SEVEN GROUPS	FOUR GRADES A Normal	B Nearly Normal	C Abnormal	D Severely Abnormal	*Group Grade A B C D
1. Effusion	• None	• Mild	• Moderate	• Severe	• • • •
2. Passive Motion Deficit					
ΔLack of extension	• <3°	• 3 to 5°	• 6 to 10°	• >10°	
ΔLack of flexion	• 0 to 5°	• 6 to 15°	• 16 to 25°	• >25°	• • • •
3. Ligament Examination (manual, instrumented, x-ray)					
ΔLachman (25° flex) (134N)	• -1 to 2mm	• 3 to 5mm(1+) • <-1 to -3	• 6 to 10mm(2+) • <-3 stiff	• >10mm(3+)	
ΔLachman (25° flex) manual max	• -1 to 2mm	• 3 to 5mm	• 6 to 10mm	• >10mm	
Anterior endpoint:	• firm		• soft		
ΔTotal AP Translation (25° flex)	• 0 to 2mm	• 3 to 5mm	• 6 to 10mm	• >10mm	
ΔTotal AP Translation (70° flex)	• 0 to 2mm	• 3 to 5mm	• 6 to 10mm	• >10mm	
ΔPosterior Drawer Test (70° flex)	• 0 to 2mm	• 3 to 5mm	• 6 to 10mm	• >10mm	
ΔMed Joint Opening (20° flex/valgus rot)	• 0 to 2mm	• 3 to 5mm	• 6 to 10mm	• >10mm	
ΔLat Joint Opening (20° flex/varus rot)	• 0 to 2mm	• 3 to 5mm	• 6 to 10mm	• >10mm	
ΔExternal Rotation Test (30° flex prone)	• <5°	• 6 to 10°	• 11 to 19°	• >20°	
ΔExternal Rotation Test (90° flex prone)	• <5°	• 6 to 10°	• 11 to 19°	• >20°	
ΔPivot Shift	• equal	• + glide	• ++ (clunk)	• +++ (gross)	
ΔReverse Pivot Shift	• equal	• glide	• gross	• marked	• • • •
4. Compartment Findings			crepitation with		
ΔCrepitus Ant. Compartment	• none	• moderate	• mild pain	• >mild pain	
ΔCrepitus Med. Compartment	• none	• moderate	• mild pain	• >mild pain	
ΔCrepitus Lat. Compartment	• none	• moderate	• mild pain	• >mild pain	
5. Harvest Site Pathology	• none	• mild	• moderate	• severe	
6. X-ray Findings					
Med. Joint Space	• none	• mild	• moderate	• severe	
Lat. Joint Space	• none	• mild	• moderate	• severe	
Patellofemoral	• none	• mild	• moderate	• severe	
Ant. Joint Space (sagittal)	• none	• mild	• moderate	• severe	
Post. Joint Space (sagittal)	• none	• mild	• moderate	• severe	
7. Functional Test					
One Leg Hop (% of opposite side)	• ≥90%	• 89 to 76%	• 75 to 50%	• <50%	
****Final Evaluation**					• • • •

* Group grade: The lowest grade within a group determines the group grade

** Final evaluation: the worst group grade determines the final evaluation for acute and subacute patients. For chronic patients compare preoperative and postoperative evaluations. In a final evaluation only the first 3 groups are evaluated but all groups must be documented. Δ Difference in involved knee compared to normal or what is assumed to be normal.

IKDC COMMITTEE AOSSM: Anderson, A., Bergfeld, J., Boland, A. Dye, S., Feagin, J., Harner, C. Mohtadi, N. Richmond, J. Shelbourne, D., Terry, G. ESSKA: Staubli, H., Hefti, F., Hoher, J., Jacob, R., Mueller, W., Neyret, P. APOSSM: Chan, K., Kurosaka, M.

administered to the patient. In addition, the IKDC SKF may be integrated with the PROMIS physical function and pain CAT for sports-related knee injury. This would be very valuable and could advance the field of measuring patient-reported outcomes for sports-related conditions.

Conclusions

The IKDC SKF was rigorously tested and found to be an instrument that was valid, reliable, and responsive and could be used to assess symptoms, function, and sports activity in patients with a variety of knee disorders including ligament and meniscal injuries, patellofemoral pain, chondral injuries [8, 10], and osteoarthritis [2, 8, 13, 14, 28]. Studies comparing IKDC SKF to other outcome measures demonstrate superior psychometric characteristics of the IKDC for meniscal [5, 33, 35], ACL [36], and cartilage repair outcomes [10].

As a result of rigorous psychometric testing, the availability of normative data, a pediatric version [28, 30, 31], and comparison to other outcome instruments, the IKDC SKF has gained worldwide recognition and popularity. It has been culturally adapted and translated in 19 languages [11, 19, 20, 29]. The forms and translated versions are available at www.sportsmed.org.

References

1. Anderson AF, Federspiel CF, Snyder RB (1993) Evaluation of knee ligament rating systems. Am J Knee Surg 6:67–74
2. Anderson AF, Irrgang JJ, Kocher MS, Mann BJ, Harrast JJ, Committee IKD (2006) The international knee documentation committee subjective knee evaluation form: normative data. Am J Sports Med 34(1): 128–135
3. Apley AG (1990) An assessment of assessment. J Bone Joint Surg 72B:957–958
4. Boykin RE, McFeely ED, Shearer D, Frank JS, Harrod CC, Nasreddine AY, Kocher MS (2013) Correlation between the child health questionnaire and the International Knee Documentation Committee score in pediatric and adolescent patients with an anterior cruciate ligament tear. J Pediatr Orthop 33(2):216–220
5. Crawford K, Briggs KK, Rodkey WG, Steadman JR (2007) Reliability, validity, and responsiveness of the IKDC score for meniscus injuries of the knee. Arthroscopy 23(8):839–844
6. Daniel DM (1991) Assessing the limits of knee motion. Am J Sports Med 19:139–146
7. Feagin JA, Blake WP (1983) Postoperative evaluation and result recording in the anterior cruciate reconstructed knee. Clin Orthop 172:143–147
8. Greco NJ, Anderson AF, Mann BJ, Cole BJ, Farr J, Nissen CW, Irrgang JJ (2010) Responsiveness of the International Knee Documentation Committee Subjective Knee Form in comparison to the Western Ontario and McMaster Universities Osteoarthritis Index, modified Cincinnati Knee Rating System, and Short Form 36 in patients with focal articular cartilage defects. Am J Sports Med 38(5):891–902. Epub 2009 Dec 31
9. Guyett G, Walter S, Norman G (1987) Measuring change over time: assessing the usefulness of evaluation instruments. J Chronic Dis 40:171–178
10. Hambly K, Griva K (2008) IKDC or KOOS? Which measures symptoms and disabilities most important to postoperative articular cartilage repair patients? Am J Sports Med 37(9):1695–1704. Epub 2008 Jun 24
11. Haverkamp D, Sierevelt IN, Breugem SJ, Lohuis K, Blankevoort L, van Dijk CN (2006) Translation and validation of the Dutch version of the International Knee Documentation Committee Subjective Knee Form. Am J Sports Med 34(10):1680–1684
12. Hefti F, Muller W, Jakob RP et al (1993) Evaluation of knee ligament injuries with the IKDC form. Knee Surg Sports Traumatol Arthrosc 1:226–234
13. Irrgang JJ, Anderson AF, Boland AL, Harner CD, Kurosaka M, Neyret P, Richmond JC, Shelborne KD (2001) Development and validation of the International Knee Documentation Committee Subjective Knee Form. Am J Sports Med 29:600–613
14. Irrgang JJ, Anderson AF, Boland AL, Harner CD, Neyret P, Richmond JC, Shelbourne KD, International Knee Documentation Committee (2006) Responsiveness of the International Knee Documentation Committee Subjective Knee Form. Am J Sports Med 34(10):1567–1573
15. Iversen MD, Lee b, Connell P, Anderson J, Anderson AF, Kocher MS. (2010) Validity and comprehensibility of the international knee documentation committee subjective knee evaluation form in children. Scand. J Med Sci Sports 20:e87–e95
16. Kirshner B, Guyett G (1985) A methodological frame work for assessing health indices. J Chronic Dis 38:27–36
17. Kocher MS, Steadman JR, Briggs KK, Sterett WI, Hawkins RJ (2004) Relationships between objective assessment of ligament stability and subjective assessment of symptoms and function after anterior cruciate ligament reconstruction. Am J Sports Med 32(3):629–634
18. Kocher MS, Smith JT, Iversen MD, Brustowicz K, Ogunwole O, Andersen J, Yoo WJ, McFeely ED, Anderson AF, Zurakowski D (2011) Reliability, validity, and responsiveness of a modified International Knee Documentation Committee Subjective Knee Form (Pedi-IKDC) in children with knee disorders. Am J Sports Med 39(5):933–939
19. Lertwanich P, Praphruetkit T, Keyurapan E, Lamsam C, Kulthanan T (2008) Validity and reliability of Thai version of the International Knee Documentation Committee Subjective Knee Form. J Med Assoc Thai 91(8):1218–1225
20. Metsavaht L, Leporace G, Riberto M, Sposito MM, Batista LA (2010) Translation and cross-cultural adaptation of the Brazilian version of the International Knee Documentation Committee Subjective Knee Form: validity and reproducibility. Am J Sports Med 38(9):1894–1899

21. Muller W, Biedert R, Hefti F, Jacob RP, Munzinger U, Staubli HU (1988) OAK knee evaluation: a new way to assess knee ligament injuries. Clin Orthop 232: 37–50
22. Nitko AJ (1983) Educational tests and measurement: an introduction. Harcourt Brace Jovanovich Inc., New York
23. Noyes FR, Barber SD, Mangine RE (1990) Bone patellar ligament bone and fascia lata allografts for reconstruction of the anterior cruciate ligament. J Bone J Surg 72A:1125–1136
24. Noyes FR, Grood ES, Torzelli PA (1989) Current concepts review: the definitions of terms for motion and position of the knee and injuries of the ligaments. J Bone Joint Surg 71A:465–472
25. Noyes FR, Cummings JF, Grood ES, Walz-Hasselfeld KA, Wroble RR (1991) The diagnosis of knee motion limits, subluxations and ligament injury. Am J Sports Med 19:163–170
26. Noyes FR, Grood ES, Cummings JF, Wroble RR (1991) An analysis of the pivot shift phenomenon: the knee motions and subluxations induced by different examiners. Am J Sports Med 19:148–155
27. Noyes FR, Barber SD, Mangine RE (1991) Abnormal lower limb symmetry determined by function hop test after anterior cruciate ligament rupture. Am J Sports Med 19:513–518
28. Oak SR, O'Rourke C, Strnad G, Andrish JT, Parker RD, Saluan P, Jones MH, Stegmeier NA, Spindler KP (2015) Statistical comparison of the pediatric versus adult IKDC Subjective Knee Evaluation Form in adolescents. Am J Sports Med 43(9):2216–2221
29. Padua R, Bondi R, Ceccarelli E, Bondi L, Romanini E, Zanoli G, Campi S (2004) Italian version of the International Knee Documentation Committee Subjective Knee Form: cross-cultural adaptation and validation. Arthroscopy 20(8):819–823
30. Schmitt LC, Paterno MV, Huang S (2010) Validity and internal consistency of the International Knee Documentation Committee Subjective Knee Evaluation Form in children and adolescents. Am J Sports Med 38(12):2443–2447
31. Slobogean GP, Mulpuri K, Reilly CW (2008) The International Knee Documentation Committee Subjective Evaluation Form in a preadolescent population: pilot normative data. Am J Sports Med 36(1):129–132
32. Snyder-Mackler L, Fitzgerald GK, Bartolozzi AR, Ciccotti MD (1997) The relationship between passive joint laxity and functional outcome after anterior cruciate ligament injury. Am J Sports Med 25:191–195
33. Tanner SM, Dainty KN, Marx RG, Kirkly A (2007) Knee-specific quality-of-life instruments: which ones measure symptoms and disabilities most important to patients? Am J Sports Med 35(9):1450–1458
34. Tegner Y, Lysholm J (1985) Rating system in the evaluation of knee ligament injuries. Clin Orthop 198:43–49
35. van de Graaf VA, Wolterbeek N, Scholtes VA, Mutsaerts EL, Poolman RW (2014) Reliability and validity of the IKDC, KOOS, and WOMAC for patients with meniscal injuries. Am J Sports Med 42(6):1408–1416
36. van Meer BL, Meuffels DE, Vissers MM, Bierma-Zeinstra SM, Verhaar JA, Terwee CB, Reijman M (2013) Knee injury and osteoarthritis outcome score or International Knee Documentation Committee Subjective Knee Form: which questionnaire is most useful to monitor patients with an anterior cruciate ligament rupture in the short term? Arthroscopy 29(4):701–715

Part III

Rotatory Knee Laxity

Static Rotational Knee Laxity Measurements

13

Caroline Mouton, Daniel Theisen, and Romain Seil

Contents

C. Mouton • R. Seil (✉)
Sports Medicine Research Laboratory, Luxembourg Institute of Health, Luxembourg City, Luxembourg

Sports Clinic, Centre Hospitalier Luxembourg – Clinique d'Eich, 76, rue d'Eich, Luxembourg City L-1460, Luxembourg
e-mail: rseil@yahoo.com

D. Theisen
Sports Medicine Research Laboratory, Luxembourg Institute of Health, Luxembourg City, Luxembourg

13.1 Introduction

Clinical assessment of knee laxity is useful prior to surgery to assist in establishing the diagnosis of knee injuries and after surgical intervention to evaluate the success of reconstruction procedures. Clinically, rotational knee laxity is evaluated by subjective manual tests, such as the dial or the pivot shift tests [27]. Whereas the former is 'static' and uniaxial, the latter is 'dynamic' and tests the knee in more than one direction [21]. There is a debate as to whether static or dynamic measurements should be preferred in the evaluation of anterior cruciate ligament (ACL) injuries [51]. While the pivot shift test is accepted to be more closely correlated with the clinical symptoms of dynamic instability ('giving way') than do static tests, it appears to be generally accepted that the latter are of interest in the diagnosis and

V. Musahl et al. (eds.), *Rotatory Knee Instability*, DOI 10.1007/978-3-319-32070-0_13

follow-up of knee soft tissue injuries [51]. Moreover, static tests induce a less complex movement of the knee in comparison to dynamic tests, which may be easier to standardise and to control with a device. Increased attention has been paid over the last decade to develop instruments measuring static rotational knee laxity. To date, few data report rotational knee laxity measurements in vivo. A systematic review reported that in 74 articles where knee rotation was measured under a controlled load, 61 used human cadavers and only 13 using living humans [31]. Preliminary data showed that rotational knee laxity measurements are of a much higher degree of complexity compared with sagittal knee laxity measurements.

The aim of the present chapter is to provide an overview of current knowledge on static rotational knee laxity measurements.

13.2 Structures Influencing Knee Rotation: What Can We Measure?

Laxity tests must be utilised with caution; there is always more than one contributing structure in one direction being tested. As a consequence, it can be challenging to isolate the structure under investigation. Between 0° and 30° of knee flexion, internal rotation is primarily restrained by the posterior oblique ligament and the iliotibial band. Secondary restraints include the ACL, the superficial fibres of the medial collateral ligament (MCL), the menisci, the popliteal tendon and the anterolateral ligament (ALL). At 60° of knee flexion, internal rotation is first restrained by the deep fibres of the MCL and the iliotibial band and then by the ACL, the menisci, the popliteal tendon and the ALL. In terms of external rotation, at full extension of the knee, it is primarily restrained by the lateral collateral ligament (LCL) and secondly by the menisci, the deep fibres of the MCL and the popliteofibular ligament complex. From 30° to 90° of knee flexion, primary restraints of external rotation are the superficial fibres of the MCL, the LCL and the popliteal tendon. Secondary restraints are the posterior cruciate ligament (PCL), the menisci and the popliteofibular ligament complex [21].

As contributing structures vary with the degree of knee flexion, patient position and/or devices to measure static rotational knee laxity must be chosen in relation to the structure(s) to be analysed. For example, cadaver studies showed that the increase of rotation related to an ACL deficiency was apparent mainly between 0° and 30° of knee flexion and disappeared with further knee flexion [6, 53, 85]. ACL-injured patients should thus be assessed at a maximal angle of 30°. In knee flexion angles below 30°, the section of the ACL lead to 2.4–4° increase more specifically in internal rotation [32, 36, 42, 53]. The same amount of increment is observed in in vivo studies (rotation of the injured knee patients with a chronic ACL injury was increased by 3° compared to the healthy knee) [40]. Given the rather limited amount of additional rotation induced by the absence of the ACL, the challenge with non-invasive measurements is to reach a high degree of precision to detect such low changes.

13.3 Static Laxity Measurements: How to Start With?

Several factors related to patient positioning, measurement methods, testing protocols and device precision deserve particular consideration to correctly understand static rotational knee laxity measurements. Patient position (i.e. knee and hip flexion angles) influences laxity measurements. At a knee flexion of 20°, greater values of knee rotation are observed when the hip is near extension compared with when the hip is flexed at 90°. On the other hand, for a similar position of the hip, knee rotation is greater at 90° of knee flexion compared with 20° [59].

Devices also differ by measurement methods (location of sensors to measure torque applied and displacement). In all reported instruments, torque is applied at the foot. Consequently, the torque may partially be absorbed by the device and other joints of the leg than the knee joint. The final torque applied to the knee may thus differ between devices depending on efficacy to immobilise the hip and ankle joints. With regard to the measurement of rotation, some devices measure knee rotation at the foot [3, 11, 37] and others directly at the tibia [49, 55, 70]. For a 10 Nm torque, Shoemaker and Markolf estimated that foot rotation represented twice the tibiofemoral rotation, i.e. two-thirds of the measured angle [59]. This aspect is specific of each device depending on the fixation of the ankles and hips. However, foot rotation may be avoided with a direct evaluation of tibial rotation via electromagnetic sensors placed on the tibia [2].

Researchers and knee surgeons should also be aware how testing protocols are standardised. The amount of torque applied usually varied between 5 and 15 Nm depending on fixation and patient comfort within the device. These amounts of torque allow for a safe test as structural integrity of the knee ligaments are only compromised for a torque greater than 35 Nm directly applied to the tibia [59]. Several researchers have shown improved reliability for total range of rotation than for internal and external rotation separately [3, 85]. Most researchers apply this torque from internal to external rotation or from external to internal rotation to obtain a complete cycle of rotation. In these cases, the hysteresis phenomenon should not be neglected as it may influence the reproducibility of the measurements. A solution to avoid this phenomenon is to perform separate measurements of internal and external rotation and includes 'preconditioning trials' [12, 44, 66]. A lack of reproducibility may also be explained by a non-reproducible starting position of the test, an aspect related to patient installation that should be carefully monitored.

All of the previously mentioned aspects influence the precision of the device, which remains poorly investigated. The determination of precision is, however, necessary to draw meaningful conclusions from any comparison study as it accounts for the measurement error. It is helpful to detect abnormalities occurring during a subject follow-up and helps to conclude if an observed difference is clinically relevant and meaningful. Studies are often limited to computations of ICCs, which depend strongly on data dispersion and do not provide a clear understanding of device precision. A conservative approach is the use of the minimum detectable change (MDC) [82]. The MDC represents the minimal required difference with a given instrument in a defined setting to be confident that a true change has indeed occurred.

13.4 Static Rotational Knee Laxity Devices: How to Measure Knee Rotation?

Knee laxity measurement devices have been specifically designed to allow for an objective and standardised evaluation of knee laxity. The authors present non-invasive devices measuring knee rotation angle in humans with a known applied torque (Fig. 13.1). Instruments associated to imaging and/or assessing complex knee movements like the pivot shift test or the rotation associated with anterior or valgus movement of the knee will not be presented. To the best of the authors knowledge, none of the devices reported below are presently commercialised.

13.4.1 Genucom Knee Analysis System (FARO Medical Technologies, Montreal, Ontario, Canada) [54]

This device was developed in the late 1980s and allows measurement of anteroposterior laxity, as well as rotational and varus-valgus laxity [54]. A six-degrees-of-freedom dynamometer indicates to the examiner the force or torque applied to the knee, and an electrogoniometer measures the displacement. The ability of the device to measure rotation has been poorly explored. This may be partly explained by a poor reproducibility. Indeed, at 20° of knee

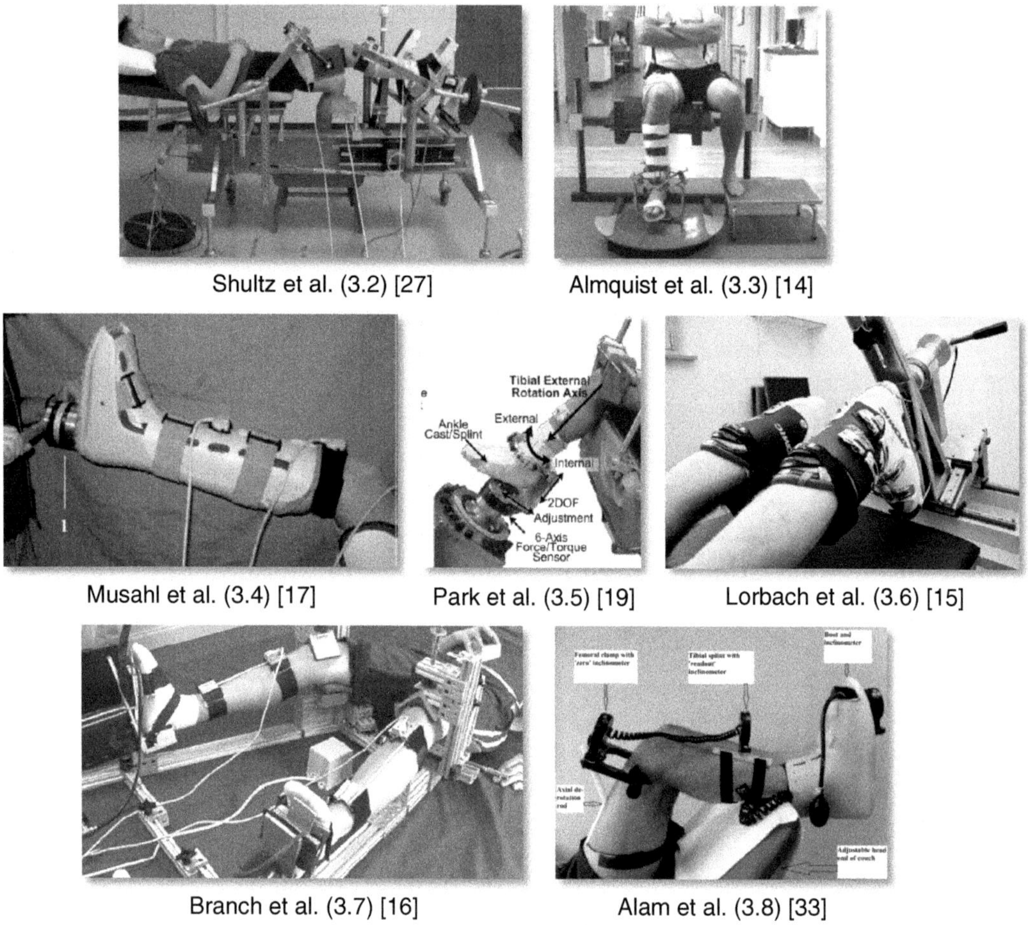

Fig. 13.1 Non-invasive devices to measure static rotational knee laxity in vivo. All devices allow applying a known amount of torque (Adapted from Refs. [14–17, 19, 27, 33])

flexion, the least significant difference reached 17.5° in tibial rotation; in other words, a change of 17.5° is required to indicate a real change in one subject's laxity [43].

13.4.2 Vermont Knee Laxity Device [77]

The Vermont knee laxity device measures anterior, rotational and varus-valgus laxity. The subject lies supine with knees flexed at 20° and hips at 10°, and the thighs are fixed with clamps at the femoral epicondyles. Rotation angle is measured on tibia through electromagnetic sensors. The intraclass correlation coefficient (ICC) is above 0.86 for internal, external and total range of rotation. The 95% confidence interval (CI) of the absolute measurement errors were evaluated to reach 5–7°, respectively, for internal and external rotation [70].

13.4.3 Rottometer [3]

The patient sits on a modified chair with knees and hips flexed to 90°. To limit artefacts and target tibiofemoral rotation, the thigh is fixed above the knee with clamps. The ankle is fixed by two screws at the calcaneus and four screws placed at the medial and lateral malleoli. An adjustable spanner is used to apply torque and a stick following the foot plate indicated the resulting degree of rotation. A comparative study using radiostereometry analysis (RSA) demonstrated that the Rottometer systematically overestimated tibiofemoral rotation by about 100% [3]. Depending on the amount of torque and degree of knee flexion, the inter-rater ICC varied between 0.49 and 0.85, with the highest ICC obtained for the highest torque (9 Nm) and the higher degree of knee flexion (90°) [4]. The 95% CI between measurements of both examiners varied between −7.9° for the lower bound and 3.8° for the upper bound [4].

13.4.4 Device by Musahl et al. [49]

This device consists of an Aircast Foam Walker boot with a 6-degrees-of-freedom moment sensor fixed on a handle bar attached to the boot. A bubble level attached to the handle bar determines the neutral rotation. To measure the relative rotation of the tibia with regard to the femur, magnetic sensors are placed on the boot, on the medial surface of the proximal tibia and on the anterior surface of the thigh. The examiner holds the leg while applying the torque, which may influence muscle relaxation and flexion angles. An initial cadaver study reported a high intra- and inter-rater ICC (>0.94) [49]. In 11 healthy subjects, inter-rater ICC was greatest at 90° of knee flexion (0.88). The 95% CI of the standard error of measurements reached 3.2° for the total range at 90° of knee flexion and 5.1° at 30° [76]. The average side-to-side difference between normal knees was reported to be 3.5° [76].

13.4.5 Device by Park et al. [55]

Park et al. [55] presented the first motorised device to measure knee rotational laxity. The patient sits in a modified chair with the hips flexed at 85° and knees at 60°. The thighs are fixed with clamps. Three LED markers were positioned on the anteromedial surface of the tibia to measure the angle of rotation. No data is available on its reproducibility.

13.4.6 Rotameter [37]

Two prototypes of the Rotameter exist. In both versions, the subject is lying prone to reproduce the dial test position. Thighs are fixed in half cones with Velcro strap band. Hips are extended and knees flexed at 30°. The subject is wearing boots (home-made boot in the first version and ski boots of appropriated size in the second version) attached to the handle bar that allows both to apply the torque and measure the degree of rotation. A cadaver study showed a high correlation (Pearson $r > 0.85$) between measurements of the first prototype and knee navigation system [36, 37]. The Rotameter, however, overestimates the total range of rotation at 5, 10 and 15 Nm in average of 5, 10 and 25°, respectively [37]. The assessment of the reliability of the first Rotameter is questionable. Greater ICC were observed for inter-tester reliability (>0.88) compared with intra-rater ICC (>0.67), suggesting that participants were not reinstalled between the measurements undertaken by the two examiners [38]. No confidence intervals for measurement errors were reported. Regarding the second version of the Rotameter, it provides lower rotation than the first device due to improvements in the standardisation of the patient installation and joint fixation. The MDC has been determined to reach 4.2° for internal rotation and 5.9° for external rotation [45]. Individualised normative references have been established considering individual characteristics [44, 45].

13.4.7 Robotic Knee Testing System [11]

Branch et al. developed a custom robotic knee system adjustable to the patient's natural lower limb alignment to avoid pretension in leg anatomical structures. The patient lies supine with knees flexed at 25°. The femur and patella are stabilised with clamps, and the ankle is stabilised in pronation and dorsiflexion to limit its rotation during the test. Rotation is measured at the foot with an inclinometer. Electromagnetic sensors placed on the proximal tibia showed that tibial rotation represented in average 48.7% of the total rotation measured at the foot [11]. The authors corrected their measurements according to these results, which may introduce bias, as this correction may vary between individuals (95 % CI: 45.3–52.1 %). Inter-rater ICC for total range of rotation reached 0.97 at a torque of 5.65 Nm [11].

13.4.8 Rotational Measurement Device [1]

This device consists of three parts: (1) a femoral clamp and (2) a tibial splint, to which inclinometers are fixed to measure rotation and (3) a boot with a torque wrench. Subjects are positioned at 90° of knee flexion. Measurements at the foot overestimate rotation in average by 136 % (95 % CI, −102 % to −171 %) compared to the rotational measurement device placed on the tibia. The latter slightly overestimated rotation (in average 2°: 95% CI −4.5° to 0.4°) when compared to electromagnetic sensors placed on the tibia [1]. Intra-rater ICC reached 0.9 [1].

Fact Box 1

- Static rotational knee laxity only assesses knee rotation. Dynamic tests constrain the knee in more than one direction (i.e. pivot shift test).
- Structures contributing to knee rotation are numerous (menisci, lateral ligaments …) and depend on the degree of knee flexion.
- Rotational knee laxity measurements are of a much higher degree of complexity compared to anterior knee laxity measurements.
- To date, eight devices have been reported with measurements of rotational knee laxity in vivo. The torque applied varies between 5 and 15 Nm. The report of their precision is insufficient for proper use in the daily practice.
- Hip flexion, knee flexion, location of sensors to measure torque applied and rotation, as well as testing protocols, critically influence rotational laxity results.

13.5 Rotational Laxity in the Normal Knee

Physiological knee laxity is the natural laxity of the knee. Recent literature reveals that physiological knee laxity may influence injury risk, as well as treatment outcomes. As such, a better understanding of physiological laxity may benefit both athletes and injured patients alike.

13.5.1 Relation with Knee Function

It is commonly accepted that knee laxity has no relation to knee function. In fact, the literature specifies that the amount of side-to-side difference in knee laxity observed after ACL reconstruction is not linked to clinical outcomes [22, 30, 56]. Nevertheless, subjects with excessive physiological knee laxity have been reported to have movement patterns associated with non-contact ACL injury mechanisms. They display greater hip and knee movements in the transverse, sagittal and frontal planes during drop landings [65, 75]. Subjects with higher anterior knee laxity also display increased knee moments [69] and delayed onset timing of muscle activation that is compensated by a higher muscle activity [60]. Moments and onset timing of muscle activation have not yet been investigated for patients with higher rotational knee laxity. These primary findings suggest that individuals may benefit from intensive neuromuscular training adapted to their laxity profile, which could have a direct impact in knee injury prevention and patient care.

13.5.2 Risk Factor for Injuries

It is well recognised that hypermobility (as defined by the Beighton score [8]) is associated with an increased risk of musculoskeletal injuries [83]. The same principle may apply to physiological rotational knee laxity. In adulthood, as for anterior knee laxity [78, 84], the healthy contralateral knee of ACL-injured patients displays, on average, greater internal rotation than healthy knees of a control group [11, 46]. Mouton et al.

set a threshold to help discriminate rotational knee laxity between healthy subjects and the healthy contralateral knee of ACL-injured patients [46]. Above the established threshold, a subject was 2.45-fold (95 % CI 1.37–4.36) more likely to be in the injured group [46]. These findings must be confirmed by prospective studies, but they suggest that prospective screening may be of interest to identify subjects at risk for non-contact ACL injuries as well as for other knee injuries.

13.5.3 Risk for Poor Reconstruction Outcomes

After ACL reconstruction with a bone-patellar tendon-bone graft, patients identified with an increased physiological rotational laxity have lower Lysholm [29] and IKDC subjective [12, 29] scores. As preoperative scores were not reported, it remains unclear whether this finding is the consequence of the ACL reconstruction or of the injury itself. Still, these results raise the question of whether patients with higher knee laxity may benefit from adapted, individualised care (i.e. graft choice) compared with other patients.

13.5.4 Influencing Factors

Previous studies have demonstrated that external rotation exceeds internal rotation by approximately 50 % [11, 38, 48, 55, 70]. However, the study of rotational knee laxity is much more complex than simply measuring internal and external rotation. Physiological laxity is indeed influenced by several individual characteristics. Females have greater rotational knee laxity than males [5, 11, 26, 44, 45, 55] and body mass appears to be inversely correlated to rotational knee laxity [44, 45, 61]. No relation has been reported between height and rotational knee laxity [44, 45].

Increased knee laxity in the paediatric population is generally well accepted [7, 17, 23]. Rotational knee laxity evolves during the adolescence and stabilises at the age of 14 years in girls and at 16 years in boys [7]. This stiffening of knee laxity coincides with the emergence of ACL injuries [14]. In adulthood, the influence of age is debated [5, 61]. Shultz et al. reported that older subjects had lower laxities. However, these researchers in their study did not include a large range of age: males were 22 ± 3 years old and females were 21 ± 3 years old [61]. In contrast, in two studies with large number of subjects and including subjects with a large range of age, no significant influence of age could be observed neither in males nor females [5, 44, 45].

While several studies suggest that anterior knee laxity may vary during the menstrual cycle of females [62, 63], the effect of the menstrual cycle on rotational knee laxity has been analysed in only one study [66]. The authors assessed rotational knee laxity in females at two different time points. Based on previous research of these authors [64], the two time points were the estimated days of minimum and maximum anterior knee laxity during menses and the early luteal phase, respectively. No increase in rotational knee laxity could be observed in females between these two time points [66].

A relation may exist between knee laxity and lower leg alignment. Healthy subjects with increased laxity compared with subjects with decreased laxity have greater navicular drop (increased: 7.1 ± 5.0 mm, decreased: 5.2 ± 3.1 mm), lower Q-angle (increased: 12.9 ± 3.9°, decreased: 11.6 ± 4.7°), lower tibial torsion (increased: 14.8 ± 7.3°, decreased: 18.6 ± 5.2°), lower quadriceps peak torque (increased: 2.3 ± 0.4 Nm/kg, decreased: 2.5 ± 0.4 Nm/kg) and shorter femur length (increased: 41.3 ± 2.6 cm, decreased: 44.5 ± 2.5 cm) [61]. Some differences are, however, minor and their clinical value has not yet been established. Another study established that subjects with foot pronation displayed higher internal rotation than subjects without pronation [13].

Physical activity has also been reported to influence rotational knee laxity. Shultz et al. measured rotational knee laxity in 59 participants during an intermittent exercise protocol [67]. The measurements were performed before and after warm-up and every 15 min during and for 1 h after the end of the exercise. The largest mean change observed was 1.7 ± 4.9° (increase of 7 % compared to before warm-up) [67]. Thirty-three percent of each sex had an increment superior to 5.2°, thereby suggesting that all participants may not respond in a similar way to an exercise. The study of Shultz et al. therefore confirms previous studies, which showed increased rotational knee laxity associated with exercise [28, 73]. Interestingly, as rotational knee laxity increases with exercise, women tend to have greater knee valgus and more absorbed energy at the knee [68]. The importance of the valgus is related to the subject's physiological knee laxity [68].

Finally, osteoarthritis may affect knee laxity. Cross-sectional studies have found that rotational laxity [80] decreased with the severity of knee osteoarthritis. It may thus be useful to consider osteoarthritis as a potential confounding factor in future studies [52].

13.5.5 Normative References

To define 'excessive' knee laxity, normative references for each device must first be established in order to define 'normal' laxity. Mouton et al. proposed a methodological approach to calculate standardised laxity scores for anterior and rotational knee laxity taking into account influencing individual characteristics [45]. For rotational knee laxity, sex and body mass were found to significantly influence its measure and to explain a non-negligible amount of the variability in internal and external rotation (46–60 %). As a consequence, the latter parameters were taken into account to calculate an individualised score. The individualisation of scores has the advantage to allow for the direct comparison of individuals, regardless of differences in sex or body mass. The final score represents the distance of the individual to the average of the healthy control group. One unit represents the standard deviation of the healthy control group. As one standard deviation has already been previously used as a threshold [78], the authors decided to use it to categorise knees as being hypo- (score < −1), normo- (score between −1 and 1) and hyperlax (score > 1) [45]. For internal and external rotation, the individualised scores follow a normal distribution (Figs. 13.2 and 13.3).

Anterior and rotational knee laxity are poorly correlated [45, 71], which suggests that they yield complementary information. A single measure of knee laxity is thus likely inappropriate to describe the static knee laxity envelope. The existence of specific knee laxity profiles has been suggested [61]. Mouton et al. showed by combining the anterior displacement to internal and external rotation that only 32 % of the participants showed a normal profile (scores > −1 and < 1 for all three directions), 33 % were concerned by hyperlaxity in at least one direction, 40 % by hypolaxity in at least one direction and 5 % by both (Fig. 13.4). The diversity of the identified laxity profiles highlights both the complexity of

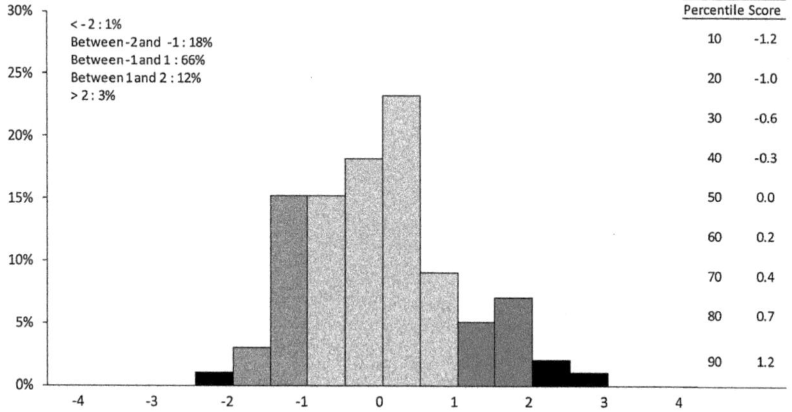

Fig. 13.2 Distribution of the knee laxity score for internal rotation at 5 Nm corrected for sex and body mass [31]

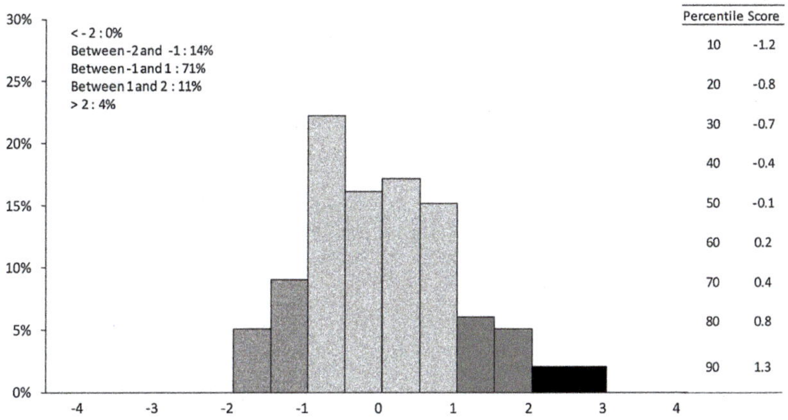

Fig. 13.3 Distribution of the knee laxity score for external rotation at 5 Nm corrected for sex and body mass [31]

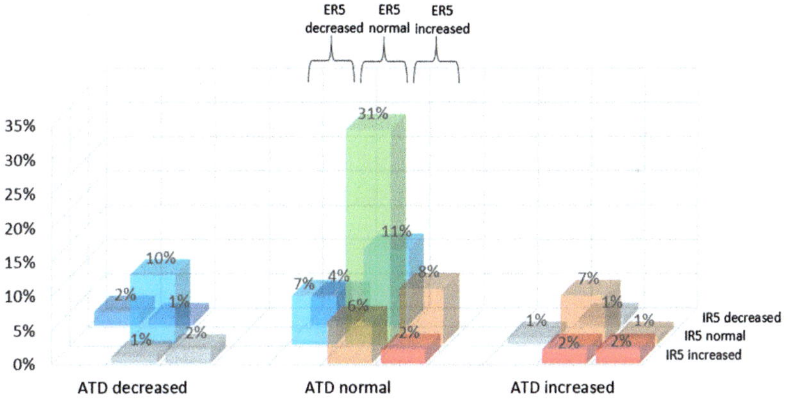

Fig. 13.4 Distribution of laxity profiles expressed in percentage (%). Decreased: laxity score < −1, normal: laxity score between −1 and 1, increased: laxity score >1. *ATD200* anterior tibial displacement at 200 N, *IR5* internal rotation at 5 Nm, *ER5* external rotation at 5 Nm [31]

the interpretation of multidirectional knee laxity and the necessity for individualised care of knee injuries and diseases.

Fact Box 2

- Subjects with excessive physiological knee laxity have been reported to display greater knee movements and moments and delayed muscle onset compensated by a higher muscle activity.
- Excessive physiological knee laxity may play a role in the risk of knee injuries and may influence outcomes after ligament, e.g. ACL reconstruction.
- External rotation has been reported to be 50 % greater than internal rotation.
- Physiological rotational knee laxity may be influenced by many individual characteristics such as sex, body mass, age, menstrual cycle, lower leg alignment, osteoarthritis, as well as exercise. These parameters can be considered in the establishment of normative references.
- A single measure of knee laxity is inappropriate to describe knee laxity. The interpretation of knee laxity profiles is complex and still at a very early stage.

13.6 Rotational Laxity in the Injured Knee

In contrast to physiological knee laxity, which only considers the healthy knee, pathological laxity typically considers the laxity of the injured knee and its difference against the contralateral knee.

Laxity measurements can be useful to establish the diagnosis of ACL injuries in complement to the clinical and imaging evaluation. Presently, the diagnosis of ACL injuries with arthrometers mainly focuses on anterior laxity measurements. However, concomitant measures of additional laxities, such as rotational knee laxity, have been proposed to refine the diagnosis of ACL injuries [16]. In cadaver studies, the section of the ACL leads to an increment of tibial internal rotation of 2.4–4° [32, 36, 42, 53]. Similar increase of 3° in tibial internal rotation could be observed in vivo [40]. More specifically, the posterolateral bundle may play a role in restraining rotation as its section induced the major increase in internal rotation [36].

To date, only the sensitivity and specificity of the Rotameter to detect an ACL injury has been reported in the literature [47]. A threshold of 3.2° for the side-to-side difference in internal rotation at 5 Nm led to correctly identify 38 % of patients (sensitivity) and reject 95 % of healthy subjects (specificity) (Fig. 13.5). Although the sensitivity of the Rotameter seems extremely low, it is still superior to the sensitivity of 24 % reported for the pivot shift test in a previous meta-analysis [9]. Moreover, compared with the common analysis of anterior displacement (side-to-side difference in anterior displacement at 200 N), further analysis of knee internal rotation increased the diagnostic sensitivity by 9 % (from 75 to 84 %) [47]. To further improve the diagnosis of ACL injuries, consideration of the slope of the curves (representative of knee stiffness) is advised as it has been shown to increase the specificity of anterior and rotational knee laxity tests to 100 %. As a result, simultaneous consideration of displacement and knee stiffness provide a test without a false positive [47].

It should be highlighted that associated injuries such as meniscal or collateral ligament injury may influence the interpretation of laxity measurements in the diagnosis of ACL injuries [25, 72, 81] but remain poorly considered. Only 40 % of ACL ruptures are, however, reported to be isolated [19].

Rotational knee laxity measurements may also be of interest in posterolateral corner injuries. These injuries induce an increase in tibial external rotation [79] of 6–14° [33, 39, 41], resulting in posterolateral rotational instability. This increment is much more important than in terms of an ACL injury and may also be easier to detect. Clinically, posterolateral corner injuries are assessed with the dial test [20]. An increment greater than or equal to 15° in the injured knee suggests a posterolateral injury [20]. The dial test does not allow for an objective assessment of posterolateral rotatory instability but to the author's knowledge, results of instrumented measurements have never been reported in such injuries.

Finally, as knee osteoarthritis affects rotational knee laxity [80], rotational knee laxity measurements may have the potential to be an indicator of the type and severity of osteoarthritis.

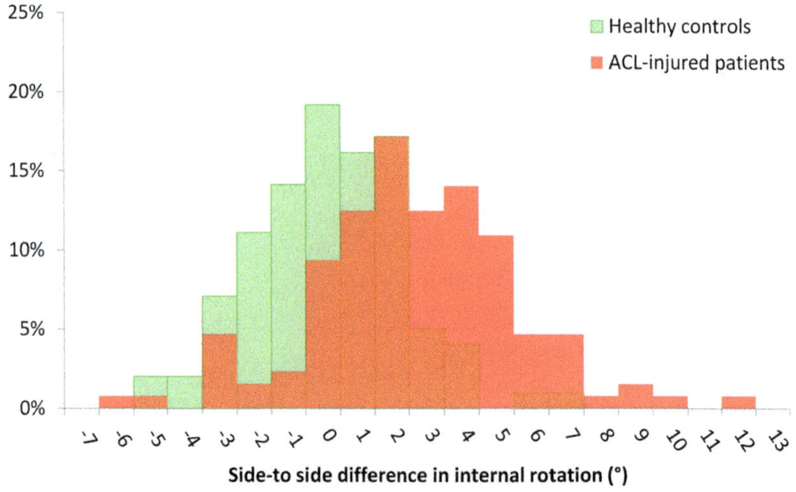

Fig. 13.5 Distribution of side-to-side difference in internal rotation at 5 Nm for healthy and ACL-injured subjects

13.7 Rotational Laxity in the Reconstructed Knee

Ideally, knee reconstruction surgery aims to restore knee laxity in all directions and prevent further degeneration of the knee joint. Therefore, knee laxity measurements are of interest after surgery as a postoperative control to follow the graft evolution and detect potential anomalies like elongation, recurrent tears, etc.

After ACL reconstruction, patient follow-up remains based on manual tests and/or on anterior knee laxity measurements. Most studies considering knee rotation analysed the pivot shift test and as such, a paucity of data exists regarding static rotational knee laxity measurements. However, these may help to detect anomalies because increased postoperative laxities may be observed in graft malpositioning [34, 57] or graft failures [18].

The effect of ACL reconstruction on rotational knee laxity and its evolution after reconstruction are not known yet. Lorbach et al. [35] reported no significant differences in static rotational knee laxity between the reconstructed and non-injured knee 27 months after ACL reconstructive surgery with a bone-patellar tendon-bone graft. Moreover, Branch et al. showed that the side-to-side differences in internal rotation did not differ between single- and double- reconstruction techniques using a semitendinosus and gracilis graft [12]. These researchers, however, did not report preoperative laxity measurements; it is thus not possible to conclude whether the ACL reconstruction reduces rotational knee laxity or whether it was already normal in these patients before surgery. Moreover, they only measured laxity at a single time point during patient follow-up.

To date, the knowledge on postoperative laxity is also insufficient to conclude on the best reconstructive technique to restore rotational knee laxity in an injured knee. With a navigation system, Bignozzi et al. demonstrated that the total range of rotation (internal and external rotation) was significantly reduced after anatomical double-bundle ACL reconstruction [10]. Moreover, Hofbauer et al. demonstrated that, using a navigation system, an anatomic double-bundle reconstruction technique reduced significantly more internal rotation (15.6°) than did an anatomic single-bundle ACL reconstruction (7.1°) [24]. A systematic review, however, showed that anatomic double-bundle ACL reconstruction did not lead neither to a lower grade of pivot shift test compared with single-bundle nor to a greater reduction in rotational knee laxity [15].

Postoperative knee laxity measurements are poorly considered after many other surgical interventions. It has, for example, been shown that medial meniscectomy will influence knee laxity [50, 58]. As for posterolateral corner injuries, Tardy et al. reported for the first time in vivo static rotational knee laxity after anatomic posterolateral corner reconstruction [74]. External rotation was in average similar to a healthy control group after reconstruction. However, the authors found a remaining significant increase in internal rotation of the tibia in 40 % of patients. They assumed that this finding was either due to the surgical technique or to associated lesions and/or unrecognised soft tissue damage at the time of injury.

Fact Box 3

- Rotational knee laxity measurements in combination with anterior knee laxity measurements improve the diagnosis of ACL injuries. They may also help to establish the diagnosis of posterolateral corner injuries.
- The diagnosis of ACL injuries may be skewed by associated injuries to structures also contributing to knee rotation.
- Rotational knee laxity measurements can improve the follow-up of knee injuries and diseases especially after knee reconstruction if used as a postoperative control (i.e. ACL or posterolateral corner injury). No prospective follow-up of patients was however reported.

Conclusions

Knee laxity measurements should be perceived as a supplement to clinical tests and imaging techniques. They should be systematically performed in order to assist the clinician with establishing a diagnosis and follow-up of knee injuries to systematically identify any abnormal evolution.

The development of arthrometers to measure static rotational knee laxity is relatively new and further studies are needed to develop further understanding. To date, we know that external rotation is greater than internal rotation and that females have greater rotational knee laxity than males. Moreover, body mass is inversely correlated to rotational knee laxity measurements. Other influencing factors remain under investigation.

The interest in physiological knee laxity is growing. Subjects with excessive physiological knee laxity are reported to have movement patterns associated with non-contact ACL injuries. This may partly explain why an increased laxity was observed in the healthy contralateral knee of ACL-injured subjects compared with a control group. This excessive physiological knee laxity may also explain inferior outcomes after an ACL reconstruction. As a consequence of this growing interest, the need for normative references has emerged. However, the analysis of either rotational or multidirectional knee laxity as well to the consideration of influencing factors lead to a high complexity of knee laxity profiles.

Recently, rotational knee laxity measurements have been shown to improve the diagnosis of ACL injuries as performed with anterior knee laxity measurements. This should encourage researchers to evaluate the diagnostic power of their own devices. The knowledge about postoperative rotational knee laxity measurements is evolving. The choice of reconstruction, the effect of reconstruction and its evolution are still insufficiently understood.

Static rotational knee laxity measurements offer the possibility to improve the understanding of physiological, pathological and reconstructed knee laxity and may help individualise the care of knee injuries and diseases.

References

1. Alam M, Bull AM, Thomas R, Amis AA (2013) A clinical device for measuring internal-external rotational laxity of the knee. Am J Sports Med 41(1): 87–94
2. Alam M, Bull AM, Thomas RD, Amis AA (2011) Measurement of rotational laxity of the knee: in vitro comparison of accuracy between the tibia, overlying skin, and foot. Am J Sports Med 39(12):2575–2581
3. Almquist PO, Arnbjornsson A, Zatterstrom R, Ryd L, Ekdahl C, Friden T (2002) Evaluation of an external device measuring knee joint rotation: an in vivo study with simultaneous Roentgen stereometric analysis. J Orthop Res 20(3):427–432
4. Almquist PO, Ekdahl C, Isberg PE, Friden T (2011) Measurements of knee rotation-reliability of an external device in vivo. BMC Musculoskelet Disord 12:291
5. Almquist PO, Ekdahl C, Isberg PE, Friden T (2013) Knee rotation in healthy individuals related to age and gender. J Orthop Res 31(1):23–28
6. Andersen HN, Dyhre-Poulsen P (1997) The anterior cruciate ligament does play a role in controlling axial rotation in the knee. Knee Surg Sports Traumatol Arthrosc 5(3):145–149
7. Baxter MP (1988) Assessment of normal pediatric knee ligament laxity using the genucom. J Pediatr Orthop 8(5):546–550
8. Beighton P, Horan F (1969) Orthopaedic aspects of the Ehlers-Danlos syndrome. J Bone Joint Surg Br 51(3):444–453
9. Benjaminse A, Gokeler A, van der Schans CP (2006) Clinical diagnosis of an anterior cruciate ligament rupture: a meta-analysis. J Orthop Sports Phys Ther 36(5):267–288
10. Bignozzi S, Zaffagnini S, Lopomo N, Fu FH, Irrgang JJ, Marcacci M (2010) Clinical relevance of static and dynamic tests after anatomical double-bundle ACL reconstruction. Knee Surg Sports Traumatol Arthrosc 18(1):37–42
11. Branch TP, Browne JE, Campbell JD, Siebold R, Freedberg HI, Arendt EA, Lavoie F, Neyret P, Jacobs CA (2010) Rotational laxity greater in patients with contralateral anterior cruciate ligament injury than healthy volunteers. Knee Surg Sports Traumatol Arthrosc 18(10):1379–1384
12. Branch TP, Siebold R, Freedberg HI, Jacobs CA (2011) Double-bundle ACL reconstruction demonstrated superior clinical stability to single-bundle ACL reconstruction: a matched-pairs analysis of instrumented tests of tibial anterior translation and internal rotation laxity. Knee Surg Sports Traumatol Arthrosc 19(3):432–440
13. Coplan JA (1989) Rotational motion of the knee: a comparison of normal and pronating subjects. J Orthop Sports Phys Ther 10(9):366–369
14. Csintalan RP, Inacio MC, Funahashi TT (2008) Incidence rate of anterior cruciate ligament reconstructions. Perm J 12(3):17–21

15. Desai N, Bjornsson H, Musahl V, Bhandari M, Petzold M, Fu FH, Samuelsson K (2014) Anatomic single- versus double-bundle ACL reconstruction: a meta-analysis. Knee Surg Sports Traumatol Arthrosc 22(5):1009–1023
16. Di Iorio A, Carnesecchi O, Philippot R, Farizon F (2014) Multiscale analysis of anterior cruciate ruptures: prospective study of 49 cases. Orthop Traumatol Surg Res 100(7):751–754
17. Flynn JM, Mackenzie W, Kolstad K, Sandifer E, Jawad AF, Galinat B (2000) Objective evaluation of knee laxity in children. J Pediatr Orthop 20(2): 259–263
18. George MS, Dunn WR, Spindler KP (2006) Current concepts review: revision anterior cruciate ligament reconstruction. Am J Sports Med 34(12):2026–2037
19. Granan LP, Forssblad M, Lind M, Engebretsen L (2009) The Scandinavian ACL registries 2004-2007: baseline epidemiology. Acta Orthop 80(5):563–567
20. Grood ES, Stowers SF, Noyes FR (1988) Limits of movement in the human knee. Effect of sectioning the posterior cruciate ligament and posterolateral structures. J Bone Joint Surg Am 70(1):88–97
21. Halewood C, Amis AA (2015) Clinically relevant biomechanics of the knee capsule and ligaments. Knee Surg Sports Traumatol Arthrosc. doi:10.1007/s00167-015-3594-8
22. Higuchi H, Terauchi M, Kimura M, Kobayashi A, Takeda M, Watanabe H, Takagishi K (2003) The relation between static and dynamic knee stability after ACL reconstruction. Acta Orthop Belg 69(3): 257–266
23. Hinton RY, Rivera VR, Pautz MJ, Sponseller PD (2008) Ligamentous laxity of the knee during childhood and adolescence. J Pediatr Orthop 28(2): 184–187
24. Hofbauer M, Valentin P, Kdolsky R, Ostermann RC, Graf A, Figl M, Aldrian S (2010) Rotational and translational laxity after computer-navigated single- and double-bundle anterior cruciate ligament reconstruction. Knee Surg Sports Traumatol Arthrosc 18(9):1201–1207
25. Hsieh HH, Walker PS (1976) Stabilizing mechanisms of the loaded and unloaded knee joint. J Bone Joint Surg Am 58(1):87–93
26. Hsu WH, Fisk JA, Yamamoto Y, Debski RE, Woo SL (2006) Differences in torsional joint stiffness of the knee between genders: a human cadaveric study. Am J Sports Med 34(5):765–770
27. Jakob RP, Staubli HU, Deland JT (1987) Grading the pivot shift. Objective tests with implications for treatment. J Bone Joint Surg Br 69(2):294–299
28. Johannsen HV, Lind T, Jakobsen BW, Kroner K (1989) Exercise-induced knee joint laxity in distance runners. Br J Sports Med 23(3):165–168
29. Kim SJ, Choi DH, Mei Y, Hwang BY (2011) Does physiologic posterolateral laxity influence clinical outcomes of anterior cruciate ligament reconstruction? J Bone Joint Surg Am 93(21):2010–2014
30. Kocher MS, Steadman JR, Briggs KK, Sterett WI, Hawkins RJ (2004) Relationships between objective assessment of ligament stability and subjective assessment of symptoms and function after anterior cruciate ligament reconstruction. Am J Sports Med 32(3): 629–634
31. Lam MH, Fong DT, Yung PS, Chan KM (2012) Biomechanical techniques to evaluate tibial rotation. A systematic review. Knee Surg Sports Traumatol Arthrosc 20(9):1720–1729
32. Lane JG, Irby SE, Kaufman K, Rangger C, Daniel DM (1994) The anterior cruciate ligament in controlling axial rotation. An evaluation of its effect. Am J Sports Med 22(2):289–293
33. LaPrade RF, Johansen S, Wentorf FA, Engebretsen L, Esterberg JL, Tso A (2004) An analysis of an anatomical posterolateral knee reconstruction: an in vitro biomechanical study and development of a surgical technique. Am J Sports Med 32(6):1405–1414
34. Lee MC, Seong SC, Lee S, Chang CB, Park YK, Jo H, Kim CH (2007) Vertical femoral tunnel placement results in rotational knee laxity after anterior cruciate ligament reconstruction. Arthroscopy 23(7):771–778
35. Lorbach O, Kieb M, Brogard P, Maas S, Pape D, Seil R (2012) Static rotational and sagittal knee laxity measurements after reconstruction of the anterior cruciate ligament. Knee Surg Sports Traumatol Arthrosc 20(5):844–850
36. Lorbach O, Pape D, Maas S, Zerbe T, Busch L, Kohn D, Seil R (2010) Influence of the anteromedial and posterolateral bundles of the anterior cruciate ligament on external and internal tibiofemoral rotation. Am J Sports Med 38(4):721–727
37. Lorbach O, Wilmes P, Maas S, Zerbe T, Busch L, Kohn D, Seil R (2009) A non-invasive device to objectively measure tibial rotation: verification of the device. Knee Surg Sports Traumatol Arthrosc 17(7): 756–762
38. Lorbach O, Wilmes P, Theisen D, Brockmeyer M, Maas S, Kohn D, Seil R (2009) Reliability testing of a new device to measure tibial rotation. Knee Surg Sports Traumatol Arthrosc 17(8):920–926
39. Markolf KL, Graves BR, Sigward SM, Jackson SR, McAllister DR (2007) Effects of posterolateral reconstructions on external tibial rotation and forces in a posterior cruciate ligament graft. J Bone Joint Surg Am 89(11):2351–2358
40. Markolf KL, Kochan A, Amstutz HC (1984) Measurement of knee stiffness and laxity in patients with documented absence of the anterior cruciate ligament. J Bone Joint Surg Am 66(2):242–252
41. McCarthy M, Camarda L, Wijdicks CA, Johansen S, Engebretsen L, Laprade RF (2010) Anatomic posterolateral knee reconstructions require a popliteofibular ligament reconstruction through a tibial tunnel. Am J Sports Med 38(8):1674–1681
42. McQuade KJ, Crutcher JP, Sidles JA, Larson RV (1989) Tibial rotation in anterior cruciate deficient knees: an in vitro study. J Orthop Sports Phys Ther 11(4):146–149

43. McQuade KJ, Sidles JA, Larson RV (1989) Reliability of the genucom knee analysis system. A pilot study. Clin Orthop Relat Res 245:216–219
44. Mouton C, Seil R, Agostinis H, Maas S, Theisen D (2012) Influence of individual characteristics on static rotational knee laxity using the Rotameter. Knee Surg Sports Traumatol Arthrosc 20(4):645–651
45. Mouton C, Seil R, Meyer T, Agostinis H, Theisen D (2014) Combined anterior and rotational laxity measurements allow characterizing personal knee laxity profiles in healthy individuals. Knee Surg Sports Traumatol Arthrosc. doi:10.1007/s00167-014-3244-6
46. Mouton C, Theisen D, Meyer T, Agostinis H, Nuhrenborger C, Pape D, Seil R (2015) Noninjured knees of patients with noncontact ACL injuries display higher average anterior and internal rotational knee laxity compared with healthy knees of a noninjured population. Am J Sports Med 43(8):1918–1923
47. Mouton C, Theisen D, Meyer T, Agostinis H, Nührenbörger C, Pape D, Seil R (2015) Combined anterior and rotational knee laxity measurements improve the diagnosis of anterior cruciate ligament injuries. Knee Surg Sports Traumatol Arthrosc. doi:10.1007/s00167-015-3757-7
48. Mouton C, Theisen D, Pape D, Nuhrenborger C, Seil R (2012) Static rotational knee laxity in anterior cruciate ligament injuries. Knee Surg Sports Traumatol Arthrosc 20(4):652–662
49. Musahl V, Bell KM, Tsai AG, Costic RS, Allaire R, Zantop T, Irrgang JJ, Fu FH (2007) Development of a simple device for measurement of rotational knee laxity. Knee Surg Sports Traumatol Arthrosc 15(8):1009–1012
50. Musahl V, Citak M, O'Loughlin PF, Choi D, Bedi A, Pearle AD (2010) The effect of medial versus lateral meniscectomy on the stability of the anterior cruciate ligament-deficient knee. Am J Sports Med 38(8):1591–1597
51. Musahl V, Seil R, Zaffagnini S, Tashman S, Karlsson J (2012) The role of static and dynamic rotatory laxity testing in evaluating ACL injury. Knee Surg Sports Traumatol Arthrosc 20(4):603–612
52. Myklebust G, Bahr R (2005) Return to play guidelines after anterior cruciate ligament surgery. Br J Sports Med 39(3):127–131
53. Nielsen S, Ovesen J, Rasmussen O (1984) The anterior cruciate ligament of the knee: an experimental study of its importance in rotatory knee instability. Arch Orthop Trauma Surg 103(3):170–174
54. Oliver JH, Coughlin LP (1987) Objective knee evaluation using the Genucom Knee Analysis System. Clinical implications. Am J Sports Med 15(6):571–578
55. Park HS, Wilson NA, Zhang LQ (2008) Gender differences in passive knee biomechanical properties in tibial rotation. J Orthop Res 26(7):937–944
56. Pollet V, Barrat D, Meirhaeghe E, Vaes P, Handelberg F (2005) The role of the Rolimeter in quantifying knee instability compared to the functional outcome of ACL-reconstructed versus conservatively-treated knees. Knee Surg Sports Traumatol Arthrosc 13(1):12–18
57. Rupp S, Muller B, Seil R (2001) Knee laxity after ACL reconstruction with a BPTB graft. Knee Surg Sports Traumatol Arthrosc 9(2):72–76
58. Salmon LJ, Russell VJ, Refshauge K, Kader D, Connolly C, Linklater J, Pinczewski LA (2006) Long-term outcome of endoscopic anterior cruciate ligament reconstruction with patellar tendon autograft: minimum 13-year review. Am J Sports Med 34(5):721–732
59. Shoemaker SC, Markolf KL (1982) In vivo rotatory knee stability. Ligamentous and muscular contributions. J Bone Joint Surg Am 64(2):208–216
60. Shultz SJ, Carcia CR, Perrin DH (2004) Knee joint laxity affects muscle activation patterns in the healthy knee. J Electromyogr Kinesiol 14(4):475–483
61. Shultz SJ, Dudley WN, Kong Y (2012) Identifying multiplanar knee laxity profiles and associated physical characteristics. J Athl Train 47(2):159–169
62. Shultz SJ, Kirk SE, Johnson ML, Sander TC, Perrin DH (2004) Relationship between sex hormones and anterior knee laxity across the menstrual cycle. Med Sci Sports Exerc 36(7):1165–1174
63. Shultz SJ, Levine BJ, Nguyen AD, Kim H, Montgomery MM, Perrin DH (2010) A comparison of cyclic variations in anterior knee laxity, genu recurvatum, and general joint laxity across the menstrual cycle. J Orthop Res 28(11):1411–1417
64. Shultz SJ, Sander TC, Kirk SE, Perrin DH (2005) Sex differences in knee joint laxity change across the female menstrual cycle. J Sports Med Phys Fitness 45(4):594–603
65. Shultz SJ, Schmitz RJ (2009) Effects of transverse and frontal plane knee laxity on hip and knee neuromechanics during drop landings. Am J Sports Med 37(9):1821–1830
66. Shultz SJ, Schmitz RJ, Beynnon BD (2011) Variations in varus/valgus and internal/external rotational knee laxity and stiffness across the menstrual cycle. J Orthop Res 29(3):318–325
67. Shultz SJ, Schmitz RJ, Cone JR, Copple TJ, Montgomery MM, Pye ML, Tritsch AJ (2013) Multiplanar knee laxity increases during a 90-min intermittent exercise protocol. Med Sci Sports Exerc 45(8):1553–1561
68. Shultz SJ, Schmitz RJ, Cone JR, Henson RA, Montgomery MM, Pye ML, Tritsch AJ (2015) Changes in fatigue, multiplanar knee laxity, and landing biomechanics during intermittent exercise. J Athl Train 50(5):486–497
69. Shultz SJ, Schmitz RJ, Nguyen AD, Levine BJ (2010) Joint laxity is related to lower extremity energetics during a drop jump landing. Med Sci Sports Exerc 42(4):771–780
70. Shultz SJ, Shimokochi Y, Nguyen AD, Schmitz RJ, Beynnon BD, Perrin DH (2007) Measurement of varus-valgus and internal-external rotational knee laxities in vivo – part I: assessment of measurement reliability and bilateral asymmetry. J Orthop Res 25(8):981–988
71. Shultz SJ, Shimokochi Y, Nguyen AD, Schmitz RJ, Beynnon BD, Perrin DH (2007) Measurement of

varus-valgus and internal-external rotational knee laxities in vivo – part II: relationship with anterior-posterior and general joint laxity in males and females. J Orthop Res 25(8):989–996
72. Slocum DB, Larson RL (2007) Rotatory instability of the knee: its pathogenesis and a clinical test to demonstrate its presence. 1968. Clin Orthop Relat Res 454:5–13; discussion 13–14
73. Stoller DW, Markolf KL, Zager SA, Shoemaker SC (1983) The effects of exercise, ice, and ultrasonography on torsional laxity of the knee. Clin Orthop Relat Res 174:172–180
74. Tardy N, Mouton C, Boisrenoult P, Theisen D, Beaufils P, Seil R (2014) Rotational profile alterations after anatomic posterolateral corner reconstructions in multiligament injured knees. Knee Surg Sports Traumatol Arthrosc 22(9):2173–2180
75. Torry MR, Myers C, Pennington WW, Shelburne KB, Krong JP, Giphart JE, Steadman JR, Woo SL (2011) Relationship of anterior knee laxity to knee translations during drop landings: a bi-plane fluoroscopy study. Knee Surg Sports Traumatol Arthrosc 19(4):653–662
76. Tsai AG, Musahl V, Steckel H, Bell KM, Zantop T, Irrgang JJ, Fu FH (2008) Rotational knee laxity: reliability of a simple measurement device in vivo. BMC Musculoskelet Disord 9:35
77. Uh BS, Beynnon BD, Churchill DL, Haugh LD, Risberg MA, Fleming BC (2001) A new device to measure knee laxity during weightbearing and non-weightbearing conditions. J Orthop Res 19(6):1185–1191
78. Uhorchak JM, Scoville CR, Williams GN, Arciero RA, St Pierre P, Taylor DC (2003) Risk factors associated with noncontact injury of the anterior cruciate ligament: a prospective four-year evaluation of 859 West Point cadets. Am J Sports Med 31(6):831–842
79. Veltri DM, Deng XH, Torzilli PA, Warren RF, Maynard MJ (1995) The role of the cruciate and posterolateral ligaments in stability of the knee. A biomechanical study. Am J Sports Med 23(4):436–443
80. Wada M, Imura S, Baba H, Shimada S (1996) Knee laxity in patients with osteoarthritis and rheumatoid arthritis. Br J Rheumatol 35(6):560–563
81. Wang CJ, Walker PS (1974) Rotatory laxity of the human knee joint. J Bone Joint Surg Am 56(1):161–170
82. Weir JP (2005) Quantifying test-retest reliability using the intraclass correlation coefficient and the SEM. J Strength Cond Res 19(1):231–240
83. Wolf JM, Cameron KL, Owens BD (2011) Impact of joint laxity and hypermobility on the musculoskeletal system. J Am Acad Orthop Surg 19(8):463–471
84. Woodford-Rogers B, Cyphert L, Denegar CR (1994) Risk factors for anterior cruciate ligament injury in high school and college athletes. J Athl Train 29(4):343–346
85. Zarins B, Rowe CR, Harris BA, Watkins MP (1983) Rotational motion of the knee. Am J Sports Med 11(3):152–156

14 The Use of Stress X-Rays in the Evaluation of ACL Deficiency

Panagiotis G. Ntagiopoulos and David H. Dejour

Contents

P.G. Ntagiopoulos, MD, PhD
Department of Hip & Knee Surgery,
Mediterraneo Hospital, Athens,
10, Ilias St., Glyfada, Athens, Greece

D.H. Dejour, MD (✉)
Department of Orthopaedics,
Lyon Ortho Clinic, 29, Avenue des Sources,
Lyon 69009, France

Clinique de la Sauvegarde, Lyon, France
e-mail: corolyon@wanadoo.fr

14.1 Introduction

Instrumented measurement of the knee laxity is a useful additional tool in both the preoperative diagnosis of anterior cruciate ligament (ACL) rupture and the postoperative evaluation of ACL reconstruction [4]. Many studies have shown their potential benefits and drawbacks from the use of arthrometry devices in the diagnosis of ACL rupture [4, 17]. The objective quantification by numerical measurement of knee laxity (e.g., laximetry) can discriminate the injured from the non-injured knee and can help identify the deficient structures [10]. Additionally, laximetry can be used as an objective tool for quantification purposes or for the validation of new reconstruction procedures [17]. But this quest for a "golden apparatus" of measuring knee laxity has been limited by the facts that their employment requires judicious interpretation of their results, and most of them are examiner dependent [4, 17].

Since the introduction of the "double-bundle" concept in the anatomy and the biomechanics of ACL reconstruction [1, 5], there has been an interest in the literature on the use of laximetry devices for two main purposes: (1) to identify complete and partial ACL ruptures and (2) to measure the rotatory laxity of ACL-deficient knees [3, 16, 21].

The original skepticism on the existence or the prevalence of partial ACL tears by some authors has been replaced by detailed reports on the diagnosis and the different available

V. Musahl et al. (eds.), *Rotatory Knee Instability*, DOI 10.1007/978-3-319-32070-0_14

treatment options of incomplete ACL tears [1–3]. The preoperative clinical diagnosis of such injuries poses difficulties even in the hands of experienced surgeons [4].

Many surgeons confirm a trend toward the application of different treatments based on the injury pattern and the ruptured bundles that include depending on the type of injury: single- or double-bundle ACL reconstruction in complete tears, augmentation of the remaining bundle in partial tears, or even conservative treatment of incomplete ACL ruptures [3, 6, 7, 15, 20, 21]. This raises the need for an accurate evaluation and measurement of ACL laxity in order to preoperatively identify the injury pattern and choose the correct treatment option [6].

Fact Box 1
The results from the addition of laximetry devices should be evaluated in combination with clinical examination and conventional imaging such as MRI.

The results from the addition of these devices should be evaluated in combination with clinical examination and conventional imaging such as magnetic resonance imaging (MRI) [4]. The need to discover tools to precisely diagnose the ACL rupture pattern is even greater when standard clinical examination tests [4, 11, 12, 14] or sophisticated imaging methods [22] fail to produce consistent results even in the hands of experienced surgeons. The use of imaging equipment seems to be insufficient when solely employed to describe the exact pattern of an ACL injury, and the results from MRI require judicious use, mainly because of the many patterns of the partial tears and because the image of a partially ruptured ACL often has similar features to complete tear or even mucoid degeneration [13–15].

Currently, there are many devices that help measure knee laxity, and among them the most popular are the well-known KT-1000™ and KT-2000™ knee ligament arthrometer (KT-1000, KT-2000; Medmetric Corp, San Diego, California), the easy-to-use Rolimeter™ (Aircast Europa, Neubeuern, Germany), and the stress radiography Telos™ device (Telos GmbH, Laubscher, Holstein, Switzerland). Many studies focus on the results of these devices in ACL laxity and compare different instrumented methods predominately to the mainstay apparatus of KT-1000™ [4, 17], although some data have questioned its efficacy [8, 17, 23]. There are also some data on different laximetry methods and partial ACL tears [2, 9, 13, 18, 19].

The importance of preoperative diagnosis of partial ACL tears arises from data that support the beneficial preservation of the ACL remnants given the synergistic effect of both bundles in knee stability [1–3]. The remaining fibers provide additional mechanical stability for the graft, especially in the immediate postoperative period [16], the vascularity of the reconstructed graft is enhanced by the remaining fibers and vessels [17], the preservation of neural mechanoreceptors in the remnants of the ACL benefits the proprioceptive function of the graft [18], and preserving the intact ACL fibers serves for a more precise tunnel positioning [5]. In cases of functional partial ACL tears, ligament augmentation results in increased stability, lower laximetry results, better proprioception, and reduced knee stiffness than single- or double-bundle reconstruction [5, 19]. The preoperative diagnosis or suspicion of such incomplete ruptures where the remaining fibers are mechanically solid and therefore functional can affect the design of the procedure (choice of graft, diagnostic arthroscopy prior to graft harvesting) and the technical aspect of certain steps, such as the arthroscopic knee analysis, the extent of debridement of the notch, the proper tunnel placement, the drill guides, and the size of the graft [1, 3, 5].

In the search of such a diagnostic approach to incomplete ACL tears, the authors designed two different studies to correlate the preoperative clinical tests and laxity measurements from stress x-rays and to test if different arthroscopically confirmed ACL injury patterns have distinctive preoperative findings in clinical tests, stress x-rays, and MRI.

14.2 Measuring Laxity with Stress X-Rays

We performed two different prospective studies where all consecutive cases of adult patients for primary isolated ACL reconstruction during a 6-month period were included. Adult patients with isolated primary ACL reconstruction and healthy contralateral knees were only included. All patients were tested clinically with the Lachman and the pivot-shift tests. Preoperative objective evaluation included bilateral Telos™ stress x-rays with the use of 15 kg. Telos™ protocol involved absolute numerical measurement of anterior tibial translation of the injured knee and the difference from the non-injured side with a test similar to Lachman under fluoroscopy. The patient was positioned in the lateral decubitus position on the evaluated side. A pressure plate was placed posteriorly at the mid-calf level with one counter bearing placed at the level of the ankle joint and the other approximately 5 cm above the patella. The patient was then instructed to relax the muscles and the knee was flexed to 20°. The stress was increased steadily and radiographs were taken after application of anteriorly directed forces of 15 kg. The anterior tibial translation was calculated by measuring the displacement of the medial compartment from the distance of a line parallel to the posterior tibial shaft cortex and tangent to the posterior contour of the medial tibial condyle (medial anterior tibial translation, MATT) to the posterior aspect of the medial femoral condyle (Fig. 14.1a). Displacement of the lateral compartment was measured with lateral anterior tibial translation (LATT) from a tangent line to the lateral tibial condyle to the posterior aspect of the lateral femoral condyle (Fig. 14.1b). Both knees were tested and the side-to-side difference was recorded.

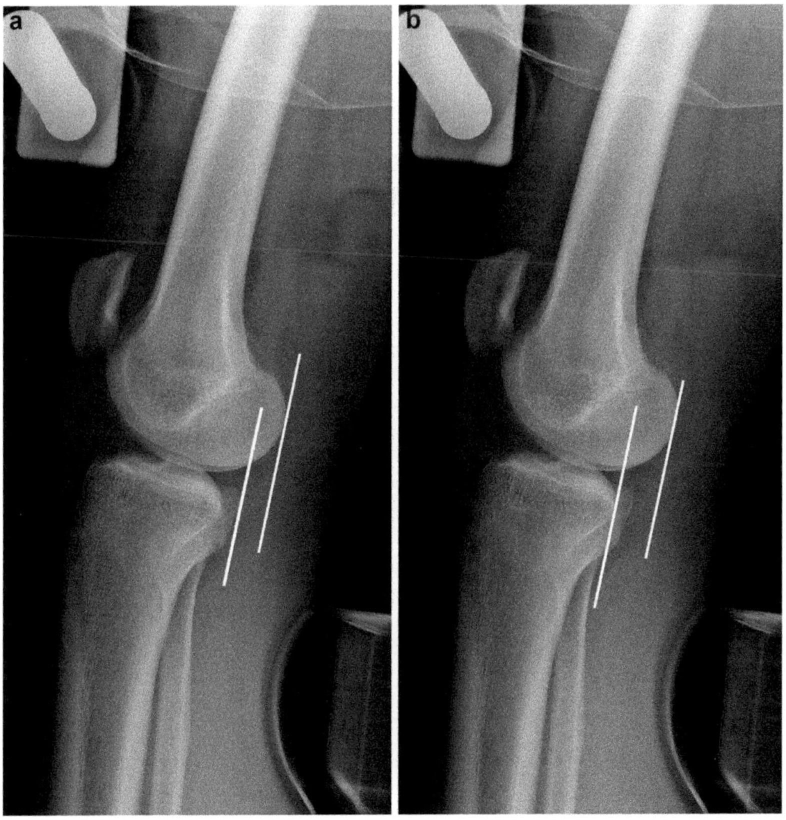

Fig. 14.1 Telos™ stress radiography lateral x-ray: (**a**) The medial anterior tibial translation (MATT) was measured from true lateral radiographs by calculating the distance of a tangent line to the posterior contour of the medial tibial condyle drawn parallel to the posterior tibial cortex and the posterior aspect of the medial femoral condyle. Side-to-side difference of anterior tibial translation from non-injured side is measured. (**b**) Displacement of the lateral compartment was measured with lateral anterior tibial translation (LATT) from a tangent line to the lateral tibial condyle to the posterior aspect of the lateral femoral condyle

14.3 Stress X-Rays Versus Rolimeter

In the first study we compared the results of stress x-rays and Rolimeter in order to quantify anterior tibial translation in complete and partial ACL tears. There was a not significant difference between the two laximetry devices, and side-to-side difference of anterior tibial translation was 6.4 ± 4.3 mm with the Telos™ and 4.5 ± 2.9 mm with the Rolimeter™ device (Spearman test $r = 0.30$, $p < .000028$). On the other hand, there was a statistically significant difference in anterior tibial translation measurement with both Telos™ and Rolimeter™ for the complete ACL tear group (7.4 ± 4.4 mm and 5.3 ± 2.6 mm, respectively) versus all types of partial ACL tear (4.0 ± 3.3 mm and 2.6 ± 2.6 mm, respectively). Telos™ results showed higher laxity values than Rolimeter, and *a threshold value of 5 mm with stress x-rays was strongly associated with differential diagnosis of complete* versus *partial tears*. Mean side-to-side difference with stress x-rays <5 mm was recorded in the majority of partial ACL tears (Fig. 14.2; Table 14.1).

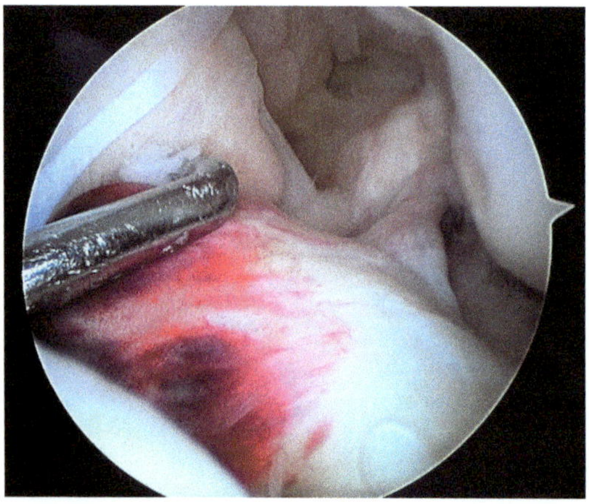

Fig. 14.2 Arthroscopic view of a complete ACL tear, where all ligament attachments have disappeared from the femoral notch

Table 14.1 Correlation between the arthroscopic ACL injury pattern and the preoperative results of Telos™ stress radiography and Rolimeter™

ACL injury pattern	Instrumented measurement of anterior tibial translation	
	Telos™	Rolimeter™
Complete tear	7.4 ± 4.3 mm*,[a]	5.3 ± 2.6 mm*,[b]
All partial tears	4.0 ± 3.3 mm[c]	2.6 ± 2.6 mm[d]
AM intact	8.0 ± 3.8 mm[NS]	5.6 ± 5.2 mm[NS]
PL intact	3.3 ± 3.1 mm[NS]	2.6 ± 1.8 mm[NS]
"PCL nurse"	2.9 ± 2.8 mm[NS]	3.4 ± 1.4 mm[NS]

NS Not significant when compared to other types of partial tears
*$p < .00001$ when compared to partial tears
[a]Interquantile range 25–75% (IQR), 4.2–10.0 mm; interquantile mean (IQM), 5.9 mm
[b]IQR, 5.3–2.6 mm; IQM, 3.5 mm
[c]IQR, 2.1–4.9 mm; IQM, 2.6 mm
[d]IQR, 1–4 mm; IQM, 3 mm

Fact Box 2
Stress x-ray results showed higher laxity values than Rolimeter, and a threshold value of 5 mm with stress x-rays was strongly associated with differential diagnosis of complete versus partial tears. Mean side-to-side difference of anterior tibial translation with stress x-rays <5 mm was recorded in the majority of partial ACL tears.

14.4 Stress X-Rays in the Diagnosis of Complete Versus Partial ACL Tears

The conclusion of the first study was that threshold values of >5 mm of anterior tibial translation with stress x-rays can confirm gross clinical laxity in cases of complete ACL tears, and when lower than 5 mm, they can raise a strong suspicion to the surgeon for the presence of a remaining ACL bundle, especially if they are accompanied with a negative pivot shift.

Fact Box 3
The conclusion of the first study was that threshold values of >5 mm of anterior tibial translation with stress x-rays can confirm gross clinical laxity in cases of complete ACL tears, and when lower than 5 mm, they can raise a strong suspicion to the surgeon for the presence of a remaining ACL bundle, especially if they are accompanied with a negative pivot shift.

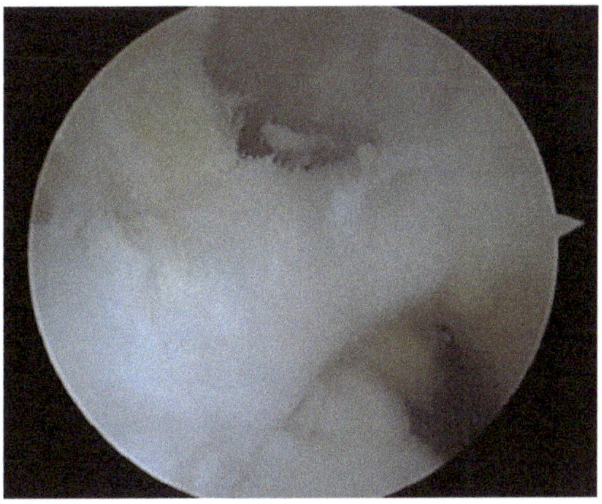

Fig. 14.3 Arthroscopic view of a "PL intact" tear

14.5 Stress X-Rays in the Diagnosis of Partial ACL Tears with Functional Remaining Fibers Versus Partial Tears with Nonfunctional Remaining Fibers

In a second study stress x-rays were performed, but also arthroscopic evaluation of the ACL rupture included the confirmation of the tear by direct vision and palpation with a probe. When the ACL was totally absent, the tear was classified as "complete," and when there was an isolated rupture of the AM bundle and the integrity of the PL bundle was verified visually and with the use of the probe in the "figure of 4" position [21], the tear was classified as "PL intact." In the case of an isolated PL bundle rupture, the tear was "AM intact," and finally when the ligamentous stump of the ACL was found "healing" on the PCL, the tear was classified as "PCL healing" (Figs. 14.3, 14.4, and 14.5). Further dynamic evaluation of the mechanical integrity of the residing fibers was performed by palpation with a probe. The remaining fibers were classified as "efficient" or "inefficient" depending on the presence of mechanically solid fibers or the ability of the examiner to further attenuate them, respectively.

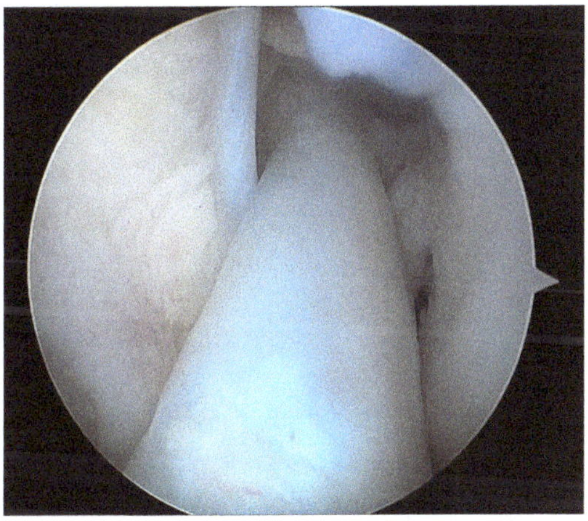

Fig. 14.4 Arthroscopic view of an "AM intact" tear

We observed a significant difference for MATT (9.1 ± 3.4 mm) and LATT (9.4 ± 4.3 mm) in complete tears versus MATT (5.2 ± 2.9 mm) and LATT (4.9 ± 3.5 mm) in all types of partial tears. The difference of anterior tibial translation among partial tears was not significantly different ($p > 0.05$) when compared to each other (Table 14.2).

We calculated the average of the anterior tibial translation for all arthroscopically confirmed efficient partial tears versus all inefficient partial tears, regardless of the injury

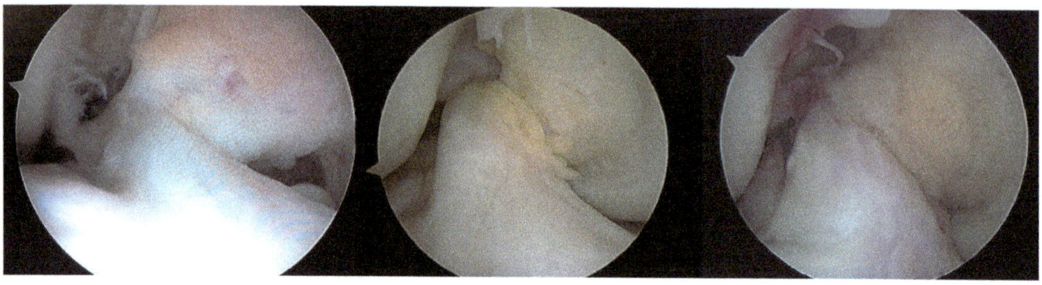

Fig. 14.5 Arthroscopic view of different cases of "PCL healing" type of partial tear. The femoral attachments have clearly disappeared from the notch but the ligamentous stump "heals" on the PCL

Table 14.2 Correlation of clinical examination results and ACL injury pattern

	Clinical examination of knee laxity					
	Lachman		Pivot			
ACL injury pattern	Delayed (<5 mm side-to-side difference)	Soft (>5 mm side-to-side difference)	Equal 0	Glide +1	Clunk +2	Gross +3
Complete tear (%)	1	99[a]	2	12	48[b]	38[b]
AM intact (%)	68	32	37	42	5	16
PL intact (%)	75	25	23	47	28	2
"PCL healing" (%)	56	44	20	65	15	0

[a] $p<.00001$ when compared with "delayed"
[b] $p<.00001$ when compared with 0 and +1

pattern (Table 14.2). *Median MATT was 9 mm in complete tears, 6 mm in inefficient partial tears, and 4 mm in efficient partial tears (p<0.00001). Median LATT was 10 mm in complete tears, 6 mm in inefficient partial tears, and 4 mm in efficient partial tears (p<0.00001).*

The combination of stress x-rays and clinical examination with the pivot shift had the following prognostic values: (*1*) *Less than 4 mm side-to-side difference* (*LATT*) *and 0 or +1 pivot shift had a 0.76 sensitivity and 0.90 specificity in the diagnosis of efficient partial ACL tears,* (2) *4–6 mm side-to-side difference and a positive pivot shift had a 0.56 sensitivity and 0.92 specificity in the diagnosis of inefficient partial ACL tears, and* (*3*) *side-to-side difference greater than 6 mm and positive pivot shift had a 0.88 sensitivity and 0.96 specificity with complete ACL tears* (*Table* 14.3).

Fact Box 4

The combination of stress x-rays and pivot shift had the following prognostic values: (1) Less than 4 mm side-to-side difference and 0 or +1 pivot shift 0 had an efficient partial ACL tear, (2) difference of 4–6 mm side-to-side difference and positive pivot shift had an inefficient partial ACL tear, and (3) side-to-side difference greater than 6 mm and positive pivot shift had a complete ACL tear.

Table 14.3 Correlation between arthroscopic ACL injury pattern and the preoperative results of side-to-side difference of anterior tibial translation from Telos™ stress radiography

ACL injury pattern	Mean side-to-side difference of anterior tibial translation (Median value)	
	MATT[a]	LATT[b]
Complete tear	9.1±3.4 mm*,[c] (9 mm)	9.4±4.3 mm*,[d] (10 mm)
All partial tears	5.2±2.9 mm[e] (5 mm)	4.9±3.5 mm[f] (5 mm)
AM intact	5.2±3.6 mm[g], NS (5 mm)	5.2±3.2 mm[h], NS (5 mm)
PL intact	5.1±2.8 mm[i], NS (5 mm)	4.7±3.7 mm[j], NS (5 mm)
"PCL healing"	7.0±2.5 mm[NS] (7 mm)	6.9±3.5 mm[NS] (7 mm)
All "efficient" partial tears	4.4±2.4 mm*,[k] (4 mm)	4.1±3.1 mm*,[l] (4 mm)
All "inefficient" partial tears	7.0±2.5 mm*,[m] (6 mm)	6.9±3.5 mm*,[n] (6 mm)

NS Not significant when compared to other partial tear groups
*$p<.00001$ when compared to partial tears
[a]Medial anterior tibial translation
[b]Lateral anterior tibial translation
[c]Interquantile range 25–75 % (IQR) = 7.0–11.0 mm
[d]IQR = 7.0–12.0 mm
[e]IQR = 3.2–7.0 mm
[f]IQR = 3.5–7.5 mm
[g]IQR = 3.7–8.0 mm
[h]IQR = 3.5–7.0 mm
[i]IQR = 3.0–7.0 mm
[j]IQR = 3.0–6.7 mm
[k]IQR = 3.0–6.0 mm
[l]IQR = 5.0–9.0 mm
[m]IQR = 2.0–6.0 mm
[n]IQR = 4.0–9.0 mm

The importance of clinical examination in the diagnostic approach of the ACL-deficient knee needs no further emphasis by the authors. But clinical tests are difficult to quantify; results often overlap among examiners and are very dependent on the examiner and suffer from a degree of intra-tester liability [14]. The pivot-shift test seems to be the most reliable testing maneuver in the identification of PL bundle tears according to Petersen and Zantop [16]. This is supported by other authors who recorded increased positive pivot-shift results in cases of PL ruptures, while the anterior drawer test and the Lachman test may be 0 or +1 [5, 14]. On the contrary, there is scarce data that the less frequent AM bundle tears result in greater laxity in Lachman test and minor laxity or even negative results in pivot-shift test [5]. But Petersen indicated that a clinical study validating the pivot-shift and the Lachman test of isolated PL and AM bundle ruptures has not been performed [13]. Our results show that great laxity in the pivot-shift test (+2 and +3) was the most consistent clinical finding in identifying complete ACL tears (86 %) versus incomplete tears (9.6 %, $p<0.0001$), yet it was not efficient to distinguish between the different types of partial ACL tear (30 % in PL tears and 21 % in AM tears, $p>0.01$). Accordingly, equal or +1 pivot shift was present in 70 % of AM tears and 79 % of PL tears in our study population. This finding is in compliance with DeFranco and Bach who identified the positive pivot shift as the mainstay of diagnosis of ACL deficiency and the need for surgery [1]. Lachman test was of similar diagnostic value since we recorded gross laxity of more than 5 mm of side-to-side difference in 99 % of complete tears versus 20.3 % ($p<0.0001$) in all cases of partial ACL tears, and the different types of partial ACL tears showed gross Lachman laxity in 75 % of AM tears versus 32 % of PL tears ($p<0.01$ when compared). This is also due to the higher prevalence of efficient PL intact cases than efficient AM intact cases.

On the other hand, instrumented methods of measuring knee laxity provide a useful numerical grading of anteroposterior laxity but are equally dependent on the patient (muscle guarding), require additional equipment and radiation exposure to the patient, provide rather static than dynamic results, and ultimately employ the same intra-tester error, especially when not used in combination with clinical examination [24, 25]. Posterolateral bundle ruptures resulted in significant lower KT-1000 results (1–3 mm difference) than complete tears according to Siebold and Fu, while AM tears had a side-to-side difference between 2 and 4 mm [5]. We recorded a statistically significant difference between anterior tibial translation in complete tears (mean MATT 9.1 mm and mean LATT 9.4 mm) and all cases of partial tears (mean MATT 5.2 mm and mean LATT 4.9 mm, $p < 0.0001$). But the different types of partial ACL tears exhibited nonsignificant differences in laximetry when compared between them, and although stress x-rays recorded higher laxity in a complete (median LATT 10 mm) than a partial ACL tear, the type of partial tear had similar laxity results. The "PCL healing" group had results smaller than the complete tear group and greater than AM or PL tear groups, but without a significant value, probably showing the degree of "pseudostability" the stump of ACL provides when it has healed on the PCL. This is also supported by Bach and Warren, who described a similar ACL tear that is attached or healing on the PCL by scar tissue, leaving a normally appearing strut of tissue that may be confused as either a complete or a partial ACL tear [22]. Instrumented laximetry can be a useful adjunct in the assessment and the quantification of anteroposterior knee laxity and can confirm a complete ACL tear or can raise a strong suspicion for the presence of efficient remaining fibers, but it is not sensitive enough to identify which bundle is injured.

We also tested the functionality of the remaining fibers by palpation with a probe. We recorded a statistically significant difference between the occurrence of "efficient" remaining PL bundles in "PL intact" group (67 %) and the "efficient" remaining fibers in "AM intact" and "PCL healing" groups (17 %, $p < 0.0001$). In our patient population, when a partial ACL tear was confirmed arthroscopically, it was predominately an AM bundle tear, and in the majority of these cases, the remaining PL bundle was functional and efficient (with a median MATT difference of 4 mm) and could be preserved for ACL augmentation (Fig. 14.6), while in the less frequent cases of PL bundle tears, the remaining fibers where

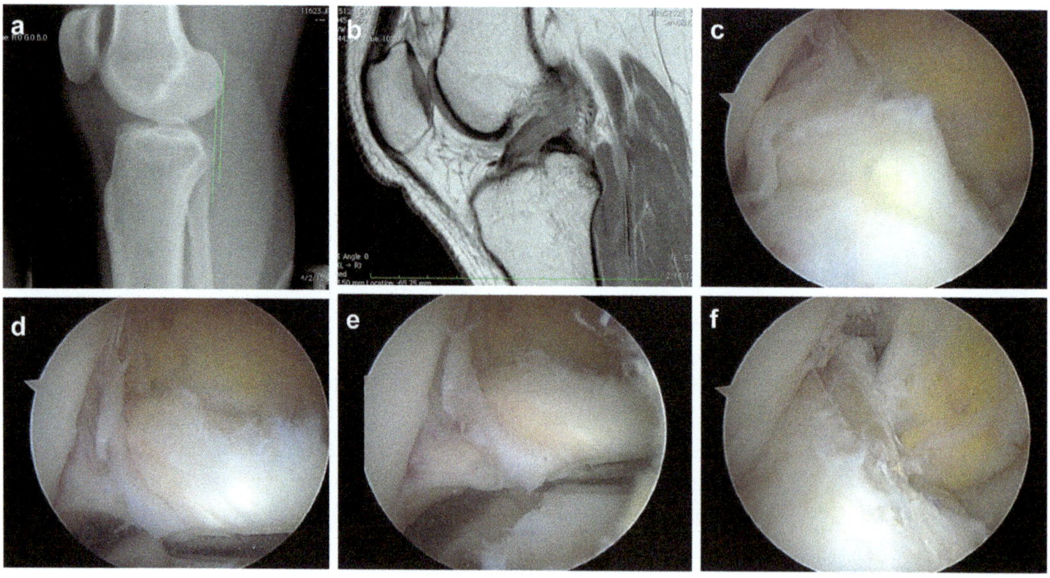

Fig. 14.6 Example of an efficient "PL intact" case where (**a**) a minor side-to-side difference of 2 mm of anterior tibial translation in Telos™ is recorded; (**b**) MRI findings show the presence of remaining fibers, but without identifying the type of injury pattern; (**c**) there are arthroscopic view and recognition of the injury type; (**d**) there is evaluation of the integrity of the remaining fibers; (**e**) there is confirmation of the mechanical integrity of the fibers in the "figure of 4" position; and (**f**) there is final view of AM bundle augmentation

mostly elongated and inefficient (median MATT difference of 6 mm) and could only serve as a guide to tunnel positioning in a standard single- or double-bundle ACL reconstruction. *From the study of our results, we recorded a threshold value of 9 mm of MATT difference in complete tears and a threshold value of 5 mm for the differentiation of efficient* versus *inefficient partial tears*.

Concomitant meniscal injuries that required some sort of further surgical treatment (i.e., partial meniscectomy or meniscal sutures) at the time of ACL reconstruction were significantly higher in patients with complete ACL tears (50 %) than all types of partial tears (32 %, $p<0.001$). Time from injury to operation was also higher in the complete tear group than all partial tears. This finding has also been supported by other authors and may be explained by the possible higher forces demanded for a complete ACL rupture or the longer time from injury to operation in cases of partial tears with a possible return to sports due to milder symptoms of instability, resulting in the progression of an undiagnosed and left untreated partial tear to a symptomatic complete ACL tear with secondary injuries to the meniscus [1].

Conclusions

In conclusion, there are different available diagnostic tools in our armamentarium for the identification of a partial ACL tear with possibly functional remaining fibers. Although the definitive diagnosis of a partial versus a complete ACL tear is not conclusive until the time of arthroscopy, the decision for operative treatment and the type of operation can be affected from grading clinical tests and from the results of instrumented laximetry. Gross pivot-shift laxity (+2 or +3) was consistent with a complete ACL tear, while 0 or +1 pivot shift was strongly related to a partial ACL tear. Laximetry with stress x-rays had increasing results in a scaled fashion from all types of partial tears to complete tears, but without identifying the injury pattern in partial tears. A partial ACL tear with efficient remaining fibers had less than 4 mm side-to-side difference in stress x-rays and 0 or +1 pivot shift, thus stressing the importance of preserving the remaining fibers during ACL surgery. Anterior tibial displacement from 4 to 9 mm side-to-side difference (MATT), especially combined with +2 or +3 pivot shift, was consistent with partial tears with inefficient remaining fibers that could serve only as landmark for tunnel position (Fig. 14.7). Side-to-side difference in laximetry greater than 9 mm (MATT) was recorded in complete ACL tears. Careful assessment of the ACL-deficient patient with the judicious use of additional tools to clinical examination such as stress x-rays can help the surgeon in the early identification of the presence of remaining functional ACL fibers before the time of operation. In such cases, the need for preserving the ligament fibers can lead to a different treatment approach or a specific surgical planning, according to the injury pattern.

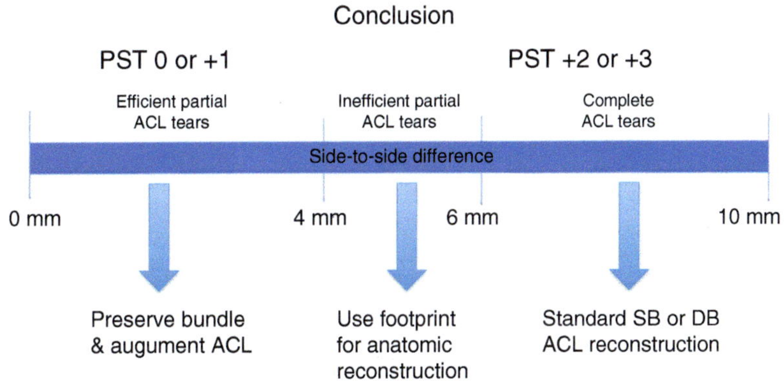

Fig. 14.7 Algorithm for the diagnosis and suggested treatment derived of different types of partial and complete ACL tears, derived from the results of the studies

References

1. Amis AA, Dawkins GP (1991) Functional anatomy of the anterior cruciate ligament. Fibre bundle actions related to ligament replacements and injuries. J Bone Joint Surg Br 73(2):260–267
2. Beldame J, Bertiaux S, Roussignol X, Lefebvre B, Adam JM, Mouilhade F, Dujardin F (2011) Laxity measurements using stress radiography to assess anterior cruciate ligament tears. Orthop Traumatol Surg Res 97(1):34–43. doi:10.1016/j.otsr.2010.08.004, S1877-0568(10)00248-3 [pii]
3. Borbon CA, Mouzopoulos G, Siebold R (2012) Why perform an ACL augmentation? Knee Surg Sports Traumatol Arthrosc 20(2):245–251. doi:10.1007/s00167-011-1565-2
4. Branch TP, Mayr HO, Browne JE, Campbell JC, Stoehr A, Jacobs CA (2010) Instrumented examination of anterior cruciate ligament injuries: minimizing flaws of the manual clinical examination. Arthroscopy 26(7):997–1004. doi:10.1016/j.arthro.2010.01.019, S0749-8063(10)00090-3 [pii]
5. Cha PS, Brucker PU, West RV, Zelle BA, Yagi M, Kurosaka M, Fu FH (2005) Arthroscopic double-bundle anterior cruciate ligament reconstruction: an anatomic approach. Arthroscopy 21(10):1275. doi:10.1016/j.arthro.2005.07.018, S0749-8063(05)01106-0 [pii]
6. Colombet P, Dejour D, Panisset JC, Siebold R, French Arthroscopy S (2010) Current concept of partial anterior cruciate ligament ruptures. Orthop Traumatol Surg Res 96(8 Suppl):S109–S118. doi:10.1016/j.otsr.2010.09.003, S1877-0568(10)00183-0 [pii]
7. Eriksson E (1997) Isolated partial rupture of the anterior cruciate ligament. Knee Surg Sports Traumatol Arthrosc 5(2):65
8. Graham GP, Johnson S, Dent CM, Fairclough JA (1991) Comparison of clinical tests and the KT1000 in the diagnosis of anterior cruciate ligament rupture. Br J Sports Med 25(2):96–97
9. Hole RL, Lintner DM, Kamaric E, Moseley JB (1996) Increased tibial translation after partial sectioning of the anterior cruciate ligament. The posterolateral bundle. Am J Sports Med 24(4):556–560
10. Hurley WL, Denegar C, Buckley WE (2008) The relationship between grading and instrumented measurements of anterior knee joint laxity. J Sport Rehabil 17(1):60–67
11. Kim SJ, Kim HK (1995) Reliability of the anterior drawer test, the pivot shift test, and the Lachman test. Clin Orthop Relat Res 317:237–242
12. Lane CG, Warren R, Pearle AD (2008) The pivot shift. J Am Acad Orthop Surg 16(12):679–688. 16/12/679 [pii]
13. Liu W, Maitland ME, Bell GD (2002) A modeling study of partial ACL injury: simulated KT-2000 arthrometer tests. J Biomech Eng 124(3):294–301
14. Musahl V, Hoshino Y, Ahlden M, Araujo P, Irrgang JJ, Zaffagnini S, Karlsson J, Fu FH (2012) The pivot shift: a global user guide. Knee Surg Sports Traumatol Arthrosc. doi:10.1007/s00167-011-1859-4
15. Oe K, Kushida T, Okamoto N, Umeda M, Nakamura T, Ikehara S, Iida H (2011) New strategies for anterior cruciate ligament partial rupture using bone marrow transplantation in rats. Stem Cells Dev 20(4):671–679. doi:10.1089/scd.2010.0182
16. Petersen W, Zantop T (2006) Partial rupture of the anterior cruciate ligament. Arthroscopy 22(11):1143–1145, S0749-8063(06)01115-7 [pii]
17. Pugh L, Mascarenhas R, Arneja S, Chin PY, Leith JM (2009) Current concepts in instrumented knee-laxity testing. Am J Sports Med 37(1):199–210. doi:10.1177/0363546508323746, 0363546508323746 [pii]
18. Rijke AM, Perrin DH, Goitz HT, McCue FC 3rd (1994) Instrumented arthrometry for diagnosing partial versus complete anterior cruciate ligament tears. Am J Sports Med 22(2):294–298
19. Robert H, Nouveau S, Gageot S, Gagniere B (2009) A new knee arthrometer, the GNRB: experience in ACL complete and partial tears. Orthop Traumatol Surg Res 95(3):171–176. doi:10.1016/j.otsr.2009.03.009, S1877-0568(09)00051-6 [pii]
20. Siebold R, Fu FH (2008) Assessment and augmentation of symptomatic anteromedial or posterolateral bundle tears of the anterior cruciate ligament. Arthroscopy 24(11):1289–1298. doi:10.1016/j.arthro.2008.06.016, S0749-8063(08)00510-0 [pii]
21. Tjoumakaris FP, Donegan DJ, Sekiya JK (2011) Partial tears of the anterior cruciate ligament: diagnosis and treatment. Am J Orthop (Belle Mead NJ) 40(2):92–97
22. Van Dyck P, Vanhoenacker FM, Gielen JL, Dossche L, Van Gestel J, Wouters K, Parizel PM (2011) Three tesla magnetic resonance imaging of the anterior cruciate ligament of the knee: can we differentiate complete from partial tears? Skeletal Radiol 40(6):701–707. doi:10.1007/s00256-010-1044-8
23. Wiertsema SH, van Hooff HJ, Migchelsen LA, Steultjens MP (2008) Reliability of the KT1000 arthrometer and the Lachman test in patients with an ACL rupture. Knee 15(2):107–110. doi:10.1016/j.knee.2008.01.003, S0968-0160(08)00008-2 [pii]
24. Dejour D, Ntagiopoulos PG, Saggin PR, Panisset JC. Arthroscopy (2013) The diagnostic value of clinical tests, magnetic resonance imaging, and instrumented laxity in the differentiation of complete versus partial anterior cruciate ligament tears 29(3):491–9
25. Panisset JC1, Ntagiopoulos PG, Saggin PR, Dejour D. (2012) A comparison of Telos™ stress radiography versus Rolimeter™ in the diagnosis of different patterns of anterior cruciate ligament tears.Orthop Traumatol Surg Res. 98(7):751–8

Classification, Diagnostics and Anatomical Considerations in Knee Dislocations

15

Jakob van Oldenrijk, Romain Seil, William Jackson, and David Dejour

Contents

J. van Oldenrijk (✉) • W. Jackson
Department of Orthopaedic Surgery, Nuffield Orthopaedic Centre, Oxford University Hospitals NHS Trust, Windmill Rd, Headington, Oxford OX3 7HE, UK
e-mail: jakobvanoldenrijk@gmail.com

R. Seil
Department of Orthopaedic Surgery, Centre Hospitalier Luxembourg, Clinique d'Eich., 78, rue d'Eich, Luxembourg City L-1460, Luxembourg

Sports Medicine Research Laboratory, Luxembourg Institute of Health, 78 rue d'Eich, Luxembourg City L-1460, Luxembourg

D. Dejour
Department of Orthopaedic Surgery, Lyon-Ortho-Clinic, 29 Avenue des Sources (BAT B), Lyon 69009, France

15.1 Introduction

Knee dislocations (KD) pose a challenge for orthopaedic surgeons. When confronted with an acute knee dislocation, whether in the field or in the emergency department, treatment begins with recognizing the severity of the injury. The extent of the injury is often not evident during the initial presentation, despite extensive multi-ligament disruptions and a high risk of limb threatening associated injuries. It is estimated that KDs account for less than 0.02–0.2 % of all orthopaedic injuries [21, 38]. High-velocity injuries account for approximately half of the KDs, particularly motorcycle injuries (18 %), motor vehicle collisions (7 %) and pedestrians struck by a car (7 %) [13]. Sports injuries are another major cause of KDs, accounting for approximately 47 % [13]. However, since patients frequently present with a reduced knee these estimations unlikely reflect the true incidence of KD. Physical examination is considered notoriously unreliable in assessing the severity of the injury [13, 15, 21, 29, 44, 47, 75, 77]. Moreover, with the rise of obesity in today's population, ultralow-velocity knee dislocations occur more frequently, with a higher incidence of associated neurovascular injuries [80]. Additionally, it is estimated that every 1-unit increase in BMI increases the odds ratio of post-operative complications after ligament reconstructions by 9.2 % [17, 62]. In morbidly obese patients, even minor injuries such as stepping of

V. Musahl et al. (eds.), *Rotatory Knee Instability*, DOI 10.1007/978-3-319-32070-0_15

a curb or a simple fall may result in a KD [80]. These patients are particularly difficult to examine.

The distinction between an acute multiligament knee injury and a true KD is difficult. It is therefore more practical to apply the same high index of suspicion to the assessment of every acute multiligament knee injury. The aim of this review is to provide a description of injury patterns after acute multiligament injuries and methods to reach a diagnosis and discuss the rationale behind the various treatment options.

15.2 Classification

Classification systems serve to determine the appropriate treatment strategy and prognosis and facilitate communication to enable comparison of cases. Kennedy classified knee dislocations based on the position of the femur relative to the tibia as: anterior, posterior, lateral, medial and rotatory [30]. Rotatory dislocations are further subdivided into anteromedial, anterolateral, posteromedial and posterolateral. The use of this classification in daily practice is however difficult if patients present with a reduced leg.

The anatomical knee dislocation classification introduced by Schenk and modified by Wascher provides a more detailed insight into the structures involved [66, 78]. A KD type I involves a torn ACL, with a functioning PCL and variable collateral involvement. A KD-II is a knee dislocation with complete disruption of both cruciates, with functional collaterals. A KD-III is an injury to both cruciate ligaments and a disruption of either the posteromedial or posterolateral ligaments, with an uppercase L indicating lateral and an uppercase M indicating medial involvement. KD-IV is associated with tears of both cruciates and both the posteromedial and the posterolateral ligaments. A KD-V is a fracture dislocation involving a multiple-ligament injury, with further subclassification to reflect the number of ligaments involved. The added uppercase C indicates circulatory damage, while the uppercase N indicates a nerve lesion.

The anatomical KD classification is relatively straightforward to use. However, determining a treatment strategy requires differentiating between lesions requiring repair (tears) and those with a good likelihood of spontaneous healing (capsuloperiosteal detachment) [4]. The distinction between a proximal, midsubstance or distal ligament detachment and a tendon disinsertion midsubstance or musculotendinous junction injury is therefore a valuable addition to the anatomical KD classification [86]. Finally, assessment of the severity of the laxity requires interpreting magnetic resonance imaging (MRI) findings in light of stability tests or stress radiographs (X-rays).

15.3 Clinical Assessment and Imaging

15.3.1 Initial Assessment

In case of a high-velocity knee dislocation, the first priority is primary assessment according to Advanced Trauma Life Support (ATLS) guidelines to rule out and treat life-threatening injuries.

If possible, reduction should be performed in the field or directly in the emergency department to avoid ischemic delays. Adjunctive examinations, such as X-rays, should not postpone reduction. After reduction, neurovascular status is assessed and X-rays are obtained to confirm an adequate reduction. CT imaging may be required to demonstrate associated fractures. Reduction may however be impossible due to impingement of soft tissues, which necessitates immediate surgical exploration. For example, during a posterolateral knee dislocation, the femoral condyle may buttonhole through the medial capsule, causing a dimple sign, an invagination of the medial structures. A true lateral dislocation or medial dislocation may however cause soft tissue impingement as well [61]. Although rarely encountered, open dislocations pose a high risk of infections and a reported neurovascular injury incidence of 63% [84]. In case of severe soft tissue compromise combined with gross instability or suspected vascular damage, immediate stabilization of the soft tissues with an MRI-compatible external fixation device may be necessary [21, 39].

Examination of knee stability in an acute situation is often impossible due to pain and swelling and should be done cautiously. The integrity of the collaterals is examined using valgus and varus stress, and the Lachman test and the posterior drawer test are performed to assess the integrity of the cruciates. More extensive stability testing using combined varus/valgus and rotatory forces is however not sensible at this stage since it may cause re-dislocation or further displacement of initially undisplaced fractures. More extensive testing should be performed cautiously under anaesthesia following initial fracture stabilization where indicated.

15.3.2 Vascular Assessment

Any patient with a PCL injury, double ligament injury or suspected knee dislocation should be examined for possible vascular damage [27]. The overall risk of vascular damage after a knee dislocation is approximately 18 % [48]. This risk may increase to 21–44 % in irreducible knee dislocations [50, 76]. Strikingly, one study reported a vascular damage rate of 41 % after ultralow-velocity knee dislocations in morbidly obese patients [1]. The highest vascular injury prevalence is with KD-IIIL injuries (33 %) and posterior dislocations (25 %) [48]. Amputation rate increases from approximately 10 % if revascularization is achieved within 6 h to 86 % if delayed more than 8 h [3, 5, 13, 21].

Vascular damage may show signs of coolness, pallor, cyanosis, absent or asymmetric distal pulses or delayed capillary refill. This situation requires urgent surgical intervention and revascularization, possibly preceded by in-theatre arteriography. The absence of distal pulses, however, is not sensitive enough to detect vascular damage and may be found in merely 30 % of knee dislocations with vascular damage [2, 5, 8, 41]. Physical exam should be accompanied by at least one adjunctive examination, although there is still debate on the optimal method. The most frequently mentioned diagnostic modality in current literature is angiography (90 %), followed by duplex ultrasonography (24 %), ankle-brachial index (ABI) (19 %) and MR angiography (9.5 %) [48].

The golden standard is still considered to be angiography, despite reported false-positive ranging from 2.4 to 7 % and considerable risks such as bleeding, thrombosis, pseudoaneurysms, arteriovenous fistulas, contrast allergic reactions and renal failure [21, 48, 70]. Stannard et al. therefore proposed an algorithm for selective angiography. If there are signs of vascular occlusion during the initial physical examination or a history of vascular abnormalities, patients will undergo angiography. In the absence of these findings, a patient is admitted to the hospital for neurovascular evaluation every 2–4 h for the first 48 h. In case of abnormalities immediate angiography is performed [21, 70].

An ABI is a fast, noninvasive, easy and inexpensive procedure to rule out vascular damage after knee dislocations. Mills et al. demonstrated a 100 % sensitivity, specificity and positive predictive value of an ABI of less than 0.9 for vascular damage after knee dislocation [50]. An ABI index may however be falsely positive in a patient with a previous history of vascular occlusive disease. In case of a well-perfused limb with an ABI of more than 0.9, some authors recommend hospital admittance for observation and repeated assessment of neurovascular status for 24 h [21, 40, 55, 56].

An ABI will however not detect a non-flow-limiting intimal tear, although its treatment is controversial, due to its unknown natural history. Progression of a minor intimal flap necessitating surgical intervention after initial conservative treatment has however been described previously [74]. However, a canine model demonstrated only 3 % of non-flow-limiting intimal tears progressed to a stenosis of more than 50 % of the lumina [65]. Currently most authors advocate a period of watchful waiting [21, 70]. Concerns for possible progression of a non-flow-limiting intimal tear have led other authors to advise angiography, CT angio or MR angio if available, on all knee dislocation patients, irrespective of the ABI [5]. Furthermore, occasionally a non-flow-limiting intimal tear may become apparent after ligament reconstructive surgery. Non-flow-limiting intimal tears may progress into complete devascularization due to the use of a tourniquet during surgery [8, 41]. In multiligament reconstructions following knee dislocations, a tourniquet should therefore be avoided, and an arterial and venous duplex should be obtained prior to surgical stabilization [40, 55, 56]. Another noninvasive and inexpensive adjunctive examination is duplex ultrasonography, although its use in knee dislocations specifically has not been studied. Bynoe et al. demonstrated a sensitivity of 95 %, specificity of 99 % and overall accuracy of 98 % in a series of 198 patients with blunt and penetration trauma of the extremities and neck [6]. Two patients with false-negative results sustained minor penetration shotgun lesions, which did not require further treatment.

15.3.3 Neurologic Assessment

Clinicians should be vigilant for nerve injuries after a knee dislocation, particularly the common peroneal nerve. Its reported overall incidence is between 13 and 40 % and it is particularly common in case of a disruption of the PCL and PLC (15–45 %) [21, 44, 53, 54]. Less than 30 % of peroneal lesions completely recover and may require neurolysis, primary repair, intercalary nerve grafting or tendon transfer [32, 51]. Mook et al. described a comprehensive treatment algorithm for suspected nerve injuries after multiligament knee injuries [53]. The first step when confronted with a suspected peroneal nerve injury in acute knee injuries is to assess the integrity of the PLC on MRI and to identify a possible surgically correctable cause. In case of a PLC injury or other correctable causes, the peroneal nerve may be explored during reconstructive surgery. Otherwise, EMG studies may be obtained 6 weeks after the injury.

15.3.4 Fractures

X-rays should carefully be assessed for subtle signs of fractures in any suspected multiligament knee injury, followed by CT scanning if necessary.

Avulsions of the tibial spine and Segond fractures are common findings in ACL injuries. Tibial spine avulsions may be very subtle and only show a small fragment in the intercondylar notch accompanied by a small cortical irregularity of the adjacent tibial eminence [18]. The Meyers and McKeever classification discerns four types of tibial spine avulsion fractures, ranging from minimally or nondisplaced type I fractures to comminuted displaced type IV fractures [49, 82]. An irregularity of the posterior tibia plateau on lateral X-rays may indicate a PCL avulsion fracture. Type I PCL avulsion fractures are nondisplaced, type II fractures are hinged with superior displacement of the posterior part of the fragment, while type III fractures are completely displaced [82].

The Segond fracture is an avulsion of the anterolateral ligament from the lateral tibia plateau and is highly associated with an anterior cruciate ligament injury [9]. The arcuate sign (or arcuate avulsion fracture) demonstrates a small elliptical avulsion of the posterolateral complex from the fibular styloid process on frontal or lateral X-rays (Fig. 15.1). It may contain the lateral collateral ligament and the biceps femoris tendon and is commonly associated with a cruciate ligament injury (Figs. 15.2 and 15.3) [18, 28]. It is usually the result of forced extension and varus and external rotation. A true varus force may cause an avulsion of the iliotibial band from its insertion on Gerdy's tubercle, although this finding is rarely seen (Fig. 15.4) [18].

Knee dislocations with associated fractures often demonstrate less extensive ligament damage than dislocations without fractures despite severe instability due to the loss of osseous support [75]. However, as in pure ligamentous dislocations, the severity of ligamentous injury in fracture dislocations often goes unrecognized. Gardner et al. showed that in patients with Schatzker II fractures with widening of more than 5 mm or a depression of more than 4 mm, the incidence of PCL and LCL injuries approached 30 %. Knee dislocations are accompanied by tibial plateau fractures in 25 % of cases and by femoral fractures in 19 % of cases [3]. Fractures resulting from a dislocation mechanism have a higher risk of ligament injuries than tibial plateau fracture resulting from

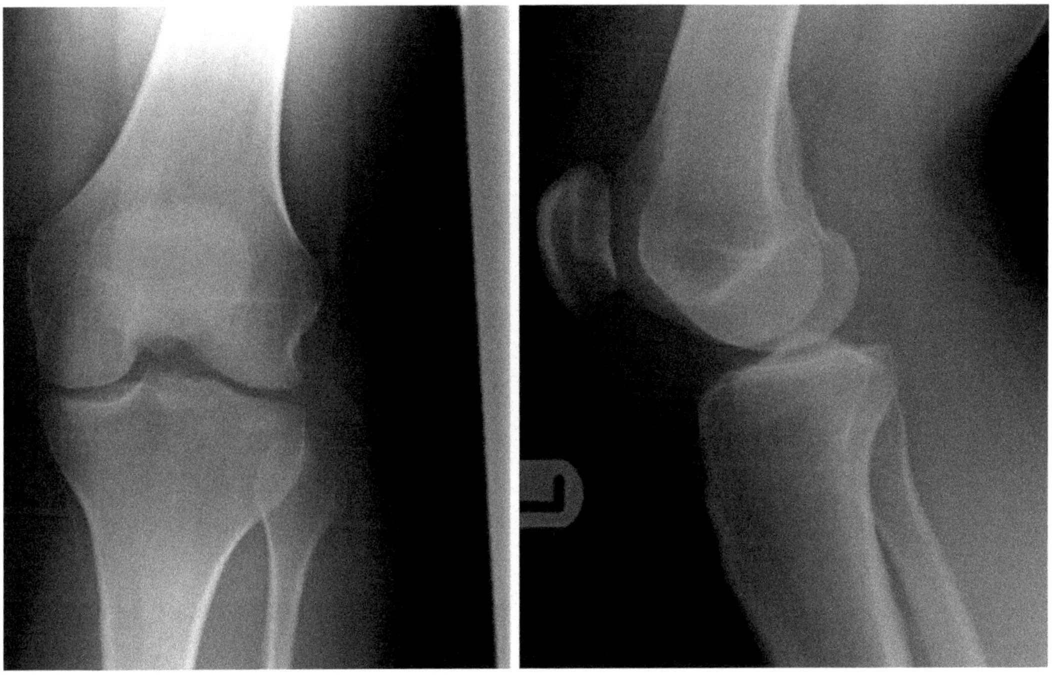

Fig. 15.1 Frontal (*left*) and lateral (*right*) knee X-ray of the left knee of a 29-year-old woman who sustained a high-velocity motorcycle injury. The X-rays clearly depict the arcuate sign: an avulsion fracture of the fibular head

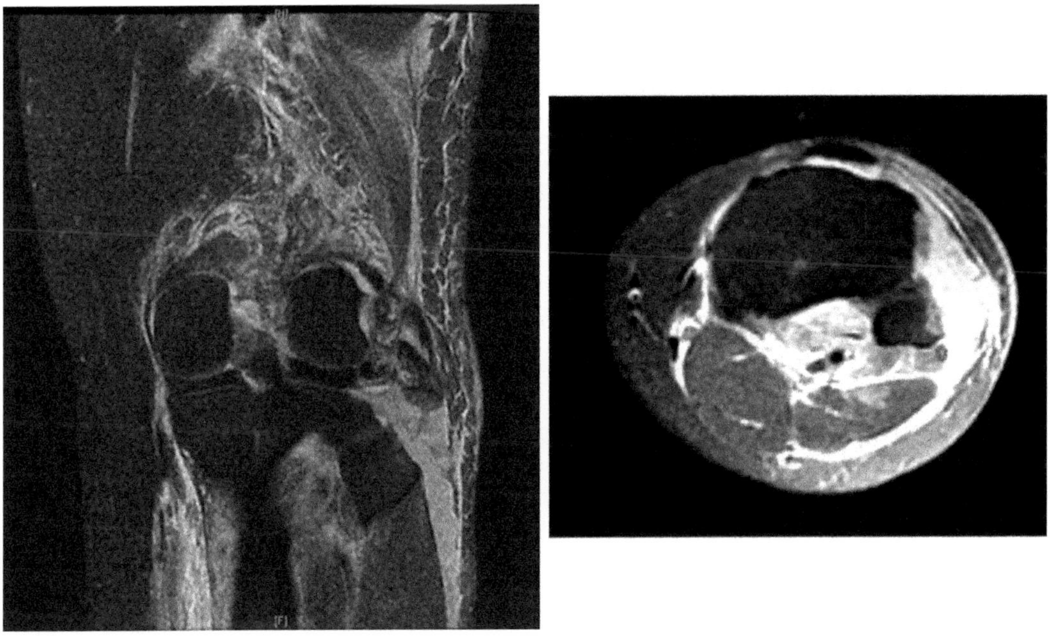

Fig. 15.2 Coronal PD FS (*left*) and axial PD FS (*right*) MRI images of the same patient confirming the fibula head avulsion fracture

strictly axial compressional forces. Tscherne and Lobenhoffer discern 5 tibial plateau fracture types which are indicative of a dislocation mechanism: D1 split fracture of the medial condyle, D2 fracture of the entire condyle, including the tibial spine, D3 a rim avulsion, D4 a rim

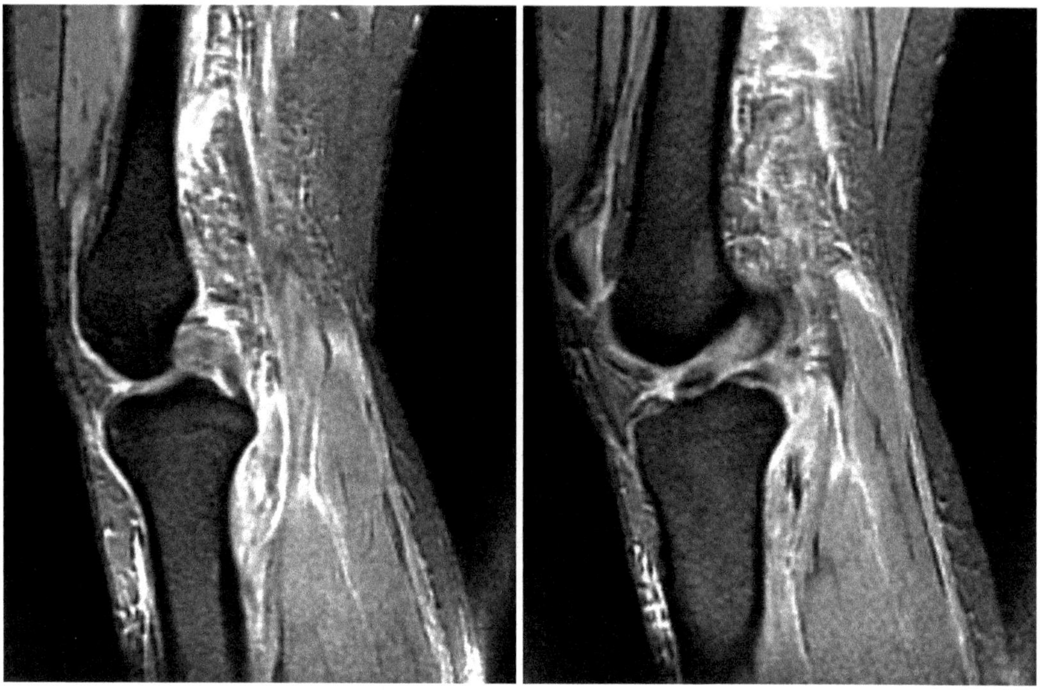

Fig. 15.3 Sagittal PD FS MRI images of the same patient demonstrating a proximal PCL tear (*left*) and a small ACL insertion avulsion fracture (*right*)

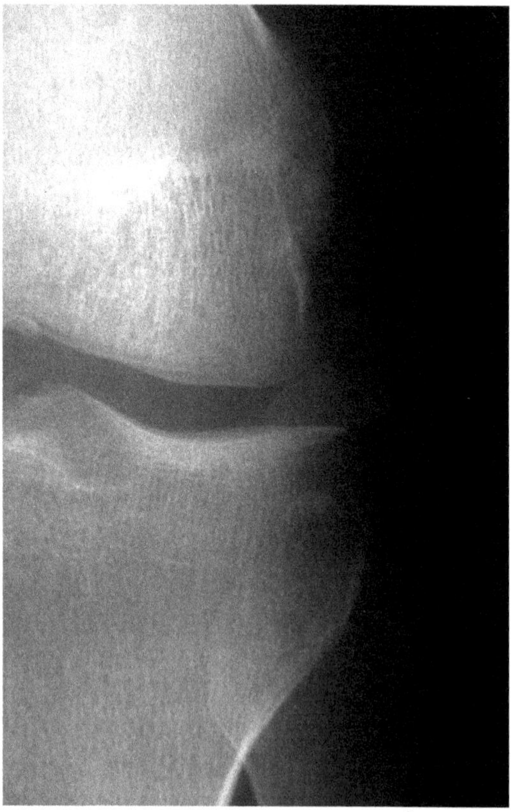

Fig. 15.4 Detail of a frontal left knee X-ray depicting an avulsion fracture of the iliotibial band from its insertion on Gerdy's tubercle

impression and D5 a 4-part fracture involving both the lateral and medial condyle as well as the tibial spine [73]. These fracture types should raise the suspicion for concomitant ligament damage.

15.3.5 Secondary Assessment

After life- and limb-saving measures during the first hours of the initial phase have been finalized, an early MRI, preferably within the first 2 weeks, enables further specifying the extent of the injury. Previous studies have shown excellent correlation between early MRI findings and intraoperative assessments [60, 75]. MRI imaging should include the fibula head. In case of suspected PLC injuries, MRI oblique coronal imaging along the entire aspect of the popliteus tendon provides a good view of the posterolateral structures [33, 36]. It is important to distinguish midsubstance tears from possible reattachable avulsions, since the latter may respond better to either early primary repair or conservative treatment in selected cases. Twaddle et al. identified the specific injury patterns and their locations in a series of 49 patients with dislocated knees [75]. The MRI diagnosis was confirmed during subsequent surgery within 3 weeks and disparities between MRI and surgical findings were noted. They found potentially reattachable ligament avulsions in 19 % of ACL injuries, 51 % of PCL injuries, 68 % of MCL injuries and 84 % of LCL injuries.

After identifying the affected structures on X-rays, CT and MRI, stability testing can be performed more judiciously. Assessing the degree of laxity and rotatory instability is valuable for determining a treatment strategy and may require examination under anaesthesia [13]. Caution is advised in highly unstable knees and stress radiographs should therefore only be performed with care by skilled surgeons. The external rotation recurvatum test is a test to assess posterolateral corner (PLC) stability [22, 34, 36]. With the leg in extension, lifting the leg by its great toe results in increase in recurvatum or hyperextension, indicative of a combined ACL and PLC injury. During this test, the amount of recurvatum is compared to the contralateral side. The examiner's other hand secures the upper leg on the table to adequately assess the amount of recurvatum, taking care to avoid dislocation in severely unstable knees. In addition to increased recurvatum, genu varum or external rotation may also be observed [22, 34]. Laprade et al. demonstrated an anterior subluxation of the tibia relative to the femur in a positive external rotation recurvatum test [34]. This explains why, in a series of 134 consecutive patients with posterolateral corner injuries, a combined ACL and PLC injury was found in all 10 patients with a positive external rotation recurvatum test. The test was found to be positive in 30 % of patients with a combined ACL and PLC injury [34].

The dial test or posterolateral rotation test can be performed in either the supine or prone position [36, 42]. With the knee flexed at either 30° or 90°, an external rotatory force is applied followed by comparison with the contralateral limb. A side-to-side increase in external rotation between 10° and 30° indicates an isolated PLC injury. Increased external rotation at 90° of flexion indicates a combined PLC and PCL injury [36, 39, 43]. The reversed pivot-shift test is another method to demonstrate PLC injuries. The knee is flexed to 90° while a valgus force and external rotation is applied. By extending the leg, the iliotibial band is tightened, thereby reducing the subluxation, producing a clunk [43]. Since it is found to be positive in approximately 35 %, a positive result must always be compared to the contralateral side [10]. The posterolateral drawer test is performed with the knee flexed at 90° and the foot externally rotated by 15°, while the posterior drawer test is performed with the foot in neutral rotation. A positive posterolateral drawer test suggests a popliteus complex injury [22, 36]. The posterior drawer test assesses the integrity of the PCL. The combination of a grade III posterior drawer test and >10 mm posterior tibial translation on stress radiographs correlates with the presence of a PLC injury and a complete rupture of the PCL [67].

Isolated superficial MCL injuries demonstrate laxity during valgus stress in 30° of flexion, while extensive valgus laxity in full extension indicates a more extensive injury often involving the posteromedial corner as well. Performing a posterior drawer test in neutral as well as in internal rotation differentiates an isolated PCL injury from a combined PCL and posteromedial corner injury. Internal rotation enables the posteromedial structures to act as a secondary restraint, which will therefore reduce posterior translation if they are preserved. In a combined injury internal rotation will not prevent anteroposterior translation and may even increase it [64, 72]. Anteromedial rotatory instability (AMRI) can be demonstrated by applying valgus stress in 30° of flexion with the foot in external rotation or an anterior drawer test in 90° of flexion in external rotation [72]. Stress radiographs under anaesthesia enable quantifying the amount of laxity. A recent systematic review by James et al. identified 10 studies on the use of stress radiographs in multiligament injuries [26]. Despite a growing number of publications with consistently high specificity and sensitivity, there is no consensus as to which technique is most appropriate.

Fact Box: Rotatory Stability Tests

Test	Pathology
External rotation recurvatum test	ACL + PLC injury
Dial test/posterolateral rotation test	
10–30° of flexion	Isolated PLC
90° of flexion	Combined PLC + PCL
Reversed pivot	PLC or normal
Posterolateral drawer test	PLC
Internal rotation posterior drawer test	Combined PCL + PMC
External rotation anterior drawer test	AMRI
External rotation valgus stress test in 30° of flexion	AMRI

15.4 Anatomical Considerations

After identifying all individual damaged anatomical structures, specifying their location and their degree of laxity, a treatment strategy can be formed, shaped to the individual expectations of each patient. Current evidence does not advocate a conservative treatment of multiligament knee injuries. Functional outcome, instability, contracture and return to activity are all in favour of surgery [21, 38, 47, 59]. Experience with conservative treatment of multiligament knee injuries is primarily based on the aggregate published outcomes of a small series of patients treated two or three decades ago, when nonoperative treatment was the standard of care [12, 59, 71].

In a multiligament injury, the question remains, which anatomical structures specifically need restoration and which structures could be treated conservatively? Treatment decisions should be based on the natural history and healing potential of the damaged structures and their combined effect on joint kinematics and long-term outcome. In case of a bicruciate injury, some surgeons may choose to treat all injuries in a single procedure, thereby facilitating rapid rehabilitation. Others may prefer a staged treatment aimed at restoring joint kinematics first and more extensive surgery only when necessary. While some cruciate and collateral injuries have a regenerative capability, additional PMC or PLC instability combined with cruciate injuries has a synergistic negative effect on joint kinematics.

15.4.1 The Cruciate Ligaments

Treatment strategies of ACL and PCL injuries in knee dislocations are still a topic of debate. Some advocate early reconstruction of the PCL together with collateral repair within 2–3 weeks, followed by delayed ACL reconstruction only if necessary [58, 85]. In two-stage surgery, the aim is to first restore knee kinematics, thereby avoiding prolonged surgery with increased fluid extravasation and possibly reducing postoperative stiffness. A later second-stage ACL reconstruction is only performed in case of functional limiting instability.

Other authors do not feel bicruciate reconstruction after knee dislocations needs to be staged and have reported good clinical results with single-stage bicruciate reconstruction [13, 14, 16, 47]. Early single-stage bicruciate reconstruction is best performed no earlier than 1 week after the injury to allow the capsule to seal, thereby reducing the risk of fluid extravasation, and no later than 2–3 weeks to avoid scarring. Single-stage early reconstruction of both cruciates may be particularly indicated in high-demand athletes, requiring fast rehabilitation. The decision to undergo a single-stage bicruciate reconstruction in athletes after a knee dislocation should be based on realistic expectations. In a series of knee dislocation with a median follow-up of 8 years by Hirschmann et al., 19 out of 24 athletes were able to return to sports after early single-stage bicruciate combined with PLC reconstruction. However, merely 8 out of 24 reached their pre-injury sports level [20]. The major obstacles were continued pain (42 %) and loss of flexion, besides invariably an altered proprioception. Outcome was affected by the timing of surgery and the injury pattern. Patients treated more than 20 days after the injury were more likely to give up their sports profession. Furthermore, patients with a KD-IIIM injury demonstrated more favourable results than with KD-IIIL and KD-IV injuries.

Some surgeons would rather avoid the challenge of single-stage bicruciate reconstruction and would prefer initial stabilization of either the ACL or the PCL. The PCL has a good regenerative capacity and may heal even in patients with multiligament injuries with limited instability [69]. Several studies demonstrated good objective and functional outcomes at long-term follow-up in patients with conservatively treated isolated PCL injuries [68]. A brace with active anterior drawer facility may be necessary during the initial healing stage to reduce posterior translation and elongation of the healing tendon [25]. The PCL plays a fundamental role in knee joint kinematics. The reported overall risk of long-term medial compartment osteoarthritis after reconstruction or conservative treatment of isolated PCL tears is approximately 41 %, with 11 % moderate to severe osteoarthritis. Reconstruction of isolated PCL injuries did not appear to reduce this risk [19, 24, 68].

Healing potential of the PCL is however insufficient in highly unstable knees due to gross collateral injuries. Mariani et al. showed that an isolated PCL or combined PCL/MCL tear with a posterior subluxation of less than 8 mm on stress radiographs corresponds to an incomplete tear that may heal spontaneously. These patients demonstrated PCL continuity and reduced posterior tibial translation on MRI after 1 year. Conversely, PCL healing was absent in patients with a PCL tear combined with an MCL and PLC injury with posterior subluxation greater than 12 mm. These patients did not regain stability [46].

Initial PCL stabilization in knee dislocations is therefore recommended in patients with displaced type II and III avulsion fractures or a PCL injury combined with a PLC or posteromedial corner (PMC) injury, as will be further explained in the next sections [52, 72, 82]. Patients with isolated PCL injuries with persistent grade III posterior drawer instability despite initial conservative treatment may benefit from delayed reconstruction.

15.4.2 Medial Structures

Due to the regenerative capacity of the MCL, most acute isolated complete and partial MCL tears can be treated conservatively with success regardless of the grade [45, 72, 83]. Treatment of medial-sided injuries as part of multiligament injuries is however more complicated. A systematic review by Kovachevich et al. did not find any studies on the conservative versus surgical treatment of MCL injuries in multiligament injuries [31].

Choosing the appropriate treatment of MCL injuries requires laxity assessment and to discern midsubstance tears from avulsions. Werner et al. considered nonoperative treatment of medial-sided injuries of KD-IV and KD-IIIM patients in case of a femoral-sided injury (Fig. 15.5), less than 5 mm side-to-side difference on stress frontal radiographs and absence

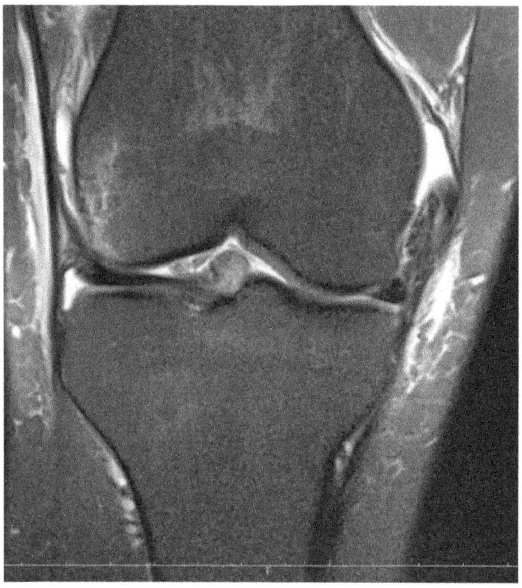

Fig. 15.5 Coronal MRI image displaying a proximal MCL detachment from the medial femoral condyle

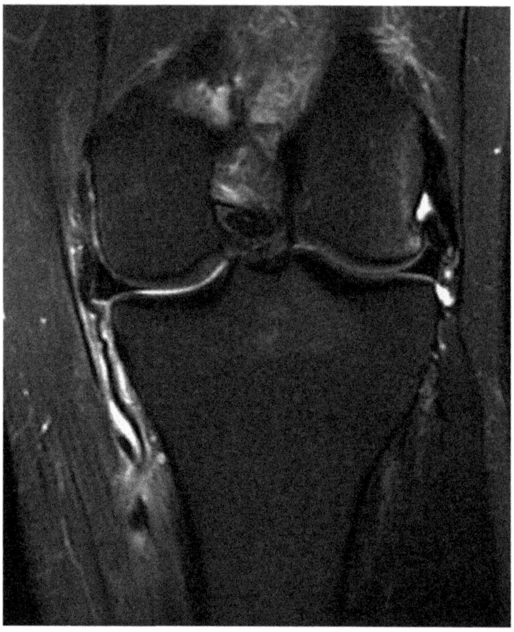

Fig. 15.6 Coronal MRI image displaying a distal MCL detachment displaced outside the pes anserine tendons

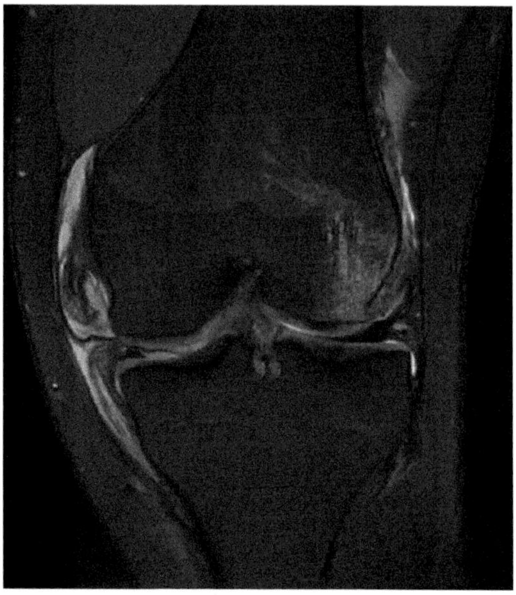

Fig. 15.7 Coronal MRI image displaying an MCL tear flipped into the joint

of valgus widening in extension. Tibial avulsions were repaired, while midsubstance tears were reconstructed [81]. Tibial avulsions more likely need surgical repair than femoral avulsions. Furthermore, if the superficial MCL is torn from its tibial insertion, it may be displaced outside the pes anserine tendons (Fig. 15.6) or even flipped into the joint (Figs. 15.7 and 15.8), thereby preventing regeneration. This situation is similar to an ulnar collateral ligament injury in the thumb or Stener lesion and requires surgical repair or reconstruction [45].

Laxity assessment in medial-sided injuries should also include rotatory testing. A large proportion of patients with KD-IIIM and KD-IV dislocations demonstrate injuries to the PMC, notably the posterior oblique ligament (64–84 %), semimembranosus tendon (38–64 %), posterior horn of the medial meniscus (38–41 %) and meniscotibial ligaments (28–50 %) [7, 81]. Injuries to the PMC may not heal without surgical repair or reconstruction, particularly when part of a multiple-ligament injury. Injury to the PMC may lead to persistent AMRI [72]. A combined lesion of the PCL and PMC is an indication for stabilization of both structures. PCL injuries result in a posterior subluxation of the medial tibial plateau, thereby changing the isometric point posteromedially, with increased risk of medial compartment osteoarthritis [79]. This posterior subluxation is greatly enhanced by

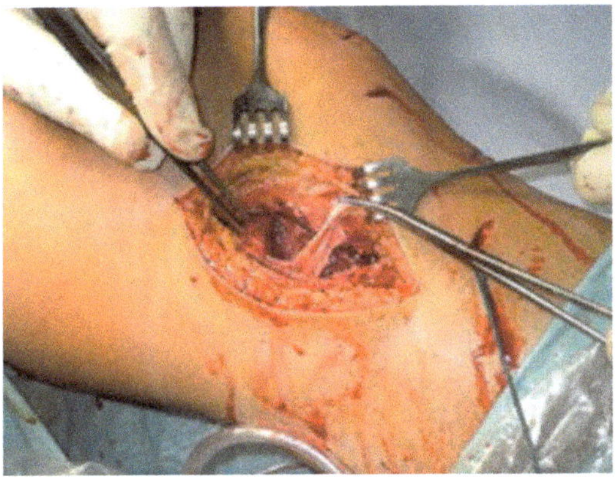

Fig. 15.8 Intraoperative image depicting an MCL tear flipped into the joint

medial-sided injuries. Therefore isolated PCL reconstruction will not completely restore stabilization [63, 68, 79]. Failure to recognize and treat associated posteromedial injuries puts additional strain on PCL reconstructions, with an increased risk of failure or long-term medial compartment osteoarthritis.

15.4.3 Posterolateral Corner

Injuries to the PLC may cause severe rotational instability and compromise the result of cruciate reconstructions [35, 57]. The PLC is very often affected in knee dislocations. Becker et al. described 43 % of multiligament knee injuries or knee dislocations involved a combination of an ACL, PCL and PLC injury [3]. On MRI a PLC injury was found in 77 % of cases, mostly demonstrating LCL (95 %), popliteus (89 %) and biceps femoris (37 %) involvement. Furthermore, peroneal nerve injury was associated with PLC injuries in 89 % of cases. Most of the LCL injuries involve an avulsion or tear from its femoral origin or distal insertion [75].

The PLC is complex and nomenclature varies with many anatomical variations described [11, 33]. Structures in the PLC can be divided into static and dynamic stabilizers. The static stabilizers include the lateral (fibular) collateral ligament (LCL), the popliteus tendon, the posterolateral capsule and the popliteofibular ligament. The dynamic stabilizers include the biceps femoris tendon, the iliotibial band and the popliteus muscle [23, 36, 39].

An isolated sectioning of the LCL will merely cause varus instability, while the combination of an LCL and the deep ligament complex will increase posterior translation and external rotation instability in response to varus stress, which is maximal at 30° of flexion. Additional PCL injury enhances posterior translation and varus external rotation [11]. High-grade PLC injuries have very little regenerative capacity and conservative treatment will often lead to poor results [11, 37]. Patients with PLC instability benefit from early surgical repair or reconstruction, preferably within the first 3 weeks [36]. This illustrates the importance of combining early MRI with specific rotatory tests to demonstrate PLC instability.

Conclusions

The diagnostic work-up of knee dislocations is summarized in Fig. 15.9. Life-threatening injuries always have the first priority in case of high-velocity injuries. If possible, reduction should be performed immediately. X-rays or CT imaging confirms the adequacy of the reduction and may reveal concomitant fractures. Severely compromised soft tissues may require a temporary external fixator to reduce swelling. Due to the high incidence of spontaneously reduced knee dislocations, clinicians should be vigilant for neurovascular damage in any multiligament knee injury. An ABI of more than 0.9 strongly suggests a preserved vascularity, although hospital admittance for 24 h and repeated assessments seem prudent. This should be accompanied with the judicious use of angiography or duplex ultrasonography when the clinician has any concerns. If a surgically correctable cause of a neurologic injury is evident on MRI, early intervention may improve symptoms. Otherwise, watchful waiting with EMG after 6 weeks is indicated. Stability testing during the first days should only be done with great care not to cause re-dislocation or displacement of nondisplaced fractures.

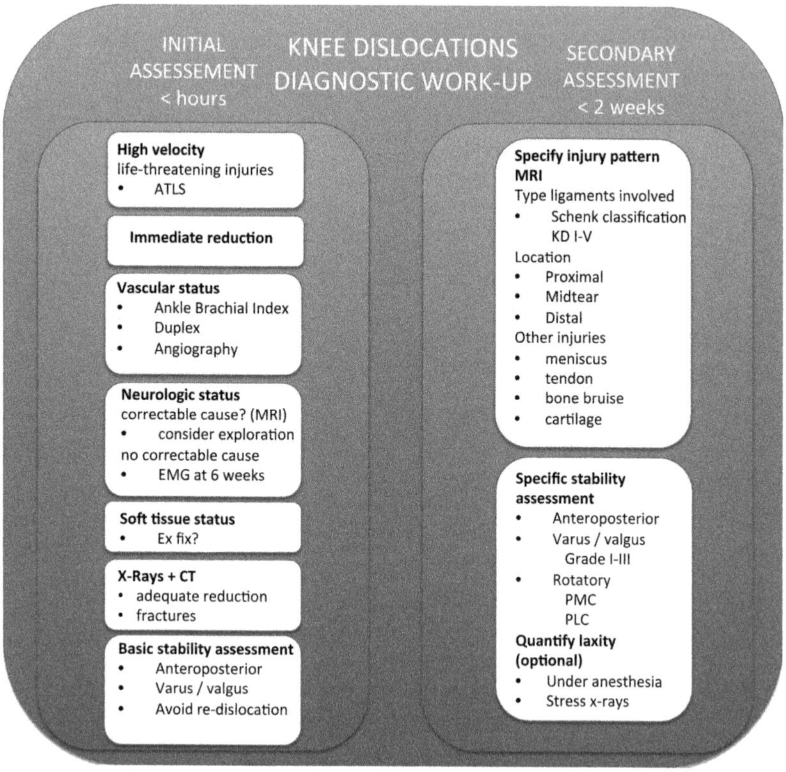

Fig. 15.9 The diagnostic work-up of knee dislocations

The injury pattern is further specified during the first 2 weeks after the injury using MRI followed by specific stability assessment. After identifying the ligaments involved, the injury is classified using the KD classification [66, 78]. Specifying the location of ligament tears into proximal or distal detachments or midtears enables identifying lesions with a good healing potential by either conservative treatment or direct repair. A distinction between high- and low-grade collateral injuries is made through laxity tests, occasionally requiring an examination under anaesthesia or stress X-rays. Rotatory stability testing is essential to reveal the negative synergistic kinematic effect of PLC or PMC injuries combined with cruciate injuries.

Determining a treatment strategy after knee dislocations requires recognizing the severity of the injury, specifying the extent and location of all damaged structures and understanding their combined effect on joint kinematics.

References

1. Azar FM et al (2011) Ultra-low-velocity knee dislocations. Am J Sports Med 39(10):2170–2174
2. Barnes CJ, Pietrobon R, Higgins LD (2002) Does the pulse examination in patients with traumatic knee dislocation predict a surgical arterial injury? A meta-analysis. J Trauma 53(6):1109–1114
3. Becker EH, Watson JD, Dreese JC (2013) Investigation of multiligamentous knee injury patterns with associated injuries presenting at a level I trauma center. J Orthop Trauma 27(4):226–231
4. Boisgard S et al (2009) Bicruciate ligament lesions and dislocation of the knee: mechanisms and classification. Orthop Traumatol Surg Res 95(8): 627–631
5. Boisrenoult P et al (2009) Vascular lesions associated with bicruciate and knee dislocation ligamentous injury. Orthop Traumatol Surg Res 95(8):621–626
6. Bynoe RP et al (1991) Noninvasive diagnosis of vascular trauma by duplex ultrasonography. J Vasc Surg 14(3):346–352
7. Chahal J et al (2010) Injury patterns to the posteromedial corner of the knee in high-grade multiligament knee injuries: a MRI study. Knee Surg Sports Traumatol Arthrosc 18(8):1098–1104

8. Chapman JA (1985) Popliteal artery damage in closed injuries of the knee. J Bone Joint Surg Br 67(3):420–423
9. Claes S et al (2014) The segond fracture: a bony injury of the anterolateral ligament of the knee. Athroscopy 30:1475–1482
10. Cooper DE (1991) Tests for posterolateral instability of the knee in normal subjects. Results of examination under anesthesia. J Bone Joint Surg Am 73(1):30–36
11. Davies H, Unwin A, Aichroth P (2004) The posterolateral corner of the knee. Anatomy, biomechanics and management of injuries. Injury 35(1):68–75
12. Dedmond BT, Almekinders LC (2001) Operative versus nonoperative treatment of knee dislocations: a meta-analysis. Am J Knee Surg 14(1):33–38
13. Engebretsen L et al (2009) Outcome after knee dislocations: a 2–9 years follow-up of 85 consecutive patients. Knee Surg Sports Traumatol Arthrosc 17(9):1013–1026
14. Fanelli GC, Edson CJ (2002) Arthroscopically assisted combined anterior and posterior cruciate ligament reconstruction in the multiple ligament injured knee: 2- to 10-year follow-up. Arthroscopy 18(7):703–714
15. Fanelli GC, Feldmann DD (1999) Management of combined anterior cruciate ligament/posterior cruciate ligament/posterolateral complex injuries of the knee. Oper Tech Sports Med 7(3):143–149
16. Gauffin H, Rockborn P (2014) Knee dislocations: is reconstruction of the posterior cruciate ligament crucial? Eur J Orthop Surg Traumatol 24(3):371–377
17. Georgiadis AG et al (2013) Changing presentation of knee dislocation and vascular injury from high-energy trauma to low-energy falls in the morbidly obese. J Vasc Surg 57(5):1196–1203
18. Gottsegen CJ et al (2008) Avulsion fractures of the knee: imaging findings and clinical significance. Radiographics 28(6):1755–1770
19. Hermans S, Corten K, Bellemans J (2009) Long-term results of isolated anterolateral bundle reconstructions of the posterior cruciate ligament: a 6- to 12-year follow-up study. Am J Sports Med 37(8):1499–1507
20. Hirschmann MT et al (2010) Surgical treatment of complex bicruciate knee ligament injuries in elite athletes: what long-term outcome can we expect? Am J Sports Med 38(6):1103–1109
21. Howells NR et al (2011) Acute knee dislocation: an evidence based approach to the management of the multiligament injured knee. Injury 42(11):1198–1204
22. Hughston JC, Norwood LA Jr (1980) The posterolateral drawer test and external rotational recurvatum test for posterolateral rotatory instability of the knee. Clin Orthop Relat Res 147:82–87
23. Ibrahim SA et al (2013) Surgical management of traumatic knee dislocation with posterolateral corner injury. Arthroscopy 29(4):733–741
24. Jackson WF et al (2008) Endoscopically-assisted single-bundle posterior cruciate ligament reconstruction: results at minimum ten-year follow-up. J Bone Joint Surg Br 90(10):1328–1333
25. Jacobi M et al (2010) Acute isolated injury of the posterior cruciate ligament treated by a dynamic anterior drawer brace: a preliminary report. J Bone Joint Surg Br 92(10):1381–1384
26. James EW, Williams BT, LaPrade RF (2014) Stress radiography for the diagnosis of knee ligament injuries: a systematic review. Clin Orthop Relat Res 472(9):2644–2657
27. Johnson ME, Foster L, DeLee JC (2008) Neurologic and vascular injuries associated with knee ligament injuries. Am J Sports Med 36(12):2448–2462
28. Juhng SK et al (2002) MR evaluation of the "arcuate" sign of posterolateral knee instability. AJR Am J Roentgenol 178(3):583–588
29. Kapur S et al (2009) Acute knee dislocation: review of an elusive entity. Curr Probl Diagn Radiol 38(6):237–250
30. Kennedy JC (1963) Complete Dislocation of the Knee Joint. J Bone Joint Surg Am 45:889–904
31. Kovachevich R et al (2009) Operative management of the medial collateral ligament in the multi-ligament injured knee: an evidence-based systematic review. Knee Surg Sports Traumatol Arthrosc 17(7):823–829
32. Krych AJ et al (2014) Is peroneal nerve injury associated with worse function after knee dislocation? Clin Orthop Relat Res 472(9):2630–2636
33. Laprade RF et al (2014) Improving outcomes for posterolateral knee injuries. J Orthop Res 32(4):485–491
34. LaPrade RF, Ly TV, Griffith C (2008) The external rotation recurvatum test revisited: reevaluation of the sagittal plane tibiofemoral relationship. Am J Sports Med 36(4):709–712
35. LaPrade RF et al (2002) The effect of injury to the posterolateral structures of the knee on force in a posterior cruciate ligament graft: a biomechanical study. Am J Sports Med 30(2):233–238
36. LaPrade RF, Wentorf F (2002) Diagnosis and treatment of posterolateral knee injuries. Clin Orthop Relat Res 402:110–121
37. LaPrade RF, Wentorf FA, Crum JA (2004) Assessment of healing of grade III posterolateral corner injuries: an in vivo model. J Orthop Res 22(5):970–975
38. Levy BA et al (2009) Decision making in the multiligament-injured knee: an evidence-based systematic review. Arthroscopy 25(4):430–438
39. Levy BA, Stuart MJ (2012) Treatment of PCL, ACL, and lateral-side knee injuries: acute and chronic. J Knee Surg 25(4):295–305
40. Levy BA et al (2005) Screening for extremity arterial injury with the arterial pressure index. Am J Emerg Med 23(5):689–695
41. Lohmann M, Lauridsen K, Vedel P (1990) Arterial lesions in major knee trauma: pedal pulse a false sign of security? Arch Orthop Trauma Surg 109(4):238–239
42. Loomer RL (1991) A test for knee posterolateral rotatory instability. Clin Orthop Relat Res 264:235–238
43. Lopez-Vidriero E, Simon DA, Johnson DH (2010) Initial evaluation of posterior cruciate ligament

injuries: history, physical examination, imaging studies, surgical and nonsurgical indications. Sports Med Arthrosc 18(4):230–237
44. Manske RC, Prohaska D (2008) Physical examination and imaging of the acute multiple ligament knee injury. N Am J Sports Phys Ther 3(4):191–197
45. Marchant MH Jr et al (2011) Management of medial-sided knee injuries, part 1: medial collateral ligament. Am J Sports Med 39(5):1102–1113
46. Mariani PP et al (2005) Evaluation of posterior cruciate ligament healing: a study using magnetic resonance imaging and stress radiography. Arthroscopy 21(11):1354–1361
47. McKee L et al (2014) Current concepts in acute knee dislocation: the missed diagnosis? Open Orthop J 8:162–167
48. Medina O et al (2014) Vascular and nerve injury after knee dislocation: a systematic review. Clin Orthop Relat Res 472(9):2621–2629
49. Meyers MH, McKeever FM (1970) Fracture of the intercondylar eminence of the tibia. J Bone Joint Surg Am 52(8):1677–1684
50. Mills WJ, Barei DP, McNair P (2004) The value of the ankle-brachial index for diagnosing arterial injury after knee dislocation: a prospective study. J Trauma 56(6):1261–1265
51. Molund M et al (2014) Posterior tibial tendon transfer improves function for foot drop after knee dislocation. Clin Orthop Relat Res 472(9):2637–2643
52. Montgomery SR et al (2013) Surgical management of PCL injuries: indications, techniques, and outcomes. Curr Rev Musculoskelet Med 6(2):115–123
53. Mook WR et al (2013) Nerve injury complicating multiligament knee injury: current concepts and treatment algorithm. J Am Acad Orthop Surg 21(6):343–354
54. Niall DM, Nutton RW, Keating JF (2005) Palsy of the common peroneal nerve after traumatic dislocation of the knee. J Bone Joint Surg Br 87(5):664–667
55. Nicandri GT, Chamberlain AM, Wahl CJ (2009) Practical management of knee dislocations: a selective angiography protocol to detect limb-threatening vascular injuries. Clin J Sport Med 19(2):125–129
56. Nicandri GT, Dunbar RP, Wahl CJ (2010) Are evidence-based protocols which identify vascular injury associated with knee dislocation underutilized? Knee Surg Sports Traumatol Arthrosc 18(8):1005–1012
57. Noyes FR, Barber-Westin SD (2005) Posterior cruciate ligament revision reconstruction, part 1: causes of surgical failure in 52 consecutive operations. Am J Sports Med 33(5):646–654
58. Ohkoshi Y et al (2002) Two-stage reconstruction with autografts for knee dislocations. Clin Orthop Relat Res 398:169–175
59. Peskun CJ, Whelan DB (2011) Outcomes of operative and nonoperative treatment of multiligament knee injuries: an evidence-based review. Sports Med Arthrosc 19(2):167–173
60. Potter HG et al (2002) Magnetic resonance imaging of the multiple-ligament injured knee. J Orthop Trauma 16(5):330–339
61. Quinlan AG, Sharrard WJ (1958) Posterolateral dislocation of the knee with capsular interposition. J Bone Joint Surg Br 40-B(4):660–663
62. Ridley TJ et al (2014) Effect of body mass index on patients with multiligamentous knee injuries. Arthroscopy 30(11):1447–1452
63. Ritchie JR et al (1998) Isolated sectioning of the medial and posteromedial capsular ligaments in the posterior cruciate ligament-deficient knee. Influence on posterior tibial translation. Am J Sports Med 26(3):389–394
64. Robinson JR et al (2006) The role of the medial collateral ligament and posteromedial capsule in controlling knee laxity. Am J Sports Med 34(11):1815–1823
65. Sawchuk AP et al (1990) The natural history of intimal flaps in a canine model. Arch Surg 125(12):1614–1616
66. Schenk R (2003) Classification of knee dislocations. Oper Tech Sports Med 11(3):193–198
67. Sekiya JK et al (2008) A clinically relevant assessment of posterior cruciate ligament and posterolateral corner injuries. Evaluation of isolated and combined deficiency. J Bone Joint Surg Am 90(8):1621–1627
68. Shelbourne KD, Clark M, Gray T (2013) Minimum 10-year follow-up of patients after an acute, isolated posterior cruciate ligament injury treated nonoperatively. Am J Sports Med 41(7):1526–1533
69. Shelbourne KD, Jennings RW, Vahey TN (1999) Magnetic resonance imaging of posterior cruciate ligament injuries: assessment of healing. Am J Knee Surg 12(4):209–213
70. Stannard JP et al (2004) Vascular injuries in knee dislocations: the role of physical examination in determining the need for arteriography. J Bone Joint Surg Am 86-A(5):910–915
71. Taylor AR, Arden GP, Rainey HA (1972) Traumatic dislocation of the knee. A report of forty-three cases with special reference to conservative treatment. J Bone Joint Surg Br 54(1):96–102
72. Tibor LM et al (2011) Management of medial-sided knee injuries, part 2: posteromedial corner. Am J Sports Med 39(6):1332–1340
73. Tscherne H, Lobenhoffer P (1993) Tibial plateau fractures. Management and expected results. Clin Orthop Relat Res 292:87–100
74. Tufaro A et al (1994) Adverse outcome of nonoperative management of intimal injuries caused by penetrating trauma. J Vasc Surg 20(4):656–659
75. Twaddle BC, Bidwell TA, Chapman JR (2003) Knee dislocations: where are the lesions? A prospective evaluation of surgical findings in 63 cases. J Orthop Trauma 17(3):198–202
76. Varnell RM et al (1989) Arterial injury complicating knee disruption. Third place winner: Conrad Jobst award. Am Surg 55(12):699–704
77. Walker RE et al (2013) Radiologic review of knee dislocation: from diagnosis to repair. AJR Am J Roentgenol 201(3):483–495

78. Wascher DC (2000) High-velocity knee dislocation with vascular injury. Treatment principles. Clin Sports Med 19(3):457–477
79. Weimann A et al (2012) Reconstruction of the posterior oblique ligament and the posterior cruciate ligament in knees with posteromedial instability. Arthroscopy 28(9):1283–1289
80. Werner BC et al (2014) Ultra-low velocity knee dislocations: patient characteristics, complications, and outcomes. Am J Sports Med 42(2):358–363
81. Werner BC et al (2014) Medial injury in knee dislocations: what are the common injury patterns and surgical outcomes? Clin Orthop Relat Res 472(9):2658–2666
82. White EA et al (2013) Cruciate ligament avulsion fractures: anatomy, biomechanics, injury patterns, and approach to management. Emerg Radiol 20(5):429–440
83. Wijdicks CA et al (2010) Injuries to the medial collateral ligament and associated medial structures of the knee. J Bone Joint Surg Am 92(5):1266–1280
84. Wright DG et al (1995) Open dislocation of the knee. J Orthop Trauma 9(2):135–140
85. Yeh WL et al (1999) Knee dislocation: treatment of high-velocity knee dislocation. J Trauma 46(4):693–701
86. Yu JS et al (1995) Complete dislocation of the knee: spectrum of associated soft-tissue injuries depicted by MR imaging. AJR Am J Roentgenol 164(1):135–139

The KneeKG System

16

Bujar Shabani, Dafina Bytyqi, Laurence Cheze, Philippe Neyret, and Sébastien Lustig

Contents

16.1 Introduction

In order to diagnose and provide effective treatment for knee conditions, the pathomechanics of injuries must be accurately described [1]. While significant information can be obtained through manual clinical examination, more precise and objective tools are needed for quantitative evaluation of the kinematics of the knee, particularly in regard to assessment of rotational laxity [2].

B. Shabani • D. Bytyqi • P. Neyret • S. Lustig (✉)
Department of Orthopaedic, Albert Trillat Center, Lyon North University Hospital, Lyon, France
e-mail: sebastien.lustig@gmail.com

L. Cheze
Laboratoire de Biomécanique et Mécanique des Chocs Université Lyon 1 - IFSTTAR, LBMC UMR_T9406, Pittsburgh, PA, USA

Gait analysis has become an innovative tool to quantify the biomechanical changes, in allowing the estimation of in vivo forces occurring at knee level.

Acquiring the movement accurately at knee level is not always simple; skin movement over the underlying bones can vary significantly over both the medial and lateral femoral condyles and is, therefore, the greatest obstacle in obtaining accurate movement data noninvasively. On the other hand, bone-mounted techniques reduce skin movement artifacts, but they are still too invasive and expensive for clinical use. Thus, establishing an objective evaluation of the kinematics of the knee in a clinically feasible way is critical to evaluate the knee function and give a valuable feedback for treatment.

Therefore, the KneeKG™ attachment system and KneeKG™ axis definition procedure were developed with the objective of providing high-reliability movement analysis.

16.2 Concept of the Device

The development of the KneeKG™ started in 1992 at the Imaging and Orthopaedics Research Laboratory in Montreal, Canada, to study the impact of tunnel positioning on ACL graft elongation, torsion, and bending. After reviewing the available scientific literature, the researchers came to the conclusion that there is a need for an assessment device to accurately quantify knee biomechanics in 3D [2].

V. Musahl et al. (eds.), *Rotatory Knee Instability*, DOI 10.1007/978-3-319-32070-0_16

As measuring the knee joint motion is limited by soft tissue artifacts, design for the new system began with a quantification of the skin-bone movement around the knee [3]. Based on this study, Sati et al. [4] proposed a system for fixing markers to the bones of the lower extremity in a semirigid manner which is composed of a femoral component, called harness, and a separate tibial component. The main objective was to develop a noninvasive instrumentation to obtain accurate in vivo knee kinematics, and the second objective was that this instrumentation should be sufficiently practical to be used on a routine basis in the clinical setting.

Using this system, called exoskeleton, the movement of markers relative to underlying bones was greatly reduced as shown by fluoroscopy [4]. This harness was shown to be accurate in obtaining 3D kinematic data that could be used to evaluate ACL and ACL graft deformation in vivo [4, 5].

The KneeKG™ system is designed to minimize floor space and maximize functionality.

Fact Box 1: KneeKG Design
An accurate 3D test of the knee
Fast examination (20 min)
Real time
Dynamic
Weight bearing
Simple
Valid
Reliable

16.3 Validation

While the soft tissue artifacts remain the main issue in assessing in vivo knee kinematics, the first step in validating the accuracy of the KneeKG™ system was to determine how accurately the semiflexible attachment system represents the motion of the underlying bones. This was evaluated by Sati et al. [4] by comparing measurements obtained with the attachment system to the actual bony motion, which was assessed with calibrated fluoroscopy. The researchers showed that within a 65° arc of motion, the system could measure knee kinematics with an average accuracy of 0.4° for knee abduction and adduction, 2.3° for axial rotation, 2.4 mm for anteroposterior translation, and 1.1 mm for axial translation.

With the goal to improve the accuracy of the system, the group developed a new exoskeleton attachment system. The accuracy of this new system was assessed using similar fluoroscopic study [6]. The results demonstrated that errors were reduced by a factor of 4.3–6.2 on average when the exoskeleton attachment was used. The accuracy of this system was assessed by Hagemeister et al. [7], and they found intra-patient reproducibility between 0.86 and 0.97 for abduction/adduction, internal/external rotation, and flexion/extension movements. In a different study, Hagemeister et al. [8] determined the repeatability of measures to range between 0.4° and 0.8° for knee rotation angles and between 0.8 and 2.2 mm for translation. It should be noted that this level of precision likely represents the best-case scenario and may not reflect actual clinical results, especially in cases of extremes of body habitus or motion patterns [2].

Labbe et al. [9] determined the intra- and interobserver reliability of the attachment system for recording 3D knee kinematics during gait. They showed that the 3D kinematic data are highly reliable with intra-class coefficient (ICC) values ranging from 0.92 (flexion/extension), 0.94 (abduction/adduction), to 0.88 (internal/external tibial rotation). The high ICC values indicate very high reliability of the exoskeleton for recording 3D knee kinematics despite reinstallation. Therefore, evaluations may be carried out by several different clinicians without impacting reliability [9]. Through comparison with cadaver studies and a perturbation analysis, the system is shown to be sufficiently accurate to predict certain in vivo ligament bending and torsion deformations [5].

Fact Box 2: kneeKG Accuracy
0.4° in frontal plane
2.3° in transverse plane
2.4 mm in AP translation

16.4 Data Collection

The KneeKG™ system is composed of a positioning system that permits the localization of a sensor embodied in a harness fixed on the knee in a quasi-rigid fashion and an infrared motion capture system (Polaris Spectra camera, Northern Digital Inc.). The harness comprises a femoral part, which is fixed on each side of the knee, and a tibial part also composed of a sensor, which is secured by means of Velcro straps (Fig 16.1). The KneeKG system also includes a data analysis and acquisition software (Emovi, Inc.) which enables real-time visualization of 3D knee movements displayed on the screen, test data results stored in hard drive, automatic printout, and results produced in customized reports. A database containing the 4 biomechanical patterns, three knee angles (flexion/extension, abduction/adduction, and internal/external tibia rotation) and anterior-posterior tibial translation, was created for each participant. During the KneeKG™ examination, the patient must wear shorts, to allow the installation of the exoskeleton. During the femoral part installation, the operator must palpate both sides of the knee, above the condyle area, to locate the lateral space in between the biceps femoris and the iliotibial band and the medial space in between the vastus medialis and the sartorius tendon. The operator can then place both orthoplasts (spring loaded) on these two sites and hold them in place while the subject wraps the elastic Velcro band around his or her thigh (Figs. 16.2 and 16.3). While in the tibial

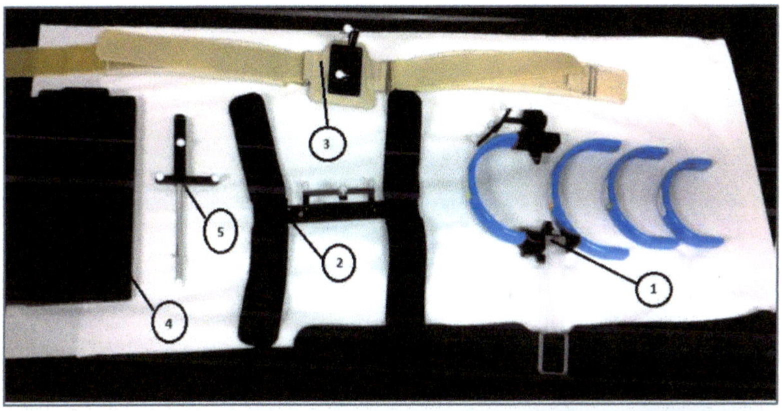

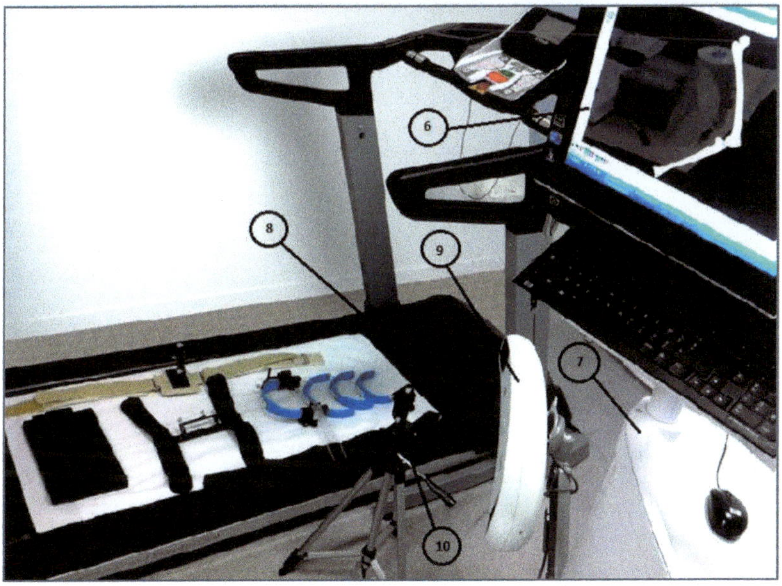

Fig. 16.1 The KneeKG™ system and its parts. *1*. Femoral harness (4 interchangeable arches), *2*. tibial harness, *3*. sacroiliac belt, *4*. feet position guide, *5*. pointer, *6*. computer, *7*. cart, *8*. treadmill, *9*. video camera, *10*. reference body

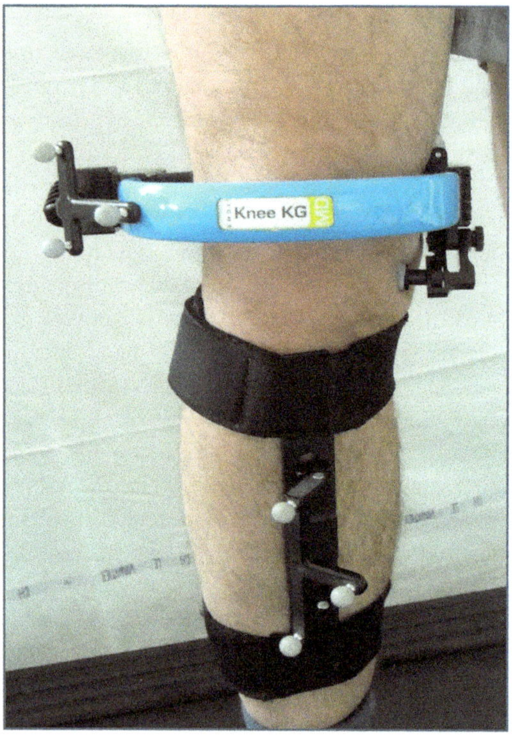

Fig. 16.2 Anterior view of a right knee fitted with the KneeKG™ tracker system

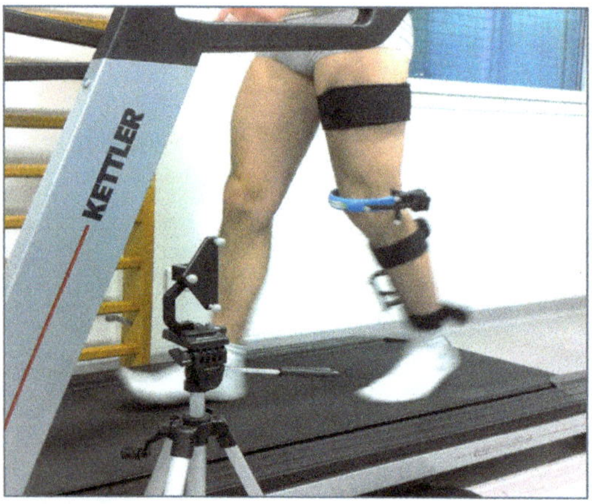

Fig. 16.3 KneeKG™ examination

part installation, the first step consists in locating the anteromedial side of the tibia, on which the operator places the tibial plate. The upper part of the plate must be situated below the tibial tuberosity, and the lower part must not be allowed to move once the ankle makes flexion/extension

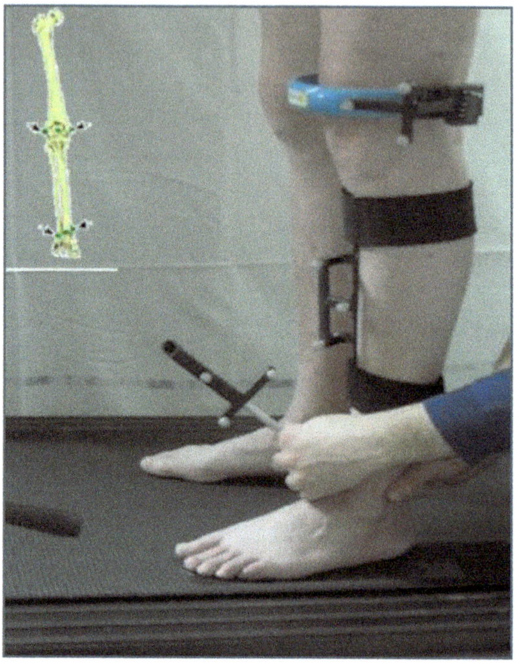

Fig. 16.4 Identification of four anatomical landmarks

movements. The operator fastens the elastic Velcro bands above and below the gastrocnemius (calf) in order to prevent muscular contraction from interfering with measurements by stretching the elastic Velcro bands (Fig 16.2). Just a few movements of flexion/extension and a short period of walking are generally sufficient to determine if the devices are properly installed on the leg.

Once the installation is finalized, the calibration procedure is done as described by Hagemeister et al. [8]. This procedure can be divided into two sections: first, the ankle, knee, and hip joint centers are defined; second, based on a predetermined posture, mediolateral, anteroposterior, and proximal-distal axes are calculated for the femur and the tibia.

The calibration begins with the identification of four anatomical sites: the medial malleolus, the lateral malleolus, the medial condyle, and the lateral condyle (Fig. 16.4).

The 3D position of the femoral head was defined using a functional method. While the subject was performing a circumduction movement of the leg, the Knee3D™ recorded

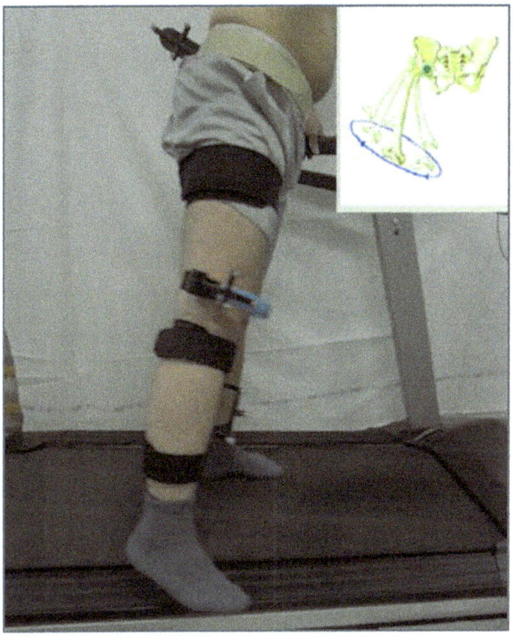

Fig. 16.5 Hip joint center definition

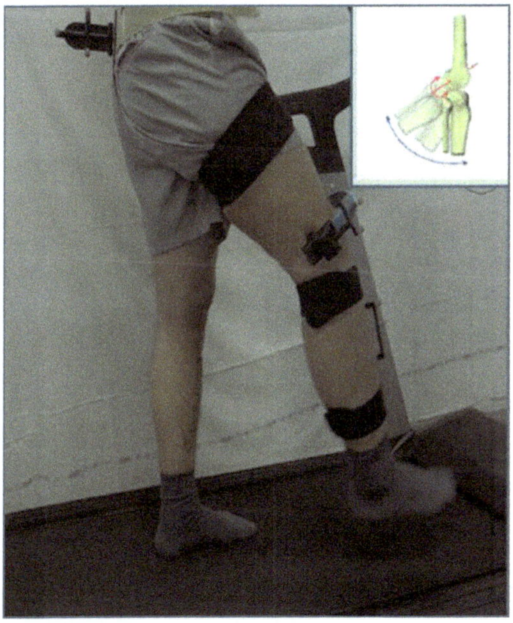

Fig. 16.6 Knee joint center definition

the motion of the sensors for a period of 5 s. The Knee3D™ then calculated the optimal point defining the center of the femoral head (Fig. 16.5).

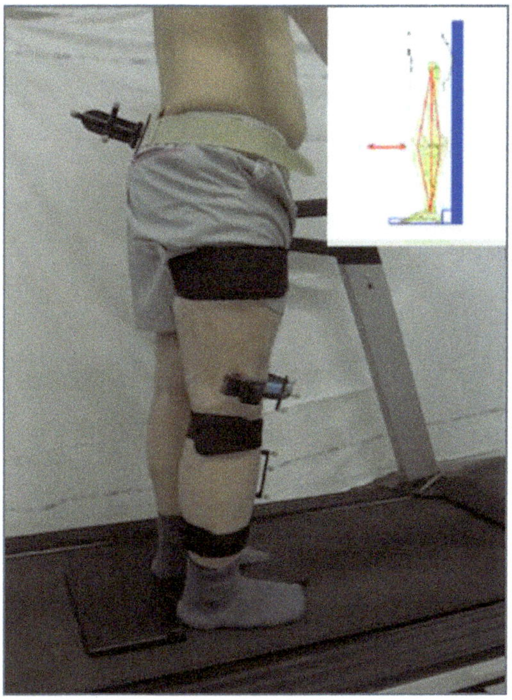

Fig. 16.7 Final step of axis definition: posture with knee in full extension

The next step of the calibration consists in defining the center of the knee in terms of 3D position (Fig. 16.6). The subject makes repetitive leg flexions/extensions (up to a maximum flexion of 60°). Once the movement has been recorded, the Knee3D™ calculates a mediolateral, middle axis for that movement. Based on this axis, the Knee3D then calculates the midpoint of the knee as well the 3D positions of the medial and lateral condyles measured in the previous steps. The middle of both condyles is projected on this axis, thereby defining the center of the knee.

The final phase of calibration is to decide the neutral transverse rotation when the knee is at 0° of flexion during a slight flexion-hyperextension movement (Fig 16.7).

The acquisition protocol takes between 15 and 20 min when performed by a trained technician. All movements are captured at a frequency rate of 60 Hz by the infrared camera. Before starting the trials collection, all patients walked 10 min to get used to walking on the treadmill. Trials are then recorded at the patient's comfortable treadmill gait speed over 45 s (Fig 16.3). During data collection, positions and orientations of the virtual models are set by the control unit in real time, allowing the user to observe the virtual bones in movement in accordance with patient's real bone movement.

Once data collection is complete, the user confirms where the gait cycle begins and confirms the automatic deletion of outliers. A report highlighting biomechanical deficiencies in all three planes of movement and during subphases of the gait cycle is automatically generated [2].

16.5 Clinical Applications

The objective visual assessment of knee joint motion provided by the KneeKG™ system may be useful in associating symptoms with specific abnormal gait mechanics [2]. It allows an accurate quantification of the knee joint function and highlights the 3D biomechanical patterns. KneeKG reports also allow you to compare two recordings (i.e., pre- and posttreatment). This section will highlight biomechanical differences between the two assessments. There are many studies that showed the capacity of this system to assess knee function in cases of ACL deficiency, ACL reconstruction, and osteoarthritis.

16.5.1 Quantitative Assessment of Patient with ACL Deficiency-Reconstruction

The precise quantitative rotational data provided by KneeKG™ make it a suitable tool for evaluation in the following situations:

- To evaluate risk factors for ACL injury
- To predict certain in vivo ligament bending and torsion deformations
- To evaluate if the knee is ready to resume contact sports after ACL reconstruction
- To illustrate the importance of 3D biomechanical evaluation in patients with ACL injuries

St-Onge et al. [10] evaluated the effect of the position of the binding pivot point and binding release characteristics on ACL strain during a phantom foot injury mechanism fall during skiing. They found out that a binding with two pivot points, one positioned in front and the other at the back, might be a solution to reduce the occurrence of the ACL injuries.

On the other hand, Fuentes et al. [11] evaluated if the knee is biomechanically ready to resume contact sports after ACL reconstruction surgery. They showed that alteration of the 3D biomechanics persists 6 months after ACL reconstruction, and this could explain why most patients do not return to their pre-injury level of activity at this time. In another study Fuentes et al. [12] evaluated gait adaptation in patients with chronic ACL deficiency to avoid anterolateral rotatory knee laxity. They hypothesized that patients with ACL-deficient knees would avoid placing their knees in a position that could potentially lead to anterolateral rotatory knee laxity during terminal stance. They were able to demonstrate that patients did adopt this "pivot-shift avoidance" gait, possibly to prevent anterolateral rotatory knee instability. Patients with ACL-deficient knees achieve this proposed gait strategy by (1) significantly reducing the internal rotation knee joint moment and (2) exhibiting a higher knee flexion angle during the terminal stance phase of the gait cycle. It is important to note here that the time from injury in this study was 22 months, which suggest that chronic ACL-deficient patients adopt a pivot-shift avoidance gait. Meanwhile, Shabani et al. [13] assessed the ACL-deficient knee behavior during all phases of gait, using a KneeKG™ system after 5.7 after injury. They presented that ACL-deficient (ACLD) knees showed a significant lower extension of the knee during gait stance phase and higher internal tibial rotation during mid-stance phase, while there was no significant difference in anteroposterior translation in any phase of the gait cycle. So, the findings in this study indicate that ACLD knees may adapt functionally to prevent excessive anterior-posterior translation, but they fail to avoid rotational instability.

In the next study, Shabani et al. [14] compared 3D kinematic patterns between patients having undergone ACL reconstruction with the healthy contralateral knee and a control group. They showed that ACL reconstruction (ACLR) knees had a significantly greater knee joint extension during the entire stance phase compared with ACLD knees. However, ACLR knees still showed a deficit of extension compared with healthy control knees. In the axial plane, there was no significant difference in the pre- and postoperative kinematic data. But, there were significant differences between ACLR knees and healthy control knees, where the ACLR knees had greater internal rotation of the tibia. There were no significant differences in anterior-posterior or coronal plane translations between the groups. It is important to note that there were biomechanical adaptations in the intact contralateral knees. While there were significant differences between ACLR and healthy control knees in both planes (sagittal, axial), there were no significant differences between ACLR and intact contralateral knees.

Conclusions

The KneeKG™ is a noninvasive, 3D, quasi-statical, real-time assessment tool that appears to provide an objective assessment of the precise biomechanical behavior of the knee. The system has the potential to improve understanding of the biomechanical consequences of injury or degenerative changes of the knee as well as more accurately quantify rotational laxity as detected by a positive pivot-shift test [2].

By understanding the pathomechanics of sports injury, biomechanics studies enhance the development of injury prevention in sports medicine.

There is the need to consistently and accurately evaluate joint throughout the continuum of care (preoperative and postoperative assessments) and minimize the flaws of the manual clinical examination.

The KneeKG™ is a noninvasive, 3D, quasi-statical, real-time assessment tool that appears to provide an objective assessment of the precise biomechanical behavior of the knee.

Published data indicates accuracy per pathology of 82.8 % for anterior cruciate ligament (ACL) and 93 % for knee osteoarthritis (OA) (sensitivity of 79 %, specificity of 100 %).

References

1. Sell TC, Ferris CM, Abt JP, Tsai YS, Myers JB, Fu FH, Lephart SM (2006) The effect of direction and reaction on the neuro- muscular and biomechanical characteristics of the knee during tasks that simulate the noncontact anterior cruciate ligament injury mechanism. Am J Sports Med 34:43–54
2. Lustig S, Magnussen RA, Cheze L, Neyret P (2012) The KneeKG system: a review of the literature. Knee Surg Sports Traumatol Arthrosc 20:633–638
3. Sati M, de Guise JA, Larouche S (1996) Quantitative assessment of skin- bone movement at the knee. Knee 3:179–190
4. Sati M, de Guise JA, Larouche S (1996) Improving in vivo knee kinematic measurements: application to prosthetic ligament analysis. Knee 3:179–190
5. Sati M, de Guise JA, Drouin G (1997) Computer assisted knee surgery: diagnostics and planning of knee surgery. Comput Aided Surg 2:108–123
6. Ganjikia S, Duval N, Yahia L, de Guise J (2000) Three-dimensional knee analyzer validation by simple fluoroscopic study. Knee 7:221–231
7. Hagemeister N, Yahia L'H, Duval N, de Guise J (1999) In vivo reproducibility of a new non-invasive diagnostic tool for the three dimensional knee evaluation. Knee 6:175–181
8. Hagemeister N, Parent G, Van de Putte M, St-Onge N, Duval N, de Guise J (2005) A reproducible method for studying three- dimensional knee kinematics. J Biomech 38:1926–1931
9. Labbe DR, Hagemeister N, Tremblay M, de Guise J (2008) Reliability of a method for analyzing three-dimensional knee kinematics during gait. Gait Posture 28:170–174
10. St-Onge N, Chevalier Y, Hagemeister N, Van De Putte M, De Guise J (2004) Effect of ski binding parameters on knee biomechanics: a three-dimensional computational study. Med Sci Sports Exerc 36:1218–1225
11. Fuentes AHHI, Sudhoff I, Fernandes J, Ranger P, de Guise JA (2007) New 3D biomechanical and imaging technologies to evaluate the effect of anterior cruciate ligament reconstructions: preliminary results. Clin J Sport Med 17:165

12. Fuentes A, Hagemeister N, Ranger P, Heron T, de Guise JA (2011) Gait adaptation in chronic anterior cruciate ligament- deficient patients: pivot-shift avoidance gait. Clin Biomech (Bristol, Avon) 26:181–187
13. Shabani B, Bytyqi D, Lustig S, Cheze L, Bytyqi C, Neyret P (2015) Gait changes of the ACL-deficient knee 3D kinematic assessment. Knee Surg Sports Traumatol Arthrosc 23:3259–3265
14. Shabani B, Bytyqi D, Lustig S, Cheze L, Bytyqi C, Neyret P (2015) Gait knee kinematics after ACL reconstruction: 3D assessment. Int Orthop 39(6):1187–1193

A Robotic System for Measuring the Relative Motion Between the Femur and the Tibia

17

Thomas P. Branch, Shaun K. Stinton, Jon E. Browne, Timothy D. Lording, Nathan K. deJarnette, and William C. Hutton

Contents

T.P. Branch, MD (✉)
University Orthopedics, Decatur, GA, USA
e-mail: doctorbranch@yahoo.com

S.K. Stinton, PhD • N.K. deJarnette, BS
ERMI Inc., Atlanta, GA, USA

J.E. Browne, MD
Orthopaedic & Sports Medicine Clinic of Kansas City, Leawood, KS, USA

T.D. Lording, MBBS, FRACS
Melbourne Orthopaedic Group, Windsor, VIC, Australia

W.C. Hutton, DSc
Department of Orthopaedics, Emory University School of Medicine, Atlanta, GA, USA

I often say that when you can measure what you are speaking about, and express it in numbers, you know something about it; but when you cannot measure it, when you cannot express it in numbers, your knowledge is of a meagre and unsatisfactory kind. Lord Kelvin (1883)

17.1 Introduction

When a patient presents with a knee injury, a clinician uses manual physical examination to determine the laxity in the knee. By anchoring the femur with one hand and manipulating the tibia with the other hand, the clinician "feels" the motion of the tibia on the involved knee and compares it to the motion of the opposite "normal" knee. This "feel" is registered by the clinician as motion in three dimensions; it is a subjective test, which is influenced by each clinician's experience. Differences in training, experience, and the

V. Musahl et al. (eds.), *Rotatory Knee Instability*, DOI 10.1007/978-3-319-32070-0_17

specific tests performed during the examination can introduce a human factor, or bias, into the manual physical examination [4, 22, 23, 25]. Thus characterizing small changes in laxity between the tibia and femur that result from a knee injury and correlating those changes with damage to a specific structure can be difficult.

During the manual examination, clinicians seek an accurate diagnosis. The goal is to determine which structures are damaged and the extent of the damage. A clinician's personal experience and physical examination skills have the greatest impact on patient outcomes. However, there are patient-related variables that can influence the findings of the manual physical examination, e.g., sickness, distraction, the demeanor of the patient, swelling, effusion, pain, patient guarding, etc. In addition, the size or shape of the patient can make the physical examination difficult, e.g., a 150 kg American football player. Testing consistently across the right and left leg of a patient can be challenging as well. Robotic testing is considered one method for limiting these confounding variables when measuring knee laxity.

In this chapter, the sequence of events that shaped the evolution of in vivo robotic testing of the knee will be explored. Several key issues that were encountered during the years of development of robotic testing will also be discussed. The first of these issues was defining the center of the knee considering both rotation and translation. The position of the center of the knee has impact on the relative translation between the femur and the tibia and, most certainly, on left-to-right comparison [12]. The three-dimensional definition of the tibial and femoral coordinate systems has a direct impact upon what is defined as 0° of tibia axial rotation and varus/valgus rotation. This kinematic setup must be consistent between limbs and across all evaluated patients in order to minimize measurement error.

The second issue is related to the manual physical exam and the evaluation of knee joint play without influencing the relative position of the tibia with respect to the femur. The tibia is an intercalary bone, i.e., the tibia is allowed to "float freely" between the ankle/foot and the femur. Typically, the femur is stationary and the tibia is held in a position determined by the examiner. Ideally, the lower leg is held at the foot, and the tibia is allowed to position itself depending upon gravity and the state of the knee ligaments. The resultant position represents an "equilibrium" state of the knee ligaments under the evaluated conditions. This represents a form of "whole-leg" testing. Care must be taken during setup to document this "initial" position or datum. Ligaments that are torn have an influence on this initial position. In essence, this initial position of the whole leg (i.e., degree of hip and knee flexion, hip abduction, and supine positioning) identifies the "equilibrium" state of the ligaments. This equilibrium state exists when the tension in all intact ligaments between the tibia and the femur sums to zero taking into account gravity at the position of evaluation. When a ligament is torn and its restraining energy/force is lost, there is a shift to a new initial or equilibrium position. It is the absolute and relative location of the tibia in this new equilibrium position that may provide the clinician with clues as to the injury. An incorrect diagnosis may result if the initial or equilibrium position is not taken into account during the analysis.

The third issue relates to the mathematical methods used to calculate the changes in motion between the tibia and the femur. Motion of the femur is restricted during testing while the tibia is positioned at a specific angle of knee flexion and allowed to move with six degrees of freedom. When a clinician examines the knee, they "feel" the motions between the tibia and the femur. This "feel" incorporates translations and rotations in all six degrees of freedom. A mathematical method should be chosen to best reflect this clinical "feel" by representing all six degrees of freedom of the tibia motion with respect to the femur.

The fourth issue is consideration of the best method to communicate these clinically felt motions in the knee during the examination. Classically, the clinician feels both the extent of the joint play and the compliance or "softness" of each end point during each test: anterior/posterior, varus/valgus, and tibial axial rotation test. When this "feel" is correlated with the force that a clinician applies throughout the examination, a full "load-deformation curve" can be produced.

By standardizing the setup, origin and coordinate system mapping, torque/load application, and mathematical analysis, multiple load-deformation curves in a study can be compared utilizing techniques from functional data analysis (FDA). These curves can be compared for both extent and shape using methods of statistical analysis providing the clinician with a visual representation of the clinical "feel" of knee ligament laxity. Dealing with these four issues, (1) the location of neutral position/rotation, (2) the impact of testing without tibia position interference or "whole-leg" testing characterizing the ligamentous equilibrium state, (3) the use of independent free body analysis to mimic the clinician's "feel" of knee laxity, and (4) the use of functional data analysis to provide a visual representation of this clinical "feel," is important in identifying knee injuries when using a robotic system for measuring the relative motion between the femur and the tibia.

Fact Box 1: Advantages of a Robotic System for Knee Laxity Testing

1. The robotic system tests the whole leg without influencing the "natural" equilibrium position of the femur and tibia.
2. It allows for a standardized application of force in a direction mimicking the physical examination during testing, thereby minimizing bias and error due to human factors.
3. This consistent application of force allows for excellent repeatability between tests on the same day and on multiple days.

17.2 The Development of Knee Laxity Testing Using a Robotic System

Standard methods for visualizing the inside of the knee include plain radiographs, CT scans, and MRI scans. The value of these "still" images when used in the diagnosis of knee ligament injuries is enhanced by applying stress to the knee using a device such as the Porto-knee testing device [3, 9, 15, 18, 19, 21, 24]. The MRI scan has the ability to show the major ligaments in the knee. A torn anterior cruciate ligament can be identified with 90 % accuracy; however, the MRI does not show how the ligaments work together in the knee as a whole. More specifically, these still images may be able to identify an individual damaged ligament, but not give the clinician insight into how a particular damaged ligament affects knee stability as a whole. While the major knee ligaments remain of great interest, damage to the smaller and less prominent ligaments may contribute significantly to the stability of the knee as a whole.

The KT-1000, in its multiple forms (e.g., KT-1000, KT-2000, and CompuKT), has been utilized in a large number of peer-reviewed studies [7, 8]. Many studies have been published reporting its validity, reliability, and reproducibility. Inconsistent results have been reported with the KT-1000 device and with other instrumented devices (e.g., Rolimeter, Stryker KT, etc.) as the "human factor" was not completely eliminated from the examination process [2, 10, 29]. In other words, these devices depend upon the examiner for setup and for control of the direction and rate of the applied force. Despite its drawbacks, the KT-1000 device is still utilized to quantify AP translation in the knee.

Kocher et al. suggested that the pivot-shift test had better correlation with overall patient satisfaction when compared to AP translation as measured by the KT-1000 [16, 17]. Since the pivot-shift maneuver appears to be a combination of tibiofemoral axial rotation, anterior/posterior translation, and varus/valgus rotation, attempts were made to quantify the tibiofemoral axial rotation component of the test [1, 20, 27, 28].

Our first attempt at quantifying tibiofemoral axial rotation in 2004 was a manual system that used a digital torque wrench and a standard scoliosis goniometer in which the patient was tested in the supine position with both knees flexed to 90° (Fig. 17.1a). The next version of the system added digital collection of the data throughout the entire tibial axial rotation test with the knee at

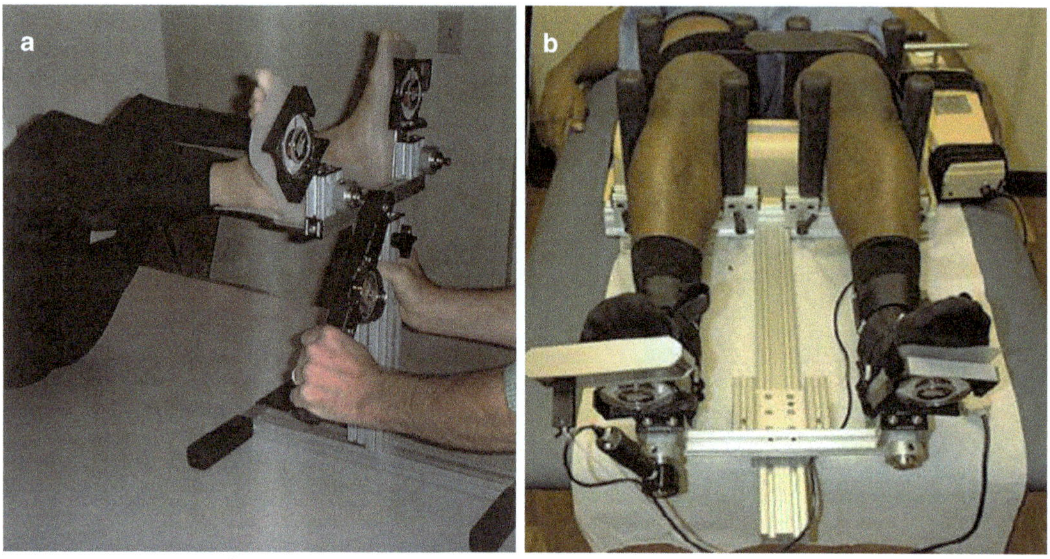

Fig. 17.1 (**a**) The first rotational knee testing system utilized manual application of force and visual reading of a goniometer. (**b**) The next version of the knee testing system utilized digital data acquisition but still required manual application of force

30° mimicking the dial test (Fig. 17.1b). We were interested in producing full load-deformation curves for analysis. With the knee at 30°, there was concern about additional rotation of the foot/ankle and the femur during the test.

In order to answer several simple questions about testing methods, multiple internal studies were completed. The first study included 10 subjects who were casted from thigh to foot. Each subject was tested under six conditions with each condition representing a reduction in casting or a change in patellar strapping. For each condition, the subject was placed into a device consisting of medial and lateral femoral pads compressing the femur proximal to the knee, a post that the distal femur rested upon, and an ankle-foot orthosis (AFO). At the distal femur, either a simple strap was used for stabilization between two posts or compression was applied to the patella with a patellar strap to help control femoral rotation. The results for rotational compliance (slope of the last 10 % of the load-deformation curve) and total axial rotation are presented in Fig. 17.2. The next study in sequence determined the effect of the speed of force application on rotational compliance. Four patients were tested using the device with data capture at four different speeds of rotation. There was significant impact on rotational compliance as the speed of force application increased (Fig. 17.2). These two studies established the importance of controlling the speed of load application and the application point during testing. Utilizing this new understanding, an improved version of the device and software was developed (Fig. 17.1b). The femur was locked medially and laterally, the patella was compressed into the trochlea, an electrogoniometer was used to measure rotation at the foot, and a digital torque wrench was used to apply the torque. Software collected the data and provided instantaneous feedback to the examiner on the speed of torque application. Since motion was measured at the level of the foot, the motion represented rotation of the lower leg and not solely the knee.

While this setup proved to be both reliable and reproducible, it did not provide measurements of the motion of the tibia with respect to the femur. The goniometer was replaced with an electromagnetic tracking system and a sensor on the tibia for measurement of tibial rotation as opposed to total lower leg rotation (Fig. 17.3). Motors were also introduced into

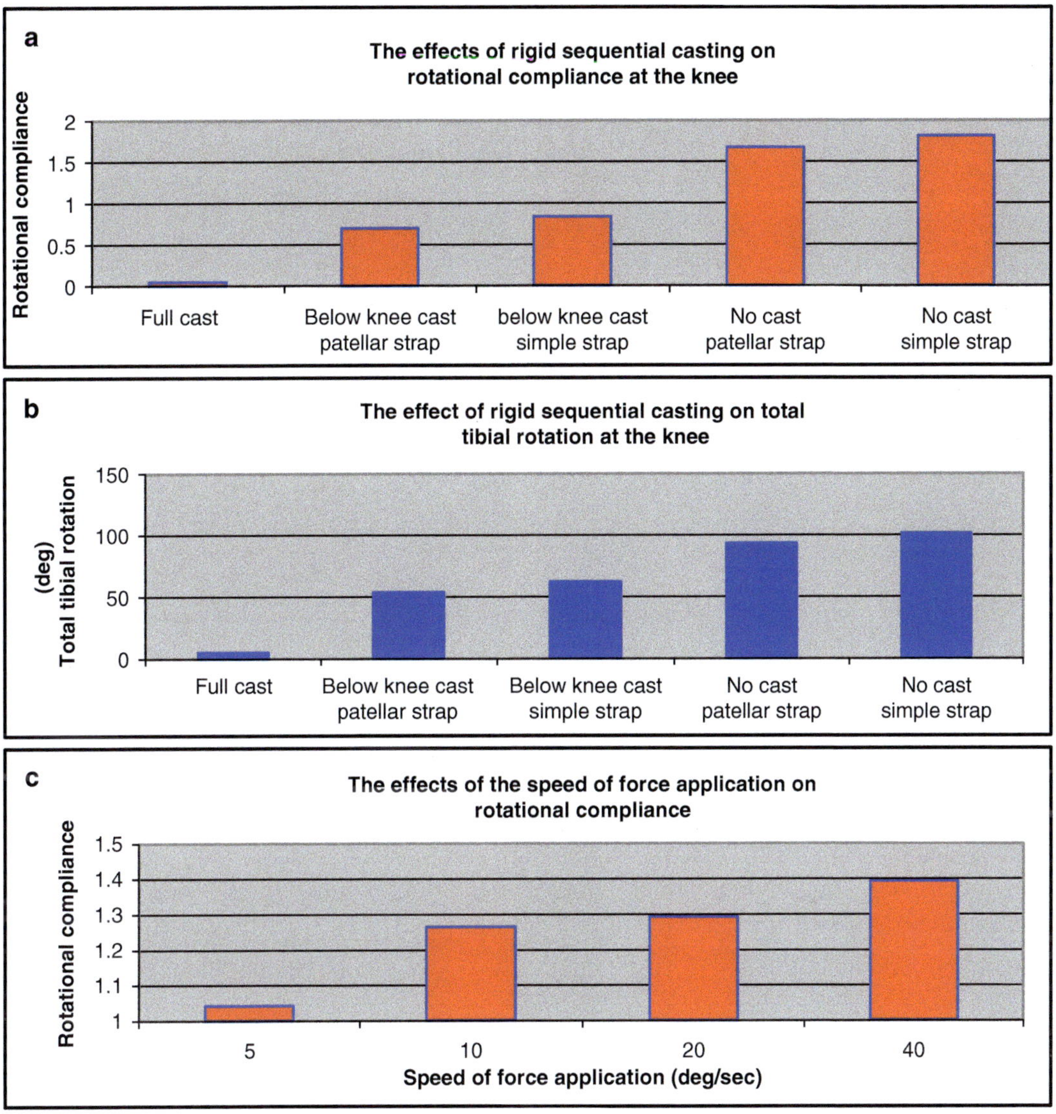

Fig. 17.2 (**a**) The effect of casting on rotational compliance of the knee (lower compliance=higher stiffness). When measuring rotation of the foot during testing, the measurement will include hip, knee, and foot/ankle rotation. (**b**) The effect of casting on total tibial rotation of the lower leg. The below-knee cast reduces motion at the ankle, while a patellar strap reduces motion of the femur. (**c**) The effect of speed of force application on rotational compliance of the knee. The change in knee compliance with varying speeds suggests that the structure is viscoelastic. Care needs to be taken during a test to use a consistent force application in terms of load and speed to reduce error

the system as a replacement for the digital torque wrench in order to standardize the magnitude and direction of the applied force. The reliability of the motorized instrument was excellent after the introduction of the electromagnetic system for motion measurement and the motors for consistent force application [5, 6]. With this system 34 patients were measured; these patients had unilateral ACL reconstructions [5, 6]. The data showed a clear correlation between patient satisfaction and lower leg axial rotation of the normal knee (Fig. 17.4). Patients with the largest total lower leg axial rotation of the normal knee (loosest knees) had

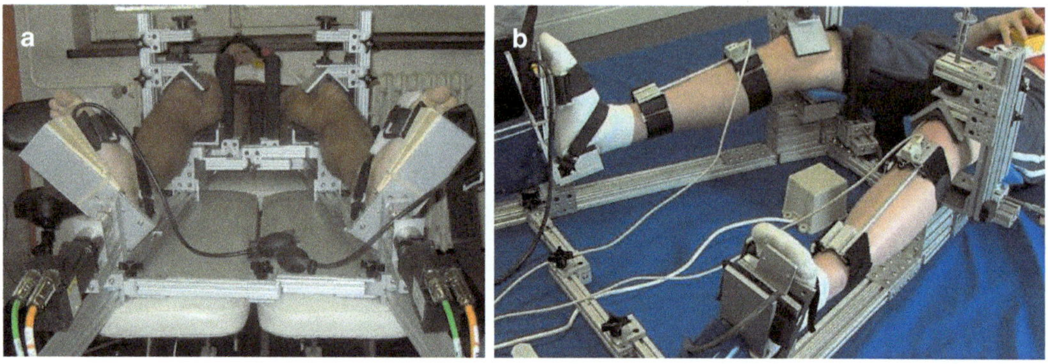

Fig. 17.3 (**a**) The knee testing system after the incorporation of motors for force application for consistency. Each patella was also locked into the trochlear groove using a patellar pad and clamp. (**b**) The knee testing system after the addition of an electromagnetic tracking system for isolated measurement of tibial rotation

Fig. 17.4 The correlation between the amount lower leg axial rotation and patient satisfaction. Patients in the lowest quartile (loosest knees) reported significantly lower patient satisfaction scores

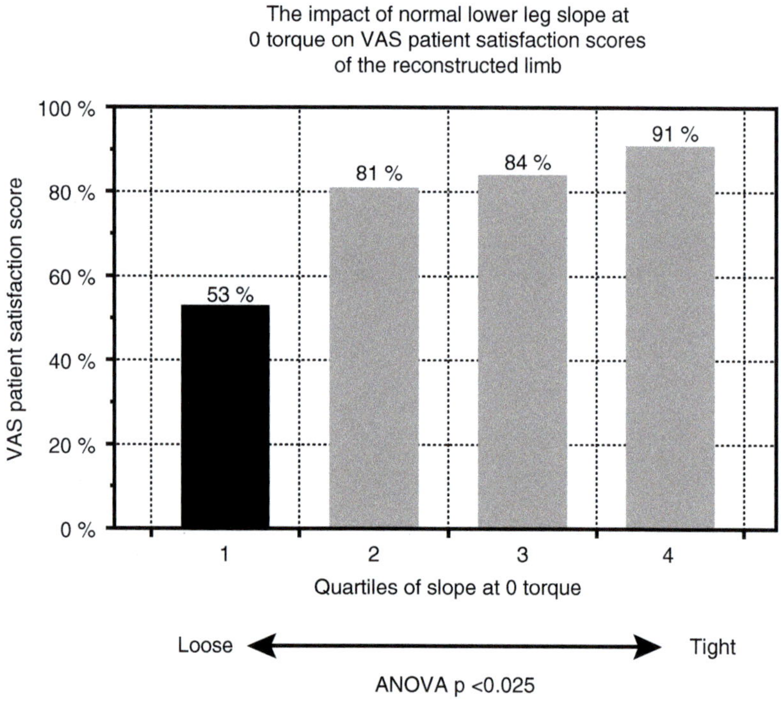

the lowest satisfaction in their reconstructed knee, as measured using the International Knee Documentation Committee (IKDC) and visual analog scale (VAS) scores. While joint play is understood to be the amount of motion between two bones in a joint, the concept of "joint play area" was introduced as a composite measure of total tibiofemoral rotation as measured by the rotation device and AP translation as measured by the KT-1000.

Based upon the reliability and reproducibility demonstrated by the device, it was concluded that additional research was warranted in the use of in vivo measured biomechanical characteristics as a means to predict future patient satisfaction [4, 6, 14]. The goal was to use biomechanical characteristics as an objective test to help clinicians identify injuries specific to tibiofemoral axial rotation while providing an acceptable level of sensitivity, specificity, positive predictive value, and negative predictive value. In order to improve the reliability and reproducibility, an error analysis was performed.

17.3 Sources of Error During Biomechanical Testing of a Knee Joint

The small changes in motion between the femur and tibia as a result of ligament damage to the knee is difficult to measure or quantify if the measurement device and methods produce error greater than the changes themselves. In order to achieve the goal of obtaining biomechanical values during knee laxity testing using the robotic system which can be used as a diagnostic test, all possible forms of error must be minimized. There are many types of error that can be introduced during testing (Table 17.1). The most important is the introduction of researcher bias, which automatically adds error to any test. Bias can be introduced any time an investigator chooses or defines an aspect of the test personally. The mathematical method chosen for description of motion between two bones can also be a potential source of error.

Table 17.1 Potential sources of error during biomechanical knee testing

Potential sources of error
1. Patient setup
2. Definition of joint center
3. Definition of coordinate systems
4. Mathematical methods
5. Spillover

17.3.1 Definition of the Joint Center

Many analysis techniques require the researcher to use radiographs to determine a center of the knee, with the researcher having to make a decision as to where on the radiograph the center is located. A ruler or a computer can be used to measure the AP width and mediolateral width of the tibia. That information can then be used to find the "middle" of the tibia, which would then be defined as the "center" of the knee. Several questions arise when attempting to pick a center of the knee in this manner: (1) Are the radiographs a "true" lateral and a "true" AP? (2) When measuring a sample of knees, are the measurements the same every time? (3) When testing in vivo, how does the clinician/technician take the radiograph measurements and apply them to the patient with skin and muscles intact? No matter the method that is used, if a researcher chooses a joint center, human error is introduced into the test.

17.3.2 Definition of Coordinate Systems

In order to determine the relative rotation between two bones, each bone must have a defined coordinate system. Typically, AP motion is defined to occur along the y-axis and internal/external axial rotation occurs around the z-axis. In order to make the coordinate system orthogonal (each axis is perpendicular to the other), the x-axis must be created in relationship to the y-axis and the z-axis. Flexion-extension around the created x-axis may not represent the true flexion-extension axis for that knee. The researcher must choose which axis is primary, which axis is secondary, and which axis is tertiary. By making this choice the researcher introduces error into the measurement. If a non-orthogonal coordinate system is chosen in order to force knee motions into a clinically friendly space, some motions between two bones become hidden by or added to one of the non-orthogonal axes [12].

17.3.3 Patient Setup and Force/Torque Application

The method a researcher uses to examine the relationship between the tibia and femur can introduce bias, and thus error, into the test. For example, if the foot is held up with the knee in full extension, some knees have a natural recurvatum. This recurvatum is the result of the knee ligament equilibrium state in that position. When the knee is flexed, the tibial position with respect to the femur may still exist in that altered ligament equilibrium state. Furthermore, the initial or equilibrium position of the tibia may reflect the end result of a damaged ligament. The recurvatum seen in the knee may represent a damaged posterolateral structure rather than a normal or healthy knee position. Devices, which rigidly hold both the tibia and femur, may influence these potential clues to ligament injury since the equilibrium position or state of the tibia with respect to the femur is influenced by this fixation. When the device holds both sides of the joint during the test, the researcher must choose the initial position of the bones, thus introducing bias and error.

Fact Box 2: Key Concepts for Analysis of Knee Laxity Data from a Robotic System

1. The position at zero torque/load is determined dynamically during testing, reducing researcher bias and error.
2. In whole-limb testing, the position at initial setup represents the "natural" equilibrium relationship between the tibia and femur.
3. Like a surgeon's clinical examination, independent free body analysis allows a full 6° of freedom (three-dimensional) understanding of the motion of the tibia with respect to the femur during testing.

17.3.4 Mathematical Methods

In 1983, Grood and Suntay developed a non-orthogonal joint coordinate system to describe the clinical motion between two bones [12]. This mathematical technique simplified the calculation of rotation and translation of one bone with respect to another bone. However, the technique accomplishes this simplification at a significant sacrifice. The position of the bones must maintain a certain consistent orientation with respect to one another. In the case of the knee, the long axis of the tibia and femur must remain parallel to one another throughout the test. If this does not occur, then the translations and rotations are contaminated by motions along other axes. When motion along or around one axis is added to or subtracted from another axis, this motion contamination is called "spillover." That is to say, if there is a change in the varus or valgus orientation of the femur with respect to the tibia, then motion in the medial and lateral direction spills over into distraction and compression of the joint. Similarly, all flexion is assumed to occur around the flexion axis of the femur, when the tibia itself can flex and extend as an independent body. The classic clinical example of "spillover" is the difference between a true lateral radiograph of the knee and one that is "off" just a little as shown in Fig. 17.5. The mathematical methods for describing motion between two bones can add to the error of the test itself.

The consequences of not managing the accumulation of error during testing are apparent in the accuracy, reliability, and reproducibility of the testing. Cumulative error during testing creates "noise" in the data such that true differences between injuries or conditions may not be readily discernible. By being careful with the sources of error, this "noise" can be reduced to a minimal level so that biomechanical characteristics can predict the presence or absence of anatomical injuries.

17.4 Management of Error During Knee Laxity Testing Using a Robotic System

The keys to the excellent accuracy, precision, reproducibility, and reliability of robotic testing of the knee lie in the choice of equipment used, the details of patient setup, the selection of mathematical methods for describing the motion between the two bones, and the means for analyzing the information produced during the test. The right equipment ensures precision in measurement of position and torque throughout the test. The setup remains critical for reducing the error

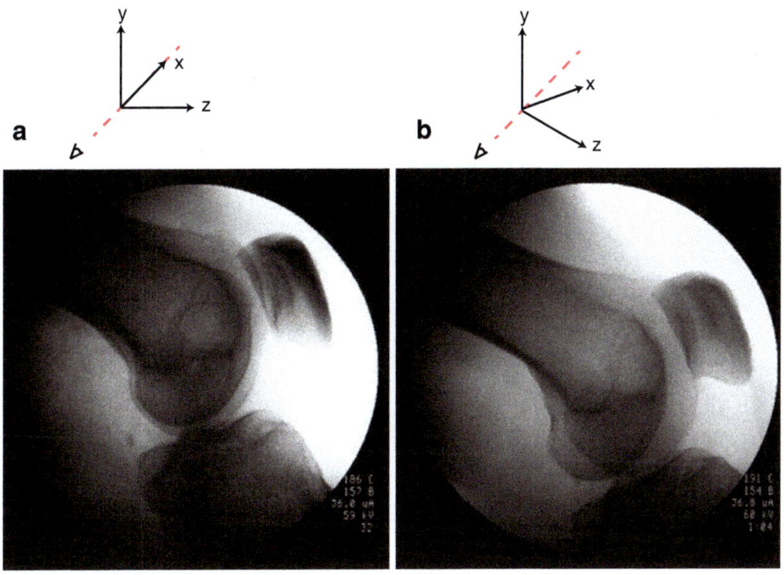

Fig. 17.5 A simple example of spillover occurs when a true lateral radiograph (**a**) is rotated slightly resulting in an offset view (**b**), thus making it harder to interpret

associated with choosing the coordinate systems and origins for the tibia and the femur. The correct mathematical method reduces the complications of unintentional "spillover" from one axis of a coordinate system to another axis in the same coordinate system. For example, the consequence of this is that some of the increased valgus rotation that is seen with an MCL injury might "spillover" and show up as increased tibial flexion during the test. Finally, the methods chosen for analysis reduce the complications of researcher bias and provide the clinician an unimpeded view of the amount of "play" between the femur and the tibia.

17.4.1 Measurement Devices

An electromagnetic tracking system to record the position of the tibia with respect to the femur was chosen. Using six degrees of freedom sensors, the system is accurate to within 0.48 mm and 0.30° based on root mean square error (0.88 mm and 0.48° 95 % CI) (Ascension Technologies, a subdivision of NDI, Bakersfield, CA, USA). Relative motion between two positions maintains the highest accuracy, while absolute position within the magnetic field has a lower accuracy. The combination of the servomotors and torque sensors can apply a force at a constant rate to a target torque with less than 1 % error.

17.4.2 Patient Setup

The methods used to set up the patient in the device and modifications made to the machine in order to make this process more reliable have been developed to minimize the error in testing (Fig. 17.6a). The patient is placed into the device in a supine position with the foot resting in a short AFO distally. The knee is placed on a pad posteriorly positioned such that the distal femur rests on the pad and the knee is flexed at 30°. The proximal tibia is off the pad and free to move. The patient's legs are positioned in 30° of femoral abduction while allowing for the femur to be centered on the posterior pad. The foot is then strapped into place such that force can be applied

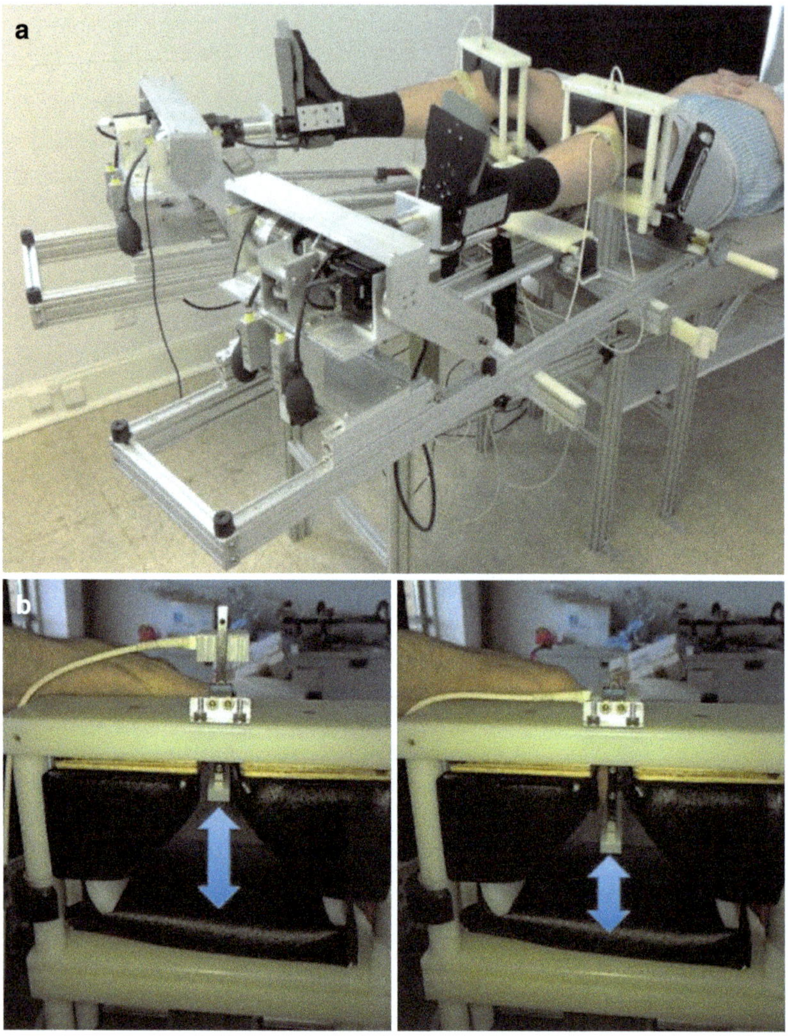

Fig. 17.6 (**a**) A patient setup in the testing device with electromagnetic sensors strapped to the proximal tibia. (**b**) A close-up view of the femoral sensor which follows femoral AP motion only. A plastic piece rests on top of the patella and a linear bearing allows for measurement of only AP motion in the direction of the arrows. The peripatellar pads consist of high-density foam for comfort

in axial rotation and in varus/valgus. Medial and lateral femoral pads are then moved into place proximal to the distal femur to aid in the reduction in femoral perturbation during testing. The distal femoral posterior pad, which can move independently in the medial/lateral direction, is then positioned such that a patellar pad can be clamped to the distal femur providing symmetrical pressure to the patella while allowing symmetrical positioning of the leg in varus/valgus. The pad is then positioned into place and the patella is clamped down into the trochlea of the distal femur with 133.5 N (30 lb) of force, which was the highest tolerable force when applied to the patella. Both femurs are locked to the machine in a similar fashion with setup methods that allow for reproducibility. Each foot is then rotated until the second toe is perpendicular to the *y*-axis and to the femoral pad where the distal femur rests. This position is used to index each motor as 0° of femoral *z*-axis rotation or tibial axial rotation with respect to the femur.

A floating femoral sensor is placed in the patellar clamp; the sensor can measure motion in the femoral *y*-axis or anterior/posterior direction during testing (Fig. 17.6b). It is referenced to the anterior patella on each knee through a rigid connection between the sensor and a plastic bar that is in direct contact with the patella. Because the femur is a bone well covered by skin, adipose, and muscle, error is introduced into measurements during axial rotation and varus/valgus rotation. Varus/valgus rotation in this setup creates a rotation around the femoral *y*-axis (AP) but also some motion around the *z*-axis (long-axis rotation). Both are measured during testing, but the *z*-axis motion is subject to the already described inability to completely control femoral rotation during testing. This is an accepted error in the in vivo evaluation. Using femoral anatomical landmarks as a means to construct both the femoral origin and coordinate system was abandoned due to the extreme variability associated with their identification through palpation in a population of patients.

A tibial sensor is placed on the medial flare of the proximal tibia in a location without interference with the force/torque application system. The skin-to-bone distance in this location is lowest on the tibia and provides excellent tracking of the tibia during the test. Points are taken on the AP midline of the medial tibial plateau and lateral tibial plateau and the AP midline of the medial malleolus and lateral malleolus, which correspond to the most prominent point on that part of the bone. While both knees are in their equilibrium position, the most anterior point on each tibial tubercle is recorded.

17.4.3 Definition of the Origin and Coordinate Systems

The origin of the tibial coordinate system is defined as the midpoint between the medial and lateral tibial plateau points that are taken during patient setup. The *z*-axis of the tibial coordinate system is constructed using the vector from the tibial origin to the midpoint of the medial and lateral malleoli. At initial setup, the *y*-axis is defined as parallel to the second toe of the foot which was previously defined to be perpendicular to the posterior distal femoral pad. Appropriate mathematical operations (cross products produce a vector perpendicular to the two other vectors that are "crossed") are used to create an orthogonal coordinate system for the tibia. The femoral origin and its coordinate system are then constructed by points on the machine itself. The femoral origin is taken from points on the machine and patellar clamp representing the overall AP depth of the distal femur. The center of these points becomes the origin of the femoral coordinate system. The *y*-axis is oriented perpendicular to the posterior femoral pad. The *z*-axis is taken from the *z*-axis of the tibial coordinate system at initial setup. Appropriate mathematical operations are again used to create an orthogonal coordinate system for the femur.

It is important to understand why the *z*-axis for the tibia is also used for the *z*-axis of the femur. As clinicians, we anchor the femur and watch or feel the movement of the tibia relative to the femur during the physical examination. Thus, the movement of the tibia is "watched" from the femur toward the top of the tibia. If the movement of the tibial plateau surface is important, then a view perpendicular to the tibial plateau surface is best for the clinician. Therefore, the *z*-axis of the tibial coordinate system projected to the femur for its *z*-axis provides the best perspective for "watching" the tibia from the femur.

This replication of the *z*-axis from the tibia to the femur should be close to the true mechanical axis. This replicated *z*-axis was used for the femur rather than the mechanical axis for several reasons. We have studied mathematical techniques available to predict the center of the femoral head by point collection during rotation of the femur. An estimation of the center of rotation of the femoral head was performed along with a three-dimensional CT scan identification of the anatomical center. The error in the prediction of the anatomical femoral head center was up to 2.5 cm from test to retest when using these mathematical methods. Subsequently, it was noted that using the *z*-axis for the tibia in both the tibial and the femoral coordinate systems allowed a reasonable estimation of the mechanical axis without the risk of measurement error associated with the estimation of the center of the femoral head. Furthermore, the tibial *z*-axis constructed from the midpoints of the malleoli and the proximal tibia provided the most consistently measurable anatomical feature in both limbs.

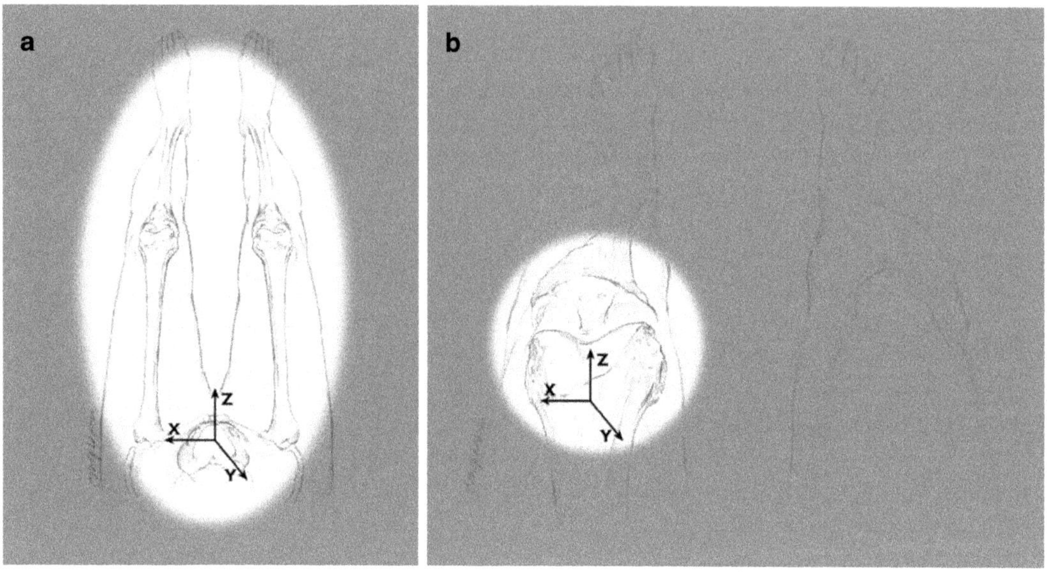

Fig. 17.7 (**a**) A representation of the world view. (**b**) A representation of the femoral view

17.4.4 Data Comparison

There are two methods available when comparing the right and left limbs of a patient. The first method relies upon the setup alone for comparison of movement in the right tibia with movement in the left tibia. It provides the examiner with a "field of view." The most important field of view when comparing the right knee with the left knee is the "world view." The world view is the view that would be seen by sitting at the head of the bed and watching two examiners move both the right knee and the left knee at the same time (Fig. 17.7a). Each knee moves in space and is recorded from this "head of the bed" perspective. The second most important field of view is from the femur of the right leg and the femur of the left leg called the "femoral view." This view is equivalent to a head sitting on each distal femur and viewing the movement of each tibia with respect to the ipsilateral femur and recording the movement separately (Fig. 17.7b). The "femoral view" of the motion of each tibia can be compared keeping in mind that the right and left motions are mirror images of each other. The accuracy of this method depends upon the ability to set up each femur in an identical but mirror opposite position in the "world view." As previously described, each tibia (right and left) will have an "initial equilibrium position" at setup. During patient setup this "equilibrium" position or state can be considered a unique feature of each tibia and should be recorded for further evaluation.

The second method for comparing between the right and the left utilizes anatomical points recorded during setup. Each set of points records the best measure of the anatomical position of the tibia and femur. As far as the best position for the femoral origin during AP translation testing, the center of the femur as described above and translated to the anterior patella is the most consistent. This eliminates the problems associated with using the AP center of the patellar clamp for the construction of the femoral origin. For the tibia, the previously described tibial origin translated anteriorly and perpendicular to the z-axis at the level of the tibial tubercle is the most consistent. Thus, when measuring the side-to-side difference in AP translation between the femur and the tibia, the relative translation between anterior patella and anterior tibial tubercle is used for consistency and reduction in error. For tibial axial rotation, the malleolar axis can be used for side-to-side comparison utilizing an anatomical measure for consistency and reduction in error. If symmetrical abduction of each femur is obtained at initial setup, then varus/valgus testing has excellent consistency.

17.4.5 Mathematical Methods

There are a number of advantages of analyzing the tibia and femur as two independent free bodies. The most important advantage is that any point on a rotating free body has the same rotation in relationship to any point on a second free body. In other words, the rotation between two free bodies is independent of any origin. The researcher cannot bias the results of a study by being forced to select an origin; thus, error is not introduced into the testing. The second advantage relates to the ease with which a chosen origin for each bone can be moved around to represent the best "world view" position for each test. The measurement of translation between two bones is dependent upon the choice of origin. This is most important for AP testing and is accommodated using the previously described anatomical techniques. This technique allows the researcher to use a rotational matrix to describe motion between the two bodies. The third advantage of this mathematical technique is that all six degrees of freedom between the femur and the tibia can be described when a load is applied (three translations – anterior/posterior, medial/lateral, compression/distraction; three rotations – roll, pitch, and yaw). The same three-dimensional "feel" that a clinician perceives during manual knee testing is recorded for evaluation during robotic testing. Flexion or extension of the tibia during testing is seen as a rotation of the tibia and not of the knee itself. The envelope of "joint play" created by an injury to the knee exists as a three-dimensional volume and can be created by any combination of motions between the two bones.

17.4.6 Data Analysis

Finally, the analysis of the data plays an important factor in the management of error during knee laxity testing using a robotic system. Data are captured by sampling at 40 Hz for both torque and position. This sampling rate surpasses the Nyquist sampling frequency for the speed of testing in the robotic system. The data that are collected are a time series of positive and negative peak torques and positions for maximum internal and external rotation from each cycle. A load-deformation curve is constructed from a single cycle (third cycle) of matched torque and position for each test. Repeated cycles have been previously evaluated, and test-retest scores over 0.96 were achieved using intraclass correlation coefficients (ICC (2,1)) with the third cycle showing the least variation. Position is calculated from the right and left "femoral views" with an appropriate mirror image transformation such that the left side can be compared to the right side. In this test, a right-handed coordinate system is applied to the left knee. Positive motion on the x-axis is lateral translation, on the y-axis is anterior translation, and on the z-axis is distraction. Similarly, positive rotation around the x-axis is flexion, around the y-axis is valgus, and around the z-axis is internal rotation. The simplest way to remember this is to place your thumb in the direction of the axis about which you rotate and your fingers will curl in the direction of positive rotation. A mirrored system is applied to the right knee such that the same rotations and translations exist for the same directions of the left knee.

Special attention must be paid to the definition of the zero position in the knee. The zero position of the knee defines the extent of internal versus external rotation, anterior versus posterior translation, and varus versus valgus rotation. It is a key biomechanical descriptor and, if chosen poorly, can introduce significant error into the analysis. Consider for a moment that the knee is like a bowling alley, with a center smooth lane and two gutters (Fig. 17.8). Now, suppose a person was asked to close their eyes and put the bowling ball in the center of the lane. Commonly an individual would put the ball in one gutter and then move the ball into the opposite gutter while gauging the distance between the two gutters. The distance is then halved and the ball is placed into the center. The center of the knee could be determined in a similar fashion considering the fact that the clinician cannot see the insides of the knee and can only "feel" where the ligaments have influence. Now imagine that only the position of the left gutter is changed. If you are blindfolded and have no knowledge of the change, figuring out that only the left gutter has moved will be difficult. If

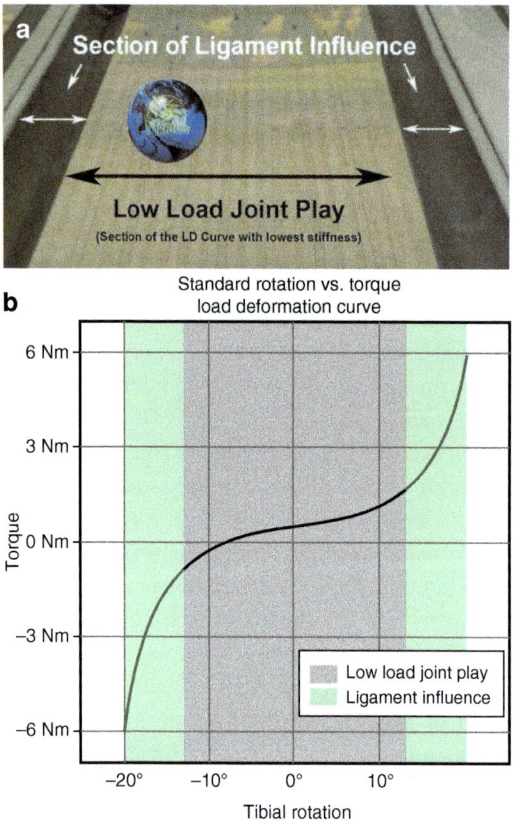

Fig. 17.8 (**a**) The analogy of comparing a knee to a bowling alley showing that the gutters represent the areas of ligament influence and the center of the lane represents the low load play region. (**b**) The correlation of the bowling lane analogy to the load-deformation curve showing the ligament influence at the end points and the flat central portion near zero torque

one considers a "center-matching" technique, when the bowling alley centers are matched to one another, both gutters will appear to have been changed. The same problem exists with the knee. If both the anterior cruciate ligament and the posterior cruciate ligament are damaged to different degrees, it is difficult to determine which of the ligaments has been compromised and by how much. Without a world view, or a reference view, one cannot determine if both gutters have moved or only one gutter has moved. In the knee, the world view provides the reference to determine which ligament was injured and by how much.

This analogy helps us to understand two important points in the analysis. The first is that peak positive torque/load must be matched with peak positive position and peak negative torque/load must be matched with peak negative position to properly represent the load-deformation curve. These maximums and minimums in the load-deformation curve are fixed "gutters" in space, in the world and femoral views. The second point is that zero position and zero torque will automatically be determined in this situation. The clinician does not have to pick those points as they define themselves. This removes bias that is introduced when the zero point for position or torque/load is picked by the clinician.

Comparison of load-deformation curves either from side to side in a single patient or across a population of patients requires further discussion. When comparing curves, it is quite tempting to "register" the curves to a specific point with "register" meaning taking a point, i.e., torque 0 or position 0, and overlapping each curve on that point. It is not uncommon for a researcher to look at curve features to find a common point of comparison between limbs or between subjects. For example, the inflection point in a load-deformation curve could be "assumed" to be torque 0 or position 0 for that limb. It is quite dangerous to assume that zero position and zero torque can be used as a reference for comparison between subjects or between right and left sides. Cumulative error exists at any point in the load-deformation curve. When the researcher assumes that one point is more important than another point, the error at the important point is propagated throughout the entire load-deformation curves. Most load-deformation curves have a long center section with two asymptotic sides. These asymptotic sides indicate the increasing torque/load as the ligament tightens and movement is limited. These end points of the load-deformation curve in which the ligament is being stretched are equivalent to the gutters of the bowling lane. The "flat" center of the load-deformation curve describes a section in which small amounts of torque can produce large changes in position (low load play region). This region is equivalent to the central, smooth portion of the bowling lane. It is the characteristics of this section that should make the researcher wary of choosing zero position or zero torque independently of the data. By choosing points at the ends of the load-deformation curve, large changes in torque produce little changes in position. Less error is introduced into the testing process.

When a load-deformation curve is constructed from data produced during knee laxity testing in the robotic system, it is produced in reference to the initial position of the tibia with respect to the femur at setup. With the tibia as an intercalary bone sitting independently between the femur and the talus, it can find its own "equilibrium" position or state. This position can be the result of a damaged or torn ligament, i.e., a posterolateral corner injury will leave the tibia in a recurvatum position. It can be confusing to compare the load-deformation curve of a "normal" or "healthy" knee with that of the injured knee due to the new position caused by the damaged ligament(s). The load-deformation curve in the injured knee is a combination of the new rotational extent and the new "equilibrium" position of the tibia with respect to the femur (Fig. 17.9). In a patient with an MCL injury, the new equilibrium position of the tibia with respect to the femur is more in valgus than the opposite extremity. Testing from this position creates the illusion that the tibia moves more into varus than the opposite extremity (Fig. 17.9a). When the initial conditions are eliminated for side-to-side comparison, the actual difference in extent becomes readily apparent (Fig. 17.9b). The patient has significant MCL laxity with valgus loading.

The preceding paragraphs have provided a systematic approach to the identification of introduced error into any system or process meant to identify small changes in motion between the tibia and the femur. It is this ability to identify sources of error that helps in producing a system that can reliably, reproducibly, precisely, and accurately identify biomechanical characteristics in the individual knee that are meaningful for diagnosis. By setting up a world view for reference between knees and a femoral view for reference within the knee, relative and absolute position changes can be identified. By allowing the biomechanics and the anatomy of the knee to define its zero position, investigator error is minimized. The goal is to provide clinicians with biomechanically based tests that will provide accurate, reliable, and reproducible predictions of specific knee injuries.

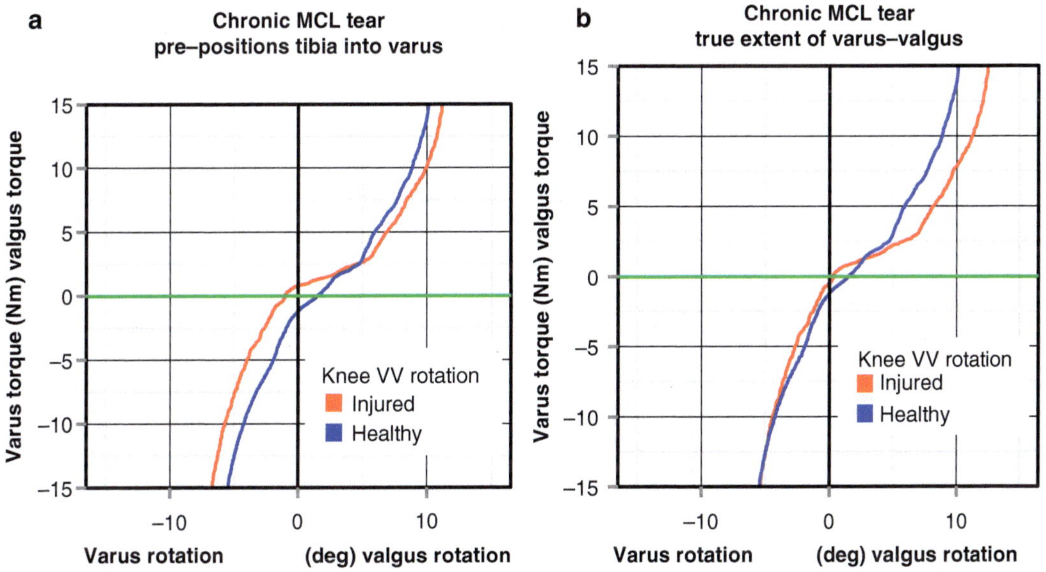

Fig. 17.9 (a) A load-deformation curve in a patient with a chronic MCL tear. (b) The load-deformation curve after normalizing to the initial position. The MCL tear becomes obvious after this preprocessing step

17.4.7 Statistical Methods

P-values from hypothesis tests tend to dominate the medical literature. This approach to scientific inquiry reduces the interpretation of the results of a study to a simple dichotomy: significant differences or nonsignificant differences. Confidence intervals are a more useful statistical approach to interpret the results of a study by giving the clinician both the magnitude of its effect and the range of its effect [11]. Confidence intervals provide separate information about the magnitude of an effect along with information about the precision of the estimate.

It is readily understood that if a p-value fails to exceed some prespecified threshold (usually 0.05), the result is significant, and while a technically proper interpretation of a p-value or a confidence interval is based on abstract statistical theory, there is a mathematical connection between them. A 95 % confidence interval for a given estimate provides a set of values of the parameter that is not rejected at the 0.05 threshold. For this reason, confidence intervals provide all the information needed for making statistical inferences and decisions.

Generally the confidence interval is computed for a single parameter of interest, and the stated confidence pertains to that single parameter. The width of the interval gives us an idea of the sampling error associated with the estimate as well as the values of the parameter that are most compatible with the data for a specified significance level. When the statistical object of interest is a function or a collection of sampled points along a curve, it is not uncommon to compute pointwise 95 % confidence intervals over the values for which the function has been defined, e.g., the mean load-deformation curve. Depending on the goals of the analysis, using bands constructed from pointwise confidence intervals may provide valuable information.

Pointwise confidence intervals are useful to give an impression of the sampling error associated with each point along the function. They can be used to pinpoint the location of specific details along a curve or for comparison between two curves (Fig. 17.10). Confidence intervals provide information about the extent of the data at each point on the curve, but they do not provide information about the shape of the curve. In addition, pointwise confi-

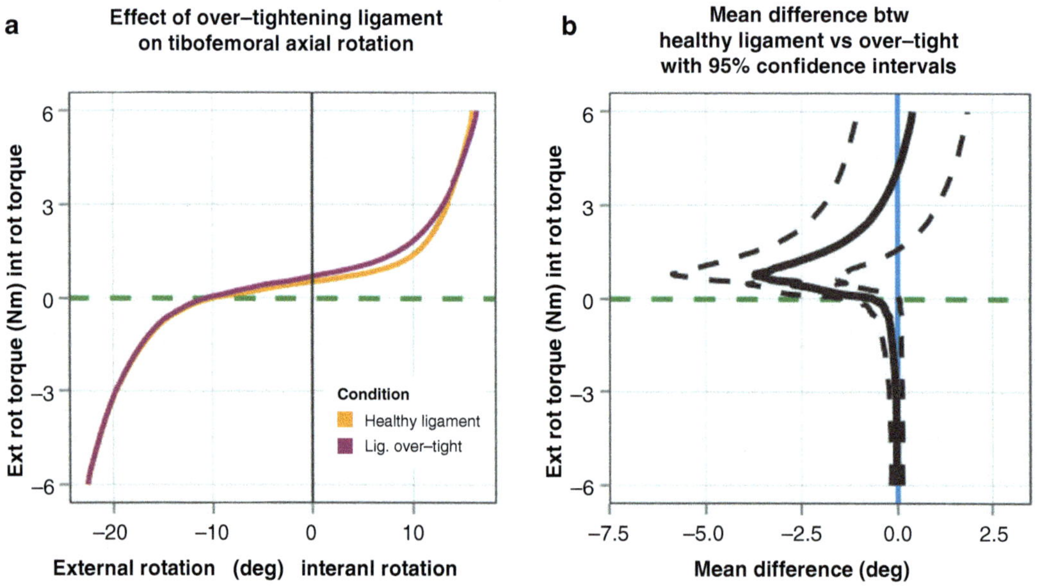

Fig. 17.10 (**a**) Load-deformation curves for two conditions. (**b**) A pointwise curve comparison with 95 % confidence intervals (*dashed lines*). Note the difference in the extent of the curve near 2 Nm. In the difference curve, both sides of the confidence interval are on the same side of zero around 2 Nm. This indicates a significant difference between the curves

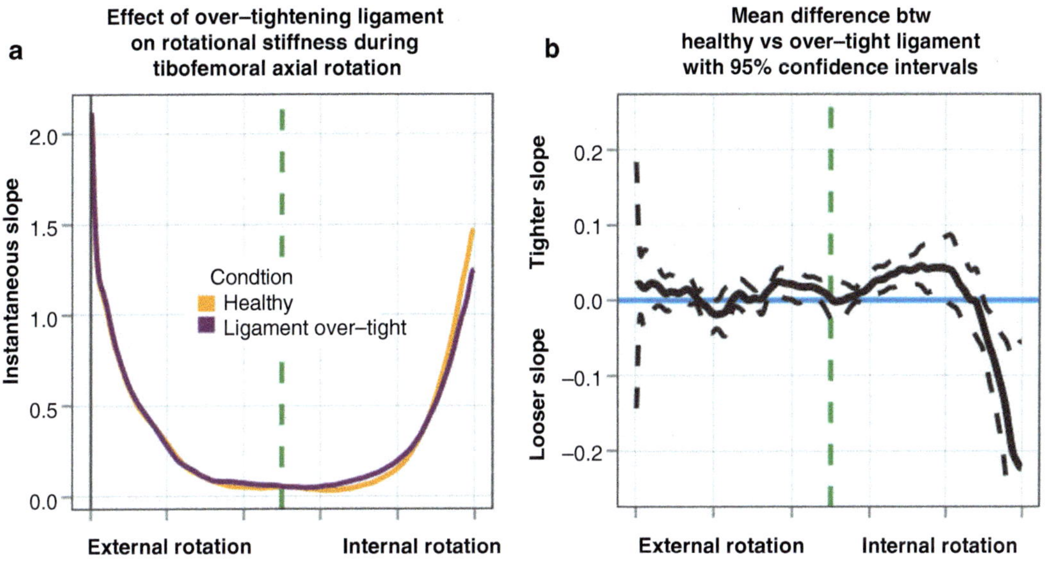

Fig. 17.11 (**a**) A first-order derivative curve calculated from the original load-deformation curve showing stiffness characteristics of a normally reconstructed ligament and an over-constrained reconstructed ligament. (**b**) A pointwise mean difference curve with 95 % confidence intervals. Note that there is a significant change in the shape of the over-tight ligament in internal rotation where both sides of the confidence interval are on the same side of zero slope

dence intervals also can provide some indication of the potential appropriateness of a functional form, i.e., a representative curve fit for a dataset.

In order to provide information about the shape of the curve, pointwise confidence intervals of the first and, perhaps, second derivative of the load-deformation curves may provide information about the shape of the curves across each point (Fig. 17.11). However, the collection of pointwise confidence intervals is not adequate for making inference about the entire function simultaneously across the whole range of values. In other words, one cannot use pointwise confidence intervals to conclude that all the points estimated along the function fall jointly within the bounds with the stated confidence upon repeated sampling. To achieve this goal one needs simultaneous confidence bands [13, 26].

In order to control the probability for a collection of points along a curve simultaneously and not just for a single point, a simultaneous confidence band may be calculated. A 95 % simultaneous confidence band is a collection of confidence intervals such that *all* of the confidence intervals simultaneously cover the true values with a probability of 0.95. To achieve the simultaneous inference, a correction or adjustment needs to be applied to each of the intervals; this will result in a widening of the original collection of single confidence intervals. The production of confidence bands treats the curve as a whole rather than specific characteristics of the curve. Bands tell us about the family of curves as a whole such that information about the curves is combined together in the representation.

Therefore, the necessity of using simultaneous confidence bands over a collection of 95 % confidence intervals for pointwise bands comes down to the intended goals of the study. In order to make inferences about all the points along a function simultaneously, for example, to decide whether it was reasonable to replace the entire data curve with a line or a polynomial, the confidence band is the appropriate tool. Similarly, confidence bands should be used to determine whether two curves are entirely different from one another with a probability of 95 %. On the other hand, pointwise 95 % confidence intervals can descriptively identify points of interest and, when combined with pointwise 95 % confidence intervals of first- and second-order derivatives, can provide useful information about the relative

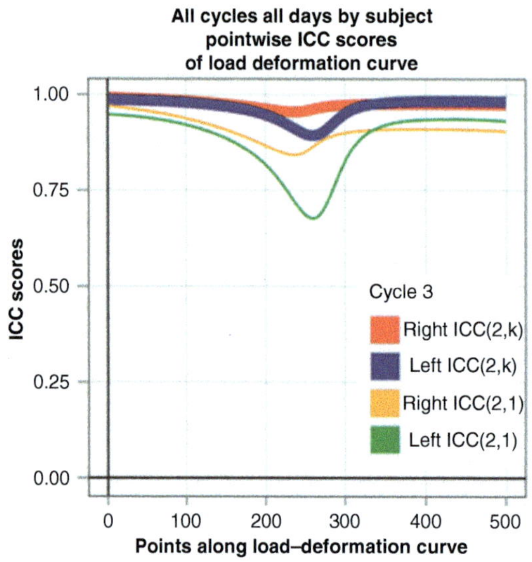

Fig. 17.12 Average pointwise ICC scores for rotational knee testing performed over 4 days on ten different subjects. ICC scores are significantly lower near torque 0 and position 0, which are near point 250 on the *x*-axis

extent and shape of the curves. It is of more value to identify specific changes in the load-deformation curves rather than to comment on the simultaneous family of curves. As such, we prefer to use pointwise 95 % confidence intervals for the evaluation of extent along with comparison of the first-order derivatives for the evaluation of slope changes between load-deformation curves.

17.5 Results of the Careful Management of Error During Knee Laxity Testing Using a Robotic System

Multiple 4-day testing sessions have been performed with the robotic system to measure the reliability and repeatability of the device as guided by our statistician. With each 4-day testing session, subjects were placed into the device at an unspecified time each day and tested. During each test, the knee was cycled four times (i.e., for tibial axial rotation, the tibia was rotated into internal and external rotation four times). Intraclass correlation coefficients (ICC) were calculated as a measure of the test-retest repeatability between cycles on a single day. Inter-day ICC values were calculated to describe day-to-day reliability of the device. An example of the tibial axial rotational ICC scores is presented in Fig. 17.12. It is important to note that the best scores (highest reliability) are at the end points of the load-deformation curve, while the worst scores (lowest reliability) center around 0 Nm of torque. This is a confirmation that the researcher should not choose 0 Nm of torque as a reference point to define zero (neutral) but should rather allow the more reliable end points to choose the zero position.

Fact Box 3: Goals for the Establishment of Standard Biomechanical Measures Using Robotic Testing

1. The use of a robotic system may establish standard measures between and among different clinicians and examiners.
2. By establishing measurable biomechanical data comparing small anatomical variations and differences between the “normal” and “injured” knee, an improved treatment plan for a patient may be developed.
3. With the development of standard and repeatable measures for comparing differences in knee biomechanics and anatomy within one patient and across a group of patients, there may be progress toward a better understanding of the impact of injury on knee biomechanics and its influence on patient symptoms.

17.6 Examples of Clinical Use of the Robotic System

In this section, two examples are presented to illustrate how robotic data were used in the clinical setting. The first example involves a 38-year-old athletic male who injured his knee while performing a deep knee squat with 90 kg. He had

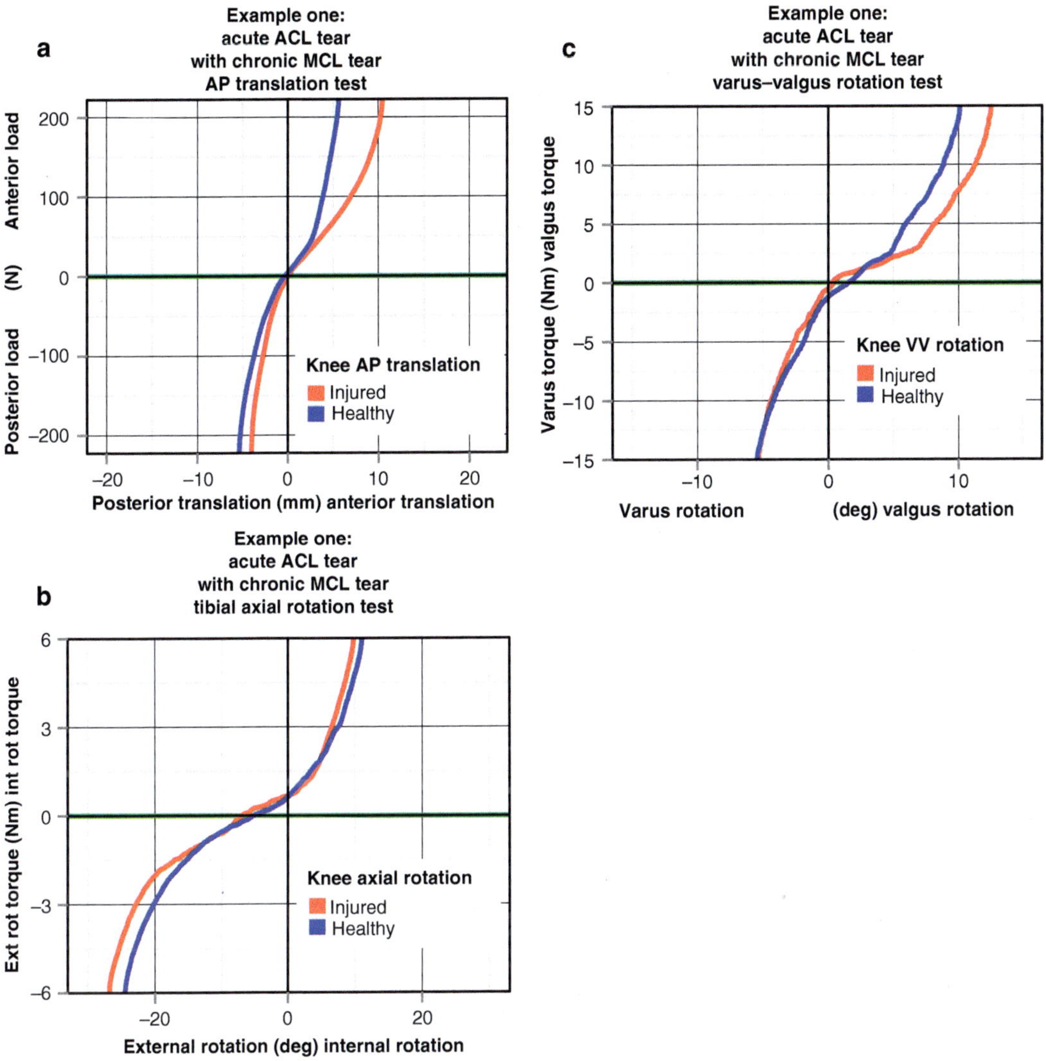

Fig. 17.13 (**a**) Anterior/posterior load-deformation curves for the injured and healthy knees showing the increased anterior translation due to an ACL tear in the right knee (*red line* on the plot). (**b**) Tibial axial rotation load-deformation curves for the injured and healthy knees. Note that the expected increase in rotation should be internal rotation, but in this case, it is external rotation. This is likely due to the MCL injury. (**c**) Varus/valgus rotational load-deformation curves for the reconstructed and healthy knees showing the significant increase in valgus extent in the injured knee suggesting chronic MCL injury

sustained a medial collateral ligament injury 11 months prior to the squatting episode. At that previous time, he was treated conservatively. He presented to our clinic with symptoms of instability. His complaints of instability occurred during ordinary walking and were described as a "wobbly" knee. On physical examination, there was a positive Lachman test, negative pivot-shift test, and grade II opening on valgus testing and increased external rotation on the dial test. The results of laxity testing using the robotic system are shown in Fig. 17.13. The robotic data clearly indicate an ACL tear in AP testing. In rotational testing, the increase in internal rotation that would be expected after an ACL tear was not evident, but rather there was an increase in external rotation in the injured knee. This is due to the chronic MCL tear. Increased valgus rotation

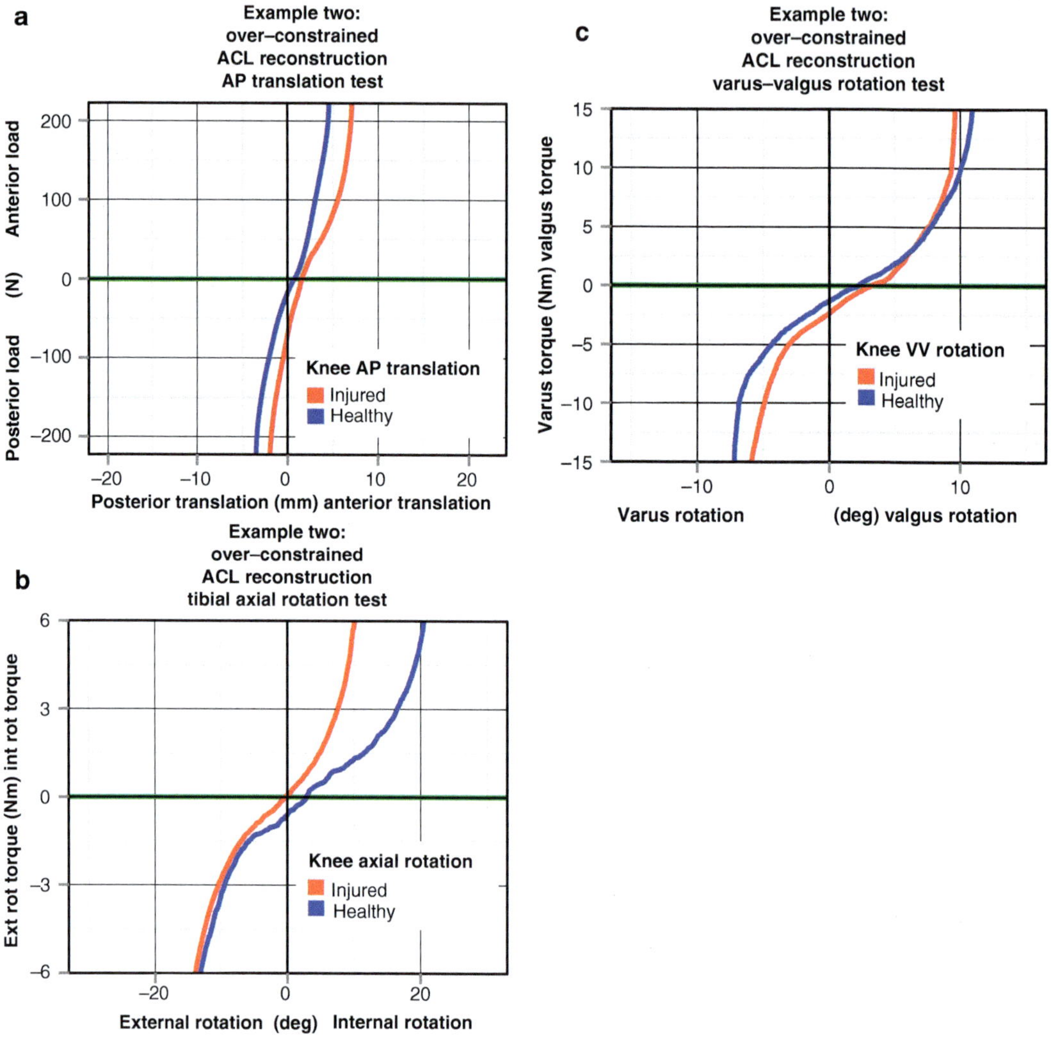

Fig. 17.14 (**a**) Anterior/posterior load-deformation curves for the reconstructed and healthy knees showing that anterior/posterior translation in the reconstructed knee was restored to the level of the healthy knee. (**b**) Tibial axial rotation load-deformation curves for the reconstructed and healthy knees showing the significant loss of internal rotation in this over-constrained knee. (**c**) Varus/valgus rotational load-deformation curves for the reconstructed and healthy knees showing the restricted varus and valgus motion in the over-constrained knee

during varus/valgus testing clearly indicates the MCL tear.

The second example involves a 49-year-old woman with a 15-year history of an ACL-deficient knee without complaint. At 17 months prior to presenting at our clinic, she twisted her knee playing tennis. The diagnosis of a medial meniscal tear was confirmed by MRI and, ultimately, surgery at an outside clinic. Since the twisting injury was felt to represent a subluxation of the knee, she chose to have a single-bundle ACL reconstruction at the time of her medial meniscectomy. Within months of the surgery, the patient reported that she felt as if something was wrong with her knee. A simple arthroscopy and an exam under anesthesia were performed, again at a different outside clinic, confirming that the ACL reconstruction was intact. The surgeon at the outside clinic suggested that her symptoms could be managed through physical therapy. At 17 months from the initial surgery, the patient continued to experience chronic lateral knee pain, tightness around the knee, and painful lack of full extension. She continued to have a quadriceps deficit and a painful limp. The patient was referred for knee laxity testing using the robotic system in order to fully characterize the biomechanics of her knees. Her load-deformation curves as recorded during laxity testing in the robotic system are shown in Fig. 17.14. The curves show good restoration of AP translation in the reconstructed knee to the level of the healthy knee. However, the reconstructed knee was shown to be over-constrained in internal rotation and varus/valgus testing. The patient went on to have her over-constraining ACL reconstruction removed during a knee arthroscopy. Within a few days, the knee was feeling "back to normal" with some residual lateral pain that resolved. The patient was able to achieve full extension without pain.

Conclusions

Considerable time was spent and care taken to develop a robotic device, data collection methods, and an analysis process to record biomechanical characteristics of the knee during whole-leg testing while minimizing the amount of error. The long-term goal of knee laxity testing using a robotic system is to provide the clinician with objective parameters (numbers and graphs) that correlate with specific injuries in the knee. These objective parameters should follow the guidelines of a diagnostic test with its associated sensitivity, specificity, positive predictive values, and negative predictive values. The results of knee laxity testing using a robotic system can provide the clinician with additional information about the injured knee to improve diagnosis and ensure that the best treatment plan for that patient is developed. The ability to improve the diagnosis of knee injuries should better allow the clinician to identify those patients that will be improved by surgical intervention and to avoid unnecessary surgery.

The goal of knee laxity testing using a robotic system is to provide the clinician with objective parameters that correlate with specific injuries in the knee. Bilateral whole-leg testing provides information on the "natural" resting position of the knee, as well as three-dimensional load-deformation curves representing the standard knee examination, i.e., anterior/posterior translation, internal/external tibial axial rotation, and varus/valgus rotation. A robotic system allows for reliable recording of biomechanical characteristics of the knee while minimizing error. The results of knee laxity testing using a robotic system can provide the clinician with additional information about an injured knee in order to ensure that the best treatment plan for that patient is developed.

References

1. Almquist PO, Ekdahl C, Isberg PE, Fridén T (2011) Measurements of knee rotation-reliability of an external device in vivo. BMC Musculoskelet Disord 12:291
2. Ballantyne BT, French AK, Heimsoth SL, Kachingwe AF, Lee JB, Soderberg GL (1995) Influence of examiner experience and gender on interrater reliability of KT-1000 arthrometer measurements. Phys Ther 75:898–906
3. Branch TP (1992) The role of knee MRI in sports medicine: a clinical commentary on magnetic resonance imaging of the knee. Emory J Med 6
4. Branch TP, Browne JE, Siebold R, Freedberg HI, Wente TM, Jacobs CA (2011) Inconsistent manual techniques make qualitative and quantitative analyses of the pivot shift test difficult in both ACL-deficient and intact knees. 8th Biennial ISAKOS congress, Rio de Janeiro, 15–19 May 2011. Available at: http://isakos.omnibooksonline.com/2011/data/papers/papers/128.htm
5. Branch T, Browne J, Campbell J (2006) Restoration of normal joint play: the correlation of axial tibial rotation, anterior laxity and patient satisfaction in the anterior cruciate reconstructed knee. Presented at the 2006 ACL study group meeting, Kohala Coast, 27 Mar 2006
6. Branch TP, Browne JE, Campbell JD, Siebold R, Freedberg HI, Arendt EA, et al (2010) Rotational laxity greater in patients with contralateral anterior cruciate ligament injury than healthy volunteers. Knee Surg Sports Traumatol Arthros 18(10):1379–1384. http://doi.org/10.1007/s00167-009-1010-y
7. Daniel DM, Stone ML, Sachs R, Malcom L (1985) Instrumented measurement of anterior knee laxity in patients with acute anterior cruciate ligament disruption. Am J of Sports Med 13(6):401–407

8. Daniel DM, Malcom LL, Losse G, Stone ML, Sachs R, Burks R (1985) Instrumented measurement of anterior laxity of the knee. J Bone Joint Surg Am 67(5):720–726
9. Espregueira-Mendes J, Pereira H, Sevivas N, Passos C, Vasconcelos JC, Monteiro A, Oliveira JM, Reis RL (2012) Assessment of rotatory laxity in anterior cruciate ligament-deficient knees using magnetic resonance imaging with Porto-knee testing device. Knee Surg Sports Traumatol Arthrosc 20:671–678
10. Forster IW, Warren-Smith CD, Tew M (1989) Is the KT1000 knee ligament arthrometer reliable? J Bone Joint Surg Br 71-B:843–847
11. Gardner MJ, Altman DJ (1996) Confidence intervals rather than P-values: estimation rather than hypothesis testing. BMJ 292:746–750
12. Grood ES, Suntay WJ (1983) A joint coordinate system for the clinical description of three-dimensional motions: application to the knee. J Biomech Eng 105(2):136–144. http://doi.org/10.1115/1.3138397
13. Hastie TJ, Tibshirani R (1994) Generalized additive model. Chapman & Hall, New York, pp P60–P64
14. Jacobs et al. (2011) Females demonstrated greater valgus laxity than males during in vivo robotic knee testing. Annual meeting of the Orthopaedic Research Society. Available at: http://www.ors.org/Transactions/57/1342.pdf
15. Kocabey Y, Tetik O, Isbell WM et al (2004) The value of clinical examination versus magnetic resonance imaging in the diagnosis of meniscal tears and anterior cruciate ligament rupture. Arthroscopy 20:696–700, PMID: 15346110
16. Kocher MS, Steadman JR, Briggs K, Zurakowski D, Sterett WI, Hawkins RJ (2002) Determinants of patient satisfaction with outcome after anterior cruciate ligament reconstruction. J Bone Joint Surg Am 84-A(9):1560–1572
17. Kocher MS, Steadman JR, Briggs KK, Sterett WI, Hawkins RJ (2004) Relationships between objective assessment of ligament stability and subjective assessment of symptoms and function after anterior cruciate ligament reconstruction. Am J Sports Med 32(3):629–634. http://doi.org/10.1177/0363546503261722
18. Liu SH, Osti L, Henry M, Bocchi L (1995) The diagnosis of acute complete tears of the anterior cruciate ligament. Comparison of MRI, arthrometry and clinical examination. J Bone Joint Surg Br 77:586–588, PMID: 76515603
19. Madhusudhan TR, Kumar TM, Bastawrous SS, Sinha A (2008) Clinical examination, MRI and arthroscopy in meniscal and ligamentous knee injuries – a prospective study. J Orthop Surg Res 3:19
20. Musahl V, Bell KM, Tsai AG et al (2007) Development of a simple device for measurement of rotational knee laxity. Knee Surg Sports Traumatol Arthrosc 15:1009–1012
21. Nikolaou VS, Chronopoulou E, Savvidou C, Plessas S, Giannoudis P, Efstathopoulos N, Papachristou G (2008) MRI efficacy in diagnosing internal lesions of the knee: a retrospective analysis. J Trauma Manag Outcomes 2:4
22. Noyes FR, Grood ES, Cummings JF, Wroble RR (1991) An analysis of the pivot shift phenomenon. The knee motions and subluxations induced by different examiners. Am J Sports Med 19:148–155, PMID: 2039066
23. Noyes FR, Cummings JF, Grood ES et al (1991) The diagnosis of knee motion limits, subluxations, and ligament injury. Am J Sports Med 19:163–171, PMID: 2039068
24. O'Shea KJ, Murphy KP, Heekin RD, Herzwurm PJ (1996) The diagnostic accuracy of history, physical examination, and radiographs in the evaluation of traumatic knee disorders. Am J Sports Med 24: 164–167, PMID: 8775114
25. Peeler J, Leiter J, MacDonald P (2010) Accuracy and reliability of anterior cruciate ligament clinical examination in a multidisciplinary sports medicine setting. Clin J Sport Med 20:80–85, PMID: 20215888
26. Poole C (1987) Beyond the confidence interval. Am J Public Health 77(20):195–199
27. Shultz SJ, Shimokochi Y, Nguyen AD et al (2007) Measurement of varus-valgus and internal-external rotational knee laxities in vivo-part I: assessment of measurement reliability and bilateral asymmetry. J Orthop Res 25(8):981–988
28. Tsai AG, Musahl V, Steckel H et al (2008) Rotational knee laxity: reliability if a simple measurement device in vivo. BMC Musculoskelet Disord 9:35
29. Tyler TF, McHugh MP, Gleim GW, Nicholas SJ (1999) Association of KT-1000 measurements with clinical tests of knee stability 1 year following anterior cruciate ligament reconstruction. J Orthop Sports Phys Ther 29(9):540–545

Part IV

The Pivot Shift

The Envelope of Laxity of the Pivot Shift Test

18

Breck Lord and Andrew A. Amis

Contents

B. Lord
Mechanical Engineering Department, Biomechanics Group, Imperial College London, London SW7 2AZ, UK

A.A. Amis (✉)
Mechanical Engineering Department, Biomechanics Group, Imperial College London, London SW7 2AZ, UK

Department of Surgery and Cancer, Musculoskeletal Surgery Group, Imperial College London School of Medicine, London W6 8RF, UK
e-mail: a.amis@imperial.ac.uk

18.1 Introduction

The pivot shift (PS) is an abnormal movement between the tibia and femur which may occur following damage of the soft tissues that stabilise the knee. The 'dynamic' PS test is accepted as being the single clinical diagnostic test that is most closely related to the functional instability that usually follows a rupture of the anterior cruciate ligament (ACL). The grade of the PS test correlates with instability symptoms [1], reduced sports activity [2] and articular cartilage and meniscal damage [3]. Although the ACL is the primary restraint to tibial anterior translation, resisting more than 80% of the drawer force [4], the PS is known as a 'rotatory instability' and that term will be explained below. The PS has been known clinically for a long time, and whilst that name was only coined relatively recently [5, 6], the concept of the 'slipping knee' instability and the resulting need for ACL reconstruction was known much earlier [7].

Despite the PS being central to clinical evaluation of knee instability, it remains resistant to efforts to arrive at standardised descriptions of the motion itself and of standardised means to elicit the instability. These aims are desirable, if clinical results are to be compared meaningfully. The variability of the PS test has been documented to result both from differences amongst examining clinicians in how they apply the test to their patients [8] and also from the wide spectrum of soft tissue damage which may occur in association with the ACL rupture. That variation

V. Musahl et al. (eds.), *Rotatory Knee Instability*, DOI 10.1007/978-3-319-32070-0_18

results in an individual surgeon eliciting a wide range of PS movements between patients [9]. It may follow from this that there may not be a single PS test method that is optimal for all patterns of soft tissue damage and that is reflected by the manner in which the examiner of a knee feels intuitively how to vary the loading and movements in order to elicit the subluxation/reduction events which characterise the PS. This review will summarise some of these aspects.

Fact Box 1
The 'envelope of laxity' is a term that describes the total pattern of laxity behaviour of a joint, across its range of motion.

The 'envelope of laxity' is a term that describes the total pattern of laxity behaviour of a joint, across its range of motion. As an example, the envelope of tibial internal-external rotation laxity is relatively narrow near to knee extension and widens with knee flexion; that pattern reflects the locking of the knee in extension when the posterior capsule tightens, followed by progressive slackening of the soft tissues as the knee flexes (Fig. 18.1). For the PS, description of the envelope of laxity is more complex, because it requires a knowledge of how the tibiofemoral joint laxity varies in two degrees-of-freedom (DoF) simultaneously with knee flexion-extension: the combination of anterior-posterior (AP) translation (translation: a linear motion without reference to rotation), plus internal-external rotations [10]. Given that the knee has 6 DoF [11], the PS test involves measuring the three simultaneously – flexion-extension and internal-external rotations, plus anterior-posterior translations – whilst ignoring the other three: medial-lateral, proximal-distal translations and varus-valgus (or abduction-adduction) rotation. In the PS test, we are concerned primarily with normal or abnormal movement of the tibia in relation to the femur in the transverse plane representing the tibial plateau, so the situation may be simplified to consideration of only the anterior-posterior (AP) translation, plus internal-external rotation.

Fact Box 2
The knee has 6 degrees-of-freedom of motion – three rotations: flexion-extension, abduction-adduction and internal-external and three translations: anterior-posterior, medial-lateral and compression-distraction. The pivot shift, in the transverse plane, involves tibial anterior-posterior translation and internal-external rotation.

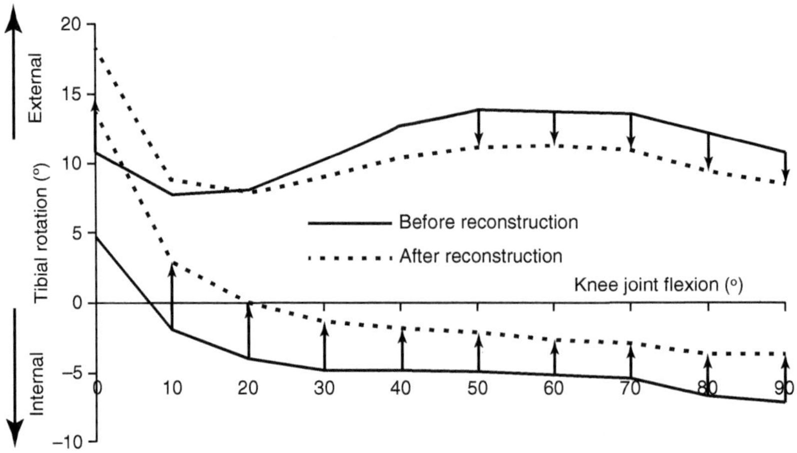

Fig. 18.1 Graph showing the mean envelope of tibial internal-external rotation laxity with manual application of torque at the foot, pre- and post-ACL reconstruction (Reproduced with permission and copyright © of the British Editorial Society of Bone and Joint Surgery Bull et al. [9])

18.2 Static Laxity Tests

18.2.1 Anterior Translation

The integrity of the ACL may be evaluated by means of the anterior draw or Lachman tests. The anterior translation caused by imposing a given anterior draw force to the proximal tibia can be assessed subjectively by feeling the 'step-off', between each of the femoral condyles and the anterior rim of the tibial plateau, and then comparing that manual examination to the (usually undamaged) contralateral knee. A subtlety in this test is that it is also possible to evaluate differences in the anterior translation between each of the medial and lateral condyles and thus obtain an impression of *coupled* rotational laxity. (Coupled motion: defined as a motion which occurs automatically in a DoF other than the principal DoF of the clinical test.) It is important to allow coupled motion to occur, because an attempt to inhibit it during the laxity test will reduce the laxity by 30 % when compared to a repeated test with the tibia free to rotate [4, 12].

The incongruence of the tibiofemoral joint also allows secondary movements, principally tibial internal-external rotations, in response to relatively low torques applied. In general, the lateral compartment is more mobile than the medial, because of the difference in the capsular attachments of their menisci. This tendency is accentuated by weight bearing, because the medial tibial plateau is concave, so the joint load stabilises the medial femoral condyle, whereas the lateral plateau is convex in the sagittal plane and so is inherently less stable. This means that there is more movement of the lateral compartment than of the medial compartment under most loading combinations. The result of this is that tibial anterior draw is normally accompanied by a 'coupled' tibial internal rotation, reported in the range 3–10° [13, 14]. Similarly, a posterior draw force causes both tibial posterior translation, plus a coupled tibial external rotation [15].

After ACL rupture there is an increase in anterior tibial translation and coupled internal tibial rotation in response to an anterior draw force [10, 14]. Due to the small moment arm about the axis of tibial rotation, the role of the cruciate ligaments in resisting internal torques is limited. However, clinically, ACL deficiency allows a significant increase in tibial internal rotation near full knee extension [16].

Because there is a wide spread of natural laxity in the population, with some intact knees having greater AP laxity than others with ACL deficiency [17], it is not appropriate simply to quote a laxity measurement in isolation: the side-to-side difference is more informative, and greater than 3 mm is often taken to be diagnostic of ACL damage [18].

Tibial anterior translation is reduced significantly if the tibia is held in fixed internal or external rotation [19]. This is because of tightness in the peripheral structures so that they can share the load with the ACL. Tibial external rotation moves the tibial attachment of the medial collateral ligament complex anteriorly; this both tightens and aligns these structures to restrain tibial anterior translation. Similarly, the iliotibial tract and lateral collateral ligament act in tibial internal rotation [4, 13, 19, 20].

18.2.2 Internal-External Rotation Laxity

The extra-articular structures are the primary restraints to tibial rotation laxity [20, 21], and so they are usually involved in ACL injuries [22, 23]. The lateral compartment is most important in tibial rotational laxity: it is more mobile than the medial, and the ACL attaches here, but there have been differing reports on the effect of isolated ACL rupture. Lipke [24] found that isolated cutting of the ACL led to a significant increase in tibial internal rotation. Andersen et al. [25] found a small but statistically significant increase in rotational laxity after isolated ACL transection near the knee extension but no measurable difference beyond 30° knee flexion. Conversely, Lane and Daniel [26] found that cutting the ACL had no significant effect on either internal or external tibial rotation laxity, so they concluded that rotational instability is not a major factor after *isolated* ACL rupture. For internal rotation laxity with anterolateral damage, Wroble et al. [27] found that cutting the anterolateral structures, which included the iliotibial tract, led to a significant increase in tibial internal rotation in the ACL-deficient knee, whilst (surprisingly) Lipke et al. [24] did not. Wang and Walker [28] also reported that tibial rotation laxity was reduced 80% after imposing a tibiofemoral joint load of 1 kN (approx 1.3 body weight).

The literature reviewed above suggested that tibial rotational laxity is not increased greatly by isolated ACL deficiency; this conflicts with the impression that ACL injury leads to rotatory instability. This divergence may be explained partly by the location of the axis of tibial rotation. In the intact knee, the axis of tibial internal-external rotation crosses the joint space near the centre of the tibial plateau [28, 29]. Therefore, tibial internal rotation causes the lateral aspect of the tibial plateau to move anteriorly, and the medial aspect to move posteriorly, by a similar distance. After ACL injury, the axis of rotation passes through the centre of the medial plateau [30] or close to the medial collateral ligament. This means that the lateral aspect is further from the axis, so the same angle of rotation will cause the lateral aspect to move further anteriorly. When this is added to the increased tibial anterior translation that follows ACL injury, there is a significantly greater anterior movement of the lateral tibia than normal. This observation led to the term 'anterolateral rotational instability' (ALRI).

18.3 Dynamic Laxity Testing

18.3.1 The Pivot Shift

Subjectively, the pivot shift is an experience of instability often associated with athletic activity and described by the patient as a 'buckling' or 'giving way'. Terry et al. [31] suggested that the pivot shift was due to the combined influence of injuries to the ACL, the mid-third capsular ligament, the lateral meniscus and its capsular attachments and the capsule-osseous and deep layers of the ITB. Most authors agree that an ACL injury is required to produce a positive PS, but an isolated ACL rupture does not necessarily result in one.

During the PS test, there may be a sudden movement between the subluxed and reduced positions [10]. A valgus moment is applied to the knee, in order to compress the lateral compartment. Because most of the PS movement occurs in the lateral compartment, the internal-external rotations occur around a medial axis [30]. When the knee is tested by flexing it from an extended posture, the lateral tibial plateau gradually subluxes anteriorly as the posterior soft tissue structures slacken and then it may suddenly reduce posteriorly [6] (Fig. 18.2). Conversely, if the knee is tested by starting in flexion, then extending it, the lateral tibial plateau remains in the correct anatomical articulation until it suddenly subluxes anteriorly, when the knee is approaching extension [32]. The movements of the lateral tibial condyle may be enhanced by applying a tibial internal rotation torque during the test, usually by grasping the foot. The sudden PS movements are usually attributed to the changing direction of the tension exerted onto Gerdy's tubercle by the ITB [33]. Near to knee extension, the tight posterior capsule holds the tibia in its correct articulation. In early flexion, the posterior capsule slackens and the lateral femoral condyle rolls 'downhill' across the sloping plateau, subluxing the lateral compartment. Then, with further flexion, the tension in the ITB acts more posteriorly in relation to the tibia, and it overcomes the 'slipping downhill' effect, resulting in a sudden tibial external rotation, pulling the lateral tibial plateau under the femoral condyle to its stable reduced configuration (Fig. 18.3).

18.3.2 The Envelope of Laxity of the Pivot Shift

The tibia is most rotationally stable in extension, due to the tightening of the posterior capsule, especially the oblique fibres of the posteromedial capsule and the arcuate ligament complex [15]. As the knee flexes, it is the lateral and medial extra-articular structures that primarily control rotation, with the ACL being a secondary restraint [22]. The pivoting mechanism of injury is the classic presentation, so there is likely to be peripheral pathology in the presence of an ACL rupture.

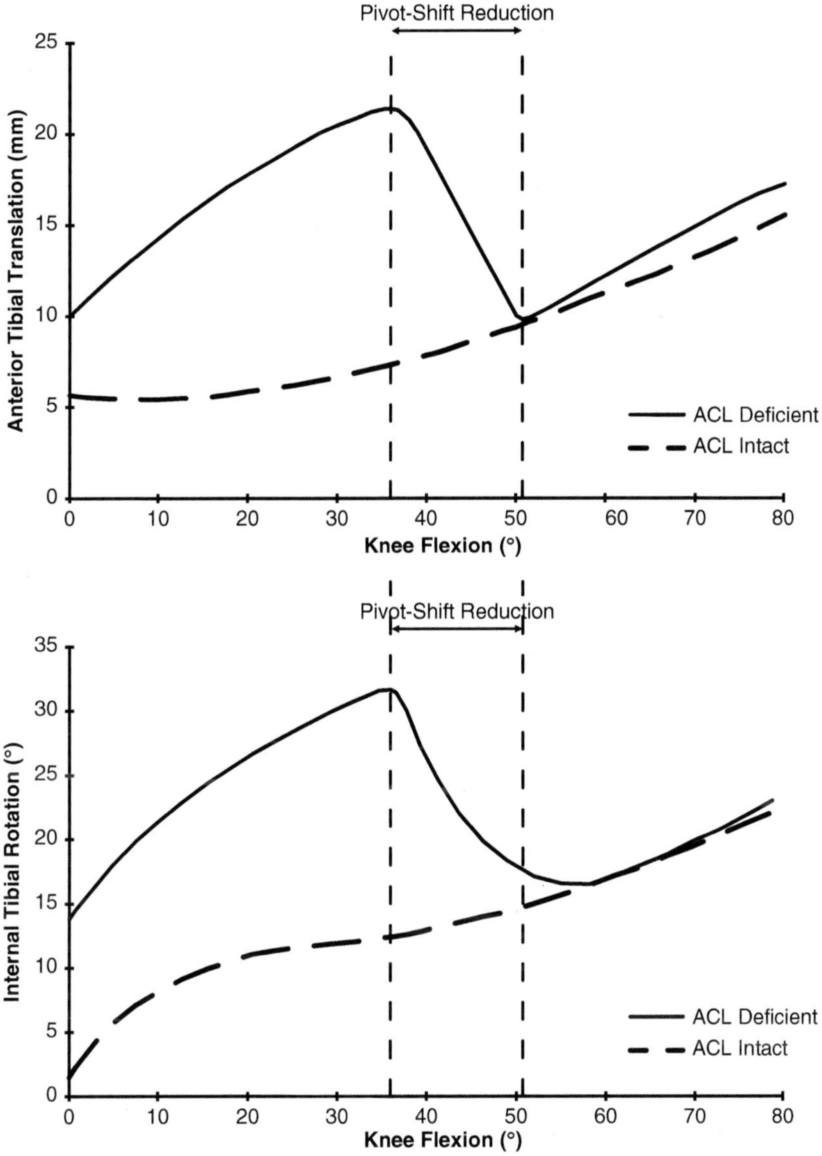

Fig. 18.2 A typical pivot shift, demonstrating the abnormal anterior tibial translation and internal rotation. These subluxations increase gradually in early knee flexion and then reduce suddenly when the tibia falls back to the anatomical position

Following isolated ACL injury, Bull et al. [9] reported the PS reduction occurring across an arc centred at a mean of 36±9° knee flexion. The reduction movement was an external rotation of 13±8° combined with a posterior tibial translation (at the centre of the plateau) of 12±8 mm. Although the exact mechanism is not yet fully understood, the tibial plateau is stable in either its 'reduced' or 'subluxed' extreme of the abnormal envelope of laxity [10] (Figs. 18.2 and 18.3). Norwood et al. [23] reported no correlation between ligament injuries and the severity of the 'pivot', whilst Terry and Hughston [31] reported that only 83 % of positive PS tests had ACL injuries.

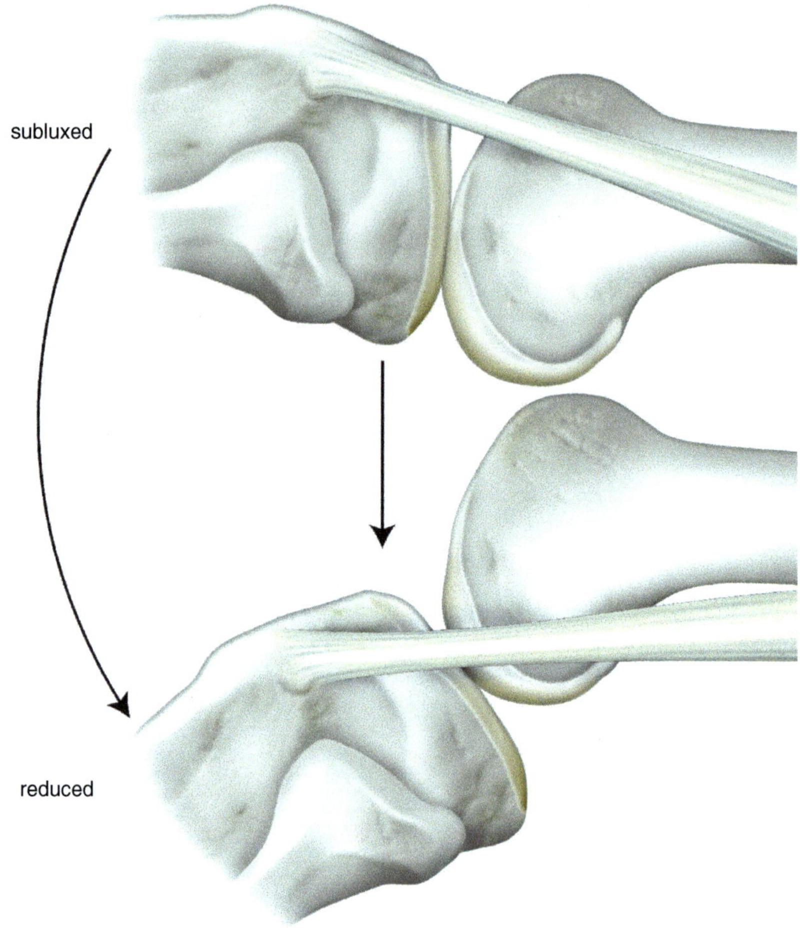

Fig. 18.3 Reduction of the lateral tibial plateau during the pivot shift. Flexion of the tibia allows the iliotibial band to externally rotate and posteriorly reduce the lateral tibial plateau. The lateral compartment of the knee is stable in subluxed or reduced positions in either side of the pivot shift

After rupture of the ACL, anterior displacement is controlled by secondary restraints on both sides of the knee, but the medial compartment is more stable than the lateral because of the articular geometry, soft tissue attachments and less meniscal mobility. The lateral compartment is therefore drawn further anteriorly than the medial, exaggerating the 'coupled' internal tibial rotation about an axis which is displaced medially (Fig. 18.4). As part of the 'unhappy triad', rupture of the medial collateral ligament is associated with some ACL injuries, and this reduces the stability of the medial compartment and the ability to elicit the PS [33].

Weight bearing has a significant effect on the PS. Following ACL rupture, the increased anterior translation in the lateral compartment moves the tibiofemoral contact point onto a 'downhill' slope at the posterior edge of the lateral tibial plateau, promoting further anterior subluxation with any increase in compressive force. Therefore, movement of the lateral compartment is exaggerated under most loading conditions. Hence, the application of a valgus moment, in addition to internal tibial torque, enhances the sensitivity of detecting PS instability. The corollary of this is that the sensitivity to subtle variations in tibiofemoral loading results in significant inter-observer variation, limiting objective comparisons between different surgeons/surgical centres [8, 10].

Multiple variations of the PS test have been described, Galway's reduction [5], Slocum's ALRI test [20] and Macintosh's lateral pivot shift test [6], and may be performed to either elicit sudden tibial reduction or subluxation [34]. It is widely accepted that the action of the ITB

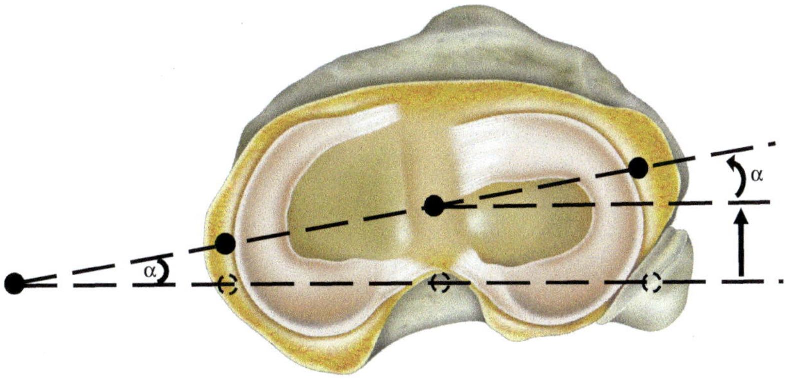

Fig. 18.4 The bony geometry and soft tissue attachments allow for more mobility within the lateral compartment under an anterior draw force, allowing for coupled anterior translation and internal rotation (α). In the case of ACL rupture, the axis of this rotation is displaced medially

accounts for the PS [33], but its exact role remains controversial. Slocum et al. [20] suggested that both the subluxation and the reduction tests require an intact ITB, which has been supported by Jakob et al., clinically [35]. Conversely, Galway and Macintosh [6] suggested that a positive PS test required an injury to the ITB whilst Bach et al. [36] suggested that the PS test was most sensitive when hip abduction reduced the tension in the ITB. In a recent biomechanical study, Kittl et al. [37] reported that the ITB was the primary restraint of isolated internal tibial rotation and the abnormal coupled displacements during the simulated PS.

18.3.3 Quantifying the Pivot Shift

Subjective grading of the PS shows large inter-observer variability [8]. The ability to objectively quantify the 'dynamic' pivot shift test pre-/postoperatively in a cost effective, repeatable manner could enable comparison of results between centres to determine the optimal technique for restoring native knee kinematics after a pivoting injury. Moreover, there is considerable variability between knees during the pivot shift in terms of how far medial the axis of external rotation is located and the magnitudes of posterior tibial translation and external rotation during reduction [9] (Fig. 18.5). This variability is likely to be a consequence of the differing patterns of soft tissue injury about the knee. Therefore, quantifying both the translational and rotational components of the PS could provide a guide for the use of, for example, a lateral extra-articular procedure.

Lopomo et al. [38] recently reviewed the literature, reporting that navigation systems [39, 40], electromagnetic devices [9, 41, 42] and acceleration devices [43] have been used to measure the components of knee kinematics during the PS. However, there is still debate as to the exact motion pattern of the manoeuvre and the combination of forces and torques that should be applied. Thus, Lopomo et al. found large variations between clinical studies: the reported anterior-posterior translations ranged from 5 ± 2 mm [44] to 20 ± 5 mm [45] and the internal-external rotations from $11 \pm 5°$ [46] to $32 \pm 3°$ [45]. Two studies had measured or calculated the translations of each compartment of the knee: Bedi et al. [47] reported a medial translation of 12 ± 2 mm and lateral 20 ± 1 mm, whilst Lopomo et al. [48] reported 5 ± 7 mm medial and 21 ± 9 mm lateral translations. In view of these measurements, Bedi et al. suggested that measurement of the movement of the lateral compartment would be most valuable when assessing the PS.

However, in vivo testing using manual manipulation has no direct control over the magnitude or direction of the forces/torques applied, so – although the clinical PS test represents a true dynamic evaluation of the constraining elements – it may not be representative of the envelope of laxity during physiological joint loading, whilst variation in the loads/torques and their speed of application may limit repeatability and comparison between individual surgeons and centres [8].

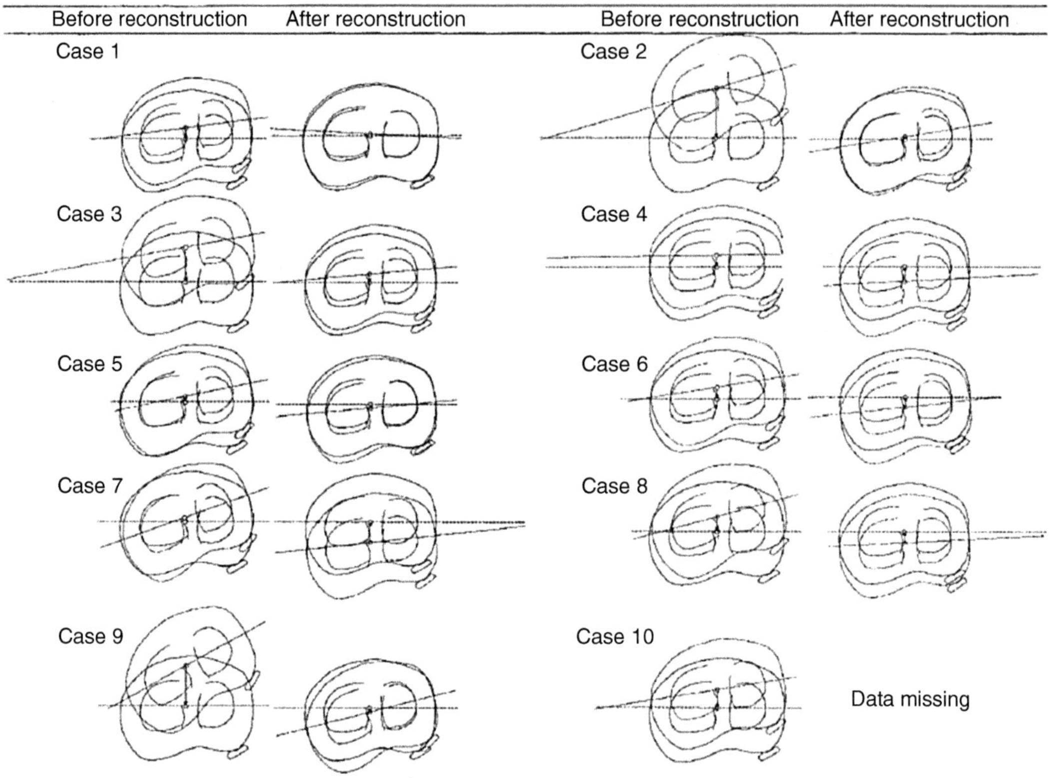

Fig. 18.5 Diagram showing movement of the tibial plateau during the pivot shift test before and after reconstruction over the same range of flexion (tracings transposed to appear to be in the right side). Some knees have mostly anterior translation, whilst others have mostly internal rotation (Reproduced with permission and copyright © of the British Editorial Society of Bone and Joint Surgery Bull et al. [9])

> **Fact Box 3**
> The lateral compartment moves more than the medial during the PS test, with mean translations of approximately 9 mm at the medial condyle and 21 mm at the lateral condyle.

18.3.4 Envelope of Motion After ACL Reconstruction

18.3.4.1 Results Post-ACL Reconstruction

Ongoing symptomatic instability has been shown to correlate with a persistent PS [1]. In postoperative assessment, persistence of abnormal secondary movements has been related to less satisfactory functional outcomes, including a failure to return to pre-injury levels of function [1]. Up to 25 % of patients have been reported to have a persistent PS following transtibial ACL reconstruction, going on to develop secondary meniscal and chondral injuries which may propagate degenerative arthrosis [49]. This led to the rotational restraint by the posterolateral (PL) bundle of the ACL being considered and the concept of anatomical double-bundle ACL reconstruction [50], but it has proven difficult to demonstrate significant reductions of residual instability [51, 52]. Bull et al. [9] and Ferretti et al. [53] examined the envelope of PS laxity using optical navigation during surgery and did not find significant differences between the single- and double-bundle reconstructions. Given the complexity of double-bundle surgery, many surgeons consider 'anatomic' single-bundle

ACL reconstruction to be the current method of choice, but the PS envelope highlights that native knee kinematics may not be fully restored: an International Knee Documentation Committee pivot grade B (often termed 'pivot glide') is a familiar concept in clinical examination and may be present in as many as 12% of patients after ACL reconstruction, even without measurable pathological anterior tibial laxity [54]. Lie et al. [55] reported the persistence of a 'mini pivot' in vitro (Fig. 18.6) after anatomically placed SB ACL reconstruction, when anterior

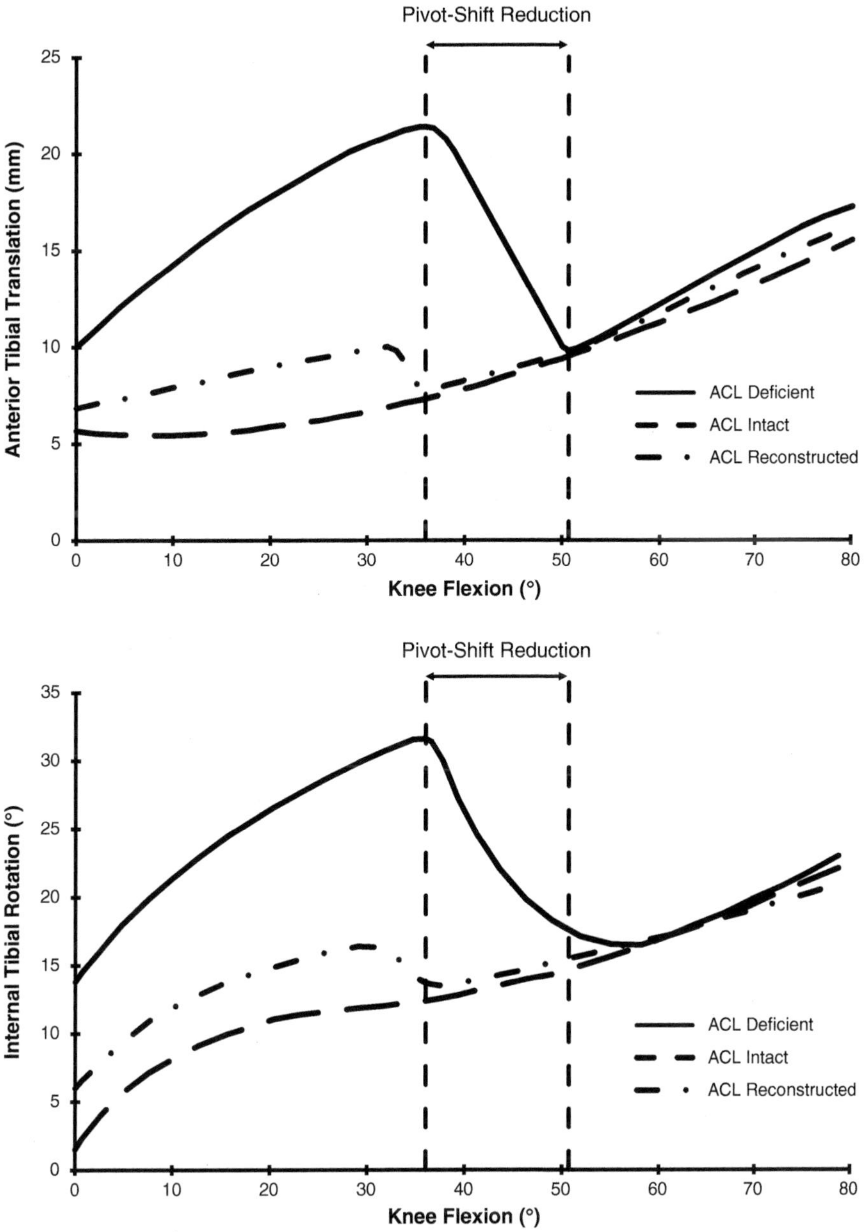

Fig. 18.6 A residual 'mini pivot shift' or 'pivot glide' after anatomically placed single-bundle ACL reconstruction. Coupled anterior then posterior tibial translation and internal then external rotation is seen in early flexion, but with reduced amplitude and velocity than when the ACL was unreconstructed

tibial translation was well controlled but rotational laxity was not eliminated by increasing graft tension.

18.3.4.2 The Role of Lateral Extra-articular Reconstructions

Combined injury to both the ACL and the lateral structures has been shown to produce a PS whilst isolated injury to either can also produce a positive test [10, 31]. Thus, a PS can remain even after an obliquely positioned ACL reconstruction [44]. The anterolateral structures have a greater mechanical advantage in the control of knee joint rotation than the ACL, and it has been suggested that injury of these structures may account for a significant proportion of ALRI [31]. Historically, instability associated with ACL deficiency was treated surgically by isolated extra-articular tenodesis such as the Lemaire [56] or Macintosh [57]. In modern practice, such procedures are being readopted in cases of high grade PS and in the context of revision. Engebretsen et al. [58] reported a 43 % decrease in the tension in an ACL graft following an iliotibial tenodesis; hence, extra-articular procedures have been adopted as 'backups' to protect ACL grafts during the early healing phase.

Studies of the lateral structures have highlighted the action of the 'Kaplan's fibres' linking the deep aspect of the ITB to the metaphysis, and the capsulo-osseous layer which forms an anterolateral sling around the lateral femoral condyle to act as a restraint to rotation [31]. Kittl et al. [37] measured the contributions of the soft tissues to the restraint of tibial internal rotation during a simulated PS using a robotic testing system. The superficial ITB fibres made a significant contribution to resisting the simulated PS at 45° of knee flexion whilst the deep ITB fibres contributed significantly at 15°, 30° and 45°; as a whole, the ITB offered 79 % of the restraint at 45° of knee flexion. In contrast, the ACL and other anterolateral structures made minimal contributions to restraining the simulated PS.

Conclusions

Native tibiofemoral joint kinematics is controlled by a complex interaction of intra- and extra-articular soft tissue restraints and the articular geometry. The exact biomechanical contributions of these structures towards the restraint of the PS are yet to be determined. The PS is a specific pattern of pathological secondary displacements associated with ACL rupture and/or injury to anterolateral structures such as the ITB attachments. The typical pathological laxity pattern during the PS test includes simultaneous tibial subluxations in anterior translation and internal rotation, which correspond to an enlarged 'envelope of laxity' in both of those degrees of freedom of motion, followed by sudden reduction of the subluxation. There is more motion in the lateral compartment, around a medially shifted axis of internal rotation with ACL deficiency. Although there are a variety of methods of quantifying the kinematics of the PS, there is as yet no clinical 'gold standard' with suitable accuracy and repeatability to measure the excessive translations and rotations. The differing patterns of rotational and translational laxities that have been reported show clearly that it is necessary to measure both, if all knees are to have their abnormal PS envelopes of laxity understood, ideally with standardised loading parameters. When that is achieved, the data should directly guide choices of surgical procedures and allow objective assessment of the return of normal envelopes of laxity and their relationship to functional knee instability.

The envelopes of tibiofemoral anterior-posterior translation and internal-external rotation are variable between knees and that may reflect the specific injured structures. Thus, it is essential to measure both translations and rotations simultaneously to gain a full understanding of the effects of surgery to treat PS instability.

References

1. Kujala UM, Nelimarkka O, Koskinen SK (1992) Relationship between the pivot shift and the configuration of the lateral tibial plateau. Arch Orthop Trauma Surg 111(4):228–229
2. Kaplan N, Wickiewicz TL, Warren RF (1990) Primary surgical treatment of anterior cruciate ligament ruptures. A long-term follow-up study. Am J Sports Med 18:354–358

3. Noyes FR, Mooar PA, Matthews DS et al (1983) The symptomatic anterior cruciate-deficient knee. Part I: the long-term functional disability in athletically active individuals. J Bone Joint Surg Am 65A:154–162
4. Butler DL, Noyes F, Grood E (1980) Ligamentous restraints to anterior-posterior drawer in the human knee. J Bone Joint Surg Am 62(2):259–270
5. Galway R, Beaupre A, MacIntosh D (1972) Pivot shift: a clinical sign of symptomatic anterior cruciate insufficiency. J Bone Joint Surg [Br] 54:763–764
6. Galway H, MacIntosh D (1980) The lateral pivot shift: a symptom and sign of anterior cruciate ligament insufficiency. Clin Orthop Relat Res 147:45–50
7. Hey Groves EW (1920) The crucial ligaments of the knee joint: their function, rupture and the operative treatment of the same. Br J Surg 7:505–515
8. Noyes FR et al (1991) An analysis of the pivot shift phenomenon the knee motions and subluxations induced by different examiners. Am J Sports Med 19(2):148–155
9. Bull AMJ, Earnshaw PH, Smith A, Katchburian MV, Hassan ANA, Amis AA (2002) Intraoperative measurement of knee kinematics in reconstruction of the anterior cruciate ligament. J Bone Jt Surg Br 84:1075–1081
10. Bull AMJ, Amis AA (1998) The pivot shift phenomenon: a clinical and biomechanical perspective. Knee 5:141–158
11. Bull AMJ, Amis AA (1998) Knee joint motion – description and measurement. Proc IMech E part H: Eng in Med 212:357–372
12. Fukubayashi T, Torzilli PA, Sherman MF et al (1982) An in vitro biomechanical evaluation of anterior-posterior motion of the knee. Tibial displacement, rotation, and torque. J Bone Joint Surg Am 64A:258–264
13. Nordt WE, Lotfi P, Plotkin E et al (1999) The in vivo assessment of tibial motion in the transverse plane in anterior cruciate ligament reconstructed knees. Am J Sports Med 27:611–616
14. Amis AA, Scammell BE (1993) Biomechanics of intraarticular and extraarticular reconstructions of the anterior cruciate ligament. J Bone Jt Surg Br 75B:812–817
15. Amis AA et al (2003) Biomechanics of the PCL and related structures: posterolateral, posteromedial and meniscofemoral ligaments. Knee Surg Sports Traumatol Arthrosc 11(5):271–281
16. Zarins B et al (1983) Rotational motion of the knee. Am J Sports Med 11(3):152–156
17. Amis AA (1989) Anterior cruciate ligament replacement knee stability and the effects of implants. J Bone Jt Surg Br 71B:819–824
18. Daniel DM, Malcom LL, Losse G et al (1985) Instrumented measurement of anterior laxity of the knee. J Bone Jt Surg Am 67A:720–726
19. Slocum DB, Larson RL (1968) Rotatory instability of the knee – its pathogenesis and a clinical test to demonstrate its presence. J Bone Jt Surg Am 50A: 211–225
20. Slocum DB et al (1976) Clinical test for anterolateral rotary instability of the knee. Clin Orthop Relat Res 118:63–69
21. Markolf KL, Mensch JS, Amstutz HC (1976) Stiffness and laxity of the knee – the contributions of the supporting structures. A quantitative in vitro study. J Bone Jt Surg Am 58A:583–594
22. Seering WP, Piziali RL, Nagel DA et al (1980) The function of the primary ligaments of the knee in varus-valgus and axial rotation. J Biomech 13(9):785–794
23. Norwood LA, Andrews JR, Meisterling RC et al (1979) Acute anterolateral rotatory instability of the knee. J Bone Jt Surg Am 61A:704–709
24. Lipke JM (1981) Role of incompetence of the anterior cruciate and lateral collateral ligaments in anterolateral and anteromedial instability. A biomechanical study of cadaver knees. J Bone Jt Surg Am 63A:954–960
25. Andersen HN, Dyhre-Poulsen P (1997) The anterior cruciate ligament does play a role in controlling axial rotation of the knee. Knee Surg Sports Traumatol Arthrosc 5:145–149
26. Lane JG, Daniel D (1994) The anterior cruciate ligament in controlling axial rotation. Am J Sports Med 22:289–293
27. Wroble RR, Grood ES, Cummings JS et al (1993) The role of the lateral extraarticular restraints in the anterior cruciate ligament-deficient knee. Am J Sports Med 21:257–263
28. Wang CJ, Walker PS (1974) Rotatory laxity of the human knee joint. J Bone Jt Surg Am 56A:161–170
29. Kaneda Y, Moriya H, Takahashi K et al (1997) Experimental study on external tibial rotation of the knee. Am J Sports Med 25:796–800
30. Mannel H, Claes L, Durselen L (2004) Anterior cruciate ligament rupture translates the axes of motion within the knee. Clin Biomech 19:130–135
31. Terry GC et al (1993) How iliotibial tract injuries of the knee combine with acute anterior cruciate ligament tears to influence abnormal anterior tibial displacement. Am J Sports Med 21(1):55–60
32. Hughston JC, Andrews JR, Cross MJ et al (1976) Classification of knee ligament instabilities. Part II. The lateral compartment. J Bone Joint Surg Am 58A:173–179
33. Matsumoto H (1990) Mechanism of the pivot shift. J Bone Jt Surg Br 72B:816–821
34. Losee RE, Johnson TR, Southwick WO (1978) Anterior subluxation of the lateral tibial plateau. A diagnostic test and operative repair. J Bone Joint Surg Am 60(8):1015–1030
35. Jakob RP, Hassler H, Staeubli HU (1981) Observations on rotatory instability of the lateral compartment of the knee. Experimental studies on the functional anatomy and the pathomechanism of the true and the reversed pivot shift sign. Acta Orthop Scand Suppl 191:1–32
36. Bach BR, Warren RF, Wickiewicz TL (1988) The pivot shift phenomenon: results and description of a modified clinical test for anterior cruciate ligament insufficiency. Am J Sports Med 16:571–576

37. Kittl C et al (2016) The role of the anterolateral structures and the ACL in controlling laxity of the intact and ACL-deficient knee. Am J Sports Med 44(2):345–354
38. Lopomo N, Zaffagnini S, Amis AA (2013) Quantifying the pivot shift test: a systematic review. Knee Surg Sports Traumatol Arthrosc 21(4):767–783
39. Lane CG et al (2008) In vivo analysis of the pivot shift phenomenon during computer navigated ACL reconstruction. Knee Surg Sports Traumatol Arthrosc 16(5):487–492
40. Zaffagnini S et al (2012) Can the pivot-shift be eliminated by anatomic double-bundle anterior cruciate ligament reconstruction? Knee Surg Sports Traumatol Arthrosc 20(4):743–751
41. Hoshino Y et al (2007) In vivo measurement of the pivot-shift test in the anterior cruciate ligament–deficient knee using an electromagnetic device. Am J Sports Med 35(7):1098–1104
42. Araki D et al (2011) A prospective randomised study of anatomical single-bundle versus double-bundle anterior cruciate ligament reconstruction: quantitative evaluation using an electromagnetic measurement system. Int Orthop 35(3):439–446
43. Lopomo N et al (2012) Quantitative assessment of pivot-shift using inertial sensors. Knee Surg Sports Traumatol Arthrosc 20(4):713–717
44. Ishibashi Y, Tsuda E, Yamamoto Y, Tsukada H, Toh S (2009) Navigation evaluation of the pivot-shift phenomenon during double-bundle anterior cruciate ligament reconstruction: is the posterolateral bundle more important? Arthroscopy 25(5):488–495
45. Colombet P, Robinson J, Christel P, Franceschi J-P, Djian P (2007) Using navigation to measure rotation kinematics during ACL reconstruction. Clin Orthop Relat Res 454:59–65
46. Bignozzi S, Zaffagnini S, Lopomo N, Fu FH, Irrgang JJ, Marcacci M (2010) Clinical relevance of static and dynamic tests after anatomical double-bundle ACL reconstruction. Knee Surg Sports Traumatol Arthrosc 18(1):37–42
47. Bedi A, Musahl V, Lane C, Citak M, Warren RF, Pearle AD (2010) Lateral compartment translation predicts the grade of pivot shift: a cadaveric and clinical analysis. Knee Surg Sports Traumatol Arthrosc 18(9):1269–1276
48. Lopomo N, Zaffagnini S, Bignozzi S, Visani A, Marcacci M (2010) Pivot-shift test: analysis and quantification of knee laxity parameters using a navigation system. J Orthop Res 28(2):164–169
49. Kocher MS et al (2004) Relationships between objective assessment of ligament stability and subjective assessment of symptoms and function after anterior cruciate ligament reconstruction. Am J Sports Med 32(3):629–634
50. Yasuda K et al (2004) Anatomic reconstruction of the anteromedial and posterolateral bundles of the anterior cruciate ligament using hamstring tendon grafts. Arthroscopy 20(10):1015–1025
51. Meredick RB et al (2008) Outcome of single-bundle versus double-bundle reconstruction of the anterior cruciate ligament: a meta-analysis. Am J Sports Med 36(7):1414–1421
52. Suomalainen P et al (2012) Double-bundle versus single-bundle anterior cruciate ligament reconstruction a prospective randomized study with 5-year results. Am J Sports Med 40(7):1511–1518
53. Ferretti A, Monaco E, Labianca L, De Carli A, Maestri B, Conteduca F (2009) Double-bundle anterior cruciate ligament reconstruction: a comprehensive kinematic study using navigation. Am J Sports Med 37:1548–1553
54. Aglietti P et al (1995) A comparison of clinical and radiological parameters with two arthroscopic techniques for anterior cruciate ligament reconstruction. Knee Surg Sports Traumatol Arthrosc 3(1):2–8
55. Lie DT, Bull AM, Amis AA (2007) Persistence of the mini pivot shift after anatomically placed anterior cruciate ligament reconstruction. Clin Orthop Relat Res 457:203–209
56. Lemaire M, Combelles F (1980) Technique actuelle de plastie ligamentaire pour rupture ancienne du ligament croisé antérieur. Rev Chir Orthop 66:523–525
57. MacIntosh D, Darby T (1976) Lateral substitution reconstruction. Proc Can Orthopaedic Asso J Bone Joint Surg Br 58:142
58. Engebretsen L, Lew WD, Lewis JL, Hunter RE (1990) The effect of an iliotibial tenodesis on intraarticular graft forces and knee joint motion. Am J Sports Med 18:169–176

Pivot Shift Test: An Evidence-Based Outcome Tool

19

Marie-Claude Leblanc, Devin C. Peterson, and Olufemi R. Ayeni

Contents

M.-C. Leblanc, MD, FRCSC
D.C. Peterson, MD, FRCSC
O.R. Ayeni, MD, MSc, FRCSC (✉)
Division of Orthopedic Surgery,
Department of Surgery, McMaster University,
Hamilton, ON, Canada
e-mail: femiayeni@gmail.com

19.1 Introduction

Anterior cruciate ligament (ACL) reconstruction is the standard of care for patients experiencing functional rotatory instability of the knee [1, 37]. Many patients report satisfactory outcomes following reconstruction; however, some continue to experience a sensation of instability, especially with pivoting and cutting activities [28]. Furthermore, ACL reconstruction does not seem to prevent knee OA, with recent studies showing that up to 50–90% of patients at 7–10 years have radiographic evidence of knee degeneration [6, 17, 19, 27, 30]. This has led researchers to search for a more complete understanding of the native and reconstructed ACLs as they relate to the role in knee biomechanics and kinematics.

Recent investigations on dynamic and rotational laxity have demonstrated that traditional ACL reconstruction fails to restore native knee kinematics [3, 4, 33]. The last decade has seen a shift toward a more anatomic ACL reconstruction technique in an attempt to improve rotational knee laxity and stability [7, 30].

Objective evaluation of rotational control requires reliable, precise, and specific outcome measurement tools and is critical in comparing different treatments of ACL injuries [7, 34]. While a variety of tools for measuring rotational laxity exist, the manual pivot shift test still remains as a valid and commonly used technique in daily clinical practice [38]. The objective of this chapter is to summarize the available evidence on the pivot shift test as an outcome measurement tool.

V. Musahl et al. (eds.), *Rotatory Knee Instability*, DOI 10.1007/978-3-319-32070-0_19

19.2 Evidence-Based Medicine and Outcome Tools

19.2.1 Evidence-Based Medicine

The principles of evidence-based medicine (EBM) were first introduced by Sackett in the early 1980s and the term later coined by Guyatt in the 1990s [35]. EBM represents the application of the scientific method into healthcare decision-making [7, 35]. The integration of best current external evidence with clinical expertise and patient values establishes the goal to optimize decision-making regarding the care of the individual patient [7, 35] (Fig. 19.1).

Best evidence is defined as clinically relevant research that provides answers to a well-defined clinical question [35]. This is not limited to high-quality randomized controlled trials, but also takes into account patient-centered clinical research and the basic sciences [13]. Well-conducted observational studies, comparative studies, systematic reviews, and meta-analysis complete the arsenal of information leading to the development of best evidence to be applied to clinical scenarios [13, 35]. EBM is not "cookbook" medicine [35]. Such evidence can inform, but never replace, individual clinical expertise regarding appropriate application evidence to inform a unique clinical scenario [35].

19.2.2 Outcome Tools and ACL Reconstruction

Improvement in surgical outcomes can only be determined when results can be accurately measured, repeated, and compared with other studies [7]. Outcome tools are essential to the evaluation of a new surgical technique, highlighting the success of known treatment and outlining the impact of surgery on patient care. Three types of outcome tools have been described: (1) general health (mental and physical), (2) disease specific, and (3) patient satisfaction [22, 41]. Accurate assessment of outcomes remains challenging, and critical characteristics for optimal outcome tools have been described: patient relevancy, user-friendliness, inexpensive, sensitive, reliable, valid, and responsiveness to clinical change [7, 36, 40, 41].

An outcome tool that can measure and validate the success of ACL surgery is very important [6]. Unfortunately, there is no consensus regarding which test or combination of tests is most appropriate [36]. A number of knee injury rating scales have been used over the years, with more than 54 outcomes measures described for ACL reconstruction alone [41]. To date, the Anterior Cruciate Ligament Quality of Life (ACL-QOL) outcome measure [29] is the only validated, disease-specific measure of health-related quality of life for ACL insufficiency [7]. Other commonly used outcome measures are the International Knee Documentation Committee (IKDC) subjective and objective forms, modified Lysholm score, Knee Injury and Osteoarthritis Outcome Score (KOOS), Cincinnati Knee Rating System, Tegner Activity Score, Marx Activity Score, Hospital for Special Surgery Score, and Knee Outcome Survey [7, 22].

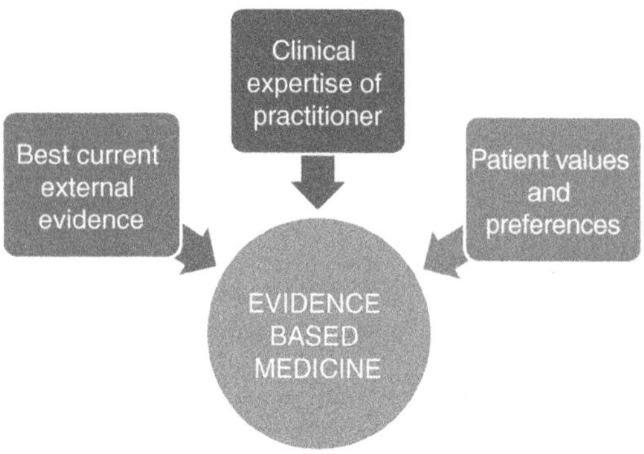

Fig. 19.1 The EBM integration

Fact Box 1

Critical characteristics for an optimal outcome tool:

1. Patient relevance
2. User-friendliness
3. Inexpensive
4. Sensitive
5. Reliable
6. Valid
7. Responsiveness to clinical change

19.3 The Pivot Shift Test: Evolution to Outcome Tool

19.3.1 Understanding the Pivot Shift Test: Origin, Terminology, Biomechanics, and Application

Origin Galway, Beaupré, and MacIntosh first described in the American literature the pivot shift test as a reduction maneuver in 1972 [20]. Given that the spontaneous reduction of the anteriorly subluxed tibial plateau could be felt by both the patient and the examiner, it was considered a clinical phenomenon giving rise to the patient's complaint of instability (giving way) as well as a physical examination sign [12, 20]. Having a relaxed patient was felt to be an essential point for its proper execution [12]. The test's name comes from axis (pivot) and dislocation (shift) [20].

Terminology Laxity is the passive response of a joint to an externally applied force or torque, representing an objective finding [31]. Stability is a functional measure and represents a symptom expressed by the patient [31] (Fig. 19.2). Two types of laxity can be assessed: static and dynamic [10]. Static laxity can be measured by applying a predetermined direct load to a still joint and measuring the resultant displacement either manually (e.g., anterior drawer, Lachman) or with an arthrometer (e.g., KT-1000-2000; Medmetric Corp., San Diego, CA, USA) [10, 21, 34, 42]. Dynamic laxity is assessed by controlled loading of the joint during movement [10]. Static laxity is easier to assess, but may not completely reflect the entire laxity envelope of the knee [33]. Dynamic laxity testing requires skill and subtle application since it can induce painful sudden motions, sometimes resulting in muscle guarding [10]. Variability from this type of testing comes from inconsistently applied and difficult to measure loads and displacements as well as subjective descriptions of the motion induced by the examiner [10]. The pivot shift is an example of a dynamic laxity test.

Biomechanics The pivot shift is a complicated motion, incorporating two components: anterior translation of the lateral tibial plateau and internal rotation of the tibia relative to the femur [3, 43]. The importance of the translational component has recently been emphasized. In ACL deficiency, the knee's pivot point shifts from its normal position centered on the medial tibial spine to an area that produces an exaggeration of anterior tibial translation from the lateral compartment, rather than rotation [32].

The mechanism of the pivot shift test is considered to be related to the geometry of the lateral compartment (convex articular surface of the lateral plateau), tension of the iliotibial tract, and the integrity of medial collateral ligament (operative arthroscopy) [34]. In the ACL intact knee, the lateral femoral condyle rests on the anterior slope of the lateral tibial plateau [34]. In the ACL-deficient knee, valgus stress combined with internal rotation and slight flexion causes anterior translation of the lateral tibial plateau resulting in the lateral femoral condyle resting on the posterior slope of the plateau [34]. At 30–40° of flexion, the tension produced by the iliotibial band forces the anteriorly subluxed lateral tibial plateau to reduce posteriorly, producing a "clunk" as the femoral condyle passes over the apex of the convex-shaped lateral tibial plateau [12, 20, 34, 39]. The dynamic nature of this test gives it

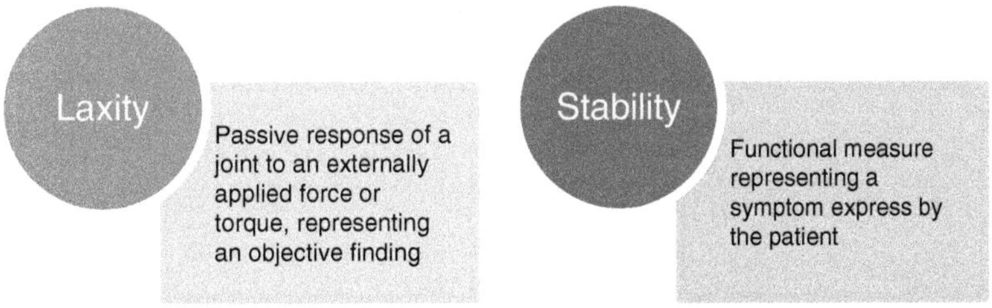

Fig. 19.2 Clinical definitions

the particular quality of assessing both laxity (objective finding of ACL deficiency) and stability (subjective feeling of giving way) [31]. A grading scheme for the pivot shift test has been proposed by the IKDC as A (normal, none), B (nearly normal, + glide), C (abnormal, ++, clunk), and D (severely abnormal, +++, gross) [21] (Fig. 19.3).

Fact Box 2
Requirement for valid interpretation of the pivot shift test:

1. Relaxed patient or under general anesthesia
2. Competent medial collateral ligament
3. Competent iliotibial band
4. Absence of displaced soft tissue (e.g., flipped meniscus, cyclops lesion, others)

Application Traditionally, the success of ACL reconstruction has been focused on effectively eliminating AP laxity, as evaluated by the Lachman test [6, 25]. However, studies have demonstrated that restoration of AP laxity does not necessarily correlate with patient satisfaction, functional outcome, and development of OA [6, 22, 25]. It has been suggested that restoration of rotational control is extremely important in obtaining a positive outcome following ACL reconstruction [4, 6, 18, 21, 22, 32, 43]. As discussed previously, the Lachman test is a static test of AP laxity and does not take into account residual rotatory laxity following ACL reconstruction [3, 23, 33]. However, the pivot shift test bridges the gap between static and dynamic laxity testing and is able to better reflect the pathological knee kinematics [18, 33]. It is the most specific, reliable, suitable, and widely used clinical tool for determining rotational dynamic laxity, making the pivot shift test an ideal outcome tool for ACL reconstruction [2, 6, 7, 9, 18, 28, 33, 42, 43].

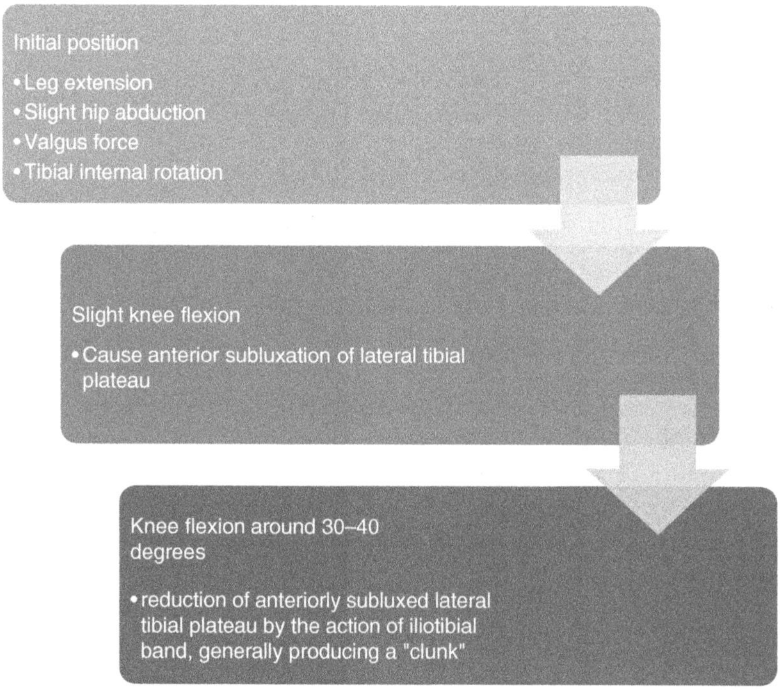

Fig. 19.3 Summary of execution for pivot shift test

19.3.2 The Pivot Shift Test as an Outcome Tool: What Is the Evidence?

The evidence correlating the pivot shift test and patient outcomes following ACL reconstruction are numerous and can be categorized as follows: patient satisfaction, subjective symptoms and instability, functional outcomes (functional instability, activities and sports limitations, overall knee function), and the development of OA [2–4, 6, 18, 21–25, 28, 32, 39, 43].

Patient Satisfaction Patient satisfaction has emerged over the last decade as an essential outcome measure [22]. It has been demonstrated to most closely follow outcome scores related to subjective symptoms and function [40, 41]. The validity of the patient reported outcome measures is often better than surgeon-based objective measures of satisfaction following treatment [40, 41]. Patient satisfaction is now an important complement to postoperative clinician-based assessment [40].

A prospective cohort study by Kocher et al. was performed to identify the determinants of patient satisfaction following ACL reconstruction [22]. Two hundred and one patients underwent primary ACL reconstruction by three surgeons with a minimum follow-up period of 2 years. A questionnaire was filled out by the patients for the subjective data and the surgeon provided the objective data. They found a significant association between a positive pivot shift test and patient dissatisfaction. However, in some cases, they noted a strong relationship between patient satisfaction and the subjective outcome measures of symptoms and function, rather than the objective measure of residual laxity. Despite this ambiguity associated with patient satisfaction and other limitations (e.g., lack of a validated patient satisfaction instrument, absence of specific details on the surgical techniques used), the study demonstrated the importance of the pivot shift sensation on patient satisfaction.

Subjective Symptoms and Functional Outcome A recent systematic review by Ayeni et al. assessed whether the pivot shift test correlated with final functional outcomes [6]. They reviewed 65 ACL-related randomized control trials, of which 47 used the pivot shift test as an outcome measure. The pivot shift test results were compared to the results of the final functional outcome scales (e.g., IKDC, Lysholm, and Tegner activity level). Forty of the studies (85 %) showed a correlation between the pivot shift test result and the final functional outcome. The authors concluded that the results of this review showed clinical evidence supporting the importance of the pivot shift test in evaluating the success of ACL surgery. Although the included studies were of respectable quality (Jadad Quality Score mean of 2.369), limitations included a lack of standardization in performing the pivot shift test in the individual studies.

> **Fact Box 3**
> **Did you know?**
> 85 % of ACL-related randomized control trials showed a correlation between the pivot shift test result and the final functional outcome, supporting the importance of this test in evaluating success of ACL surgery [6].

A retrospective cohort study by Kocher et al. examined the relationship between the objective assessment of ligament laxity and subjective symptoms and function following ACL reconstruction [21]. The investigators reviewed 202 primary ACL reconstruction patients with a minimum of 2-year follow-up. Contrary to instrumented knee laxity and Lachman examination, patients with positive pivot shift were found to have a negative association with satisfaction with outcome, partial and full giving way, difficulty cutting and twisting, activity limitation, knee function, sports participation, and the Lysholm score. Patients with higher grade pivot shift had less satisfaction with outcome, more activity and sports limitations, lower overall knee function, and lower Lysholm scores. These findings support the functional importance of the pivot shift phenomenon and the clinical relevance of the pivot shit test. Limitation of this study included selective nature of the cohort, multiple physical examiners, and the absence of specific details on the surgical technique used.

Jonsson et al. in 2004 and Streich et al. in 2011 also evaluated the significant relationship between the pivot shift test and clinical assessment score [18, 38]. Their results supported those of Kocher et al. and demonstrated that patients with a negative pivot shift test had significantly better results in functional subjective outcome (IKDC subjective score, Lysholm score, Tegner activity scale, and one-leg hop).

Development of OA Jonsson et al. studied the association between degree of knee laxity 2 years after surgery and signs of OA at 5–9-year follow-up [18]. Sixty-eight patients were assessed at 2 years and again at 5–9 years after primary ACL reconstruction. Knee laxity was assessed for both AP (radiostereometric technique) and rotational laxity (pivot shift test). Degenerative status of the knee was evaluated with scintigraphic bone studies and radiographs (weightbearing AP and lateral views in flexion) at the latest follow-up. They found that patients with a positive pivot shift 2 years after their ACL reconstruction had greater differences in bone scintigraphic uptake in the subchondral bone of the entire knee at the 5–9-year follow-up. This suggests a positive relationship may exist between the pivot shift and knee joint degeneration. However, the radiographic Fairbank grading at the latest follow-up was not affected by the presence or absence of the pivot shift test either at 2 years or at the latest follow-up. They also found that a pivot shift test that was only first recorded at the 5–9-year follow-up could not predict scintigraphic uptake result or signs of OA. Limitations of this study included patients lost to follow-up, a small simple size, a relatively short follow-up period, and the use of both anatomic and nonanatomic ACL reconstructions without separation of the results. Furthermore, many other factors impact the development of OA such as concomitant cartilage and meniscal damage, activity levels, and body mass index.

A recent retrospective study done by Streich et al. showed the results on a matched-pair long-term follow-up comparing reconstructive vs. nonreconstructive (physiotherapy) treatment for ACL insufficiency [38], in which patients with arthroscopically confirmed ACL tears were followed for 15 years. They found a significant relationship between a positive pivot shift test at follow-up and the IKDC radiographic grading of OA, while patients with negative pivot shift tests showed significantly less signs of radiographic OA. The surgical technique used was an anatomical footprint using transtibial drilling for the femoral tunnel and autograft bone-patellar tendon-bone.

Limitations of the Pivot Shift Test Unfortunately, the pivot shift test is not standardized and is subjective. There have been numerous techniques reporting how to perform it, thus increasing its variability and decreasing reproducibility [5, 7, 11, 23, 25, 30, 39, 42]. A meta-analysis by Benjamisne et al. on clinical diagnosis of ACL injury showed that the pivot shift had a reported pooled sensitivity of 24 % and a specificity of 98 % [9]. Another systematic review focusing on more recent literature also looked at determining the diagnostic accuracy of clinical testing for ACL insufficiency [26]. Due to insufficient data, only the pooled sensitivity was calculated. During awake evaluation, the pivot shift showed a sensitivity of 86 % for complete rupture, 67 % for partial rupture, and an overall sensitivity of 79 % for all ACL injuries (partial and complete).

There are a number of general factors that potentially explain the variability in rotational laxity measurement: examiner experience, presence of knee effusion, muscle spasms, thigh circumference, type of rupture (complete versus partial), presence of concomitant intra-articular and extra-articular injuries, individual anatomy of the knee (slope and condyle), and whether the examination is performed with the patient awake or under anesthesia [26]. Finally, the constitutional laxity of the patient plays a role [32]. Despite these limitations, the pivot shift test still remains the best clinical test available to assess rotational knee laxity [28, 33, 42, 43].

Fact Box 4

Summary of evidence for pivot shift test as an outcome measure:

1. Patient satisfaction
   (a) Significant association between a positive pivot shift test and patient dissatisfaction
2. Subjective symptom and functional outcome
   (a) Significant association between a positive pivot shift test and:
      (i) Partial and full giving way
      (ii) Difficulty cutting
      iii. Difficulty twisting
      (iv) Activity limitation
      (v) Lower knee function
      (vi) Limitation in sports participation
      (vii) Lower Lysholm score
   (b) Significant association between a negative pivot shift test and better results in functional subjective outcome (IKDC subjective score, Lysholm score, Tegner activity scale, and one-leg hop).
   (c) Significant association between grade of pivot shift test and level of patient "disabilities"
   (d) Significant correlation between the pivot shift test result and the final functional outcome
   (e) Limited association between the pivot shift test result and knee function scoring if only done at mid- to long-term follow-up
3. Development of OA
   (a) Significant association between a positive pivot shift test at 2 years after surgery and subchondral bone scintigraphic uptake at 5–9 years of follow-up
   (b) Controversial evidence regarding association of a positive pivot shift test and radiographic changes of OA

19.3.3 Futures Directions

The variable nature of the current methods of performing the pivot shift test has raised questions about the ability and the practicality of using this test as an outcome measure [6]. However, the available evidence outlines the importance of the pivot shift test in evaluating rotational laxity associated with ACL incompetence. Research is ongoing regarding ways to improve the accuracy of this critical test.

Techniques for examining the anterior tibial translation and acceleration of the tibial reduction have emerged and show promise as a more consistent method in evaluating the pivot shift test [5]. Excellent correlation has been found between the amount of lateral compartment translation and clinical grade of the pivot shift [8, 32, 34, 39].

Future focus is being concentrated into methods to accurately, simply, and reproducibly measure this value in the clinical setting, enabling the clinician to rigorously evaluate residual rotatory laxity after ACL reconstruction. In order to eliminate human variability on test execution, research has been directed toward the use of technological support. Skin sensors placed on specific bony landmarks with computer analysis of the relationship between those sensors while executing the pivot shift test is one method undergoing evaluation [5, 14–16, 32]. This would allow for precise measurement of lateral compartment anterior displacement without relying on the examiner's impression of displacement.

Hoshino et al. in 2011 combined the idea of using a standardized manual technique to execute the pivot shift test with the technological advantage being precise measurement of the tibial translation and acceleration [14]. Twelve expert surgeons performed on a cadaveric specimen the pivot shift test using first their preferred technique, then the standardized technique. The standardized technique was design on the basis of Galway and MacIntosh procedure, and an instructional video was use to teach the technique. Measurement of anterior tibial translation and acceleration during the reduction was calculated by electromagnetic tracking. They showed that performing the pivot shift test with a standardized technique significantly decreased the variation of the acceleration. There was no difference regarding the tibial translation.

Conclusion

The pivot shift test is the most specific, reliable, suitable, and widely used clinical tool for assessing rotational dynamic laxity. It bridges the gap between static and dynamic laxity testing while eliciting patient instability symptoms. It has been proven to correlate with patient satisfaction and functional outcome; however, the relationship between a positive pivot shift and OA remains controversial. Unfortunately, the pivot shift test suffers from a lack of standardization, the subjective nature of the assessment, and the variability arising from patient-derived factors. This has led to the development of more reliable and reproducible techniques. Adjuncts such as skin sensors on specific bony landmarks coupled with computer analysis have the potential to bring about the necessary objectiveness required.

References

1. Abrams GD, Harris JD, Gupta AK, McCormick FM, Bush-Joseph CA, Verma NN, Cole BJ, Bach BR (2014) Functional performance testing after anterior cruciate ligament reconstruction: a systematic review. Orthop J Sports Med 2:1–10
2. Ahldén M, Araujo P, Hoshino Y, Samuelsson K, Middleton KK, Nagamune K, Karlsson J, Musahl V (2012) Clinical grading of the pivot shift test correlates best with tibial acceleration. Knee Surg Sports Traumatol Arthrosc 20:708–712
3. Ahldén M, Hoshino Y, Samuelsson K, Araujo P, Musahl V, Karlsson J (2012) Dynamic knee laxity measurement devices. Knee Surg Sports Traumatol Arthrosc 20:621–632
4. Amis AA (2012) The functions of the fibre bundles of the anterior cruciate ligament in anterior drawer, rotational laxity and the pivot shift. Knee Surg Sports Traumatol Arthrosc 20:613–620
5. Araujo PH, Ahlden M, Hoshino Y, Muller B, Moloney G, Fu FH, Musahl V (2012) Comparison of three non-invasive quantitative measurement systems for the pivot shift test. Knee Surg Sports Traumatol Arthrosc 20:692–697
6. Ayeni OR, Chahal M, Tran MN, Sprague S (2012) Pivot shift as an outcome measure for ACL reconstruction: a systematic review. Knee Surg Sports Traumatol Arthrosc 20:767–777
7. Ayeni OR, Evaniew N, Ogilvie R, Peterson DC, Denkers MR, Bhandari M (2013) Evidence-based practice to improve outcomes of anterior cruciate ligament reconstruction. Clin Sports Med 32:71–80
8. Bedi A, Musahl V, Lane C, Citak M, Warren RF, Pearle AD (2010) Lateral compartment translation predicts the grade of pivot shift: a cadaveric and clinical analysis. Knee Surg Sports Traumatol Arthrosc 18:1269–1276
9. Benjaminse A, Gokeler A, van der Schans CP (2006) Clinical diagnosis of an anterior cruciate ligament rupture: a meta-analysis. J Orthop Sports Phys Ther 36:267–288
10. Bull AM, Amis AA (1998) The pivot-shift phenomenon: a clinical and biomechanical perspective. Knee 5:141–158
11. Engebretsen L, Wijdicks CA, Anderson CJ, Westerhaus B, LaPrade RF (2012) Evaluation of a simulated pivot shift test: a biomechanical study. Knee Surg Sports Traumatol Arthrosc 20:698–702
12. Galway HR, MacIntosh DL (1980) The lateral pivot shift: a symptom and sign of anterior cruciate ligament insufficiency. Clin Orthop 147:45–50
13. Greenhalgh T, Howick J, Maskrey N, for the Evidence Based Medicine Renaissance Group (2014) Evidence based medicine: a movement in crisis? BMJ 348:g3725
14. Hoshino Y, Araujo P, Ahlden M, Moore CG, Kuroda R, Zaffagnini S, Karlsson J, Fu FH, Musahl V (2012) Standardized pivot shift test improves measurement accuracy. Knee Surg Sports Traumatol Arthrosc 20:732–736
15. Hoshino Y, Araujo P, Ahldén M, Samuelsson K, Muller B, Hofbauer M, Wolf MR, Irrgang JJ, Fu FH, Musahl V (2013) Quantitative evaluation of the pivot shift by image analysis using the iPad. Knee Surg Sports Traumatol Arthrosc 21:975–980
16. Hoshino Y, Araujo P, Irrgang JJ, Fu FH, Musahl V (2012) An image analysis method to quantify the lateral pivot shift test. Knee Surg Sports Traumatol Arthrosc 20:703–707
17. Johnson DL (2011) Outcome measurement tools for ACL reconstruction: we must do better. Orthopedics 34:417–418
18. Jonsson H, Riklund-Ahlström K, Lind J (2004) Positive pivot shift after ACL reconstruction predicts later osteoarthrosis 63 patients followed 5-9 years after surgery. Acta Orthop 75:594–599
19. Junkin DM Jr, Johnson DL, Fu FH, Miller MD, Willenborg M, Fanelli GC, Wascher DC (2009) Chapter 12: Knee ligaments injuries. In: Kibler WB (ed) Orthopaedic knowledge update: sports medicine, 4th edn. American Academy of Orthopaedic Surgeons, Rosemont, pp 135–154
20. Kirchhoff C, Brucker PU, Imhoff AB (2013) Chapter 69: Evolving concepts in tunnel placement for Acl

reconstruction. In: Johnson DH (ed) Oper. Arthrosc. 4th edn. Wolters Kluwer Health/Lippincott Williams & Wilkins, Philadelphia, pp 772–777
21. Kocher MS (2004) Relationships between objective assessment of ligament stability and subjective assessment of symptoms and function after anterior cruciate ligament reconstruction. Am J Sports Med 32:629–634
22. Kocher MS, Steadman JR, Briggs K, Zurakowski D, Sterett WI, Hawkins RJ (2002) Determinants of patient satisfaction with outcome after anterior cruciate ligament reconstruction. J Bone Joint Surg 84:1560–1572
23. Kopf S, Kauert R, Halfpaap J, Jung T, Becker R (2012) A new quantitative method for pivot shift grading. Knee Surg Sports Traumatol Arthrosc 20: 718–723
24. Kuroda R, Hoshino Y, Araki D, Nishizawa Y, Nagamune K, Matsumoto T, Kubo S, Matsushita T, Kurosaka M (2012) Quantitative measurement of the pivot shift, reliability, and clinical applications. Knee Surg Sports Traumatol Arthrosc 20:686–691
25. Lane CG, Warren R, Pearle AD (2008) The pivot shift. J Am Acad Orthop Surg 16:679–688
26. Leblanc M-C, Kowalczuk M, Andruszkiewicz N, Simunovic N, Farrokhyar F, Turnbull TL, Debski RE, Ayeni OR (2015) Diagnostic accuracy of physical examination for anterior knee instability: a systematic review. Knee Surg Sports Traumatol Arthrosc 23:2805–13
27. Leiter JRS, Gourlay R, McRae S, de Korompay N, MacDonald PB (2013) Long-term follow-up of ACL reconstruction with hamstring autograft. Knee Surg Sports Traumatol Arthrosc 22:1061–1069
28. Lopomo N, Signorelli C, Bonanzinga T, Marcheggiani Muccioli GM, Neri MP, Visani A, Marcacci M, Zaffagnini S (2014) Can rotatory knee laxity be predicted in isolated anterior cruciate ligament surgery? Int Orthop 38:1167–1172
29. Mohtadi N (1998) Development and validation of the quality of life outcome measure (questionnaire) for chronic anterior cruciate ligament deficiency. Am J Sports Med 26:350–359
30. Mouton C, Theisen D, Pape D, Nührenbörger C, Seil R (2012) Static rotational knee laxity in anterior cruciate ligament injuries. Knee Surg Sports Traumatol Arthrosc 20:652–662
31. Musahl V, Hoshino Y, Becker R, Karlsson J (2012) Rotatory knee laxity and the pivot shift. Knee Surg Sports Traumatol Arthrosc 20:601–602
32. Musahl V, Kopf S, Rabuck S, Becker R, van der Merwe W, Zaffagnini S, Fu FH, Karlsson J (2012) Rotatory knee laxity tests and the pivot shift as tools for ACL treatment algorithm. Knee Surg Sports Traumatol Arthrosc 20:793–800
33. Musahl V, Seil R, Zaffagnini S, Tashman S, Karlsson J (2012) The role of static and dynamic rotatory laxity testing in evaluating ACL injury. Knee Surg Sports Traumatol Arthrosc 20:603–612
34. Okazaki K, Tashiro Y, Izawa T, Matsuda S, Iwamoto Y (2012) Rotatory laxity evaluation of the knee using modified Slocum's test in open magnetic resonance imaging. Knee Surg Sports Traumatol Arthrosc 20:679–685
35. Sackett DL, Rosenberg WM, Gray JA, Haynes RB, Richardson WS (1996) Evidence based medicine: what it is and what it isn't. BMJ 312:71
36. Shaw T, Chipchase LS, Williams MT (2004) A users guide to outcome measurement following ACL reconstruction. Phys Ther Sport 5:57–67
37. Spindler KP, Parker RD, Andrish JT, Kaeding CC, Wright RW, Marx RG, McCarty EC, Amendola A, Dunn WR, Huston LJ, Harrell FE, MOON Group (2013) Prognosis and predictors of ACL reconstructions using the MOON cohort: a model for comparative effectiveness studies. J Orthop Res 31:2–9
38. Streich NA, Zimmermann D, Bode G, Schmitt H (2011) Reconstructive versus non-reconstructive treatment of anterior cruciate ligament insufficiency. A retrospective matched-pair long-term follow-up. Int Orthop 35:607–613
39. Tanaka M, Vyas D, Moloney G, Bedi A, Pearle AD, Musahl V (2012) What does it take to have a high-grade pivot shift? Knee Surg Sports Traumatol Arthrosc 20:737–742
40. Webster KE, Feller JA (2014) Use of the short form health surveys as an outcome measure for anterior cruciate ligament reconstruction. Knee Surg Sports Traumatol Arthrosc 22:1142–1148
41. Wright RW (2009) Knee injury outcomes measures. J Am Acad Orthop Surg 17:31–39
42. Zaffagnini S, Marcheggiani Muccioli GM, Lopomo N, Signorelli C, Bonanzinga T, Musiani C, Vassilis P, Nitri M, Marcacci M (2012) Can the pivot-shift be eliminated by anatomic double-bundle anterior cruciate ligament reconstruction? Knee Surg Sports Traumatol Arthrosc 20:743–751
43. Zampeli F, Pappas E, Giotis D, Hantes ME, Georgoulis AD (2012) Kinematic predictors of subjective outcome after anterior cruciate ligament reconstruction: an in vivo motion analysis study. Knee Surg Sports Traumatol Arthrosc 20:785–792

Navigating the Pivot-Shift Test

20

Stefano Zaffagnini, Cecilia Signorelli, Francisco Urrizola, Alberto Grassi, Federico Raggi, Tommaso Roberti di Sarsina, Tommaso Bonanzinga, and Nicola Lopomo

Contents

S. Zaffagnini (✉) • A. Grassi • F. Raggi
T. Roberti di Sarsina • T. Bonanzinga
Laboratorio di Biomeccanica e Innovazione Tecnologica, Istituto Ortopedico Rizzoli, Bologna, BO, Italy
e-mail: stefano.zaffagnini@unibo.it

Clinica Ortopedica e Traumatologica II, Istituto Ortopedico Rizzoli, Bologna, BO, Italy

C. Signorelli
Laboratorio di Biomeccanica e Innovazione Tecnologica, Istituto Ortopedico Rizzoli, Bologna, BO, Italy

F. Urrizola
Servicio Traumatologia y Ortopedia, Hospital Las Higueras, Talcahuano, Chile

N. Lopomo
Laboratorio di Biomeccanica e Innovazione Tecnologica, Istituto Ortopedico Rizzoli, Bologna, BO, Italy

Dipartimento di Ingegneria dell'Informazione, Università degli Studi di Brescia, Brescia, BS, Italy

20.1 Introducing the Navigation

Approximately 7 % of orthopedics procedures are computer assisted [9]. Computer-assisted surgery (CAS) was used for the first time in spinal surgery around 20 years ago. The main objective of this tool is to optimize surgical outcomes by decreasing intraoperative mistakes and providing real-time information about the procedure to the surgeon. It can be used in several different procedures, including knee surgeries [37]. The first computer-assisted anterior cruciate ligament (ACL) reconstructive surgery was performed in 1995 by Dessene et al. [13]. Since then, with the development of more surgeon-friendly systems combined with the evolution of softwares for computer-based ACL surgery, the interest in this field during the last decades has increased. This increase was especially due to research applications. Analysing the literature it can be seen that the number of CAS ACL publications is low compared to the overall number of ACL publications per year (1–3 %) [33] (Fig. 20.1).

Most of the presented articles are in vivo case series or controlled laboratory studies. There are more in vivo than in vitro studies, which are related to the fact that navigation has been specifically designed for surgery [48].

One of the main CAS systems is represented by the intraoperative navigation system. There are several kinds of navigation systems available. First of all they could be active (when they

V. Musahl et al. (eds.), *Rotatory Knee Instability*, DOI 10.1007/978-3-319-32070-0_20

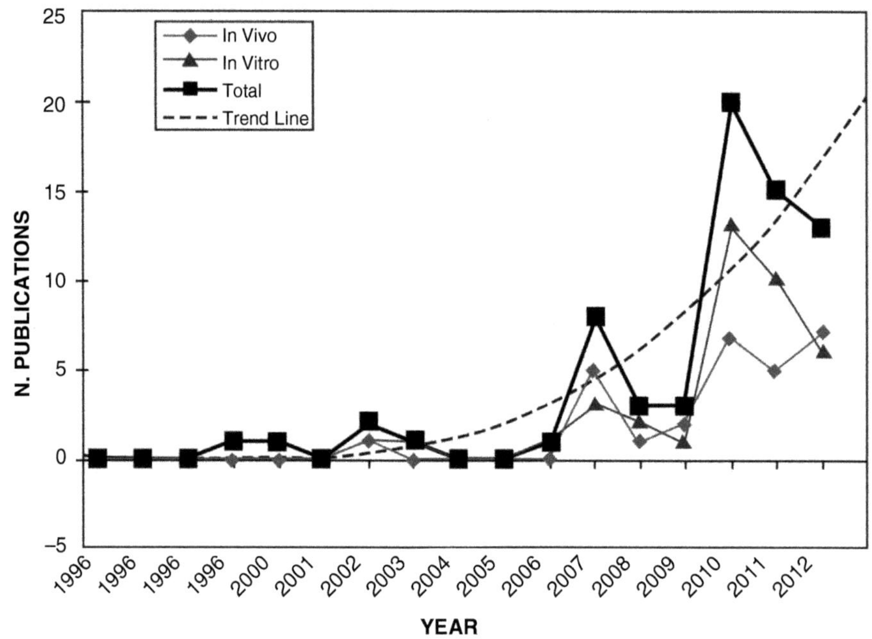

Fig. 20.1 Publications found in Medline and PubMed databases about DB and CAS ACL reconstruction in the last years

perform surgical tasks or prohibit predefined zone) or passive (when they provide intraoperative information) [37]. The main disadvantage of this method is related to the fact that it is invasive, restricting its use to the injured limb and to the clinical practice to evaluate preoperative and postoperative laxities [32, 48].

During the first navigated reconstructive ACL surgeries, the main goal of the procedures was to improve the positioning of the graft tunnels using anatomic references and graft isometry during the range of motion. Subsequently the goal of CAS quickly changed to measure knee laxity in 3D conditions. This has vastly improved the understanding of such pathologies [8, 10, 21, 42, 43, 48].

The first author who studied the reliability and the precision of the CAS system was Pearl in 1997 by comparing an image-free navigation system to a robotic/UFS testing system in an in vitro study [41]. The results demonstrated that the accuracy is in the range of ±0.1 mm for linear measurements and ±0.1° for angular measurements. It has been also highlighted the possibility to objectively measure the residual laxity and improve the evaluation of ACL reconstruction [34]. In fact, navigation systems allow precise intraoperative measurements considering different degrees of freedom. Improved surgical accuracy that combined with intraoperative measurements has the potential to upgrade biomechanics research and introduce new surgical techniques for knee-joint disease [5, 18, 21, 25, 38, 43].

20.2 The Pivot-Shift Test

ACL insufficiency is normally diagnosed using clinical manual tests. Several manual tests are described including the most widely used Lachman and pivot-shift tests [4, 6, 23]. These tests not only allow for a better surgical approach for patients but are also used to measure outcomes after ACL reconstruction. For many years, the goal of surgical treatment for ACL reconstruction was to achieve anterior-posterior stability. It was used the KT-1000 as a benchmark to control knee laxity [12, 16]. In the 1970s, Slocum and Larson (1976) were the first to describe the rotational instability of the knee. They proposed that one of the most important issue was the pathological external rotation of the tibial plateau with respect to the femur. Given that, they performed a variation of the anterior drawer test by adding internal and external rotation while stressing anteriorly the joint [44]. Four years later, Galway (1980) was the first to describe the pivot-shift phenomenon and related this to dynamic instability, the clinical symptom of giving way and also with later degenerative changes in the injured knee [15]. From there, many maneuvers were described to detect this important phenomenon making the PS test the most specific maneuver for the detection of dynamic instability. The PS test is considered difficult to perform, subjective, and limited by examiner's experience. Additionally, many different versions have been described [40]. Moreover, pathological knee laxity resulting from ACL injury is complex and multidirectional, this makes important the evaluation performed by the PS test [7]. During such test a complex rotational and translational stress is applied to the tibiofemoral joint to determine knee status. This has been shown to be correlated with reduced sport activity and a complete or partial ACL tear. A positive PS test can also help to predict the onset of osteoarthritis [4, 15, 22, 26, 31].

A recent systematic review summarized 42 in vitro studies [33].

Fact Box

1. Navigation system is considered the gold standard for knee laxity evaluation. In conjunction with the pivot-shift test, it allows for its different parameters to be intraoperatively quantified.
2. The pivot-shift test is the most specific maneuver for ACL injury. In particular, it is the lateral tibial compartment that is mainly affected by the phenomenon.
3. Highly precise quantification of the pivot-shift phenomenon may enable an improved and more individualized approach to surgery.

20.3 Quantitative Instrumented Evaluation of Knee Rotational Dynamic Laxity

The PS test is widely used for the objective assessment of joint laxity in the most common clinical scores for ligament laxity, such as the International Knee Documentation Committee (IKDC) score [17]. Complex systems requiring footplates [1], magnetic resonance imaging [45], markers [11], and robotic technology [14] have been developed to quantify PS outcome. While electromagnetic sensors were dedicated to quantitatively evaluate PS test [2, 19, 20, 27–29], unfortunately they present with complicated equipment (wires, specific surgical instrumentation, and setup) and costs that are incompatible with office practice. In particular, it has been found that both acceleration and velocity during PS test could be indicative parameters for dynamic laxity which is also correlated with clinical grade of PS [28, 29]. An electromagnetic device was used to evaluate PS test acceleration [3, 19, 20].

Computer-assisted surgery (CAS) has been used to assess knee kinematics and laxity. It is still considered the gold standard for this.

Comparison of the previously reported systems has been summarized (Table 20.1).

20.4 Quantitative Parameters for Pivot-Shift Test Quantification

The following parameters can be considered as a decomposition of the pivot-shift test in translation, rotation, and acceleration or velocity.

The following list (Table 20.2) summarizes the parameters reported in the literature [33].

20.5 Quantitative PS Test Parameter During Intraoperative Navigation

The use of navigation for evaluating translational and rotational uniplanar joint laxities under stress

Table 20.1 Dynamic laxity devices comparison

	RSA	DSX	Electromagnetic sensors	MRI	CAS
Accuracy	•	•			•
Non invasive		•	•	•	
Iosilateral side only	•				•
No radiation			•		•
Costly	•	•	•	•	•
Labor-intensive	•	•			

Table 20.2 Parameters for PS test quantification

Translational parameters	
AP	Peak or range of translation in anterior-posterior direction of the origin of the femoral or tibial anatomical reference system usually with respect to a specific reference motion or position Reported in (mm)
AP-L	Peak or range of translation in anterior-posterior direction of the lateral compartment of the femur or tibia usually with respect to a specific reference motion or position. Reported in (mm)
AP-M	Peak or range of translation in anterior-posterior direction of the medial compartment of the femur or tibia usually with respect to a specific reference motion or position. Reported in (mm)
ML	Peak or range of translation in medial/lateral direction of the origin of the femoral or tibial anatomical reference system usually with respect to a specific reference motion or position. Reported in (mm)
DISP-3D	Peak or range of three-dimensional translation of the origin of the femoral or tibial anatomical reference system usually with respect to a specific reference motion or position. Reported in (mm)
Rotational parameters	
IE	Axial internal, external, or range of rotation of the tibial or femur. Reported in degrees (°)
VV	Varus, valgus, or range of rotation of the tibial or femur. Reported in degrees (°)
Acceleration and velocity parameters	
ACC-AP	Peak of acceleration of the tibial or femur in anterior-posterior direction during PS reduction. Reported in (mm/s^2)
VEL-AP	Peak of velocity of tibia or femur in anterior-posterior direction during reduction in PS test Reported in (mm/s)
ACC-ML	Peak of acceleration in anterior-posterior direction of tibia or femur during PS reduction. Reported in (mm/s^2)
VEL-ML	Peak of velocity of tibia or femur in medial/lateral direction during reduction in PS test. Reported in (mm/s)
ACC-3D	Peak of three-dimensional acceleration of tibia or femur during PS reduction. Reported in (mm/s^2)
VEL-IE	Peak of angular velocity of tibia or femur in internal/external rotation. Reported in (°/s)
VEL-3D	Peak of three-dimensional velocity of femur or tibia during reduction in PS test. Reported in (mm/s)
ACC-IE	Peak of acceleration in anterior-posterior direction during PS reduction. Reported in (°/s^2)
VEL-VV	Peak of angular velocity of tibia or femur in varus/valgus rotation. Reported in (°/s)
ACC-VV	Peak of acceleration in anterior-posterior direction during PS reduction. Reported in (°/s^2)
ACC-TIB	Peak of three-dimensional acceleration measured only on the tibia during PS test. Reported in (mm/s^2)
Areas and other parameters	
AREA-AP	Area included by the curves of anterior-posterior displacement of tibia or femur during flexion and extension in PS test. Reported in (mm*°)
AREA-AP-L	Area included by the curves of anterior-posterior displacement of lateral compartment of tibia of femur during flexion and extension in PS test. Reported in (mm*°)
AREA-IE	Area included by the curves of internal/external rotation during flexion and extension in PS test. Reported in (°^{2})
AREA-AP-M	Area included by the curves of anterior-posterior displacement of medial compartment of tibia or femur during flexion and extension in PS test. Reported in (mm*°)
AREA-VV	Area included by the curves of VV rotation during flexion/extension in PS test. Reported in (°^{2})
P-ANGLE	Angle measured between the arc of motion with the lateral tibia subluxed anteriorly and internally rotated and the arc of motion obtained from a reference motion path in the sagittal plane (passive flexion/extension). Reported in (°)
CI	Colombet's Index: translation/rotation ratio during PS test. Reported in (mm/°)

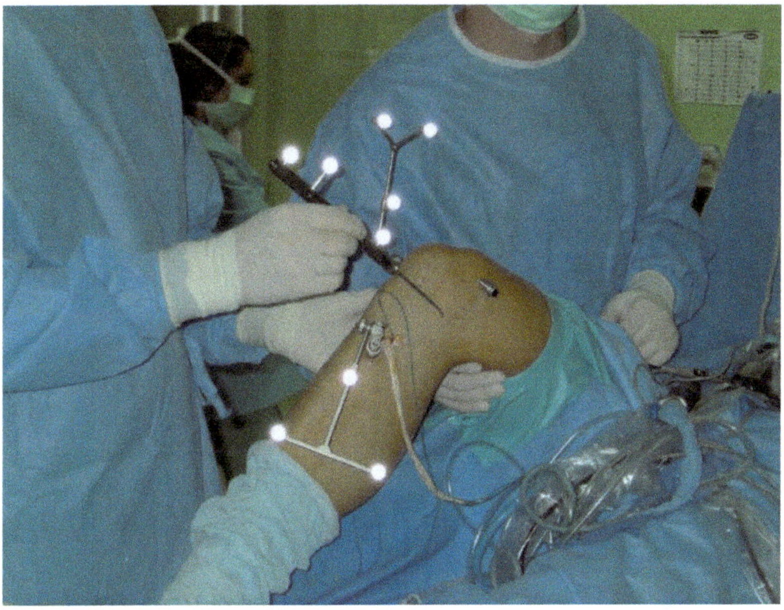

Fig. 20.2 Intraoperative setup for laxity quantification: probe, tibial, and femoral trackers are highlighted

has only been reported since 2006. It has been validated an in vivo setup with a high intersurgeon and intrasurgeon repeatability of the maneuvers [36, 47]. The setup used in the operating room for intraoperative laxity evaluation has been reported (Fig. 20.2).

During the analysis of the PS test attention should be focused on the lateral tibial compartment which has been demonstrated to be the one most affected by the pivot-shift phenomenon [34, 35]. Now most of the studies are focused on the anterior-posterior translation, internal/external rotation, and anterior-posterior acceleration of lateral compartment.

Using an optoelectronic system, the pivot-shift phenomenon has been studied and a new concept has been introduced: the P angle [30]. They observed a P-shaped pattern of motion created by the lateral tibia internally rotated and anteriorly subluxed and the arc of motion once the tibia reduces as compared to the reference motion path in the sagittal plane.

A strong correlation was found between the clinical grade of the PS test and the angle of P. This angle was statistically significant between all clinical grade groups in the study.

Later on, the pivot-shift phenomenon was decomposed in a set of new parameters at determined limb flexion/extension angles (at 0°, 30°, and 90° degrees of flexion) using a commercial surgical navigation system (BLU-IGS, Orthokey, Lewes, DE) equipped with a software focused on kinematics acquisition (KLEE; Orthokey, Lewes, DE) [32].

The pivot-shift phenomenon can be represented in the following scheme (Fig. 20.3).

In particular it is possible to analyze the anterior-posterior translation of the knee in the lateral, central, and medial compartment, internal/external rotation, and varus/valgus rotation (Figs. 20.4 and 20.5).

The study found good correlation between preoperative PS grade and the following areas: anterior-posterior translation in the lateral and central compartments, internal/external rotation, and varus/valgus rotation. However, clinical correlation was not found with regard to the anterior-posterior translation of the medial compartment tibial.

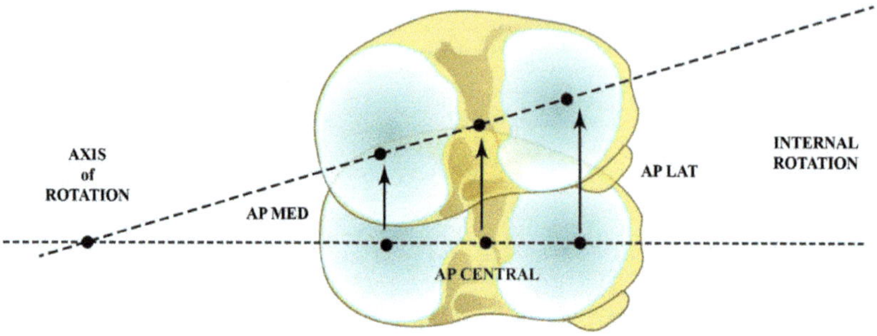

Fig. 20.3 Schematic representation of the parameters used to describe the PS. Note the important displacement of the lateral compartment

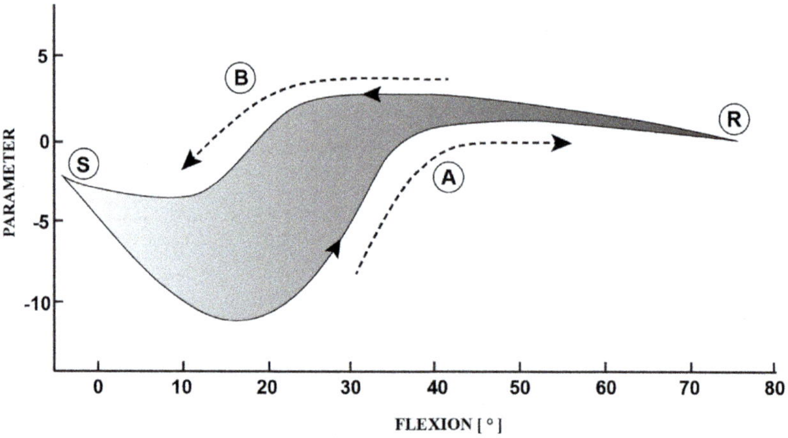

Fig. 20.4 The limb is fully extended at the beginning of the PS test. The tibia starts to subluxate (*S*); pivot-shift maneuver is then performed; (*A*) the tibia is subluxated with respect to the femur until 60°–70° of flexion, where the reduction occurs (*R*); then limb is normally extended (*B*)

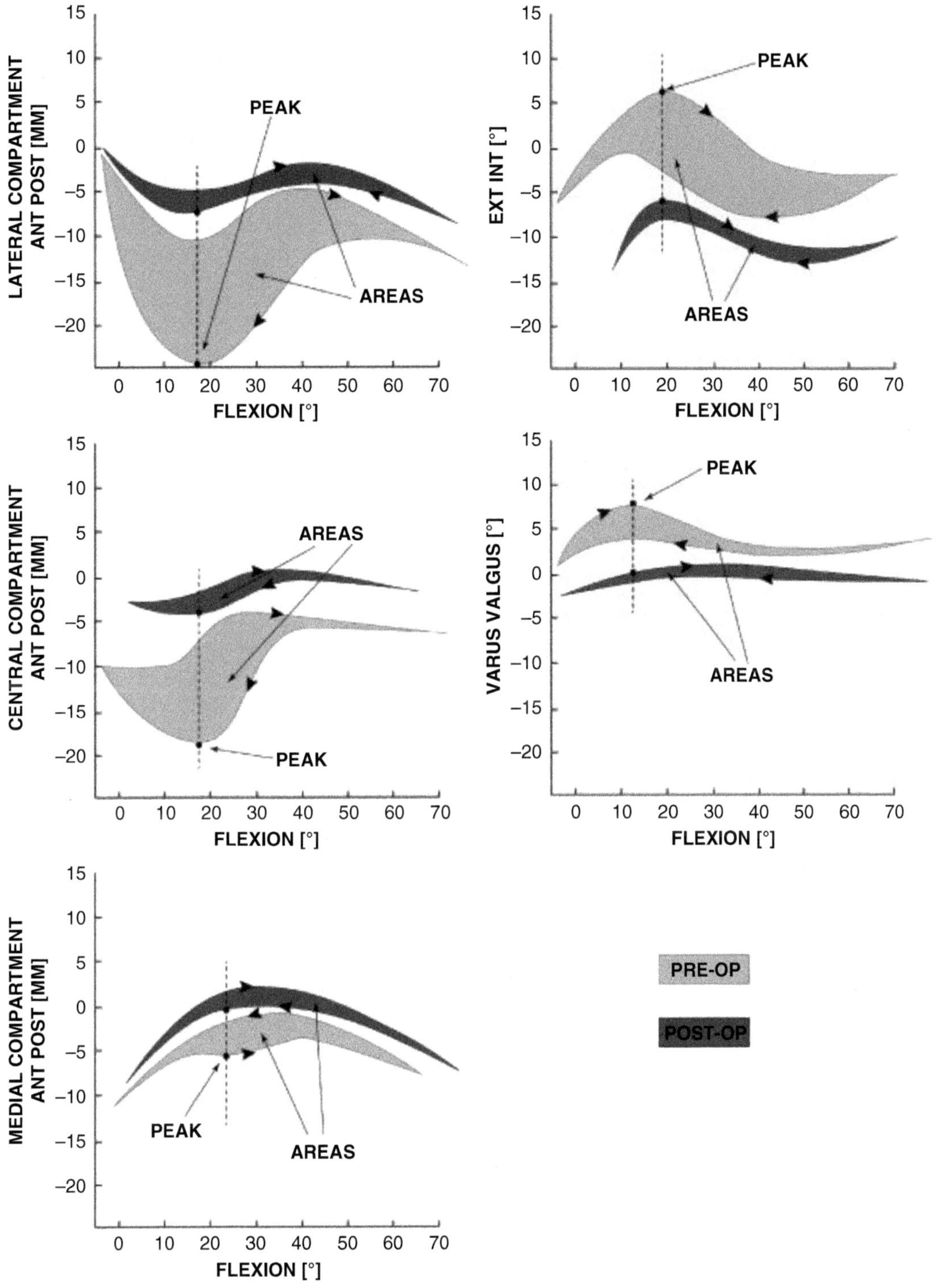

Fig. 20.5 Pivot-shift decomposition in lateral, medial end central tibial compartment translation and internal/external, varus/valgus rotation. Comparison of pre- to postoperative values has been reported

Conclusions

The PS test, nowadays, is the most important clinical exam evaluating dynamic laxity of the knee in the assessment of an ACL injury. ACL reconstruction surgery often controls the anterior-posterior translation of the tibia, but rotational instability may persist [46]. The pivot shift test is now considered the gold standard for postoperative follow-up: its results predicts the success of the surgery [4, 6, 15, 22–24, 26, 31]. In fact, its presence is related with poor outcomes, with limited sport activities, and also with degenerative changes and meniscal lesions.

The main disadvantage of this exam is related to the complexity of the maneuver applied to the joint; moreover many different forms have been described to perform the pivot-shift test.

In the last years, expert surgeons standardized such test to improve the accuracy of the quantitative measurements [39].

Using the navigation system, quantitative measurements were possible allowing a better understanding of the knee's kinematic. During the last 20 years, the PS test was decomposed into many different parameters.

Navigation systems have proven to be highly precise and reliable for quantifying knee laxity after ACL injury. Given this, it is considered the gold standard for laxity quantification, and validation of new noninvasive devices must be related to it.

Both the knowledge acquired by using this tool for quantifying the pivot shift test and its disadvantages motivated the development of new accurate and noninvasive systems that can be used outside the operating room allowing preoperative and postoperative evaluations and also comparative analysis with the non-injured limb. All of these advances will allow for a better and individualized approach to surgery.

References

1. Amis A, Bull A, Lie D (2005) Biomechanics of rotational instability and anatomic anterior cruciate ligament reconstruction. Oper Tech Orthop 15(1):29–35
2. Amis AA, Cuomo P, Rama RBS, Giron F, Bull AMJ, Rhidian T, Aglietti P (2008) Measurement of knee laxity and pivot-shift kinematics with magnetic sensors. Oper Tech Orthop 18(3):196–203
3. Araujo PH, Ahlden M, Hoshino Y, Muller B, Moloney G, Fu FH, Musahl V (2012) Comparison of three noninvasive quantitative measurement systems for the pivot shift test. Knee Surg Sports Traumatol Arthrosc 20(4):692–697
4. Benjaminse A, Gokeler A, van der Schans CP (2006) Clinical diagnosis of an anterior cruciate ligament rupture: a meta-analysis. J Orthop Sports Phys Ther 36(5):267–288
5. Bignozzi S, Zaffagnini S, Lopomo N et al (2009) Does a lateral plasty control coupled translation during antero-posterior stress in single-bundle ACL reconstruction? An in vivo study. Knee Surg Sports Traumatol Arthrosc 17:65–70
6. Bull AM, Amis AA (1998) Knee joint motion: description and measurement. Proc Inst Mech Eng H 212(5):357–372
7. Bull AM, Amis AA (1998) The pivot-shift phenomenon: a clinical and biomechanical perspective. Knee 5:141–158
8. Bull AMJ, Earnshaw PH, Smith A et al (2002) Intraoperative measurement of knee kinematics in reconstruction of the anterior cruciate ligament. J Bone Joint Surg Br 84:1075–1081
9. Catani F, Zaffagnini S (eds) (2013) Knee surgery using computer assisted surgery and robotics. doi: 10.1007/978-3-642-31430-8, © ESSKA
10. Colombet P, Robinson J, Christel P et al (2007) Using navigation to measure rotation kinematics during ACL reconstruction. Clin Orthop Relat Res 454:59–65
11. Csintalan RP, Ehsan A, Mc Garry MH, Fithian DF, Lee TQ (2006) Biomechanical and anatomical effects of an external rotational torque applied to the knee: a cadaveric study. Am J Sport Med 34(10):1623–1629
12. Daniel DM, Malcom LL, Losse G, Stone ML, Sachs R, Burks R (1985) Instrumented measurement of anterior laxity of the knee. J Bone Joint Surg Am 67:720–726
13. Dessene V, Lavallé S, Julliard R et al (1995) Computer-assisted knee anterior cruciate ligament reconstruction: First clinical test. J Image Guide Surg 1:59–64
14. Diermann N, Schumacher T, Schanz S, Raschke MJ, Petersen W, Zantop T (2009) Rotational instability of the knee: internal tibial rotation under a simulated pivot shift test. Arch Orthop Trauma Surg 129(3): 353–358
15. Galway HR, MacIntosh DL (1980) The lateral pivot shift: a symptom and sign of anterior cruciate ligament insufficiency. Clin Orthop Relat Res 147:45–50
16. Graham GP, Johnson S, Dent CM, Fairclough JA (1991) Comparison of clinical tests and the KT1000 in the diagnosis of anterior cruciate ligament rupture. Br J Sports Med 25(2):96–97
17. Hefti F, Müller W (1993) Current state of evaluation of knee ligament lesions. The new IKDC knee evaluation form. Orthopade 22:351–362

18. Ho JY, Gardiner A, Shah V et al (2009) Equal kinematics between central anatomic single-bundle and double-bundle anterior cruciate ligament reconstructions. Arthroscopy 25:464–472
19. Hoshino Y, Kuroda R, Nagamune K (2007) In vivo measurement of the pivot-shift test in the anterior cruciate ligament-deficient knee using an electromagnetic device. Am J Sports Med 35:1098–1104
20. Hoshino Y, Kuroda R, Nagamune K, Araki D, Kubo S, Yamaguchi M, Kurosaka M (2011) Optimal measurement of clinical rotational test for evaluating anterior cruciate ligament insufficiency. Knee Surg Sports Traumatol Arthrosc 21:975–980
21. Ishibashi Y, Tsuda E, Yamamoto Y et al (2009) Navigation evaluation of the pivot-shift phenomenon during double-bundle anterior cruciate ligament reconstruction: Is the posterolateral bundle more important?". Arthroscopy 25:488–495
22. Jakob RP, Stäubli HU, Deland JT (1987) Grading the pivot shift. Objective tests with implications for treatment. J Bone Joint Surg Br 69:294–299
23. Jensen K (1990) Manual laxity tests for anterior cruciate ligament injuries. J Orthop Sports Phys Ther 11(10):474–481
24. Jonsson H, Riklund-Ahlström K, Lind J (2004) Positive pivot shift after ACL reconstruction predicts later osteoarthrosis: 63 patients followed 5–9 years after surgery. Acta Orthop Scand 75(5):594–599
25. Kanaya A, Ochi M, Deie M et al (2009) Intraoperative evaluation of anteroposterior and rotational stabilities in anterior cruciate ligament reconstruction: Lower femoral tunnel placed single-bundle versus double-bundle reconstruction. Knee Surg Sports Traumatol Arthrosc 17:907–913
26. Kocher MS, Steadman JR, Briggs KK, Sterett WI, Hawkins RJ (2004) Relationships between objective assessment of ligament stability and subjective assessment of symptoms and function after Anterior Cruciate Ligament reconstruction. Am J Sports Med 32(3):629–634
27. Kuroda R, Hoshino Y, Nagamune K, Kubo S, Nishimoto K, Araki D, Yamaguchi M, Yoshiva S, Kurosaka M (2008) Intraoperative measurement of pivot shift by electromagnetic sensors. Oper Tech Orthop 18(3):190–195
28. Labbe DR, de Guise JA, Godbout V, Grimard G, Baillargeon D, Lavigne P, Fernandes J, Masse V, Ranger P, Hagemeister N (2010) Accounting for velocity of the pivot shift test manoeuvre decreases kinematic variability. Knee 18(2):88–93
29. Labbe DR, de Guise JA, Mezghani N, Godbout V, Grimard G, Baillargeon D, Lavigne P, Fernandes J, Ranger P, Hagemeister N (2010) Feature selection using a principal component analysis of the kinematics of the pivot shift phenomenon. J Biomech 43(16):3080–3084
30. Lane CG, Warren RF, Stanford FC et al (2008) In vivo analysis of the pivot shift phenomenon during computer navigated ACL reconstruction. Knee Surg Sports Traumatol Arthrosc 16:487–492
31. Leitze Z, Losee RE, Jokl P, Johnson TR, Feagin JA (2005) Implications of the pivot shift in the ACL-deficient knee. Clin Orthop Relat Res 436:229–236
32. Lopomo N, Zaffagnini S, Bignozzi S et al (2010) Pivot-shift test: analysis and quantification of knee laxity parameters using a navigation system. J Orthop Res 28:164–169
33. Lopomo N, Zaffagnini S, Amis AA (2013) Quantifying the pivot shift test: a systematic review. Knee Surg Sports Traumatol Arthrosc 21:767–783
34. Martelli S, Zaffagnini S, Falcioni B, Motta M (2001) Determination of an optimal kinematic protocol for computer-assisted evaluation of anterior cruciate ligament deficiency. Ann Biomed Eng 29(12): 1112–1121
35. Martelli S, Zaffagnini S, Bignozzi S et al (2007) Description and validation of a navigation system for intra-operative evaluation of knee laxity. Comput Aided Surg 12:181–188
36. Martelli S, Zaffagnini S, Bignozzi S et al (2007) KIN-Nav navigation system for kinematic assessment in anterior cruciate ligament reconstruction: features, use, and perspectives. Proc Inst Mech Eng H 221: 725–737
37. Mavrogenis AF, Savvidou OD, Mimidis G, Papanastasiou J, Koulalis D, Demertzis N, Papagelopoulos PJ (2013) Computer-assisted navigation in orthopedic surgery. Orthopedics 36(8):631–642
38. Monaco E, Labianca L, Conteduca F, De Carli A, Ferretti A (2007) Double bundle or single bundle plus extraarticular tenodesis in ACL reconstruction? A CAOS study. Knee Surg Sports Traumatol Arthrosc 15:1168–1174
39. Musahl V, Hoshino Y, Ahlden M, Araujo P, Irrgang JJ, Zaffagnini S, Karlsson J, Fu FH (2012) The pivot shift: a global user guide. Knee Surg Sports Traumatol Arthrosc 20(4):724–731
40. Noyes FR, Grood ES, Cummings JF, Wroble RR (1991) An analysis of the pivot shift phenomenon. The knee motions and subluxations induced by different examiners. Am J Sports Med 19(2):148–155
41. Pearle AD, Solomon DJ, Wanich T et al (2007) Reliability of navigated knee stability examination: A cadaveric evaluation. Am J Sports Med 35: 1315–1320
42. Robinson J, Carrat L, Granchi C, Colombet P (2007) Influence of anterior cruciate ligament bundles on knee kinematics: clinical assessment using computer-assisted navigation. Am J Sport Med 35:2006–2013
43. Seon JK, Park SJ, Lee KB et al (2009) Stability comparison of anterior cruciate ligament between double- and single-bundle reconstructions. Int Orthop 33: 425–429
44. Slocum DB, James SL, Larson RL, Singer KM (1976) Clinical test for anterolateral rotary instability of the knee. Clin Orthop Relat Res 118:63–69
45. Tashiro Y, Okazaki K, Miura H, Matsuda S, Yasunaga T, Hashizume M, Nakanishi Y, Iwamoto Y (2009) Quantitative assessment of rotatory instability after

anterior cruciate ligament reconstruction. Am J Sports Med 37(5):909–916
46. Tashman S, Collon D, Anderson K, Kolowich P, Anderst W (2004) Abnormal rotational knee motion during running after anterior cruciate ligament reconstruction. Am J Sports Med 32(4):975–983
47. Zaffagnini S, Bignozzi S, Martelli S, Imakiire N, Lopomo N, Marcacci M (2006) New intraoperative protocol for kinematics evaluation of ACL reconstruction: preliminary results". Knee Surg Sports Traumatol Arthrosc 14:811–816
48. Zaffagnini A, Klos TV, Bignozzi S (2010) Computer-assisted anterior cruciate ligament reconstruction: an evidence- based approach of the first 15 years. Arthroscopy 26(4):546–554

21 Mechanizing the Pivot Shift Test

Jelle P. van der List and Andrew D. Pearle

Contents

J.P. van der List • A.D. Pearle (✉)
Computer Assisted Surgery Center, Department of Orthopaedic Surgery, Hospital for Special Surgery, 535 East 70th Street, New York, NY 10021, USA
e-mail: vanderlistj@hss.edu; pearlea@hss.edu

21.1 Introduction

In 1968, Slocum and Larson described anterolateral rotational instability of the tibia during the anterior drawer test of ACL-deficient knees [46]. A few years later, Galway and Macintosh found this observation to be pathognomonic for ACL deficiency, causing the "giving way" experience that patients describe. This maneuver was emphasized as not purely rotational but with both anterior translation and internal rotation given the small anterior translation of the medial compartment and large translation of the lateral compartment [17, 18]. In an attempt to objectify the pivot shift test, Jakob et al. classified the anterior subluxation as none (grade 0), glide (grade I), clunk (grade II), or gross (grade III). Despite this, the test remained subjective [20]. This test is widely used due to its high specificity [54] and predictive value in knee stability and outcomes after ACL reconstruction [26, 31], but variability among examiners is high [41]. The subjectivity and high interobserver variability are among the reasons for the quest to objectify the pivot shift test.

Many human cadaveric studies have been performed with a simulated pivot shift test to measure kinematic forces, thereby attempting to objectify the pivot shift. Kanamori et al. performed a simulated pivot shift test with 10 Nm (Nm) of internal rotation and 10 Nm of valgus force throughout the flexion–extension arc. They found that both anterior subluxation (in millimeter) and internal rotation (in degrees) were higher

V. Musahl et al. (eds.), *Rotatory Knee Instability*, DOI 10.1007/978-3-319-32070-0_21

in ACL-deficient knees [21]. These findings were further confirmed by other studies [22, 57]. Furthermore, the simulated pivot shift test was used to objectify the effect of different ACL reconstruction techniques [14, 15, 35, 52, 59].

Despite the value of these studies in assessing the kinematics and forces in the pivot shift test, study designs are unusable in developing a test with clinical application. The purpose of the mechanized pivot shift test was to develop an objective pivot shift test that has high accuracy and can be clinically useful in the future [39].

21.2 The Mechanized Pivot Shift Test

In order to objectify the pivot shift test and lower its interobserver variability, it is important to standardize the methodology of the test. The cadaveric preparations, measurement methods, and the actual performance of the test were standardized, as detailed below.

21.2.1 Cadaveric Preparations

All cadaveric specimens were human, fresh frozen, hip-to-toe lower extremity cadavers; the preparation procedures of which were equal in all studies. Prior to the testing procedure, the cadavers were thawed at room temperature for 24 h. The specimens were placed supine on an operating room table (Maquet, Rastatt, Germany) and the pelvis was secured proximally. The setup was such that it allowed full and unrestricted range of motion of both the hip and the knee. Specimens were excluded if there were signs of gross ligamentous laxity at the knee, advanced arthritis, gross malalignment, or evidence of previous surgery.

21.2.2 Measurement Methods

The Praxim Medivision Surgetics navigation system (Praxim, Grenoble, France) was used to measure alignment, kinematics, and morphologic characteristics [23, 24]. This measurement technique utilizes an infrared passive optical sensor to detect the relative positions of two rigid bodies. These rigid bodies are threaded Steinmann pins placed in the proximal femur and distal tibia with reflective markers enabling the sensor to track the marker positions. The leg was subsequently rotated through the hip joint to determine the center of rotation of the lower extremity. Malalignment was determined through placing surface landmarks on the tibial plateau, distal femur, and medial and lateral malleoli. Intra-articular surface geometry was mapped and a three-dimensional (3D) model was created. From this 3D model, the anterior tibial translation (ATT) and the internal tibial rotation could be calculated. This measurement system has been proven accurate within 1 mm (mm) and within 1° (°) when compared with a six-degrees-of-freedom (DOF) robotic universal force moment sensor testing system [12, 42].

The measurement system reports ATT and internal tibial rotation during the pivot shift test in the different positions within the flexion arc, as presented by Lane et al. [30]. In this study, a P-shaped motion is evident in the sagittal plane during the pivot shift. This means that, in early flexion, the tibia is anteriorly translated, which is followed by reduction of this translation when the knee is further flexed. This P-shaped motion pattern is pathognomonic for a positive pivot shift test and can be displayed with the Surgetics navigation system [12, 30].

21.2.3 The Test

Before the mechanized pivot shift is performed and recorded, the cadaver must be positioned and secured and the setup completed. A continuous passive motion (CPM) machine is secured to the operating room table at a 45° angle. The foot is placed in a custom-made foot holder (Fig. 21.1, number 6) and fixed in a position so that there is an internal rotation moment at the knee. A valgus moment is then applied with the use of a three-degrees-of-freedom (3-DOF) arm, to which an axial load cell is attached to measure the exact load (Fig. 21.1, numbers 7 and 8, respectively). A

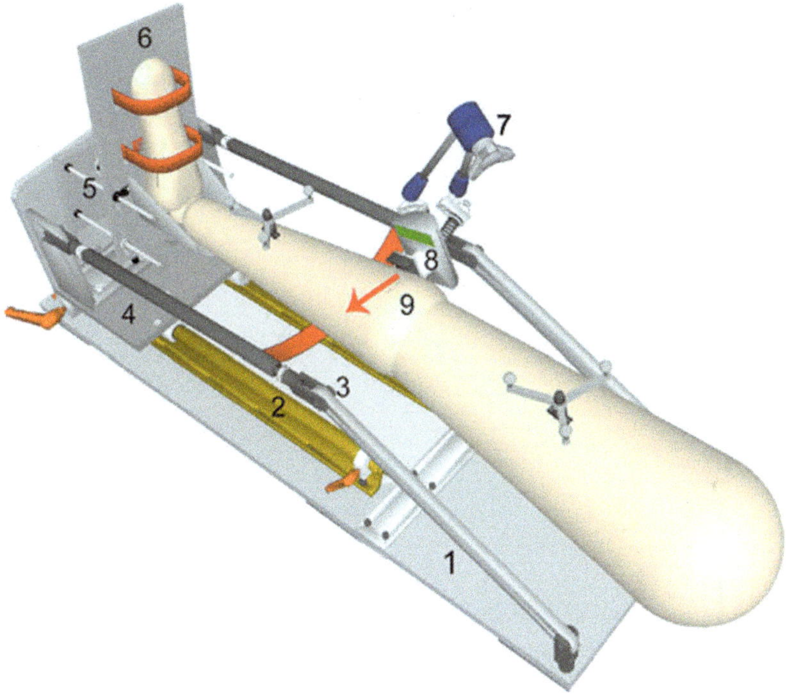

Fig. 21.1 Second-generation pivot shifter: *1* base plate, *2* linear bearing rail system, *3* joint, *4* leg driver component, *5* threaded rod, *6* fixation device for the foot, *7* three-degree-of-freedom arm, *8* axial load cell, *9* axial load (Reprinted from Citak et al. [11] with kind permission of Springer Science and Business Media)

band is attached at the posterior side of the proximal tibia to assist the leg through the motion of extension to flexion. Thigh supports were removed, and the tibia was fixed at the foot holder in order to enable free motion of the proximal tibia and femur in relation to each other. The leg is flexed as the 3-DOF arm and axial load cells move along with the leg, so the valgus forces are stable during flexion (Fig. 21.2). With this setup, there is a continuous torque and valgus force while the knee is moved through the flexion–extension arc and simulates the pivot shift test, as described by Galway et al. [17] and with hip in abduction, as described by Bach et al. [3].

21.3 Reliability of Mechanized Pivot Shift Test

Before the mechanized pivot shift test could be used, it was important to measure the intra-class correlation coefficient (ICC) and compare this test to the manual pivot shift test. Subsequently, some changes were made, thereby resulting in the second-generation test.

21.3.1 Comparison to Manual Pivot Shift

The purpose of the mechanized pivot shift test was to simulate the test in a clinical setting and to lower the subjectivity and interobserver variability of the pivot shift test. In the first study with the mechanized pivot shift test, 12 cadavers were used. The purpose of the study was to measure test intra-class correlation coefficient (ICC) [39]. The outcomes of the pivot shift test, ATT, and internal rotation were compared between the mechanized pivot shift test and the manual pivot shift test that was performed by a single examiner. It was found that the mechanized pivot shift test had a higher ICC than the manual pivot shift test in the intact knee for both ATT (0.78 vs. 0.75, respectively) and internal rotation (0.97 vs. 0.74, respectively). In the ACL-deficient knee, the ICC in the mechanized test was higher for translation (0.92 vs. 0.76, respectively), but lower for internal rotation (0.82 vs. 0.89, respectively). However, the standard error of measurements was lower in the mechanized test for both translation and rotation. Furthermore, in this study, the

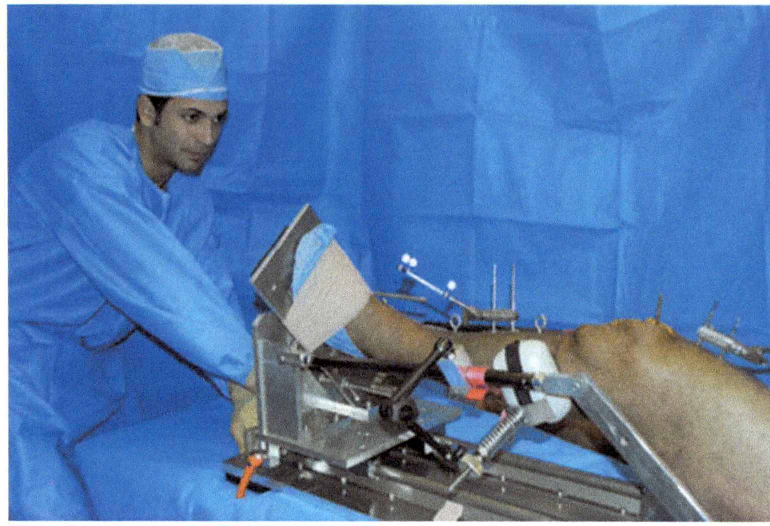

Fig. 21.2 The examiner pushes the handle of the foot driver component, while pulling the handle of the base plate. Note that the foot is not yet in internal rotation (Reprinted from Citak et al. [11] with kind permission of Springer Science and Business Media)

mechanized pivot shift underestimated ATT and internal rotation by approximately one-third.

21.3.2 Second Generation

Due to the underestimation of the initial design, improvements were made regarding the valgus forces. In the initial design, there was no 3-DOF with load cells used for the valgus force and this was added. With the second-generation tester, Citak et al. found no statistical difference in ATT between manual performed pivot shift and the second-generation mechanized pivot shift test, and the ICC for the mechanized pivot shift was increased to 0.99 [11]. With these results, the mechanized pivot shift was proven to have a high reliability in ATT and no differences in magnitude between the manual pivot shift test and the mechanized pivot shift test.

The difference between the first- and second-generation test is explained by the change in design regarding the valgus force. Markolf et al. described that in order to produce a positive pivot shift, it is necessary that valgus moments and iliotibial band forces be applied accurately [35]. However, the authors described that the loading conditions to produce a pivot shift in the ACL-deficient knee varied among specimens and represented a delicate equilibrium between applied valgus moment and iliotibial force. This could indicate that in the clinical setting, different amounts of valgus moment and rotational torque have to be applied in patients to obtain a positive pivot shift; thus, the exact performance of the pivot shift must be individualized.

Citak et al. [10] performed a study with the mechanized pivot shift test in which they assessed the amount of valgus forces necessary to cause a positive pivot shift. Using these load cells, they applied a stepwise increase of valgus forces during the mechanized pivot shift and measured the ATT in the lateral compartment. In this regard, there was a difference in lateral ATT of 6.6 mm between 0 and 1 kg of valgus force during the pivot shift. However, there was no significant difference by further increasing valgus forces up to 5 kg. Therefore, valgus force is a necessary part of the pivot shift, but the amount of lateral ATT does not increase with further application of forces over 1 kg.

21.4 Results

With this high reliability test, many studies were performed to answer various questions: (I) Are the medial ATT, the lateral ATT, and the internal rotation outcomes useful in measuring the pivot shift? (II) What amount of ATT in millimeters is necessary to get a positive pivot shift grade? (III) What are the influences of the so-called secondary stabilizers on the outcomes of the pivot shift test? (IV) How do several ACL reconstruction techniques, such as single bundle and double bundle, as well as different tunnel positions differ in the pivot shift outcomes? The current authors sought to answer these questions, among others.

Fact Box 1: Different Pivot Shift Grades
Minimal lateral ATT for a pivot shift grade:

Grade 1: 6 mm
Grade 2: 12 mm
Grade 3: 20 mm

21.4.1 Objectifying the Pivot Shift

First, an attempt was made to objectify the pivot shift and solidify when different grades of the manual pivot shift are reached and thus, when a pivot shift is considered positive. Subsequently, we assessed distribution values of the pivot shift in both intact and ACL-deficient knees.

21.4.1.1 Positive Pivot Shift

The mechanized pivot shift test was utilized to assess the correlation between the exact ATT in mm and the grade of pivot shift. Grade 0 indicated a normal finding, grade I as a glide, grade II as a clunk, and grade III as a gross clunk with locking [20, 29]. The mechanized pivot shift was used to assess this correlation by studying 77 cadavers [5]. In order to create different pivot shift grades, the ACL, medial meniscus, and/or lateral meniscus were removed in some knees. After the dissection, 20 knees were grade 0, 19 were grade 1, 18 were grade 2, and 20 were grade 3 with a manual pivot shift test. Thereafter, a manual pivot shift was performed with the measurement system installed. The examiner graded the pivot as 0, 1, 2, or 3 and was blinded for the outcomes of the measurement system. Then, the mechanized pivot shift was performed. There were three different outcomes: the grade of the manual pivot shift, the ATT of the manual pivot shift, and the ATT of the mechanized pivot shift. The ATT of both the medial compartment and the lateral compartment were measured.

It was determined that the ATT in the lateral compartment predicted the pivot shift grade test for the first three grades. Grade 0 correlated with a lateral ATT of -2.1 mm (±8.1 mm), grade 1 correlated with 11.1 mm (±2.2 mm), and grade 2 correlated with 19.6 mm (±2 mm). Furthermore, a threshold value of 6–7 mm was found to differentiate between a negative (grade 0) and a positive (grade ≥1) pivot shift (Fig. 21.3). It is therefore possible to use this threshold value in the future. Neither ATT of the medial compartment nor the internal rotation could be correlated with different grades of the pivot shift. The lack of correlation of the medial compartment with pivot shift grades could be explained by the smaller magnitude of anterior tibial translation on the medial side [17, 34], and these smaller differences could not be used to distinguish the different grades. Problems with identifying differences in internal rotation in the different pivot shift grades can be explained by the inconsistent

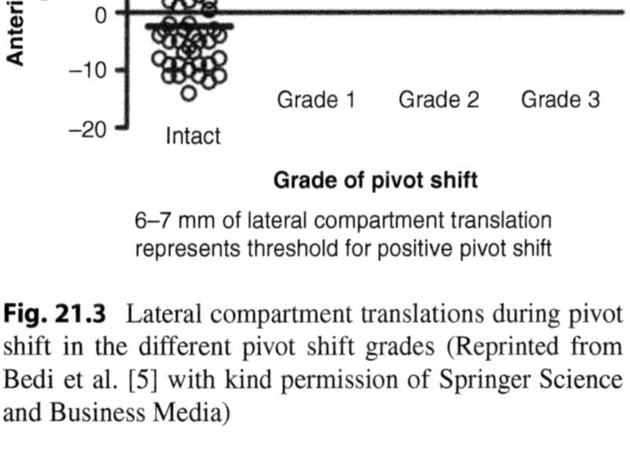

Fig. 21.3 Lateral compartment translations during pivot shift in the different pivot shift grades (Reprinted from Bedi et al. [5] with kind permission of Springer Science and Business Media)

Fact Box 2: Mean (± SD) of Anterior Tibial Translation (ATT) and Internal Rotation in Different Pivot Shift Grades of the Mechanized Pivot Shift

	Lateral ATT	Medial ATT	Internal rotation
Grade 0	-0.2 mm (±2.1)	-1.2 mm (±5.1)	12.4° (±4.5)
Grade 1	9.5 mm (±0.9)	0.0 mm (±6.3)	16.9° (±6.9)
Grade 2	14.7 mm (±0.9)	3.7 mm (±8.7)	19.5° (±7.7)
Grade 3	20.5 mm (±1.3)	8.1 mm (±7.9)	19.0° (±5.5)
Correlation between grades	$R^2=0.88$ ($p<0.001$)	$R^2=0.50$ ($p<0.001$)	$R^2=0.39$ ($p<0.004$)

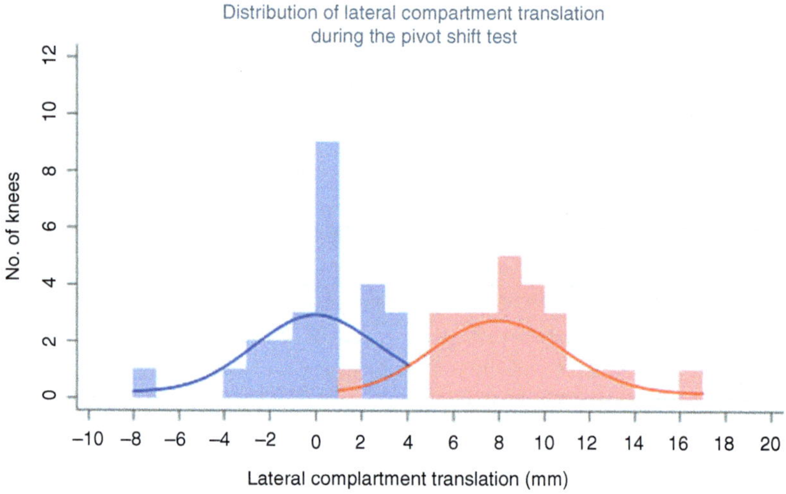

Fig. 21.4 Variability in the magnitude of translation of the lateral compartment for ACL-intact knees (*blue*) and ACL-deficient knees (*red*) during a mechanized pivot shift test (Reprinted from Dawson et al. [13] with kind permission of Springer Science and Business Media)

data of internal rotation [8, 28] and the lower ICC found in our first study [39]. This study demonstrates that, for the manual pivot shift and the mechanized pivot shift, the lateral ATT should be used to discriminate between different grades.

21.4.1.2 Normal Distributions

With the use of the mechanized pivot shift test, it is possible to distinguish between the ACL-intact and the ACL-deficient knees since the threshold value of 6–7 mm between ACL-intact (grade 0) and ACL-deficient knees (grade ≥1) is known. These differences were assessed by comparing the ATT in the lateral compartment in the ACL-intact knee with the ACL-deficient knee with the mechanized pivot shift test [13].

The ATT in the lateral compartment in the intact knee was -0.2 mm (±2.6 mm) and after dissection of the ACL, the ATT in the lateral compartment increased to an average of 8.2 mm (±3.1 mm) after transection of the ACL. The ACL-deficient knee had an average of 8.4 mm larger lateral ATT than the ACL-intact knee (Fig. 21.4). This difference of 8.4 mm is enough to convert a grade 0 pivot shift to a grade 1 pivot shift (threshold value of 6–7 mm), but it does not explain in all cases how a grade 2 or grade 3 is reached. It seems that deficiency of solely the ACL does not cause a grade 2–3 pivot shift, and there seems to be other bony and ligamentous structures – so-called secondary stabilizers – that play a role in ATT.

Fact Box 3: The Mechanized Pivot Shift Test

Cadaver preparation

Hip-to-toe lower extremity

No comorbidity in the lower extremities

Measurement

Two Steinmann pins in femur and tibia

Reflective markers attached to pins

3-D model to measure P-shaped pattern

Pivot shift

Foot in internal rotation

Valgus load with axial load cells

Move knee through extension–flexion arc

High repeatability (ICC 0.99)

21.4.2 Secondary Stabilizers

There are several secondary stabilizers of the knee in addition to the ACL [49]. Of all the ligaments in the knee, the ACL is considered the primary stabilizer [9, 16], and many other factors have been suggested as having additional influence in knee stability and the pivot shift. With the mechanized pivot shift, it is possible to examine these secondary stabilizers.

21.4.2.1 Meniscus

In 1982, Levy et al. reported a correlation between medial meniscectomy and increased anterior–posterior laxity of the knee [33]. A few years later, the correlation between the lateral meniscectomy and anterior–posterior laxity was reported [32]. In 48 % of the ACL reconstructions, a meniscus tear was found that required meniscectomy [47], although a lower frequency (40 %) was found in young athletes [25]. These frequencies show the relevance of assessing the relationship between meniscectomy and ATT in the ACL-deficient knee.

A study was performed comparing the difference between the ATT in the mechanized pivot

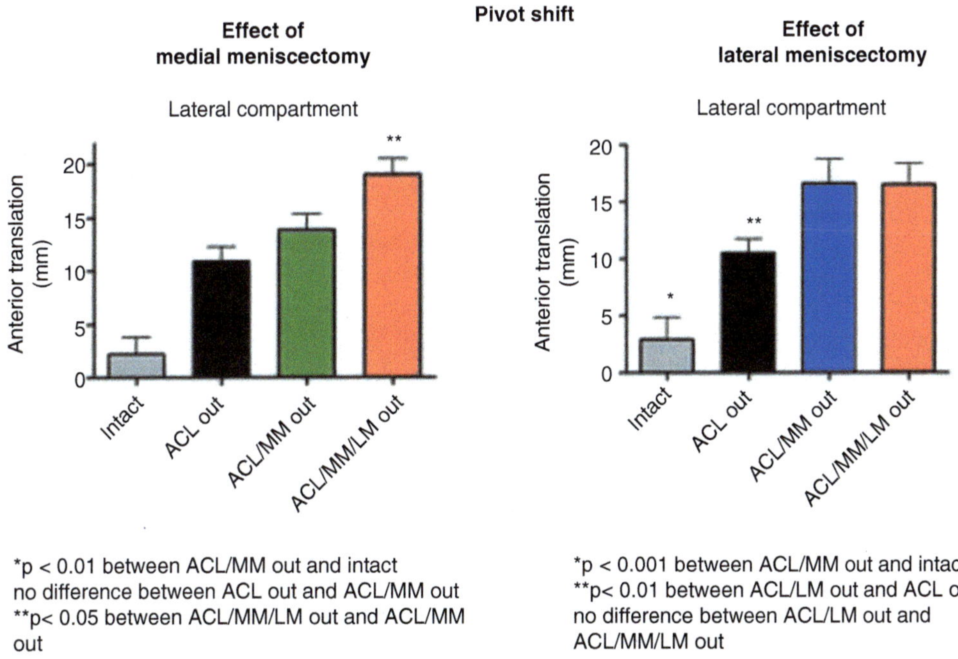

Fig. 21.5 The effect of medial meniscectomy (MM) and lateral meniscectomy (LM) in response to pivot shift test. Anterior tibial translation in the lateral compartment for the intact knee, isolated ACL deficiency (ACL out), ACL with single meniscectomy (ACL/LM out and ACL/MM out), and ACL-double meniscectomy (ACL/LM/MM-D) is shown (Reprinted from Musahl et al. [38] with kind permission of *American Journal of Sports Medicine*)

shift in ACL-deficient knees with the menisci intact, ACL-deficient knees with medial meniscectomy, ACL-deficient knees with lateral meniscectomy, and ACL-deficient knees with bilateral meniscectomy [38]. Medial meniscectomy did not play a role in anterior–posterior stability of the knee, but a lateral meniscectomy increased the ATT significantly in the ACL-deficient knee and in the ACL-deficient knee with medial meniscectomy in situ. The lateral meniscectomy increased the ATT in the mechanized pivot shift test with approximately 5–6 mm (Fig. 21.5). Recently, Shybut et al. confirmed this increase of the ATT in a biomechanical study of specimens with lateral meniscus deficiency. A simulated pivot shift was performed in knees that underwent arthroscopic posterior root detachment of the lateral meniscus and found a 2.1 mm increase of the lateral ATT in these knees with ACL deficiency and posterior lateral meniscus release [45].

21.4.2.2 Iliotibial Band

Slocum et al. suggested a role of the influence of the iliotibial band (ITB) on the pivot shift in their first study [46]. Bach et al. [3] found that performing the pivot shift test with the hip in abduction caused a more significant ATT and contributed this to the relaxation of the ITB. More recently, Yamamoto et al. [58] confirmed the role of the ITB in the pivot shift in a biomechanical study in which they applied several forces to the ITB in the ACL-deficient knee. They reported that a higher force of the ITB reduced the ATT in the pivot shift.

With the mechanized pivot shift, the role of the ITB on lateral ATT in ACL-deficient knees was assessed, and hip abduction was varied to find the optimal degree of hip abduction for the pivot shift [48]. Deficiency of the ITB caused a significantly greater lateral ATT compared to the knee with an intact ITB (from 8.1 mm to 10.8 mm); this corresponds to the finding of Yamamoto et al. [58]. Interestingly, in the ACL-deficient knee with both an intact and dissected ITB, there was no difference in lateral ATT between the different hip abduction angles (0°, 15°, and 30°). In this study, we could not confirm the findings of Bach et al. [3] that hip abduction increased the subjective outcome of the pivot shift test. However, these data indirectly support that relaxation of the ITB (with dissection in this study) cause more ATT in hip abduction. It should be stated that these studies differ in clinical patients versus cadavers and objective (mechanized pivot shift) versus subjective (manual pivot shift) measurement. The assessment of optimal hip abduction should be tested with the mechanized pivot shift test in clinical patients in the future.

21.4.2.3 Tibial Slope

Brandon et al. retrospectively measured the posterior–inferior tibial slope on radiographs of patients with isolated ACL deficiencies and found that a higher posterior–inferior tibial slope was associated with higher pivot shift grade [7]. In addition, the study by Ristic et al. confirmed this correlation between a higher posterior tibial slope and ACL deficiency [43], and Hashemi et al. considered this increased posterior tibial slope as a major risk factor for ACL injury [19].

We performed a cadaveric study with the mechanized pivot shift test to assess the role of a 5° increase or 5° decrease of the posterior–inferior tibial slope on the lateral ATT in ACL-deficient knees [56]. A 5° increase of the posterior–inferior slope increased the ATT by 2.2 mm, and a 5° decrease of the tibial slope reduced the lateral ATT by 3.0 mm. However, these changes were not significant. These results point in the direction of a relationship between the tibial slope and ATT, but further clinical research is necessary to assess if the tibial slope can contribute to the risk prediction or treatment in a specific patient group.

Fact Box 4: Factors Influencing Lateral ATT (in Millimeters)

This box shows the amount of additional lateral ATT when a primary or secondary structure is deficient and the amount of reduction of lateral ATT with different reconstruction techniques.

Deficiency of secondary stabilizers is in addition to ACL deficiency

Primary stabilizer	
ACL	+ 8.4 mm
Secondary stabilizers	
Lateral meniscus	+ 5–6 mm
Iliotibial band	+ 2.8 mm
Tibial slope	+ 2–5 mm
AP length lateral tibia	positive
Valgus force (0/1 kg) in test	+ 6.6 mm
Surgical restorations of ATT	
Single-bundle nonanatomic	−5.3 mm
Single-bundle anatomic	−7.9 mm
Double bundle	−11.4 mm (risk of overconstrain)

21.4.3 Comparing Surgical Techniques

The mechanized pivot shift test can also be used to compare the outcomes in knee laxity in different surgical techniques for ACL reconstruction. Different positions of the tibial tunnel, different bundle techniques, and the influence of meniscectomy on the outcomes of different surgical techniques were assessed.

21.4.3.1 Tibial Tunnel Placement

Malpositioning of the tunnels is considered to be the most common causative factor for ACL graft failure. It is estimated that tunnel malpositioning contributes to ACL graft failure in 50–80 % of cases [1, 51]. With the mechanized pivot shift, we tried to assess the role of tibial tunnel placement on the pivot shift [4]. Three different tibial tunnel positions were compared, and these positions were over the top (anterior aspect of proximal tibial epiphysis), anterior (anteromedial (AM) aspect of tibial footprint), and posterior (posterolateral (PL) aspect of tibial footprint). The tunnel in the over-the-top (OTT) position translated 1.7 mm more anteriorly than the intact ACL, the anterior tunnel position 4.1 mm more anteriorly, and the posterior tunnel position translated 8.0 mm more anteriorly than the intact knee. However, graft impingement in the notch was significant in the OTT position in 40° flexion, in the anterior position in 20° flexion, and in the posterior position in 10° flexion. Although more studies focus on the femoral position of the tunnel, this study shows that tibial position is important in single-bundle ACL reconstruction.

In a separate study, four different graft positions were compared with the mechanized pivot shift test [55]. These graft positions were AM (tibial AM footprint position to femoral AM footprint), horizontal (tibial AM footprint to femoral posterolateral footprint), conventional (PL tibial footprint to AM femoral footprint), and PL (tibial PL footprint to femoral PL footprint). Results showed that in ACL reconstruction, all grafts reduced the ATT, but the tibial AM footprint tunnels (AM and horizontal graft) caused less ATT and internal rotation than the tibial PL footprint (PL and conventional graft). Furthermore, they found that the tibial PL footprint graft did not control the internal rotation when compared to the intact ACL. In other words, anterior positioning in the tibial footprint is important in both reducing the ATT as the reduction of the internal rotation and that the PL tibial footprint is less effective in restoring the knee to its native kinematics.

21.4.3.2 Single Versus Double Bundle

Several systematic reviews and meta-analyses have been published to assess differences between single-bundle (SB) and double-bundle (DB) ACL reconstruction techniques [6, 27, 36, 50, 53]. The general conclusion is that the DB technique provides improved rotational stability and reduces the pivot shift test. Both techniques do not seem to differ with respect to clinical outcomes and failure rates. The current group performed a study with the mechanized pivot shift to compare two single-bundle techniques with the double-bundle ACL reconstruction [40], of which the single-bundle techniques were the AM graft (tibial AM footprint to femoral AM footprint) and the conventional graft (tibial PL footprint to femoral AM footprint). When comparing the three techniques, it was found that all techniques restored the ATT compared to the ACL-deficient knee. The DB technique provided significantly more reduction to an ATT of -1.7 mm compared to the AM SB technique (ATT of 1.8 mm) and the conventional SB technique (ATT of 4.4 mm), while the intact knee had a 1.7 mm ATT. However, internal rotational laxity was reduced in the DB and AM SB technique but was not reduced in the conventional technique compared to the ACL-deficient knee. This supports the earlier findings that tibial PL footprint position does not fully restore the internal rotation and can cause knee laxity. Moreover, it supports the findings of superiority of the DB technique in reducing rotational laxity in the systematic reviews.

The results also show that there is possible overconstraint associated with the DB technique. The ATT was reduced 3.4 mm when compared to the intact knee. A biomechanical study by Anderson et al. showed that the angle of flexion in which both the AM and the PL bundles are tensioned in the DB technique are of influence with respect to the amount of overconstraining or underconstraining of the graft [2]. In our study, all bundles were constrained in 20° of flexion, and the study by Anderson et al. demonstrated overconstraining when both the AM and the PL were constrained at the same degrees (e.g., 0–0°, 30–30°, 60–60°, and 90–90°). This could further explain the overconstraining of the DB technique in ATT in our study.

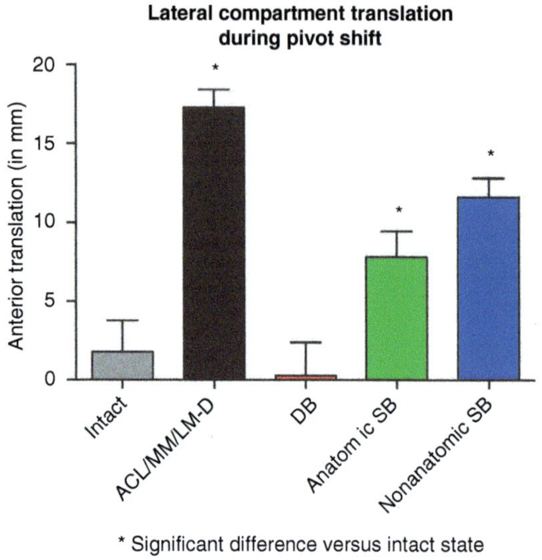

Fig. 21.6 Anterior tibial translations in the lateral compartment in different knee conditions. ACL/LM/MM-D indicates anterior cruciate ligament deficient and lateral and medial meniscus deficient; *DB* double bundle, *SB* single bundle (Reprinted from Musahl et al. [37] with kind permission of *American Journal of Sports Medicine*)

21.4.3.3 Bundle Technique with Meniscectomy

In a previously mentioned study by Musahl et al., it was demonstrated that lateral meniscectomy caused an increase in lateral ATT [38]. It was also shown that ATT was reduced in all graft techniques (nonanatomic SB, anatomic SB, and DB technique) but that the DB technique caused more of decrease in ATT with the risk of overconstraining [40]. Because meniscectomy is a commonly indicated procedure in patients with ACL reconstruction [25, 47], it is important to compare these different graft techniques in the meniscus-deficient knees as well.

The nonanatomic SB, anatomic SB, and DB ACL reconstruction techniques were compared in knees lacking the medial and lateral meniscus using the mechanized pivot test [37]. In this study, the single-bundle techniques differed significantly from the intact knee in the anterior translation shift test, while the double-bundle technique restored ATT to the intact knee. It appears better to restore the ACL-deficient knee with the DB technique when a meniscectomy is necessary or already performed (Fig. 21.6). In the 1980s, Levy et al. showed in biomechanical studies that medial and lateral meniscectomies both increased ATT in ACL-deficient knees with the pivot shift [32, 33], and the current group showed in previous studies that the lateral meniscus plays a more important role than the medial meniscus [38]. However, to our knowledge, it was not previously described that meniscectomy in ACL-deficient knees influences the ACL reconstruction technique. As a result of this cadaveric study, more clinical research is necessary to confirm this relationship and evaluate the different ACL techniques.

Conclusions

With the mechanized pivot shift test and its high reliability, it was possible to perform studies in ACL-deficient knees and objectify the pivot shift using a standardized method (Fact Box 1). A tibial translation of 6–7 mm corresponds to a subjective grade 1 in the manual pivot shift test and the mean ATT in the ACL-deficient knee was 8.2 mm, which exceeds this grade 1 in most cases.

The so-called secondary stabilizers are factors that cause an increase in ATT in addition to the increase by ACL deficiency [49]. With the mechanized pivot shift, lateral meniscectomy, the iliotibial band, and an increased posterior–inferior tibial slope were identified as factors that influenced ATT (Fact Box 2).

In the studies performed with the mechanized pivot shift, different tunnel positions and graft techniques were compared. Studies showed that the tibial tunnel should be placed in the footprint of the anteromedial bundle to optimize the reduction of the ATT without causing notch impingement. With the different graft techniques, the DB technique caused the greatest reduction of the ATT, but that this can potentially overconstrain the knee joint. In addition, in meniscus-deficient knees, there may be a preference for the double-bundle technique over single-bundle techniques.

For future clinical application, the need to place invasive pins to track the kinematics of the tibia and femur is a major limitation, and it is necessary to use noninvasive reference markers for future application of the mechanized pivot shift test. These noninvasive markers have been used by Russell et al. and showed similar test–retest repeatability [44], so combining the mechanized pivot shift test with these markers would bring us a step closer to clinical application.

In conclusion, the mechanized pivot shift has allowed many questions about the subjectivity of the pivot shift test to be investigated and answered. The primary and secondary stabilizers of the knee were quantified, and the outcomes of different tibial placements and surgical techniques for ACL reconstruction were shown. The mechanized pivot shift test is not yet optimized for clinical use, but has clarified issues about knee instability and the pivot shift test.

References

1. Allen CR, Giffin JR, Harner CD (2003) Revision anterior cruciate ligament reconstruction. Orthop Clin North Am 34(1):79–98
2. Anderson CJ, Westerhaus BD, Pietrini SD, Ziegler CG, Wijdicks CA, Johansen S, Engebretsen L, Laprade RF (2010) Kinematic impact of anteromedial and posterolateral bundle graft fixation angles on double-bundle anterior cruciate ligament reconstructions. Am J Sports Med 38(8):1575–1583. doi:10.1177/0363546510364841
3. Bach BR Jr, Warren RF, Wickiewicz TL (1988) The pivot shift phenomenon: results and description of a modified clinical test for anterior cruciate ligament insufficiency. Am J Sports Med 16(6):571–576
4. Bedi A, Maak T, Musahl V, Citak M, O'Loughlin PF, Choi D, Pearle AD (2011) Effect of tibial tunnel position on stability of the knee after anterior cruciate ligament reconstruction: is the tibial tunnel position most important? Am J Sports Med 39(2):366–373. doi:10.1177/0363546510388157
5. Bedi A, Musahl V, Lane C, Citak M, Warren RF, Pearle AD (2010) Lateral compartment translation predicts the grade of pivot shift: a cadaveric and clinical analysis. Knee Surg Sports Traumatol Arthrosc Off J ESSKA 18(9):1269–1276. doi:10.1007/s00167-010-1160-y
6. Bjornsson H, Desai N, Musahl V, Alentorn-Geli E, Bhandari M, Fu F, Samuelsson K (2015) Is double-bundle anterior cruciate ligament reconstruction superior to single-bundle? A comprehensive systematic review. Knee Surg Sports Traumatol Arthrosc Off J ESSKA 23(3):696–739. doi:10.1007/s00167-013-2666-x
7. Brandon ML, Haynes PT, Bonamo JR, Flynn MI, Barrett GR, Sherman MF (2006) The association between posterior-inferior tibial slope and anterior cruciate ligament insufficiency. Arthrosc J Arthrosc

Relat Surg Off Publ Arthrosc Assoc North Am Int Arthrosc Assoc 22(8):894–899. doi:10.1016/j.arthro.2006.04.098
8. Bull AM, Earnshaw PH, Smith A, Katchburian MV, Hassan AN, Amis AA (2002) Intraoperative measurement of knee kinematics in reconstruction of the anterior cruciate ligament. J Bone Joint Surg 84(7):1075–1081
9. Butler DL, Noyes FR, Grood ES (1980) Ligamentous restraints to anterior-posterior drawer in the human knee. A biomechanical study. J Bone Joint Surg Am 62(2):259–270
10. Citak M, O'Loughlin PF, Citak M, Suero EM, Bosscher MR, Musahl V, Pearle AD (2012) Influence of the valgus force during knee flexion in neutral rotation. Knee Surg Sports Traumatol Arthrosc Off J ESSKA 20(8):1571–1574. doi:10.1007/s00167-011-1767-7
11. Citak M, Suero EM, Rozell JC, Bosscher MR, Kuestermeyer J, Pearle AD (2011) A mechanized and standardized pivot shifter: technical description and first evaluation. Knee Surg Sports Traumatol Arthrosc Off J ESSKA 19(5):707–711. doi:10.1007/s00167-010-1289-8
12. Colombet P, Robinson J, Christel P, Franceschi JP, Djian P (2007) Using navigation to measure rotation kinematics during ACL reconstruction. Clin Orthop Relat Res 454:59–65. doi:10.1097/BLO.0b013e31802baf56
13. Dawson CK, Suero EM, Pearle AD (2013) Variability in knee laxity in anterior cruciate ligament deficiency using a mechanized model. Knee Surg Sports Traumatol Arthrosc Off J ESSKA 21(4):784–788. doi:10.1007/s00167-012-2170-8
14. Diermann N, Schumacher T, Schanz S, Raschke MJ, Petersen W, Zantop T (2009) Rotational instability of the knee: internal tibial rotation under a simulated pivot shift test. Arch Orthop Trauma Surg 129(3):353–358. doi:10.1007/s00402-008-0681-z
15. Engebretsen L, Wijdicks CA, Anderson CJ, Westerhaus B, LaPrade RF (2012) Evaluation of a simulated pivot shift test: a biomechanical study. Knee Surg Sports Traumatol Arthrosc Off J ESSKA 20(4):698–702. doi:10.1007/s00167-011-1744-1
16. Fukubayashi T, Torzilli PA, Sherman MF, Warren RF (1982) An in vitro biomechanical evaluation of anterior-posterior motion of the knee. Tibial displacement, rotation, and torque. J Bone Joint Surg Am 64(2):258–264
17. Galway HR, MacIntosh DL (1980) The lateral pivot shift: a symptom and sign of anterior cruciate ligament insufficiency. Clin Orthop Relat Res 147:45–50
18. Galway R, Beaupre A, MacIntosh D (1972) Pivot shift: a clinical sign of symptomatic anterior cruciate insufficiency. J Bone Joint Surg 54:763–764
19. Hashemi J, Chandrashekar N, Mansouri H, Gill B, Slauterbeck JR, Schutt RC Jr, Dabezies E, Beynnon BD (2010) Shallow medial tibial plateau and steep medial and lateral tibial slopes: new risk factors for anterior cruciate ligament injuries. Am J Sports Med 38(1):54–62. doi:10.1177/0363546509349055
20. Jakob RP, Staubli HU, Deland JT (1987) Grading the pivot shift. Objective tests with implications for treatment. J Bone Joint Surg 69(2):294–299
21. Kanamori A, Woo SL, Ma CB, Zeminski J, Rudy TW, Li G, Livesay GA (2000) The forces in the anterior cruciate ligament and knee kinematics during a simulated pivot shift test: a human cadaveric study using robotic technology. Arthrosc J Arthrosc Relat Surg Off Publ Arthrosc Assoc North Am Int Arthrosc Assoc 16(6):633–639. doi:10.1053/jars.2000.7682
22. Kanamori A, Zeminski J, Rudy TW, Li G, Fu FH, Woo SL (2002) The effect of axial tibial torque on the function of the anterior cruciate ligament: a biomechanical study of a simulated pivot shift test. Arthrosc J Arthrosc Relat Surg Off Publ Arthrosc Assoc North Am Int Arthrosc Assoc 18(4):394–398
23. Kendoff D, Bogojevic A, Citak M, Citak M, Maier C, Maier G, Krettek C, Hufner T (2007) Experimental validation of noninvasive referencing in navigated procedures on long bones. J Orthop Res Off Publ Orthop Res Soc 25(2):201–207. doi:10.1002/jor.20318
24. Kendoff D, Citak M, Pearle A, Gardner MJ, Hankemeier S, Krettek C, Hufner T (2007) Influence of lower limb rotation in navigated alignment analysis: implications for high tibial osteotomies. Knee Surg Sports Traumatol Arthrosc Off J ESSKA 15(8):1003–1008. doi:10.1007/s00167-007-0308-x
25. Kilcoyne KG, Dickens JF, Haniuk E, Cameron KL, Owens BD (2012) Epidemiology of meniscal injury associated with ACL tears in young athletes. Orthopedics 35(3):208–212. doi:10.3928/01477447-20120222-07
26. Kocher MS, Steadman JR, Briggs KK, Sterett WI, Hawkins RJ (2004) Relationships between objective assessment of ligament stability and subjective assessment of symptoms and function after anterior cruciate ligament reconstruction. Am J Sports Med 32(3):629–634
27. Kongtharvonskul J, Attia J, Thamakaison S, Kijkunasathian C, Woratanarat P, Thakkinstian A (2013) Clinical outcomes of double- vs single-bundle anterior cruciate ligament reconstruction: a systematic review of randomized control trials. Scand J Med Sci Sports 23(1):1–14. doi:10.1111/j.1600-0838.2011.01439.x
28. Kubo S, Muratsu H, Yoshiya S, Mizuno K, Kurosaka M (2007) Reliability and usefulness of a new in vivo measurement system of the pivot shift. Clin Orthop Relat Res 454:54–58. doi:10.1097/BLO.0b013e31802b4a38
29. Lane CG, Warren R, Pearle AD (2008) The pivot shift. J Am Acad Orthop Surg 16(12):679–688
30. Lane CG, Warren RF, Stanford FC, Kendoff D, Pearle AD (2008) In vivo analysis of the pivot shift phenomenon during computer navigated ACL reconstruction. Knee Surg Sports Traumatol Arthrosc Off J ESSKA 16(5):487–492. doi:10.1007/s00167-008-0504-3
31. Leitze Z, Losee RE, Jokl P, Johnson TR, Feagin JA (2005) Implications of the pivot shift in the ACL-deficient knee. Clin Orthop Relat Res 436:229–236

32. Levy IM, Torzilli PA, Gould JD, Warren RF (1989) The effect of lateral meniscectomy on motion of the knee. J Bone Joint Surg Am 71(3):401–406
33. Levy IM, Torzilli PA, Warren RF (1982) The effect of medial meniscectomy on anterior-posterior motion of the knee. J Bone Joint Surg Am 64(6):883–888
34. Lopomo N, Zaffagnini S, Amis AA (2013) Quantifying the pivot shift test: a systematic review. Knee Surg Sports Traumatol Arthrosc Off J ESSKA 21(4):767–783. doi:10.1007/s00167-013-2435-x
35. Markolf KL, Park S, Jackson SR, McAllister DR (2008) Simulated pivot-shift testing with single and double-bundle anterior cruciate ligament reconstructions. J Bone Joint Surg Am 90(8):1681–1689. doi:10.2106/JBJS.G.01272
36. Mascarenhas R, Cvetanovich GL, Sayegh ET, Verma NN, Cole BJ, Bush-Joseph C, Bach BR Jr (2015) Does Double-Bundle Anterior Cruciate Ligament Reconstruction Improve Postoperative Knee Stability Compared With Single-Bundle Techniques? A Systematic Review of Overlapping Meta-analyses. Arthrosc J Arthrosc Relat Surg Off Publ Arthrosc Assoc North Am Int Arthrosc Assoc. doi:10.1016/j.arthro.2014.11.014
37. Musahl V, Bedi A, Citak M, O'Loughlin P, Choi D, Pearle AD (2011) Effect of single-bundle and double-bundle anterior cruciate ligament reconstructions on pivot-shift kinematics in anterior cruciate ligament- and meniscus-deficient knees. Am J Sports Med 39(2):289–295. doi:10.1177/0363546510385422
38. Musahl V, Citak M, O'Loughlin PF, Choi D, Bedi A, Pearle AD (2010) The effect of medial versus lateral meniscectomy on the stability of the anterior cruciate ligament-deficient knee. Am J Sports Med 38(8):1591–1597. doi:10.1177/0363546510364402
39. Musahl V, Voos J, O'Loughlin PF, Stueber V, Kendoff D, Pearle AD (2010) Mechanized pivot shift test achieves greater accuracy than manual pivot shift test. Knee Surg Sports Traumatol Arthrosc Off J ESSKA 18(9):1208–1213. doi:10.1007/s00167-009-1004-9
40. Musahl V, Voos JE, O'Loughlin PF, Choi D, Stueber V, Kendoff D, Pearle AD (2010) Comparing stability of different single- and double-bundle anterior cruciate ligament reconstruction techniques: a cadaveric study using navigation. Arthrosc J Arthrosc Relat Surg Off Publ Arthrosc Assoc North Am Int Arthrosc Assoc 26(9 Suppl):S41–S48. doi:10.1016/j.arthro.2010.01.028
41. Noyes FR, Grood ES, Cummings JF, Wroble RR (1991) An analysis of the pivot shift phenomenon. The knee motions and subluxations induced by different examiners. Am J Sports Med 19(2):148–155
42. Pearle AD, Solomon DJ, Wanich T, Moreau-Gaudry A, Granchi CC, Wickiewicz TL, Warren RF (2007) Reliability of navigated knee stability examination: a cadaveric evaluation. Am J Sports Med 35(8):1315–1320. doi:10.1177/0363546507300821
43. Ristic V, Maljanovic M, Pericin B, Harhaji V, Milankov M (2014) The relationship between posterior tibial slope and anterior cruciate ligament injury. Med Pregl 67(7-8):216–221. doi:10.2298/mpns1408216r
44. Russell DF, Deakin AH, Fogg QA, Picard F (2014) Repeatability and accuracy of a non-invasive method of measuring internal and external rotation of the tibia. Knee Surg Sports Traumatol Arthrosc Off J ESSKA 22(8):1771–1777. doi:10.1007/s00167-013-2812-5
45. Shybut TB, Vega CE, Haddad J, Alexander JW, Gold JE, Noble PC, Lowe WR (2015) Effect of lateral meniscal root tear on the stability of the anterior cruciate ligament-deficient knee. Am J Sports Med 43(4):905–911. doi:10.1177/0363546514563910
46. Slocum DB, Larson RL (1968) Rotatory instability of the knee. Its pathogenesis and a clinical test to demonstrate its presence. J Bone Joint Surg Am 50(2): 211–225
47. Sri-Ram K, Salmon LJ, Pinczewski LA, Roe JP (2013) The incidence of secondary pathology after anterior cruciate ligament rupture in 5086 patients requiring ligament reconstruction. Bone Joint J 95-B(1):59–64. doi:10.1302/0301-620X.95B1.29636
48. Suero EM, Njoku IU, Voigt MR, Lin J, Koenig D, Pearle AD (2013) The role of the iliotibial band during the pivot shift test. Knee Surg Sports Traumatol Arthrosc Off J ESSKA 21(9):2096–2100. doi:10.1007/s00167-012-2257-2
49. Tanaka M, Vyas D, Moloney G, Bedi A, Pearle AD, Musahl V (2012) What does it take to have a high-grade pivot shift? Knee Surg Sports Traumatol Arthrosc Off J ESSKA 20(4):737–742. doi:10.1007/s00167-011-1866-5
50. Tiamklang T, Sumanont S, Foocharoen T, Laopaiboon M (2012) Double-bundle versus single-bundle reconstruction for anterior cruciate ligament rupture in adults. Cochrane Database Syst Rev 11:CD008413. doi:10.1002/14651858.CD008413.pub2
51. Trojani C, Sbihi A, Djian P, Potel JF, Hulet C, Jouve F, Bussiere C, Ehkirch FP, Burdin G, Dubrana F, Beaufils P, Franceschi JP, Chassaing V, Colombet P, Neyret P (2011) Causes for failure of ACL reconstruction and influence of meniscectomies after revision. Knee Surg Sports Traumatol Arthrosc Off J ESSKA 19(2):196–201. doi:10.1007/s00167-010-1201-6
52. Tsai AG, Wijdicks CA, Walsh MP, Laprade RF (2010) Comparative kinematic evaluation of all-inside single-bundle and double-bundle anterior cruciate ligament reconstruction: a biomechanical study. Am J Sports Med 38(2):263–272. doi:10.1177/0363546509348053
53. van Eck CF, Kopf S, Irrgang JJ, Blankevoort L, Bhandari M, Fu FH, Poolman RW (2012) Single-bundle versus double-bundle reconstruction for anterior cruciate ligament rupture: a meta-analysis--does anatomy matter? Arthrosc J Arthrosc Relat Surg Off Publ Arthrosc Assoc North Am Int Arthrosc Assoc 28(3):405–424. doi:10.1016/j.arthro.2011.11.021
54. van Eck CF, van den Bekerom MP, Fu FH, Poolman RW, Kerkhoffs GM (2013) Methods to diagnose acute anterior cruciate ligament rupture: a meta-analysis of physical examinations with and without anaesthesia. Knee Surg Sports Traumatol Arthrosc Off J ESSKA 21(8):1895–1903. doi:10.1007/s00167-012-2250-9

55. Voos JE, Musahl V, Maak TG, Wickiewicz TL, Pearle AD (2010) Comparison of tunnel positions in single-bundle anterior cruciate ligament reconstructions using computer navigation. Knee Surg Sports Traumatol Arthrosc Off J ESSKA 18(9):1282–1289. doi:10.1007/s00167-010-1162-9
56. Voos JE, Suero EM, Citak M, Petrigliano FP, Bosscher MR, Citak M, Wickiewicz TL, Pearle AD (2012) Effect of tibial slope on the stability of the anterior cruciate ligament-deficient knee. Knee Surg Sports Traumatol Arthrosc Off J ESSKA 20(8):1626–1631. doi:10.1007/s00167-011-1823-3
57. Woo SL, Kanamori A, Zeminski J, Yagi M, Papageorgiou C, Fu FH (2002) The effectiveness of reconstruction of the anterior cruciate ligament with hamstrings and patellar tendon.A cadaveric study comparing anterior tibial and rotational loads. J Bone Joint Surg Am 84-A(6):907–914
58. Yamamoto Y, Hsu WH, Fisk JA, Van Scyoc AH, Miura K, Woo SL (2006) Effect of the iliotibial band on knee biomechanics during a simulated pivot shift test. J Orthop Res Off Publ Orthop Res Soc 24(5):967–973. doi:10.1002/jor.20122
59. Zantop T, Herbort M, Raschke MJ, Fu FH, Petersen W (2007) The role of the anteromedial and posterolateral bundles of the anterior cruciate ligament in anterior tibial translation and internal rotation. Am J Sports Med 35(2):223–227. doi:10.1177/0363546506294571

Development of Electromagnetic Tracking for the Pivot Shift

22

Ryosuke Kuroda, Yuichi Hoshino, Takehiko Matsushita, Kouki Nagamune, and Masahiro Kurosaka

Contents

R. Kuroda (✉) • T. Matsushita • M. Kurosaka
Department of Orthopaedic Surgery,
Graduate School of Medicine, Kobe University,
7-5-2 Kusunoki-chi, Chuo-ku, Kobe 650-0017, Japan
e-mail: kurodar@med.kobe-u.ac.jp

Y. Hoshino
Department of Orthopaedic Surgery,
Kobe Kaisei Hospital, Kobe, Japan

K. Nagamune
Department of Human and Artificial Intelligent Systems, Graduate School of Engineering,
University of Fukui, Fukui, Japan

22.1 Introduction

Anterior cruciate ligament (ACL) insufficiency is clinically diagnosed by manual tests, such as the pivot-shift [11, 20, 34, 47] and the Lachman tests [50, 52]. These manual tests are used not only for diagnosing a primary ACL injury but also as an outcome measure after ACL reconstruction. Performing an accurate, dynamic functional evaluation is necessary for outcome measurement after ACL reconstruction. The pivot-shift test is commonly used for assessing dynamic laxity in ACL-insufficient knees and is related to subjective knee function [24]. Static load displacement measurement, such as the Lachman test and KT measurement, is unrelated to the dynamic knee function of ACL insufficiency [24, 48]. Any residual pivot shift after ACL reconstruction is a crucial factor related to poor clinical outcome. One clinical follow-up study showed the presence of a pivot-shift phenomenon after ACL reconstruction related to functional impairment and poor patient satisfaction [24]. Jonsson et al. [22] reported patients with positive pivot-shift results showed increased scintigraphic activity in the subchondral bone, while long-term studies [8, 10, 22] have shown radiographic signs of osteoarthritis at follow-up do not correlate with AP knee laxity. Residual knee laxity can be detected by the pivot-shift test in ACL-reconstructed knees in which anterior laxity has been successfully restored. As a result of the ability to evaluate a dynamic and a rotational component of the

V. Musahl et al. (eds.), *Rotatory Knee Instability*, DOI 10.1007/978-3-319-32070-0_22

knee stability, postoperative laxity evaluation should include the pivot-shift test. Moreover, quantitative evaluation for the pivot-shift test has been sought after analogous to the KT-1000 arthrometer [9] or other instruments [12, 42, 45], which can provide objective values to evaluate the anterior laxity.

22.2 Pivot-Shift Test

The pivot-shift phenomenon [11], which consists of a tibial anterior dislocation and a subsequent reduction of lateral compartment of the knee joint, is a dynamic instability of the knee with ACL deficiency which can be reproduced and described by the pivot-shift test [11, 34]. The pivot-shift test was first reported in the American literature by Galway and McIntosh [11] in which the hip was abducted and the knee was passively flexed from full extension with internal tibial torque and valgus stress applied manually to the knee to make a subluxation of the lateral component. Subsequently, sudden reduction spontaneously occurs at around 20–40° of knee flexion. The magnitude of the pivot shift during the test is normally graded only by the examiner's subjective impression [18, 28, 41], and the mechanism of the dynamic laxity measurement has not been strictly defined. Although three-dimensional (3D) kinematic assessment of the pivot-shift phenomenon has been attempted to explore how the knee moves during the pivot-shift test in previous studies, this methodology cannot be utilized in current clinical settings [2, 3, 13, 37]. Knee kinematic measurements of the pivot-shift test have been introduced in order to measure the 3D displacement of the tibia with respect to the femur as a potential objective parameter for the pivot-shift test [7, 13, 17, 35]. Furthermore, it has been suggested that 3D acceleration should represent the dynamism of the pivot-shift phenomenon and can be related to the dynamic knee laxity evaluated by the pivot-shift test [30, 33, 36]. Recent advancement in the pivot-shift measurement provides more dynamic and more clinically meaningful assessment of ACL-deficient and ACL-reconstructed knees.

22.3 Noninvasive Methods of Monitoring Knee Kinematics with an Electromagnetic Device

A noninvasive in vivo measurement system that uses an electromagnetic tracking device (FASTRAK or LIBERTY, Polhemus, Colchester, VT, USA) has been introduced to measure the 6 degrees-of-freedom knee kinematics during the pivot-shift test with a high sampling rate (FASTRAK 60 Hz and LIBERTY 240 Hz) [15, 16, 27]. It enables monitoring of instantaneous 3D tibial displacement relative to the femur and calculates 3D acceleration of the motion. The electromagnetic device consists of a transmitter that produces an electromagnetic field and three electromagnetic receivers. Two of the receivers, which are used for motion measurement of the tibia and femur, are attached to a plastic brace by a circumferential Velcro strap placed 10 cm above the patella on the thigh and 7 cm below the tibial tubercle on the lower leg. A third receiver used to register the 3D position data of the anatomic landmarks is attached to a specially made stylus. Seven anatomical bony landmarks include three on the femur, the major trochanter, the medial epicondyle, and the lateral epicondyle, and four for the tibia, the intersection of the medial collateral ligament and the knee joint line, the fibula head, and the medial and the lateral malleoli of the ankle. Based on the 3D positional relationship between the anatomic landmarks and the two receivers for motion measurement, a 3D coordinate system of the knee joint can be configured and provide the 6 degrees-of-freedom kinematics according to a modified 3-cylinder open-chain mechanism proposed by Grood and Suntay [14]. This system has a root mean square (RMS) accuracy of 0.03 mm for position and 0.15° for orientation (Fig. 22.1).

22.4 Quantitative Assessment of the Pivot-Shift Test

The 6 degrees-of-freedom measurement during passive flexion with the tibia held externally rotated is performed and used as the referral movement for comparing the 3D position displacement during the pivot-shift test. The external rotational stress is applied to stabilize rotation during passive flexion of the tibia. The same 6 degrees-of-freedom measurement is taken during the pivot-shift test, and the relative displacement of the tibial AP translation is calculated as the coupled anterior tibial translation (c-ATT). c-ATT and the acceleration of the tibial reduction from anterior subluxation to the original normal position (the acceleration of posterior translation, APT) are potential parameters for quantitative evaluation of the pivot-shift test [15, 28, 29, 33]. Since the tibial anteroposterior translation normally occurs during the flexion–extension movement, the anterior tibial translation during the pivot-shift test should be taken as a relative position to a reference movement or a hysteresis of the movement [6] to eliminate the effect of the natural tibial anteroposterior (AP) movement. This c-ATT could be regarded as a parameter that evaluates the magnitude of the tibial anterior translation, or the tibial anterior subluxation, during a dynamic motion. The c-ATT might be categorized as a load displacement measurement like KT-1000 arthrometer measurement [9] or Rolimeter [45], which has been reported to have poor correlation with subjective symptom and knee function [24, 48]. On the other hand, APT (the acceleration of posterior translation), which jumps at the moment of changing the direction of tibial anterior translation to the posterior, could represent the dynamism of the pivot shift and can also be regarded as a parameter that represents the dynamism of the pivot-shift phenomenon [15, 30, 33, 36]. The increased APT during the pivot-shift test could be detected in ACL-deficient knees along with the increased c-ATT, and this increment was correlated with the clinical grading [15]. The acceleration is closely related to the force according to basic physics. It can be assumed that the change of force in the knee can be represented by the increment of the acceleration and induce the feeling of giving way when the force was large enough. A slight posterior tibial translation and its acceleration could also be monitored even in ACL intact knees which cannot be captured by the clinician's hands and graded as none. It could be considered that the examiner's hand is not sensitive enough to detect such a small acceleration, but this can be measured by advanced measurement technology (Fig. 22.2).

22.5 Intact Knees Versus ACL-Deficient Knees

Seventy unilateral ACL-injured patients were examined to obtain the baseline data for the diagnosis of the ACL insufficiency. c-ATT was measured by an electromagnetic tracking device in the patients in both injured and contralateral intact knees prior to the ACL reconstruction. All of the ACL ruptures were diagnosed preoperatively by clinical findings and MRI and confirmed arthroscopically. There were significant differences ($p < 0.01$) in the peak c-ATTs between intact knees and injured knees. The mean tibial acceleration during the pivot-shift test was larger in the ACL-injured knee, 1.9 ± 1.2 m/sec^2, than in the contralateral intact knee, which registered 0.8 ± 0.3 m/sec^2. There were also significant differences ($p < 0.01$) in the APT between intact knees and injured knees. The ratio of patients with APTs of less than 1 m/s^2 was 83.3 % in the intact knees and 3.3 % in the ACL-deficient knees [unpublished data from Kobe University].

22.6 Quantitative Evaluation of the Pivot-Shift Test for Comparison Between Double-Bundle and Single-Bundle Reconstruction

The goal of ACL reconstruction is to restore the normal function of the native ACL. Recent studies suggest conventional single-bundle reconstructive procedures may not restore the native physiological kinematics of the knee, even when satisfactory AP laxity is restored, thereby resulting in residual impairment [6, 23, 31, 32, 44, 49]. It has been reported in biomechanical studies that anatomic reconstruction of both the

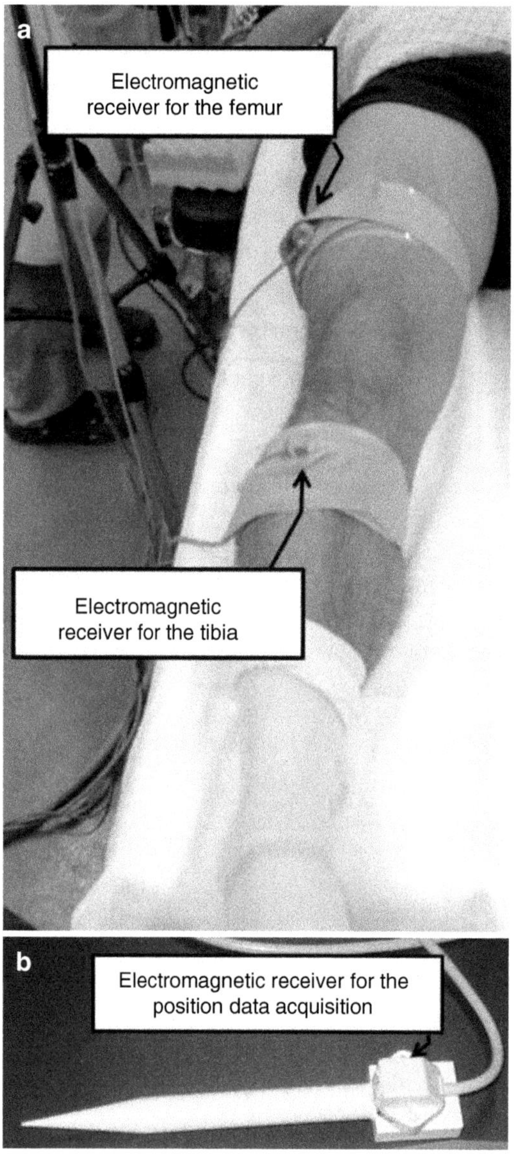

Fig. 22.1 Electromagnetic sensor setup. (**a**) Two sensors are attached onto the thigh and the lower leg. (**b**) Third receiver is attached to the original stylus which can be used to digitize the 3D position data of bony landmarks

anteromedial (AM) and posterolateral (PL) bundles can better restore knee stability than a single-bundle reconstruction [35, 53] Additionally, clinical studies with a 2-year follow-up period showed a significantly superior outcome after anatomic double-bundle ACL reconstruction in terms of anterior laxity restoration, as measured with KT-1000 arthrometer, or rotational laxity restoration, as evaluated by the pivot-shift test when compared to single-bundle ACL reconstruction [21, 25, 39, 46, 55]. In contrast, clinical results of anatomic double-bundle ACL reconstruction did not detect any significant improvement over the conventional single-bundle procedure [1]. A meta-analysis of single-bundle versus double-bundle ACL reconstruction techniques from Meredick et al. [38] also supported these results. They reported that double-bundle reconstruction did not result in clinically significant differences in the KT-1000 measurements or with clinical manual evaluation with the pivot-shift test. However, the pivot-shift test results in this report were later reanalyzed in detail and demonstrated better outcomes with respect to restoring a normal pivot shift in double-bundle procedure compared to the single bundle [19]. This controversy might highlight the difficulty of the clinical pivot-shift test evaluation and interpretation. Therefore, to assess whether these modifications provide functional improvement, postoperative laxity evaluations should be objective and meticulous, considering both a dynamic and a rotational component of the knee movement, rather than simple static measurement and rough manual examination. Currently, there are an increasing number of studies in which single-bundle and double-bundle ACL reconstructions are being compared by examining tibial anterior translation, combined rotatory load, or simulated pivot-shift test using multiple techniques [5, 26, 40, 43, 51]. Most of them have reported that double-bundle reconstruction provides better restoration of laxity than single-bundle reconstruction and can restore the laxity parameters more closely to the normal knees. Most surgeons now recognize the importance of the pivot-shift test that can be used to assess both rotational and dynamic laxities [6, 22–24, 30]. Yagi et al. [54] analyzed rotational laxity using an electromagnetic tracking device with 3 reconstruction techniques in 60 consecutive patients who were randomly divided into 3 groups (double bundle, anteromedial single bundle, posterolateral single bundle) and found that anatomical double-bundle ACL reconstruction can improve rotational laxity [54]. Araki et al. [4] conducted a prospective randomized study of anatomical single-bundle versus double-bundle ACL reconstructions using

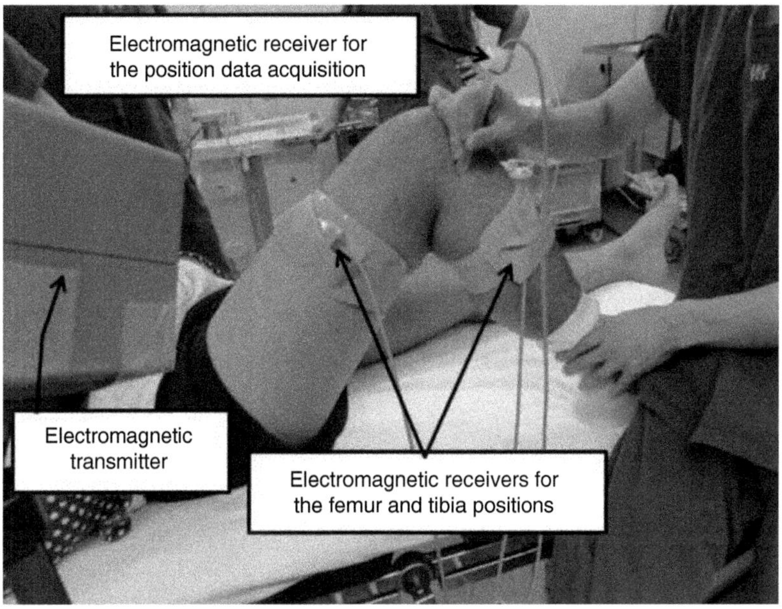

Fig. 22.2 Digitization of the 3D position data of the bony landmarks. Three receivers, two for the femur and the tibia and one for the digitization of bony landmarks, are located within the electromagnetic field which is generated from the electromagnetic transmitter (*on the left*)

Table 22.1 Tibial acceleration measured by the electromagnetic system

	ACL-reconstructed knees	Contralateral intact knees
Single bundle	940 ± 524 mm/sec^{2a}	640 ± 138 mm/sec^2
Double bundle	701 ± 226 mm/sec^2	685 ± 262 mm/sec^2

Comparison between double-bundle and single-bundle ACL reconstructions

[a]Statistical significance achieved compared to the contralateral knees, $p < 0.05$

hamstrings tendons. Twenty patients with unilateral ACL deficiency were randomized into two groups. Two bone tunnels of the femur were created at the position of the original insertion of the anteromedial bundle footprint and posterolateral bundle footprint in the anatomic double-bundle group, and one tunnel was created at the central position between these two bundles in the anatomic single-bundle group. All the patients were tested before ACL reconstruction and 1 year after surgery. Single-bundle reconstruction could not fully restore the tibial acceleration during the pivot-shift test to the intact knee level, while double-bundle ACL reconstruction could reduce the rotational laxity to the normal level (Table 22.1). The electromagnetic tracking device data showed that the anatomical double-bundle ACL reconstruction tended to be biomechanically superior to the anatomic single-bundle reconstruction [4] (Fig. 22.3).

22.7 Limitations of the Measurement System

There are limitations to this measurement system, inherent in which is that the pivot-shift test has wide variability among examiners [28, 41]. In the pivot-shift test, the speed of test procedure, the angle of hip abduction during the test, and the magnitude of force applied to the knee are not exactly the same in each test and among the examiners. Although valgus stress is a requisite for the pivot-shift test, there is a mixed opinion as to which, internal or external, rotational stress should be applied for the pivot-shift test. In this regard, internal rotational stress is more advocated than external rotational stress [28], and these variables could possibly affect the result. It is possible to improve consistency and accuracy of the measurement by limiting the number of examiners or designing the testing procedure more strictly. Additionally, since this measurement system assesses the pivot-shift phenomenon, which is provoked by a manual test, muscular resistance or improper test procedure could suppress the pivot-shift phenomenon.

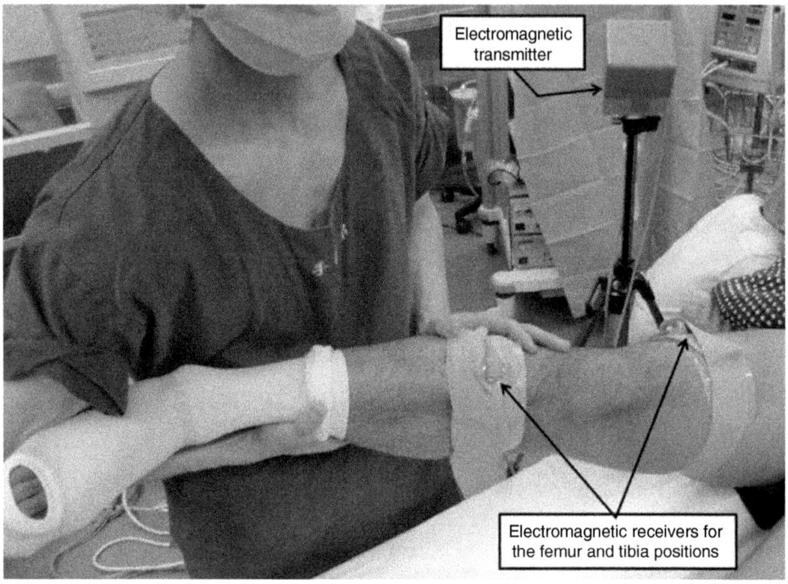

Fig. 22.3 Recording the knee kinematics data during the pivot-shift test

Fact Box
- Electromagnetic measurement system can measure 6 degrees-of-freedom knee kinematics during the pivot-shift test with a high sampling rate.
- The tibial anterior translation and the tibial acceleration during the pivot-shift test can be calculated from the 6 degrees-of-freedom knee kinematics data.

Conclusion

The electromagnetic tracking system can be used to monitor the 6 degrees-of-freedom knee kinematics during the pivot-shift test. Using this system, increased tibial anterior translation during the pivot-shift test can be observed in the pivot-shift-positive knees, while boosted acceleration of the following tibial reduction can also be monitored. The electromagnetic system can be used to provide quantitatively measurable data of the rotational laxity tested by the pivot-shift test. The measured laxity can be used to consider the surgical options of the ACL reconstruction, such as single-bundle, double-bundle, and augmentation procedure for partial tears or additional lateral tenodesis. At the same time, such objective measurements can provide fair comparison between different types of the ACL treatments for research purposes and to improve outcomes for patients.

References

1. Adachi N, Ochi M, Uchio Y et al (2004) Reconstruction of the anterior cruciate ligament. Single- versus double-bundle multistranded hamstring tendons. J Bone Joint Surg Br 86(4):515–520
2. Allum R, Jones D, Mowbray MA et al (1984) Triaxial electrogoniometric examination of the pivot shift sign for rotatory instability of the knee. Clin Orthop Relat Res 183:144–146
3. Andersson C, Gillquist J (1990) Instrumented testing for evaluation of sagittal knee laxity. Clin Orthop Relat Res 256:178–184
4. Araki D, Kuroda R, Kubo S et al (2011) A prospective randomised study of anatomical single-bundle versus double-bundle anterior cruciate ligament reconstruction: quantitative evaluation using an electromagnetic measurement system. Int Orthop 35(3):439–446
5. Bedi A, Musahl V, O'Loughlin P et al (2010) A comparison of the effect of central anatomical single-bundle anterior cruciate ligament reconstruction and double-bundle anterior cruciate ligament reconstruction on pivot-shift kinematics. Am J Sports Med 38(9):1788–1794
6. Bignozzi S, Zaffagnini S, Lopomo N et al (2010) Clinical relevance of static and dynamic tests after anatomical double-bundle ACL reconstruction. Knee Surg Sports Traumatol Arthrosc 18(1):37–42

7. Bull AM, Earnshaw PH, Smith A et al (2002) Intraoperative measurement of knee kinematics in reconstruction of the anterior cruciate ligament. J Bone Joint Surg Br 84(7):1075–1081
8. Daniel DM, Stone ML, Dobson BE (1994) Fate of the ACL-injured patient. A prospective outcome study. Am J Sports Med 22(5):632–644
9. Daniel DM, Malcom LL, Losse G et al (1985) Instrumented measurement of anterior laxity of the knee. J Bone Joint Surg Am 67(5):720–726
10. Ferretti A, Conteduca F, De Carli A et al (1991) Osteoarthritis of the knee after ACL reconstruction. Int Orthop 15(4):367–371
11. Galway HR, MacIntosh DL (1980) The lateral pivot shift: a symptom and sign of anterior cruciate ligament insufficiency. Clin Orthop Relat Res 147:45–50
12. Ganko A, Engebretsen L, Ozer H (2000) The rolimeter: a new arthrometer compared with the KT-1000. Knee Surg Sports Traumatol Arthrosc 8(1):36–39
13. Gillquist J, Messner K (1995) Instrumented analysis of the pivot shift phenomenon after reconstruction of the anterior cruciate ligament. Int J Sports Med 16(7):484–488
14. Grood ES, Suntay WJ (1983) A joint coordinate system for the clinical description of three-dimensional motions: application to the knee. J Biomech Eng 105(2):136–144
15. Hoshino Y, Kuroda R, Nagamune K et al (2007) In vivo measurement of the pivot-shift test in the anterior cruciate ligament-deficient knee using an electromagnetic device. Am J Sports Med 35(7):1098–1104
16. Hoshino Y, Kuroda R, Nagamune K et al (2012) Optimal measurement of clinical rotational test for evaluating anterior cruciate ligament insufficiency. Knee Surg Sports Traumatol Arthrosc 20(7):1323–1330
17. Hoshino Y, Araujo P, Ahlden M et al (2013) Quantitative evaluation of the pivot shift by image analysis using the iPad. Knee Surg Sports Traumatol Arthrosc 21(4):975–980
18. Irrgang JJ, Anderson AF, Boland AL et al (2001) Development and validation of the international knee documentation committee subjective knee form. Am J Sports Med 29(5):600–613
19. Irrgang JJ, Bost JE, Fu FH (2009) Re: outcome of single-bundle versus double-bundle reconstruction of the anterior cruciate ligament: a meta-analysis. Am J Sports Med 37(2):421–422; author reply 422
20. Jakob RP, Staubli HU, Deland JT (1987) Grading the pivot shift. Objective tests with implications for treatment. J Bone Joint Surg Br 69(2):294–299
21. Jarvela T, Moisala AS, Sihvonen R et al (2008) Double-bundle anterior cruciate ligament reconstruction using hamstring autografts and bioabsorbable interference screw fixation: prospective, randomized, clinical study with 2-year results. Am J Sports Med 36(2):290–297
22. Jonsson H, Riklund-Ahlstrom K, Lind J (2004) Positive pivot shift after ACL reconstruction predicts later osteoarthrosis: 63 patients followed 5–9 years after surgery. Acta Orthop Scand 75(5):594–599
23. Kanamori A, Zeminski J, Rudy TW (2002) The effect of axial tibial torque on the function of the anterior cruciate ligament: a biomechanical study of a simulated pivot shift test. Arthroscopy 18(4):394–398
24. Kocher MS, Steadman JR, Briggs KK, et al (2004) Relationships between objective assessment of ligament stability and subjective assessment of symptoms and function after anterior cruciate ligament reconstruction. Am J Sports Med 32(3):629–634
25. Kondo E, Yasuda K, Azuma H et al (2008) Prospective clinical comparisons of anatomic double-bundle versus single-bundle anterior cruciate ligament reconstruction procedures in 328 consecutive patients. Am J Sports Med 36(9):1675–1687
26. Kondo E, Merican AM, Yasuda K et al (2010) Biomechanical comparisons of knee stability after anterior cruciate ligament reconstruction between 2 clinically available transtibial procedures: anatomic double bundle versus single bundle. Am J Sports Med 38(7):1349–1358
27. Kubo S, Muratsu H, Yoshiya S et al (2007) Reliability and usefulness of a new in vivo measurement system of the pivot shift. Clin Orthop Relat Res 454:54–58
28. Kuroda R, Hoshino Y, Kubo S et al (2012) Similarities and differences of diagnostic manual tests for anterior cruciate ligament insufficiency: a global survey and kinematics assessment. Am J Sports Med 40(1): 91–99
29. Kuroda R, Hoshino Y, Araki D et al (2012) Quantitative measurement of the pivot shift, reliability, and clinical applications. Knee Surg Sports Traumatol Arthrosc 20(4):686–691
30. Labbe DR, de Guise JA, Mezghani N et al (2010) Feature selection using a principal component analysis of the kinematics of the pivot shift phenomenon. J Biomech 43(16):3080–3084
31. Logan MC, Williams A, Lavelle J et al (2004) Tibiofemoral kinematics following successful anterior cruciate ligament reconstruction using dynamic multiple resonance imaging. Am J Sports Med 32(4):984–992
32. Loh JC, Fukuda Y, Tsuda E et al (2003) Knee stability and graft function following anterior cruciate ligament reconstruction: Comparison between 11 o'clock and 10 o'clock femoral tunnel placement. 2002 Richard O'Connor Award paper. Arthroscopy 19(3):297–304
33. Lopomo N, Zaffagnini S, Signorelli C et al (2012) An original clinical methodology for non-invasive assessment of pivot-shift test. Comput Methods Biomech Biomed Engin 15(12):1323–1328
34. Losee RE (1983) Concepts of the pivot shift. Clin Orthop Relat Res 172:45–51
35. Mae T, Shino K, Miyama T et al (2001) Single- versus two-femoral socket anterior cruciate ligament reconstruction technique: Biomechanical analysis using a robotic simulator. Arthroscopy 17(7):708–716
36. Maeyama A, Hoshino Y, Debandi A et al (2011) Evaluation of rotational instability in the anterior cruciate ligament deficient knee using triaxial accelerom-

eter: a biomechanical model in porcine knees. Knee Surg Sports Traumatol Arthrosc 19(8):1233–1238
37. Matsumoto H (1990) Mechanism of the pivot shift. J Bone Joint Surg Br 72(5):816–821
38. Meredick RB, Vance KJ, Appleby D et al (2008) Outcome of single-bundle versus double-bundle reconstruction of the anterior cruciate ligament: a meta-analysis. Am J Sports Med 36(7):1414–1421
39. Muneta T, Koga H, Mochizuki T et al (2007) A prospective randomized study of 4-strand semitendinosus tendon anterior cruciate ligament reconstruction comparing single-bundle and double-bundle techniques. Arthroscopy 23(6):618–628
40. Musahl V, Voos JE, O'Loughlin PF et al (2010) Comparing stability of different single- and double-bundle anterior cruciate ligament reconstruction techniques: a cadaveric study using navigation. Arthroscopy 26(9 Suppl):S41–S48
41. Noyes FR, Grood ES, Cummings JF et al (1991) An analysis of the pivot shift phenomenon. The knee motions and subluxations induced by different examiners. Am J Sports Med 19(2):148–155
42. Oliver JH, Coughlin LP (1987) Objective knee evaluation using the genucom knee analysis system. Clinical implications. Am J Sports Med 15(6):571–578
43. Plaweski S, Grimaldi M, Courvoisier A et al (2011) Intraoperative comparisons of knee kinematics of double-bundle versus single-bundle anterior cruciate ligament reconstruction. Knee Surg Sports Traumatol Arthrosc 19(8):1277–1286
44. Ristanis S, Giakas G, Papageorgiou CD, et al (2003) The effects of anterior cruciate ligament reconstruction on tibial rotation during pivoting after descending stairs. Knee Surg Sports Traumatol Arthrosc 11(6):360–365
45. Schuster AJ, McNicholas MJ, Wachtl SW, et al (2004) A new mechanical testing device for measuring anteroposterior knee laxity. Am J Sports Med 32(7):1731–1735
46. Siebold R, Dehler C, Ellert T (2008) Prospective randomized comparison of double-bundle versus single-bundle anterior cruciate ligament reconstruction. Arthroscopy 24(2):137–145
47. Slocum DB, James SL, Larson RL et al (1976) Clinical test for anterolateral rotary instability of the knee. Clin Orthop Relat Res 118:63–69
48. Snyder-Mackler L, Fitzgerald GK, Bartolozzi AR 3rd et al (1997) The relationship between passive joint laxity and functional outcome after anterior cruciate ligament injury. Am J Sports Med 25(2):191–195
49. Tashman S, Collon D, Anderson K et al (2004) Abnormal rotational knee motion during running after anterior cruciate ligament reconstruction. Am J Sports Med 32(4):975–983
50. Torg JS, Conrad W, Kalen V (1976) Clinical diagnosis of anterior cruciate ligament instability in the athlete. Am J Sports Med 4(2):84–93
51. Tsai AG, Wijdicks CA, Walsh MP et al (2010) Comparative kinematic evaluation of all-inside single-bundle and double-bundle anterior cruciate ligament reconstruction: a biomechanical study. Am J Sports Med 38(2):263–272
52. Weiss JR, Irrgang JJ, Sawhney R et al (1990) A functional assessment of anterior cruciate ligament deficiency in an acute and clinical setting. J Orthop Sports Phys Ther 11(8):372–373
53. Yagi M, Wong EK, Kanamori A, et al (2004) Biomechanical analysis of an anatomic anterior cruciate ligament reconstruction. Am J Sports Med 30(5):660–666
54. Yagi M, Kuroda R, Nagamune K et al (2007) Double-bundle ACL reconstruction can improve rotational stability. Clin Orthop Relat Res 454:100–107
55. Yasuda K, Kondo E, Ichiyama H et al (2006) Clinical evaluation of anatomic double-bundle anterior cruciate ligament reconstruction procedure using hamstring tendon grafts: comparisons among 3 different procedures. Arthroscopy 22(3):240–251

Quantifying the "Feel" of the Pivot Shift

23

Nicola Lopomo and Stefano Zaffagnini

Contents

N. Lopomo, PhD (✉)
Dipartimento di Ingegneria dell'Informazione, Università degli Studi di Brescia, Via Branze, 38, Brescia, BS 25123, Italy

Laboratorio di Biomeccanica e Innovazione Tecnologica, Istituto Ortopedico Rizzoli, Via di Barbiano, 1/10, Bologna, BO 40136, Italy
e-mail: n.lopomo@biomec.ior.it

S. Zaffagnini, MD
Laboratorio di Biomeccanica e Innovazione Tecnologica, Istituto Ortopedico Rizzoli, Via di Barbiano, 1/10, Bologna, BO 40136, Italy

Dipartimento di Scienze Biomediche e Neuromotorie, Università degli Studi di Bologna, Via Pupilli, 1, Bologna, BO 40136, Italy

23.1 Introduction

The clinical assessment of the knee joint is considered a mandatory step during the diagnostic phase of anterior cruciate ligament (ACL) injury, as well as in the evaluation process of surgical outcomes after reconstruction. In this regard, various physical and clinical tests have been used to date in the outpatient setting [7, 29, 31, 57, 61]. More specifically, in the clinical practice concerning ACL injury, both *static* and *dynamic* joint laxity are usually evaluated [11].

In mechanical terms, *statics* is related to the analysis of loads and torque on physical systems in a state of equilibrium. However, in the clinical setting, *static* instead refers to the fact that the evaluation occurs only in one plane or in one direction with known loads and without considering accelerations or changes in velocity due to coupled stress conditions applied to the limb. Static laxity can be measured, in general, by means of a direct evaluation of abnormal increased joint values of translation or rotation, applying known loads and measuring the corresponding displacement and rotation. For instance, static laxity is evaluated through Lachman and drawer tests in the sagittal plane (Fig. 23.1). The problem of evaluating static laxity is that different structures can contribute at different levels to the overall restraining force (i.e., primary and secondary restraints). Therefore, it can prove difficult to clearly identify which ligament or structures are injured. Moreover, given that this type

V. Musahl et al. (eds.), *Rotatory Knee Instability*, DOI 10.1007/978-3-319-32070-0_23

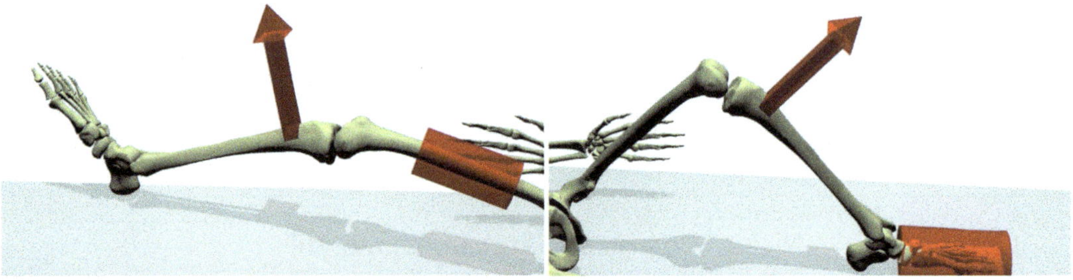

Fig. 23.1 Examples of static laxity: Lachman (*left*) and drawer (*right*)

of test is considered to be static only, it is impossible to demonstrate the joint's functional behavior by applying proper stress conditions.

By comparison to statics, *dynamics* is related to the study of forces and torques, and their effect on motion. Isaac Newton defined the fundamental physical laws, which govern dynamics. In particular, his second law of motion correlates to applied forces and obtained accelerations through the term "mass." Here, from a clinical perspective, dynamic laxity of the knee (from the patient's perspective, often referred to as instability in the form of "giving way") results in one of the most common clinical symptoms associated with ACL injury. "Dynamic" is appropriate in the sense that the limb is subjected to varying loads and torques, which leads to an overall stress condition that is supported by the involved structures. For these reasons, several clinical tests have been implemented to mimic these symptoms by controlling loads/movements of the joint, thereby recreating the "giving way" phenomenon.

Fact Box 1

In orthopedics, *statics* is related to linear or angular displacement while maintaining the joint in a condition of "equilibrium," whereas *dynamics* is associated with complex loading conditions, i.e., forces and moments applied to the joint.

Dynamic assessment represents the basis of the analysis in terms of rotatory knee laxity and the contribution to the clinical examination related to the "pivot shift" test. In fact, dynamic instability is often highlighted clinically via the pivot shift test, which results from complex rotational and translational loading applied to the tibiofemoral joint (Fig. 23.2).

In the 1970s–1980s, Slocum and Jakob were one of the first who underlined the necessity of systematically highlighting anterolateral instability of the knee, i.e., when the lateral tibial plateau subluxates anteriorly on the femur [27, 28, 62]. This subluxation was found to be followed by a reduction phenomenon, which is felt as the knee passes through 25°–40° of flexion: the pivot shift phenomenon! This "clunking" phenomenon was then identified as one of the classic clinical signs of ACL insufficiency.

However, this sudden "clunk" or "thud" that occurs when the iliotibial tract reduces the lateral femoral condyle is neither simple nor easily clinically identified. Moreover, it is not easily quantified or measured. For these reasons, the examiners experience and perception of the "clunk" still plays a fundamental role in the clinical assessment. During the last several years, several technologies have been introduced to quantify the pivot shift test.

23.2 Biomechanical Insights of the "Feel"

From a biomechanical perspective, the pivot shift phenomenon has been widely investigated due to its inherent importance to the behavior of the knee joint.

Using both in vivo and in vitro conditions, several studies have been performed in an effort to highlight kinematic patterns and the influence of joint anatomy and ligamentous structures as a

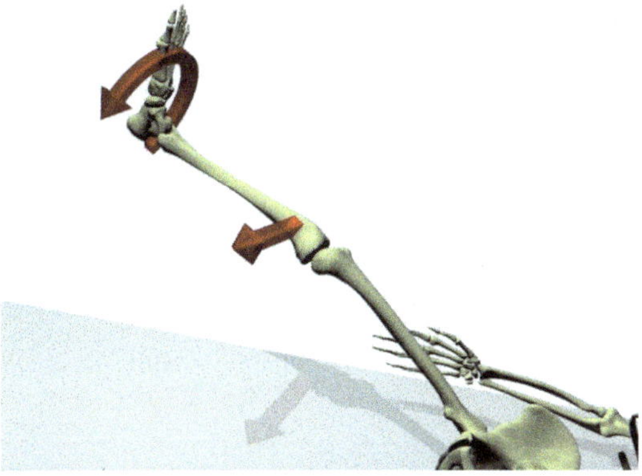

Fig. 23.2 Lateral pivot shift test [21]. Internal rotation and valgus stress are highlighted. As the stress is applied, the knee is slowly flexed

means of eliciting the phenomenon [6, 20, 28, 36, 37, 51, 55]. All of these factors have been reported as fundamental to understanding the means by which this phenomenon can be "felt" by the examiner and how the "feel" can be translated to enhance the perception of what is happening within the knee joint during the specific maneuver of pivot shift test.

In terms of kinematics, the pivot shift phenomenon presents both a rotational component of the tibia about its long axis and a translational component related to the anterior subluxation of the lateral tibial plateau, followed by its sudden reduction (Fig. 23.3). Intuitively, both of these components are linked [11, 12, 14].

As reported in a biomechanical study by Bull and Amis, the pivot shift is most probably caused by a functional insufficiency of primary restraints to anterior displacement of the lateral tibial plateau and to internal rotation of the tibia [11, 14]. An ACL injury appears to represent a necessary condition for the pivot shift to occur [22, 33, 52, 57, 59]. Moreover, injuries located on the lateral structures, including the iliotibial band, can also contribute to elicitation of the phenomenon, whereas tears of the medial collateral ligament can reduce it, altering the rotatory pattern of the knee [11, 14].

Moreover, also the complex anatomy of the knee joint can modify findings related to the pivot shift. For instance, several studies have reported how sudden movement during this phenomenon is due not only to the lack of ligamentous constraint but also to the complex interaction between the geometry of the knee and applied torques [36, 55].

Fact Box 2
The pivot shift phenomenon is related to the complex interaction among the anatomy of the knee, the native and residual function of the ligamentous structures and the applied loads.

For these reasons, the "feel" is fundamental in terms of both eliciting the phenomenon and qualitatively grading the pivot shift. Recent understanding that the "feel" is strictly associated to the amount of "clunk" that the knee presents under the maneuver has been quantified by means of systems and devices able to measure the acceleration and velocity reached by the tibia during the reduction phase.

23.3 Clinical Perspective of the "Feel"

The pivot shift test has been historically utilized in the clinical evaluation of ACL deficiency and the assessment of knee laxity [21, 27, 28], including, for instance, in the International Knee Documentation Committee (IKDC) score [24]. The result of the pivot shift test is correlated with reduced sporting activity and a complete or partial tear of the ACL [21, 28]. These findings have shown how this dynamic maneuver is correlated to the "feel" that the patient perceives in loading conditions of his/her joint.

From a historical perspective, this clinical necessity of mimicking these specific loading conditions led to the definition of several types of tests able to stress the joint and elicit the pivot shift phenomenon, thereby defining the dynamic laxity of the joint.

Following this concept related to knee joint dynamics, Slocum et al. [62] described a physical test intended to describe anterolateral instability of the knee as early as 1976. In 1979, using an

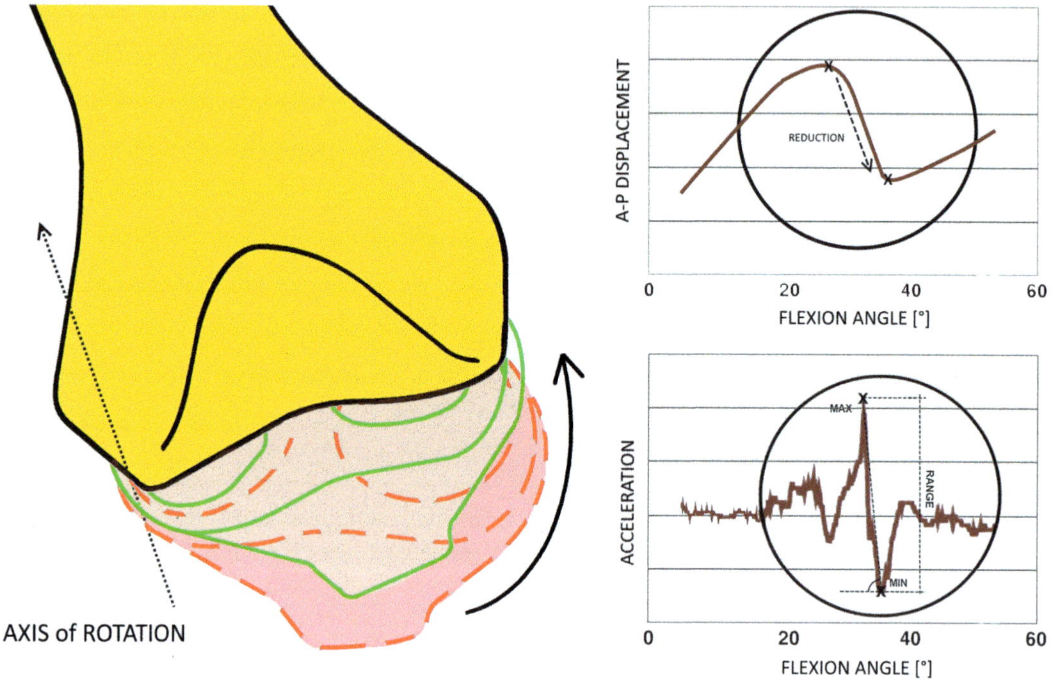

Fig. 23.3 Kinematic patterns of the pivot shift phenomenon. *On left side*: after subluxation (*red dashed line*), the lateral plateau reduces (*green continuous line*); the coupled rotation happens around a specific axis [11, 14]. *On the right side*: an example of kinematic analysis with anteroposterior displacement obtained during reduction and the corresponding acceleration

in vitro experiment, Fetto and Marshall [20] defined the pathomechanism that is necessary to produce the pivot shift sign, demonstrating that it was correlated to a tear of the ACL. This specific phenomenon was subsequently more precisely identified by Galway and MacIntosh in 1980 [21] as the "lateral pivot shift" and demonstrated the subluxation of the lateral tibial plateau and the sudden "clunk" that occurred as the iliotibial tract reduced the lateral femoral condyle. Larson [44] highlighted in 1983 the physical tests used in the diagnosis of the anterolateral rotatory instability (ALRI) related to ACL deficiency. In the same year, Losee [51] demonstrated how the pivot shift is a sign of ACL, as well as lateral and posterolateral capsular deficiency, clinically demonstrated by a subluxation or reduction combined with an impingement of the lateral compartment of the knee. All these studies were based on the ability of catching the sudden reduction of the tibia during the maneuver: the "feel" of the pivot shift!

Moreover, the capacity of correctly defining this "feel" associated with ACL insufficiency has since been analyzed in further detail. Lucie et al. [53] assessed the reliability of the pivot shift test in patients with acute ACL injuries under anesthesia. Losee [52], who defined a specific maneuver, described how the pivot shift is fundamental in demonstrating that knee instability is associated with chronic injuries. In 1986, Sandberg et al. [60] highlighted the problem of limited clinical reliability of the pivot shift test compared with the Lachman test and anterior drawer sign. They analyzed 182 knees with ligamentous injuries and emphasized its clinical usefulness only under anesthesia. Conversely, Katz and Fingeroth [31] reported high sensitivity and specificity of the pivot shift test in detecting an ACL injury, regardless of comparison with the Lachman or anterior drawer tests, both in acute and chronic lesions. These different findings may reflect different techniques which may be used to perform the pivot shift: a more rigorous or "dynamic" technique may cause discomfort and consequent muscle spasm, which contribute to reduce the sensitivity of the tester to grade the "feel."

For this reason, the importance of the pivot shift in identifying knee laxity was studied by Jakob et al. [28], who developed a joint laxity test by simply providing evidence of the existence of ACL deficiency to an effective grading of the phenomenon. They defined three grades of the pivot shift based on objective measurement of the AP displacements of each of the medial and lateral condyles, supported by radiographic evaluation. This kind of grading was not yet thought to be correlated to the "feel" of that "clunk" that happens during the joint reduction. For this reason, the historical grading system is presently of limited value [56].

Scholten et al. [61] also described the high predictive value of the pivot shift test to identify an ACL lesion compared with the good negative value of the Lachman test. In 2006, Ostrowski et al. [57] and Prins et al. [59] reported, using arthrotomy and arthroscopy as reference standards, that the Lachman test had a higher sensitivity than the drawer and pivot shift test, while the pivot shift test had a higher specificity than the drawer and Lachman tests. Benjaminse et al. [7] performed a meta-analysis on the clinical diagnosis of ACL rupture and identified the Lachman test as the most valid test, showing good specificity and sensitivity, whereas the pivot shift revealed the highest specificity, but poor sensitivity, both in the acute or chronic conditions. The effects on the pivot shift phenomenon conferred by anesthesia or pathology other than an isolated complete tear of the ACL were investigated by Donaldson et al. [19]. They specifically showed that the accuracy of the pivot shift test in detecting an ACL tear decreased dramatically without anesthesia. They also found that the pivot shift sign was reduced in the presence of a rupture of the medial collateral ligament or if the ACL was only partially ruptured. These results were later confirmed by Harilainen et al. [23], who performed laxity assessments on 350 consecutive patients by means of clinical examination and examination under anesthesia. They described the importance of performing the pivot shift test under anesthesia in order to detect the anterolateral rotatory instability arising from acute ligamentous injuries.

Fact Box 3

There are several factors that can reduce the sensitivity in quantifying the "feel" during pivot shift maneuver: associated lesions, muscular guarding, and limb position.

In addition to anesthesia, there are several other parameters which can potentially influence the pivot shift sign and subsequent grading. Bach et al. [6] proposed a modified clinical pivot shift test, which was able to account for the position of the hip and rotation of the tibia. They found that the degree of pivot shift correlated strongly with the position of the hip, regardless of tibial rotation; hip abduction produced a higher degree of pivot shift. This is unexpected, because the sudden reduction of motion of the tibia during the pivot shift is caused partly by the tension in the iliotibial tract, a structure which is slackened by hip abduction. In 1992, Kujala et al. [36] analyzed the influence of anatomical parameters on the pivot shift test. Specifically, the authors reported good correlation between the convexity of the lateral tibial plateau, the pivot shift test, and the history of unexpected knee instability of the patients. In 1993, Terry et al. [64] analyzed the influence of injuries of the iliotibial tract in combination with ACL lesions and found that they were highly correlated with the variation in grades of anterior tibial translation instabilities.

Kim and Kim [33] subsequently analyzed the reliability of the anterior drawer, Lachman and pivot shift tests in detecting chronic ACL injury in 147 patients under anesthesia. The Lachman and pivot shift tests were the most sensitive for the diagnosis of chronic ACL injuries, but the outcome of the pivot shift test was more influenced by other factors, including reattachment of the end of the torn ACL in combination with meniscal tears. Kurosaka et al. [37] then confirmed the efficacy of the pivot shift maneuver to detect menis-

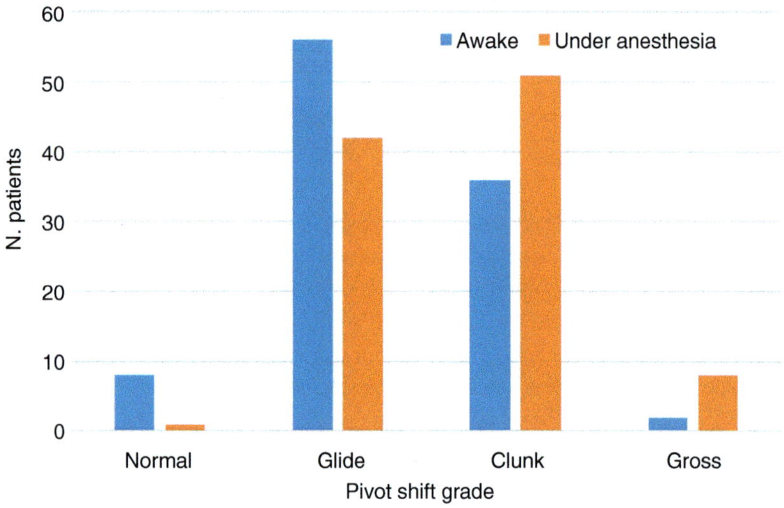

Fig. 23.4 Influence of anesthesia on pivot shift grading (unpublished materials, courtesy of ISAKOS PIVOT Study Group)

cal tears, by means of an axially loaded pivot shift test. The diagnostic value was high. Kocher et al. [34] reported that an objective measurement of anterior laxity using the Lachman test did not significantly correlate with any subjective evaluation, whereas the pivot shift test could be correlated significantly with subjective satisfaction, overall knee function, and sports participation. Later, Jain et al. [26] confirmed that the pivot shift test had the highest sensitivity and specificity to establish the diagnosis of an ACL lesion under anesthesia. Muscular guarding plays a fundamental role in the grading of the "feel" (Fig. 23.4).

The presence of a residual positive pivot shift sign during the follow-up period after ACL reconstruction was demonstrated by Jonsson et al. in 2004 to be a better predictor of development of osteoarthritis of the knee than an anteroposterior laxity assessment [30]. Moreover, Leitze et al. [45] showed that the presence of a pivot shift postoperatively was related to poor subjective evaluations by the patients and poor scoring outcomes, and Lie et al. [46] found residual "mini pivots" persisted at the conclusion of ACL reconstruction surgery, using electromagnetic sensors attached directly to the bones.

All of these studies have clearly underlined the importance of analyzing the presence of the pivot shift phenomenon in ACL functional insufficiency, keeping in mind all the factors that can influence the sensitivity of the test and its reliability. The scientific literature seems to support, from both a clinical and a biomechanical point of view, that that the pivot shift can present different characteristics that are associated to the "feel" perceived by the tester and to that "giving way" (i.e., the "clunk" highlighted during reduction) symptom perceived by the patient.

23.4 How to Quantitatively Catch the "Feel"

Although the pivot shift has been widely investigated, a lack of a systematic assessment and objective quantification of the exact pattern of motion components remains. The main problem is that the test itself is a combined loading of the joint, inducing movements in more than one degree of freedom during knee flexion-extension motion, which makes it difficult to derive a single quantitative parameter that is sufficient to synthetize the pivot shift test. Moreover, this measurement has to be strictly correlated with the clinical evaluation of the joint itself, which is associated with the "feel."

Nevertheless, the pivot shift test remains the most relevant test in the analysis of tibiofemoral knee dynamic laxity. Recent reviews [2, 42, 66] have all described the importance of the pivot shift maneuver in the assessment of ACL injuries in clinical practice and have acquired quantitative data. These reviews summarized the differences among descriptions of the clinical maneuver and the proposed pathomechanism of the phenomenon.

Historically, quantifying the pivot shift required complex systems requiring markers [16], footplates [3], robotic technology [18], and magnetic resonance imaging [63] which have been proposed. Moreover, navigation systems have been used to measure the kinematic components associated with the pivot shift phenomenon [32]. Colombet et al. used a navigation system to measure pivot shift kinematics before and after ACL reconstruction [15]. Lane et al. also used an optical navigation system to define the exact parameters of the pivot shift intraoperatively [43] and so have Lopomo et al. [49]. The pivot shift in vivo has also been investigated by using less-invasive electromagnetic devices [13, 25, 39], even if they presented with complicated equipment (wires, specific surgical instrumentation, and setup) and high costs that are incompatible with office practice.

Recently, the important feature to quantify the "feel" in the outpatient setting had led to the development of less-invasive methodologies able to directly measure the "clunk" of the joint during the reduction phase. In the last several years, substantial efforts have been made in order to establish noninvasive systems based on inertial sensors in quantifying the pivot shift test, thus allowing a quantitative assessment in both surgical and outpatient settings, where CAS technology still presents major limitations.

As a result of the use and development of noninvasive technologies, several parameters have been subsequently identified, as reported by Lopomo et al. [48]. Some of these parameters can be considered as directly correlated with the "feel," such as the acceleration and the velocity measured during joint reduction (Table 23.1).

Using a principal component analysis of the kinematics associated with the pivot shift phenomenon and extracting the most significant features, Labbe et al. [39] suggested that efforts to quantify the pivot shift should focus more on the velocity and acceleration of tibial translation and less on the traditionally accepted parameters related to posterior translation and external tibial rotation.

Table 23.1 Parameters reported by scientific literature and correlated to the "feel"

Acceleration	Peak of relative linear acceleration in anterior-posterior direction Peak of relative linear acceleration in mediolateral direction Peak of relative angular acceleration associated to internal-external rotation Peak of relative angular acceleration associated to varus-valgus rotation Peak of linear three-dimensional acceleration Peak of linear three-dimensional acceleration measured only on the tibia
Velocity	Peak of relative linear velocity in anterior-posterior direction Peak of relative linear velocity in mediolateral direction Peak of relative angular velocity associated to internal-external rotation Peak of relative angular velocity associated to varus-valgus rotation Peak of relative linear three-dimensional velocity

In greater detail, these parameters can be directly quantified by means of different technologies, specifically, accelerometers and gyroscopes, which are usually integrated in inertial sensors. These sensors can be used in a single mode (Fig. 23.5), as reported by Lopomo et al. [47, 50], or coupled (Fig. 23.6). In this latter modality, the tester is able to acquire information coming from both tibia and femur and thereby estimate the kinematic pattern during the maneuver.

Accelerometers were specifically used to directly measure the sudden "clunk" felt by the tester, whereas the gyroscope is able to define factors associated with the velocity reached by the limb during the test. Several recent studies have reported the use of single or coupled inertial sensors to quantify the pivot shift test. Expanding on this, an in vivo study by Lopomo et al. set the basis for the use of a single inertial sensor in quantifying the pivot shift test [47, 50], which

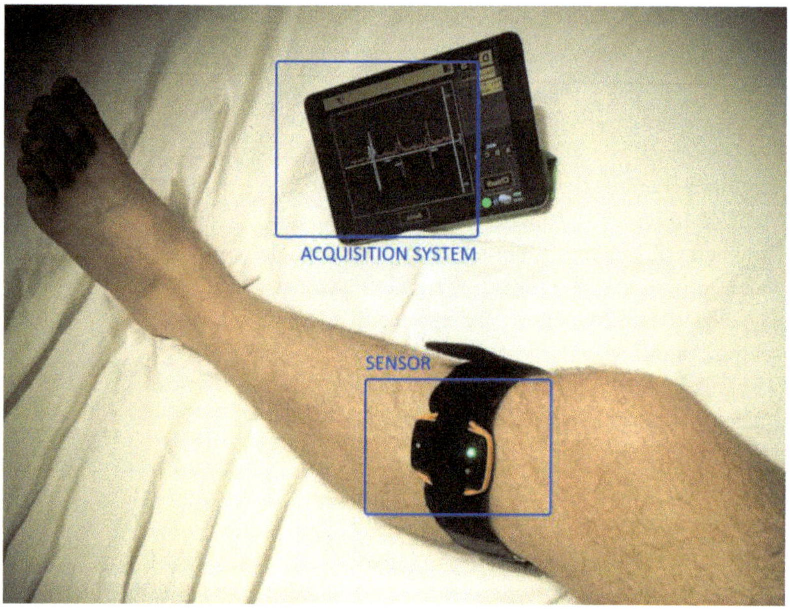

Fig. 23.5 Example of inertial sensor and acquisition system used in pivot shift assessment [47, 50]

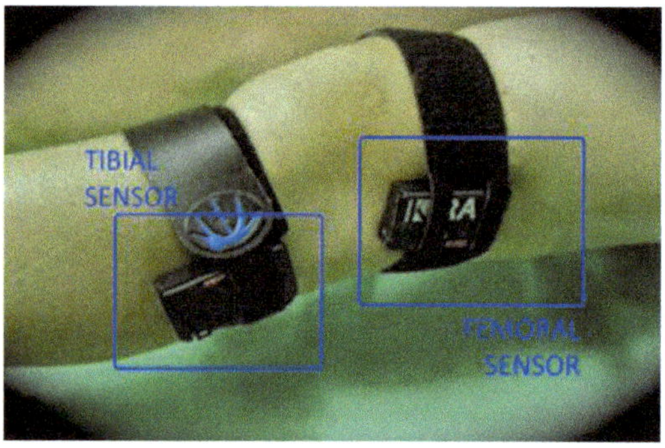

Fig. 23.6 Example of coupled inertial sensors

was followed by Berruto et al. [8] and Zaffagnini et al. [65]. Specifically, Maeyama et al. [54] and Debandi et al. [17] used a triaxial accelerometer in a porcine model to assess the rotational instability associated to ACL deficiency and reconstruction. Asai et al. [5] used the same methodology in an in vitro experimental study to describe the differences between single-bundle and over-the-top ACL reconstruction techniques, thus underlining the possibility to use this kind of technology even to appreciate differences in ACL reconstruction techniques. Extensive in vitro experiments by Ahldén et al. [1] and Araujo et al. [4] described that the clinical grading of the pivot shift test correlates best with tibial acceleration, more than with displacement of the lateral compartment, thus highlighting the importance of the "feel."

Since acceleration and velocity can take into account different aspects of joint behavior and test performance, both of these components were recently used to quantify and grade the pivot shift.

Kopf et al. [35] presented a new quantitative method for pivot shift grading based on coupled inertial sensors and a classification system based on acceleration parameters. In a cadaver study, Petrigliano et al. proposed measuring the tibial rotation during a simulated pivot shift maneuver by using a gyroscopic sensor [58]. Similarly, Borgstrom et al. reported the use of a gyroscopic sensor in an in vivo study to quantify tibial motion during the pivot shift test [9]. Labbe et al. used an inertial sensor coupling accelerometer and gyroscopes to improve the test outcome and variability [38]. The same group also proposed a first attempt of objectively grading the pivot shift phenomenon using a support vector machine based on acceleration and velocity data [40] and, more recently, reported the use of combined inertial and magnetic sensing to grade the phenomenon [41]. Furthermore, Borgstrom et al. [10] proposed a decision support system able to use these information sources summarized in 23 different parameters to predict pivot shift grade during preoperative testing.

Conclusions

The pivot shift phenomenon appears to represent two phenomena: one is related to the amount of displacement of the lateral compartment during subluxation, while the other is related to the "clunk" perceived during the reduction phase. These two phenomena have been reflected in the technologies and methodologies used to quantify the phenomenon itself.

This chapter describes several methodologies and technologies utilized in analyzing and quantifying the "feel" related to the pivot shift phenomenon. All of these methods concern the possibility of measuring the "clunk" that occurs during reduction phase, which is more related to the perception that the tester has of the phenomenon by using only his own hands. More specifically, in all of the reported in vivo studies – where the dynamics of the limb can be properly controlled and acquired – the pivot shift should be correctly considered a dynamic maneuver, and accordingly specific dynamic parameters, such as velocity and acceleration, should be used in its overall assessment.

It is worth mentioning that all these methods have specific advantages and disadvantages, but clinicians continue to seek a standardized, "gold standard" method by which dynamic laxity can be quantified. The work is ongoing …

Fact Box 4

Although the concept of "feel" can be associated with acceleration and velocity and appear to be related to a strictly subjective assessment, only the widespread adoption of a standardized pivot shift maneuver and a common measurement method will allow meaningful comparison outcomes obtained during ACL assessment.

The "feel" perceived by the tester during the execution of pivot shift maneuver is one of the main motivations that has led to the development of a novel set of noninvasive methodologies and technologies able to quantify that phenomenon in terms of acceleration and velocity, i.e., joint dynamics. These systems have allowed both preoperative and postoperative assessment of the injured joint with respect to the contralateral one, which is fundamental in the clinical assessment of ACL injury. These methodologies are contributing to improving the treatment and to individualize the surgical and rehabilitative approaches.

References

1. Ahldén M, Araujo P, Hoshino Y, Samuelsson K, Middleton KK, Nagamune K, Karlsson J, Musahl V (2012) Clinical grading of the pivot shift test correlates best with tibial acceleration. Knee Surg Sport Traumatol Arthrosc 20:708–712
2. Ahldén M, Hoshino Y, Samuelsson K, Araujo P, Musahl V, Karlsson J (2012) Dynamic knee laxity measurement devices. Knee Surg Sport Traumatol Arthrosc 20:621–632
3. Amis AA, Bull AMJ, Lie DTT (2005) Biomechanics of rotational instability and anatomic anterior cruciate ligament reconstruction. Oper Tech Orthop 15:29–35
4. Araujo PH, Ahlden M, Hoshino Y, Muller B, Moloney G, Fu FH, Musahl V (2012) Comparison of three non-invasive quantitative measurement systems for the pivot shift test. Knee Surg Sport Traumatol Arthrosc 20:692–697
5. Asai S, Maeyama A, Hoshino Y, Goto B, Celentano U, Moriyama S, Smolinski P, Fu FH (2014) A comparison of dynamic rotational knee instability between anatomic single-bundle and over-the-top anterior cruciate ligament reconstruction using triaxial accelerometry. Knee Surg Sport Traumatol Arthrosc 22:972–978
6. Bach BR, Warren RF, Wickiewicz TL (1988) The pivot shift phenomenon: Results and description of a modified clinical test for anterior cruciate ligament insufficiency. Am J Sports Med 16:571–576
7. Benjaminse A, Gokeler A, van der Schans CP (2006) Clinical diagnosis of an anterior cruciate ligament rupture: a meta-analysis. J Orthop Sports Phys Ther 36:267–288
8. Berruto M, Uboldi F, Gala L, Marelli B, Albisetti W (2013) Is triaxial accelerometer reliable in the evaluation and grading of knee pivot-shift phenomenon? Knee Surg Sport Traumatol Arthrosc 21:981–985
9. Borgstrom PH, Markolf KL, Foster B, Petrigliano FA, McAllister DR (2013) Use of a gyroscope sensor to

quantify tibial motions during a pivot shift test. Knee Surg Sport Traumatol Arthrosc 22:2064–2069
10. Borgstrom PH, Markolf KL, Wang Y, Xu X, Yang PR, Joshi NB, Yeranosian MG, Petrigliano FA, Hame SL, Kaiser WJ, McAllister DR (2015) Use of inertial sensors to predict pivot-shift grade and diagnose an ACL injury during preoperative testing. Am J Sports Med 43(4):857–864
11. Bull AM, Amis AA (1998) Knee joint motion: description and measurement. Proc Inst Mech Eng H 212:357–372
12. Bull AM, Andersen HN, Basso O, Targett J, Amis AA (1999) Incidence and mechanism of the pivot shift. An in vitro study. Clin Orthop Relat Res 363:219–231
13. Bull AMJ, Earnshaw PH, Smith A, Katchburian MV, Hassan ANA, Amis AA (2002) Intraoperative measurement of knee kinematics in reconstruction of the anterior cruciate ligament. J Bone Joint Surg Br 84:1075–1081
14. Bull AMJ, Amis AA (1998) The pivot-shift phenomenon: a clinical and biomechanical perspective. Knee 5:141–158
15. Colombet PD, Robinson JR (2008) Computer-assisted, anatomic, double-bundle anterior cruciate ligament reconstruction. Arthroscopy 24:1152–1160
16. Csintalan RP, Ehsan A, McGarry MH, Fithian DF, Lee TQ (2006) Biomechanical and anatomical effects of an external rotational torque applied to the knee: a cadaveric study. Am J Sports Med 34:1623–1629
17. Debandi A, Maeyama A, Hoshino Y, Asai S, Goto B, Smolinski P, Fu FH (2013) The effect of tunnel placement on rotational stability after ACL reconstruction: evaluation with use of triaxial accelerometry in a porcine model. Knee Surg Sport Traumatol Arthrosc 21:589–595
18. Diermann N, Schumacher T, Schanz S, Raschke MJ, Petersen W, Zantop T (2009) Rotational instability of the knee: internal tibial rotation under a simulated pivot shift test. Arch Orthop Trauma Surg 129:353–358
19. Donaldson WF, Warren RF, Wickiewicz T (1985) A comparison of acute anterior cruciate ligament examinations: initial versus examination under anesthesia. Am J Sports Med 13:5–10
20. Fetto JF, Marshall JL (1979) Injury to the anterior cruciate ligament producing the pivot-shift sign. J Bone Joint Surg Am 61:710–714
21. Galway HR, MacIntosh DL (1980) The lateral pivot shift: a symptom and sign of anterior cruciate ligament insufficiency. Clin Orthop Relat Res 147:45–50
22. Graham GP, Johnson S, Dent CM, Fairclough JA (1991) Comparison of clinical tests and the KT1000 in the diagnosis of anterior cruciate ligament rupture. Br J Sports Med 25(2):96–97
23. Harilainen A (1987) Evaluation of knee instability in acute ligamentous injuries. Ann Chir Gynaecol 76:269–273
24. Hefti E, Müller W, Jakob RP, Stäubli HU (1993) Evaluation of knee ligament injuries with the IKDC form. Knee Surg Sport Traumatol Arthrosc 1:226–234
25. Hoshino Y, Kuroda R, Nagamune K, Yagi M, Mizuno K, Yamaguchi M, Muratsu H, Yoshiya S, Kurosaka M (2007) In vivo measurement of the pivot-shift test in the anterior cruciate ligament-deficient knee using an electromagnetic device. Am J Sports Med 35:1098–1104
26. Jain DK, Amaravati R, Sharma G (2009) Evaluation of the clinical signs of anterior cruciate ligament and meniscal injuries. Indian J Orthop 43:375–378
27. Jakob RP, Hassler H, Staeubli HU (1981) Observations on rotatory instability of the lateral compartment of the knee. Experimental studies on the functional anatomy and the pathomechanism of the true and the reversed pivot shift sign. Acta Orthop Scand Suppl 191:1–32
28. Jakob RP, Stäubli HU, Deland JT (1987) Grading the pivot shift. Objective tests with implications for treatment. J Bone Joint Surg Br 69:294–299
29. Jensen K (1990) Manual laxity tests for anterior cruciate ligament injuries. J Orthop Sports Phys Ther 11:474–481
30. Jonsson H, Riklund-Ahlström K, Lind J (2004) Positive pivot shift after ACL reconstruction predicts later osteoarthrosis: 63 patients followed 5-9 years after surgery. Acta Orthop Scand 75:594–599
31. Katz JW, Fingeroth RJ (1986) The diagnostic accuracy of ruptures of the anterior cruciate ligament comparing the Lachman test, the anterior drawer sign, and the pivot shift test in acute and chronic knee injuries. Am J Sports Med 14:88–91
32. Kendoff D, Citak M, Voos J, Pearle AD (2009) Surgical navigation in knee ligament reconstruction. Clin Sports Med 28:41–50
33. Kim SJ, Kim HK (1995) Reliability of the anterior drawer test, the pivot shift test, and the Lachman test. Clin Orthop Relat Res 317:237–242
34. Kocher MS, Steadman JR, Briggs KK, Sterett WI, Hawkins RJ (2004) Relationships between objective assessment of ligament stability and subjective assessment of symptoms and function after anterior cruciate ligament reconstruction. Am J Sports Med 32:629–634
35. Kopf S, Kauert R, Halfpaap J, Jung T, Becker R (2012) A new quantitative method for pivot shift grading. Knee Surg Sport Traumatol Arthrosc 20:718–723
36. Kujala UM, Nelimarkka O, Koskinen SK (1992) Relationship between the pivot shift and the configuration of the lateral tibial plateau. Arch Orthop Trauma Surg 111:228–229
37. Kurosaka M, Yagi M, Yoshiya S, Muratsu H, Mizuno K (1999) Efficacy of the axially loaded pivot shift test for the diagnosis of a meniscal tear. Int Orthop 23:271–274
38. Labbe DR, de Guise JA, Godbout V, Grimard G, Baillargeon D, Lavigne P, Fernandes J, Massé V, Ranger P, Hagemeister N (2011) Accounting for velocity of the pivot shift test manoeuvre decreases kinematic variability. Knee 18:88–93
39. Labbe DR, de Guise JA, Mezghani N, Godbout V, Grimard G, Baillargeon D, Lavigne P, Fernandes J, Ranger P, Hagemeister N (2010) Feature selection

using a principal component analysis of the kinematics of the pivot shift phenomenon. J Biomech 43:3080–3084
40. Labbe DR, de Guise JA, Mezghani N, Godbout V, Grimard G, Baillargeon D, Lavigne P, Fernandes J, Ranger P, Hagemeister N (2011) Objective grading of the pivot shift phenomenon using a support vector machine approach. J Biomech 44:1–5
41. Labbé DR, Li D, Grimard G, de Guise JA, Hagemeister N (2014) Quantitative pivot shift assessment using combined inertial and magnetic sensing. Knee Surg Sport Traumatol Arthrosc 23(8):2330–2338
42. Lane CG, Warren R, Pearle AD (2008) The pivot shift. J Am Acad Orthop Surg 16:679–688
43. Lane CG, Warren RF, Stanford FC, Kendoff D, Pearle AD (2008) In vivo analysis of the pivot shift phenomenon during computer navigated ACL reconstruction. Knee Surg Sport Traumatol Arthrosc 16:487–492
44. Larson RL (1983) Physical examination in the diagnosis of rotatory instability. Clin Orthop Relat Res 172:38–44
45. Leitze Z, Losee RE, Jokl P, Johnson TR, Feagin JA (2005) Implications of the pivot shift in the ACL-deficient knee. Clin Orthop Relat Res 436:229–236
46. Lie DTT, Bull AMJ, Amis AA (2007) Persistence of the mini pivot shift after anatomically placed anterior cruciate ligament reconstruction. Clin Orthop Relat Res 457:203–209
47. Lopomo N, Signorelli C, Bonanzinga T, Muccioli GMM, Visani A, Zaffagnini S (2012) Quantitative assessment of pivot-shift using inertial sensors. Knee Surg Sport Traumatol Arthrosc 20:713–717
48. Lopomo N, Zaffagnini S, Amis AA (2013) Quantifying the pivot shift test: a systematic review. Knee Surg Sport Traumatol Arthrosc 21:767–783
49. Lopomo N, Zaffagnini S, Bignozzi S, Visani A, Marcacci M (2010) Pivot-shift test: analysis and quantification of knee laxity parameters using a navigation system. J Orthop Res 28:164–169
50. Lopomo N, Zaffagnini S, Signorelli C, Bignozzi S, Giordano G, Marcheggiani Muccioli GM, Visani A (2011) An original clinical methodology for non-invasive assessment of pivot-shift test. Comput Methods Biomech Biomed Engin 15(12):1323–1328
51. Losee RE (1983) Concepts of the pivot shift. Clin Orthop Relat Res 172:45–51
52. Losee RE (1985) Diagnosis of chronic injury to the anterior cruciate ligament. Orthop Clin North Am 16:83–97
53. Lucie RS, Wiedel JD, Messner DG (1984) The acute pivot shift: clinical correlation. Am J Sports Med 12:189–191
54. Maeyama A, Hoshino Y, Debandi A, Kato Y, Saeki K, Asai S, Goto B, Smolinski P, Fu FH (2011) Evaluation of rotational instability in the anterior cruciate ligament deficient knee using triaxial accelerometer: a biomechanical model in porcine knees. Knee Surg Sport Traumatol Arthrosc 19:1233–1238
55. Matsumoto H (1990) Mechanism of the pivot shift. J Bone Joint Surg Br 72:816–821
56. Musahl V, Hoshino Y, Ahlden M, Araujo P, Irrgang JJ, Zaffagnini S, Karlsson J, Fu FH (2012) The pivot shift: a global user guide. Knee Surg Sport Traumatol Arthrosc 20:724–731
57. Ostrowski JA (2006) Accuracy of 3 diagnostic tests for anterior cruciate ligament tears. J Athl Train 41:120–121
58. Petrigliano FA, Borgstrom PH, Kaiser WJ, McAllister DR, Markolf KL (2014) Measurements of tibial rotation during a simulated pivot shift manoeuvre using a gyroscopic sensor. Knee Surg Sport Traumatol Arthrosc 23(8):2237–2243
59. Prins M (2006) The Lachman test is the most sensitive and the pivot shift the most specific test for the diagnosis of ACL rupture. Aust J Physiother 52:66
60. Sandberg R, Balkfors B, Henricson A, Westlin N (1986) Stability tests in knee ligament injuries. Arch Orthop Trauma Surg 106:5–7
61. Scholten RJPM, Opstelten W, van der Plas CG, Bijl D, Deville WLJM, Bouter LM (2003) Accuracy of physical diagnostic tests for assessing ruptures of the anterior cruciate ligament: a meta-analysis. J Fam Pract 52:689–694
62. Slocum DB, James SL, Larson RL, Singer KM (1976) Clinical test for anterolateral rotary instability of the knee. Clin Orthop Relat Res 118:63–69
63. Tashiro Y, Okazaki K, Miura H, Matsuda S, Yasunaga T, Hashizume M, Nakanishi Y, Iwamoto Y (2009) Quantitative assessment of rotatory instability after anterior cruciate ligament reconstruction. Am J Sports Med 37:909–916
64. Terry GC, Norwood LA, Hughston JC, Caldwell KM (1993) How iliotibial tract injuries of the knee combine with acute anterior cruciate ligament tears to influence abnormal anterior tibial displacement. Am J Sports Med 21:55–60
65. Zaffagnini S, Lopomo N, Signorelli C, Marcheggiani Muccioli GM, Bonanzinga T, Grassi A, Visani A, Marcacci M (2013) Innovative technology for knee laxity evaluation: clinical applicability and reliability of inertial sensors for quantitative analysis of the pivot-shift test. Clin Sports Med 32:61–70
66. Zaffagnini S, Muccioli GMM, Lopomo N, Signorelli C, Bonanzinga T, Musiani C, Vassilis P, Nitri M, Marcacci M (2012) Can the pivot-shift be eliminated by anatomic double-bundle anterior cruciate ligament reconstruction? Knee Surg Sport Traumatol Arthrosc 20:743–751

Quantifying "the Look" of the Pivot Shift

24

Paulo H. Araujo, Bruno Ohashi, and Maurício Kfuri Jr

Contents

P.H. Araujo, MD, PhD (✉)
Department of Biomechanics, Medicine and Rehabilitation of Locomotor System - Ribeirao Preto Medical School, São Paulo University, Pittsburgh, PA, USA

Department of Orthopaedic Surgery, University of Pittsburgh, Pittsburgh, PA, USA
e-mail: pauloaraujo@hotmail.com

B. Ohashi, MD
Department of Orthopaedic Surgery, University of Pittsburgh, Pittsburgh, PA, USA

M. Kfuri Jr, MD, PhD
Department of Biomechanics, Medicine and Rehabilitation of Locomotor System - Ribeirao Preto Medical School, São Paulo University, Pittsburgh, PA, USA

24.1 Introduction

The dynamic instability attributed to the pivot-shift phenomenon is still subject of discussion including the structures involved in producing a positive pivot shift [8]. The lack of a standardized pivot-shift maneuver makes its interpretation extremely subjective and dependent on examiner's experience [5, 21, 23, 33, 35].

Systems for clinical grading of the pivot-shift test, such as the ones used in the International Knee Documentation Committee (IKDC) and described as a glide, clunk, or gross pivot shift, are used for estimating the surgeons' feeling during test execution [12, 13, 21, 23, 35]. The introduction of objective pivot-shift measurement techniques is needed for a more precise documentation of cases in the pre-, peri-, and postsurgery segment and for clinical research protocols with the objective of comparison between different knee rotatory instability patterns and surgical techniques.

There are a number of historical techniques to objectively measure the pivot-shift test. Jakob et al. [21], in 1987, compared radiographic measurements of anterior tibial translation under stress caused by an anterior drawer with subjective clinical grading of the pivot-shift test. The authors demonstrated a positive correlation between anterior tibial translation and the clinical grading attributed to the pivot-shift test. Although useful and ahead of its time, this article was not able to quantitatively document the rotational instability. Correlations of pivot-shift measurements to the measurements of

V. Musahl et al. (eds.), *Rotatory Knee Instability*, DOI 10.1007/978-3-319-32070-0_24

anterior tibial translation obtained through the anterior draw test were provided.

In 1991, Noyes et al. [35] studied the execution of the pivot-shift test by 11 different surgeons on a cadaveric specimen and found large variations on knee kinematics of each test. In this study, measurements were performed by a computerized device coupled to an articulated instrumentation system fixed to the femur and tibia. Concluding, the authors emphasize that the test execution technique should be standardized and that the development of instruments, which would allow the quantification of the pivot shift, would be of great value.

Despite the pivot-shift test being deemed of great relevance for the diagnosis and prognosis of knee instability in patients with anterior cruciate injury, this test presents some limitations.

Since its first description in the English literature published by Galway et al. [11], other maneuvers for the test were described [10, 18, 30] and other techniques, not described in literature and that derive from these first ones, are also performed [33] considering a great variety of maneuvers for performing the test and provoking the pivot-shift phenomenon. This great variety of maneuvers generates difficulties in the comparison of results obtained for the pivot-shift test, and as a consequence in the analysis of post-ACL reconstruction results, when different surgeons perform the test, each one with his/her technique of preference.

The pivot-shift test grading is subjective and dependent on the experience and interpretation of the surgeon performing it [5, 21, 23, 33, 35]. The lack of objectivity for defining results of the pivot-shift test and also the variety of existing techniques for its performance provoke limitations for the diagnosis of ACL injuries and for comparisons of postsurgical results.

In a review of the pivot-shift test published in 2008, Lane et al. [25] stated that the objective quantification of pivot-shift test kinematics could provide the basis for an individualized approach to the treatment of ACL injuries based on the elimination of the rotational knee laxity. However, decomposing the pivot shift into quantifiable parameters is not an easy task. The pivot-shift phenomenon is a complex movement that is composed of a six degree-of-freedom tibial internal–external (i–e) rotation, varus–valgus (v–v) rotation, and anterior–posterior (a–p) translation [8], and this is the primary reason for the difficulty to establish an evaluation system for the test.

In this chapter, we will discuss the mechanisms to objectively quantify what we call "the look" of the pivot shift, that is, the amount of shifting, or more specifically, the tibial translation perceived in the lateral aspect of the knee during the pivot-shift test. It is important to differentiate "the look" from "the feeling" of the pivot shift, where the first is related to the amount of tibial dislocation and the second to the force or the severity of shifting.

24.2 Pivot-Shift Measuring Devices

The three-dimensional measurement of the tibial displacement in relation to the femur, as verified through the pivot-shift phenomenon, was the object of studies in the literature [6, 7, 9, 17, 24, 26, 28, 31, 36].

Research on the objective evaluation of the pivot-shift test demonstrated that either tibial translation or acceleration of the tibial reduction could provide a quantitative measure for the pivot-shift test [2, 7, 14, 17, 20, 22, 23, 26–29, 31]. Other studied parameters, such as rotation measurements, were not consistent, even if analyzed in tests performed by the same examiner [9, 16].

Many devices were developed with the capability of objectively measuring the pivot-shift test [1] such as navigation systems, electromagnetic tracking systems, accelerometers, and methods based on radiologic images (radiostereometric (RSA) and dynamic stereo radiograph system (DSX)). However, these devices are not universally available. Other limitations present in many of these devices are the invasiveness and considerable costs.

24.3 Image Analysis System

Bedi et al. [6] showed a good correlation between anterior translation of the lateral compartment of the knee and the clinical grading of the pivot-shift test using a navigation system. The authors

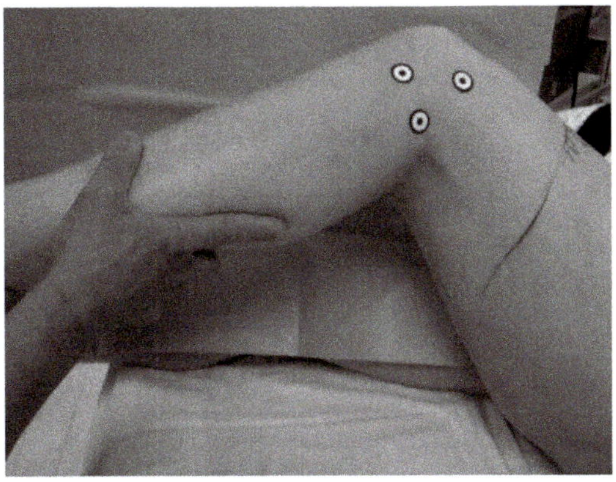

Fig. 24.1 Video image capture of the lateral side of the knee with markers highlighting bony landmarks (lateral epicondyle, fibular head and Gerdy's tubercle) during the pivot-shift test for posterior measurement of the anterior tibial translation through the image analysis method

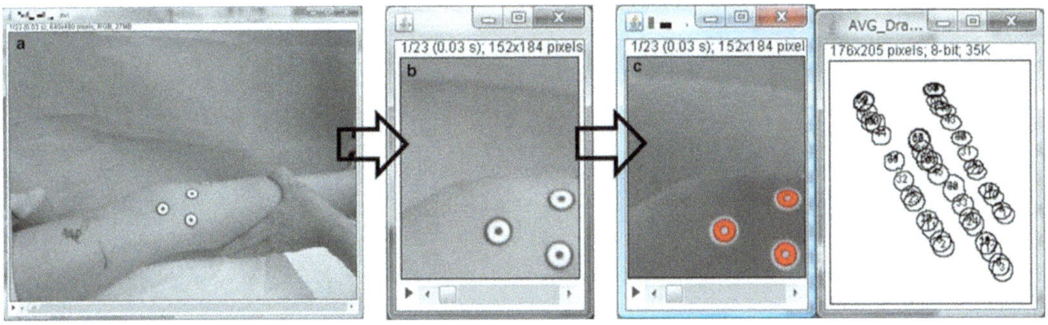

Fig. 24.2 Processing of images from the video capture undergoing adjustments for grey scale up to the adhesive centroids space location on a XY graph with the use of the "Image J" program

demonstrated that each clinical grade correlated to an increment of approximately 6 mm to the lateral compartment translation [6]. The findings of this study suggested that the anterior translation of the lateral compartment of the knee could reflect the clinical grading of the pivot-shift test.

With this concept in mind, the idea of using video images from the pivot-shift test taken from the lateral side of the knee emerged as a possible technique to quantify the anterior translation of the lateral side of the knee during the pivot-shift test. Noteworthy, this new method would also have the advantage of being universally available and with a low cost, therefore capable for a clinical usage.

24.3.1 Description of the Method

Three 14-mm-diameter target-shaped markers (Staples, Inc., Framingham, MA, USA) are placed on the skin above bony landmarks of the knee: Gerdy's tubercle, fibular head, and lateral epicondyle. The distance between the center of the markers over the Gerdy's tubercle and fibular head is measured with a malleable ruler.

A video of the lateral knee side comprising the three markers is recorded during the manual performance of the pivot-shift test (Galway et al.'s technique [11]) with a conventional digital camera (Fig. 24.1).

The images are then analyzed using the "Image J" (NIH, Bethesda, MD, USA) program.

The three markers should be visible at each video frame of the video so the tibial translation could be measured. The centroids from the markers are then detected, located, and plotted on an XY graph, frame by frame. The centroids' space variation is used to calculate the anterior tibial translation on the lateral knee compartment (Fig. 24.2).

24.3.2 Calculation of Tibial Lateral Compartment Translation

At each frame, the point of intersection, pivot point (P), between the line connecting the centroid of the marker over Gerdy's tubercle (G) and the centroid of the marker over the fibular head (F) (horizontal tibial line) with the perpendicular line from the centroid of the marker over the lateral epicondyle (L) up to the horizontal tibial line is calculated on an XY graph (Fig. 24.3).

The ratio of the perpendicular offset distance of the point from the lateral epicondyle to Gerdy's tubercle (distance "b" on Fig. 24.3) to the length of the horizontal tibial line (distance "a" on Fig. 24.3) is calculated from XY graph data. The femur's anteroposterior position in relation to Gerdy's tubercle can be calculated multiplying the ratio obtained by the distance of the 2 tibial points obtained on measurement preliminary to the test. At the moment of pivot-shift reduction, the lateral plateau moves posterior to the lateral femur condyle, which is noted in a reverse manner as an anterior movement of the lateral femoral condyle in relation to the lateral plateau. Thus, the distance between the femoral point most posterior position before the pivot shift and the most anterior after the pivot shift is calculated as lateral translation providing a distance over time graph (Fig. 24.4).

24.3.3 Precision of the Image Analysis Method

A preliminary validation of the lateral compartment translation measured by the image analysis method was performed on the knee of a cadaveric specimen comparing with results

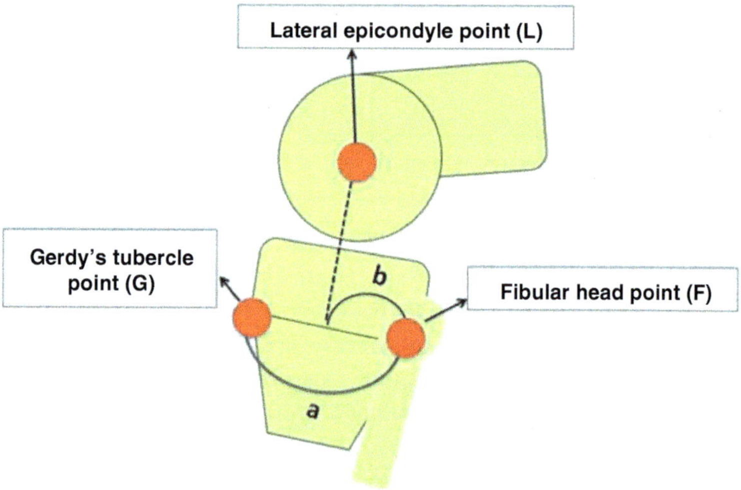

Fig. 24.3 A perpendicular line is drawn from the lateral femur epicondyle (*L*) up to line "*a*". The intersection between the two lines is called "pivot" point (P). A third line is drawn from the two points (*G*) and (P) is called line "*b*". The position of the distal femur is calculated from lines "*a*" and "*b*"

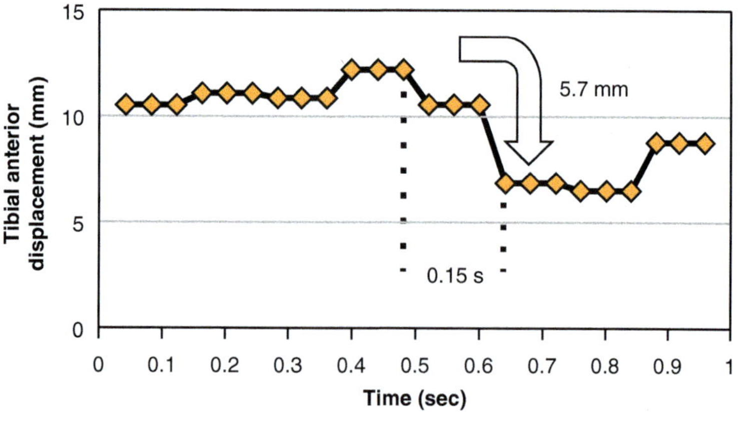

Fig. 24.4 Graph showing the distal anteroposterior femur translation (*y axis*) during the pivot-shift test per time (*x axis*). A sudden anterior translation (5.7 mm) of the distal femur occurred within 0.15 s (*arrow*) during the phase of reduction of the manual test of the pivot shift

obtained with the measurement performed by electromagnetic sensors tracking device fixed to the femur and tibia bones [9, 16, 34]. On the specimen tested with total ACL section, the lateral compartment translation during the pivot-shift test was 3.0 ± 0.8 mm for three consecutive tests, while the bone movement given by the device fixed to the bone was 22.8 ± 0.4 mm. The values obtained by the image analysis method were smaller than the bony movement, but the lateral compartment translation was consistently observed.

In another laboratory study [2], the image analysis system measurements were compared to a reference measuring device attached to the femur and tibia, i. e., electromagnetic tracking system. A cadaveric specimen was prepared to have a positive pivot shift by sectioning the ACL and the anterior horn of the lateral meniscus. Twelve surgeons performed the pivot shift according to their preferred technique and according to a standardized technique. A positive correlation was found between the image analysis system and the reference method when the standardized technique was used to reproduce the pivot-shift phenomenon.

Fact Box 1

The image analysis system was capable of detecting and measuring the lateral tibial compartment on ACL-deficient knees in a consistent manner and represents a simple, reliable, accessible method for the quantitative measurement of the pivot-shift test.

24.4 iPad Technology for Image Analysis

Despite being a low cost and universally available method for measuring the pivot-shift test, the results processing through the image analysis system is quite time consuming, because the pivot-shift video has to be analyzed frame by frame by the examiner, requiring more than 2 h processing time.

In order to obtain the objective results of the lateral compartment translation automatically and immediately, an application for iPad® was developed to avoid the frame-by-frame manual processing performed on the image analysis system [15].

24.4.1 Image Analysis Using the iPad Technology

The same steps performed in the image analysis system are also required to achieve the lateral compartment translation measurements in the iPad app. Therefore, three yellow circular markers, ¾ inches in diameter (Color Coding Labels, Avery Dennison Corporation, Pasadena, CA, USA), should be attached to the skin, over bony landmarks including Gerdy's tubercle, fibular head, and femur lateral epicondyle.

The images of the pivot-shift test should be captured using the video function of the iPad technology. An assistant holds the iPad in a fixed position perpendicular to the lateral side of the knee at approximately 1 m of distance from the tested knee. The assistant makes sure the skin markers did not leave the video field during the entire test. A monochromatic sheet is used behind the tested knee in order to diminish possible distortions on the captured images (Fig. 24.5).

After adjusting the iPad® in an adequate position, the pivot-shift test should be performed with the standardized technique [13, 33] based on the description of the pivot-shift test (Galway et al) [11].

Similarly to that described for the image analysis system [15], however automatically, the process of measurement of the tibial lateral compartment translation is obtained by the technology. The typical result of the translation obtained by the iPad technology is shown on Fig. 24.6.

During the pivot-shift reduction, the lateral plateau moves posterior to the lateral femoral condyle, which is observed in reverse as an anterior movement of the lateral femoral condyle related to the lateral plateau. So, the distance between the most posterior position of the femur before the pivot shift and the most anterior after the pivot shift is calculated as the lateral translation.

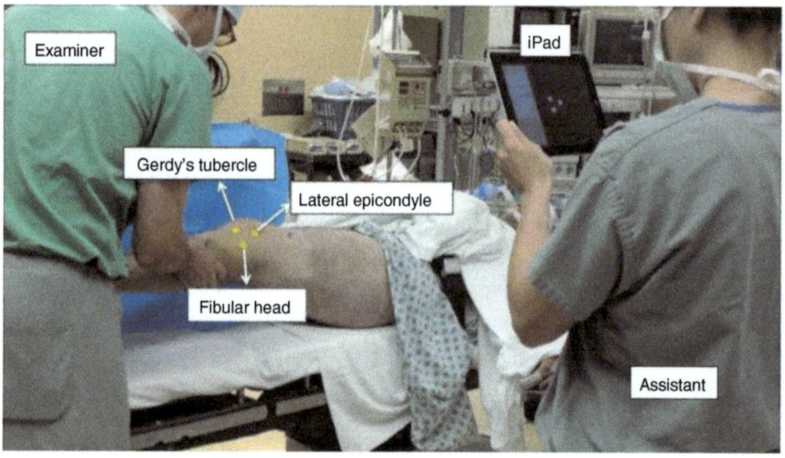

Fig. 24.5 Acquisition of images of the pivot-shift test with the iPad application

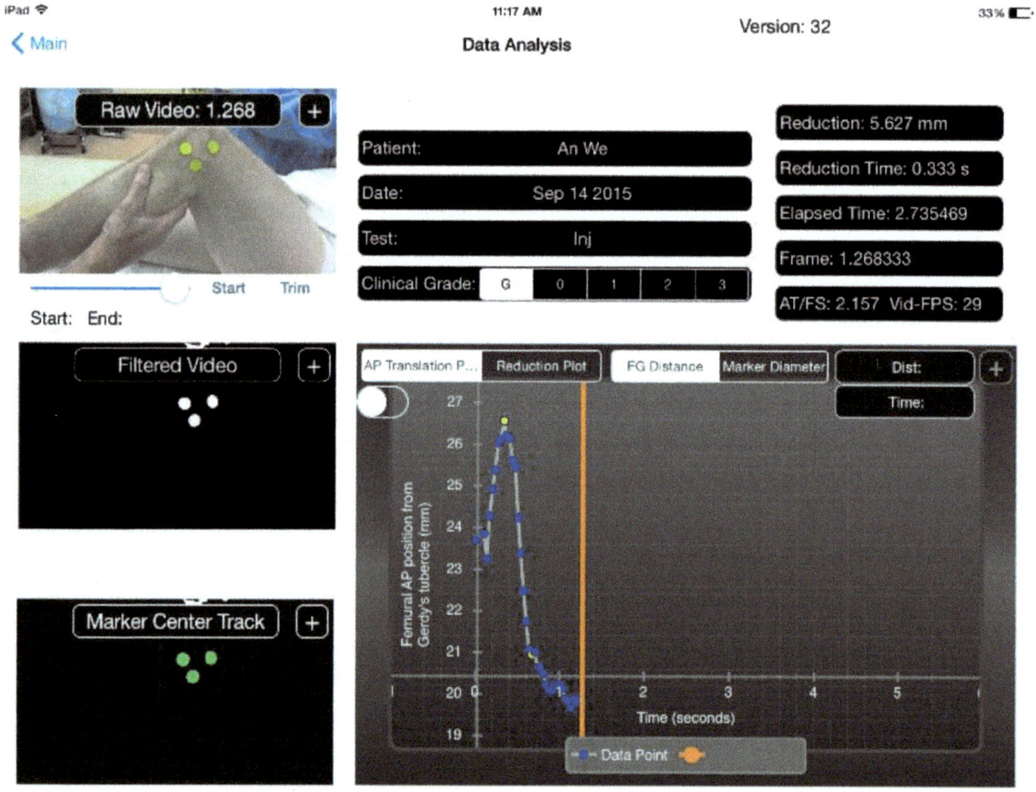

Fig. 24.6 iPad application screen. The video of the pivot-shift test appears *on the top to the left*; the tracking of the markers is shown below the video. The anteroposterior femoral translation starting from Gerdy's tubercle (in mm) per time (in seconds) is shown on the graph below to the *right*; the sudden decrease (anterior femur translation or the tibial reduction) is shown on the *arrow*. The calculated numerical results are shown on the *top to the right* (5.627 mm)

24.5 iPad Technology Validation

A clinical study [14] analyzing 34 consecutive patients with unilateral ACL injury was performed. The pivot-shift test was performed on each knee with the standardized technique [13, 33] and filmed using the iPad technology. Before knowing the measurement result through the application, the surgeon attributed a degree to the performed test according to IKDC [19].

The highest value of the lateral translation in two consecutive pivot-shift tests was used for posterior analysis. The average of the lateral translation of the ACL-deficient knees and ACL-intact knees was compared. The lateral translation of the knees was also compared with ACL injury that had different degrees of pivot shift attributed by the surgeon.

The tests that did not detect the translation of the lateral compartment on ACL-deficient knees and knees where tests evidenced lateral translation greater than 10 mm due to the obvious discrepancy between the result of the average and the observed translation were excluded.

The early results showed that valid results were only observed in 20 of the 34 patients with ACL insufficiency (59 %). Of these, 18 patients had valid results for the non-injured knee. For the remaining 14 patients, no reduction of the pivot shift was detected in 10 patients, and in 4 an excessive lateral translation was detected. The arthroscopic evaluation verified the complete ACL injury in all 34 patients. However, the updated versions (2.0 and 3.0) have increased the accuracy to over 90 % [4, 32].

The difference of the average of the lateral translation between ACL-deficient knees and ACL-intact knees and lateral translation of ACL-deficient knees that had different degrees of pivot shift attributed by the surgeon is shown on Table 24.1.

Table 24.1 Average of the lateral translation between ACL-deficient knees and ACL-intact knees and lateral translation of ACL-deficient knees that had different degrees of pivot shift attributed by the surgeon

	Knee with injury	Contralateral knee	Difference between sides
Pivot shift +/3+	2.7 ± 0.6 ($n = 10$)	1.4 ± 1.9 ($n = 9$)	1.3 ± 2.0 ($n = 9$)
Pivot shift ++/3+	3.6 ± 1.2^a ($n = 10$)	1.0 ± 1.5 ($n = 8$)	2.5 ± 2.0 ($n = 8$)
Total ($n = 17$)	3.2 ± 1.0^b	1.3 ± 1.7	1.9 ± 2.1

[a]Significantly higher compared to patients with pivot shift +/3+ ($p < 0.05$)

[b]Significantly higher compared to contralateral knees ($p < 0.01$)

24.6 Summary

The sudden shift of the lateral compartment of the knee was successfully detected by the iPad technology. The increase of lateral translation was detected by the iPad technology on ACL-deficient knees compared to ACL-intact knees and also in relation to knees with higher degree attributed to the pivot-shift test. However, differences between sides were not detected among patients that had different degrees attributed to the pivot shift. This is a method still underdevelopment, and new software versions must implement the precision of the pivot-shift analysis.

Fact Box 2

The iPad technology for image analysis is effective to detect the anterior translation of the lateral compartment in ACL-deficient knees with the advantage of providing automatic and immediate results compared to the image analysis system.

24.7 Future Perspectives

Quantitative analysis of pivot-shift test can aid in the establishment of treatment algorithms for ACL reconstruction [3]. This will ultimately lead to more individualized surgery, thereby with fewer ACL graft re-ruptures and improved clinical outcomes for patients. The main purpose of the iPad app is the pre- and postoperative assessment of rotatory knee laxity to improve ACL reconstruction. Large databases are currently being collected, ultimately helping to categorize different rotatory knee instability patterns and preventing failure of ACL reconstruction in patients.

Patients that have persistent rotatory knee instability could be better served with an individualized approach at the time of initial ACL reconstruction surgery. This approach would warrant quantitative diagnosis of the ACL-deficient knees using, e.g., the iPad app. The clinician could then modify his/her surgical approach according to the quantitative amount ("look") of rotatory knee instability recorded by the iPad technology, e.g., performing an augmentation surgery in cases of small anterior displacements or adding an extra-articular tenodesis in cases of larger anterior displacements.

In addition, clinical follow-up evaluation could be enhanced by the iPad technology. Potentially, quantitative analysis of the pivot-shift test during clinical follow-up can give information on knee function that can otherwise not be obtained by noninvasive means.

These new noninvasive technologies could be used for patient-individualized and functional treatment of ACL injury. The long-term goal of these technologies is the establishment of a kinematics-based diagnosis and treatment algorithm for patients with ACL injuries.

Conclusion

The anterior translation of the lateral compartment of the knee is a consistent parameter to measure the pivot-shift test. The analysis of videos of the pivot-shift test taken from the lateral side of the knee consists of a simple, cheap, and reliable method, and therefore a possible tool for the clinical practice, to measure the pivot-shift test. The ultimate goal of these new technologies for the pivot-shift measurements is the establishment of treatment algorithms for the individualized treatment for the ACL-deficient knees.

References

1. Ahldén M, Hoshino Y, Samuelsson K, Araujo P, Musahl V, Karlsson J (2012) Dynamic knee laxity measurement devices. Knee Surg Sports Traumatol Arthrosc 20(4):621–632
2. Araujo PH, Ahldén M, Hoshino Y, Muller B, Moloney G, Fu FH, Musahl V (2012) Comparison of three non-invasive quantitative measurement systems for the pivot shift test. Knee Surg Sports Traumatol Arthrosc 20(4):692–697
3. Araujo PH, Kfuri Junior M, Ohashi B, Hoshino Y, Zaffagnini S, Samuelsson K et al (2014) Individualized ACL reconstruction. Knee Surg Sports Traumatol Arthrosc 22(9):1966–1975
4. Arila F, Rahnemai-Azar A, Scott B, Yacuzzi C, Guenther D, Fu F, Debski R, Musahl V (2015) Reliability of a 2D simple image analysis method to predict 3D bony motion of the lateral. Poster presentation at Orthopaedic Research Society, Las Vegas
5. Bach BR, Warren RF, Wickiewicz TL (1988) The pivot shift phenomenon: results and description of a modified clinical test for anterior cruciate ligament insufficiency. Am J Sports Med 16(6):571–576
6. Bedi A, Musahl V, Lane C, Citak M, Warren RF, Pearle AD (2010) Lateral compartment translation predicts the grade of pivot shift: a cadaveric and clinical analysis. Knee Surg Sports Traumatol Arthrosc 18(9):1269–1276
7. Bignozzi S, Zaffagnini S, Lopomo N, Fu FH, Irrgang JJ, MarCASci M (2010) Clinical relevance of static and dynamic tests after anatomical double-bundle ACL reconstruction. Knee Surg Sports Traumatol Arthrosc 18(1):37–42
8. Bull AMJ, Amis AA (1998) The pivot-shift phenomenon: a clinical and biomechanical perspective. Knee 5(3):141–158
9. Bull AMJ, Earnshaw PH, Smith A, Katchburian MV, Hassan AN, Amis AA (2002) Intraoperative measurement of knee kinematics in reconstruction of the anterior cruciate ligament. J Bone Joint Surg Br 84(7):1075–1081
10. Slocum DB, James SL, Larson RL, Singer KM (1976) Clinical test for anterolateral rotary instability of the knee. Clin Orthop Relat Res. Jul–Aug (118):63–69
11. Galway R, Beaupre A, MacIntosh D (1972) Pivot shift: a clinical sign of symptomatic anterior cruciate insufficiency. J Bone Joint Surg Br 54(4):763–764
12. Hefti F, Müller W, Jakob RP, Stäubli HU (1993) Evaluation of knee ligament injuries with the IKDC form. Knee Surg Sports Traumatol Arthrosc 1(3–4):226–234
13. Hoshino Y, Araujo P, Ahldén M, Moore CG, Kuroda R, Zaffagnini S et al (2012) Standardized pivot shift test improves measurement accuracy. Knee Surg Sports Traumatol Arthrosc 20(4):732–736
14. Hoshino Y, Araujo P, Ahldén M, Samuelsson K, Muller B, Hofbauer M et al (2013) Quantitative evaluation of the pivot shift by image analysis using the iPad. Knee Surg Sports Traumatol Arthrosc 21(4):975–980
15. Hoshino Y, Araujo P, Irrgang JJ, Fu FH, Musahl V (2011) An image analysis method to quantify the lateral pivot shift test. Knee Surg Sports Traumatol Arthrosc 20(4):703–707
16. Hoshino Y, Kuroda R, Nagamune K, Nishimoto K, Yagi M, Mizuno K et al (2007) The effect of graft ten-

sioning in anatomic 2-bundle ACL reconstruction on knee joint kinematics. Knee Surg Sports Traumatol Arthrosc 15(5):508–514
17. Hoshino Y, Kuroda R, Nagamune K, Yagi M, Mizuno K, Yamaguchi M et al (2007) In vivo measurement of the pivot-shift test in the anterior cruciate ligament-deficient knee using an electromagnetic device. Am J Sports Med 35(7):1098–1104
18. Hughston JC, Andrews JR, Cross MJ, Moschi A (1976) Classification of knee ligament instabilities. Part I The medial compartment and cruciate ligaments. J Bone Joint Surg Am 58(2):159–172
19. Irrgang JJ, Anderson AF, Boland AL, Harner CD, Kurosaka M, Neyret P et al (2001) Development and validation of the international knee documentation committee subjective knee form. Am J Sports Med 29(5):600–613
20. Ishibashi Y, Tsuda E, Yamamoto Y, Tsukada H, Toh S (2009) Navigation evaluation of the pivot-shift phenomenon during double-bundle anterior cruciate ligament reconstruction: is the posterolateral bundle more important? Arthroscopy 25(5):488–495
21. Jakob RP, Stäubli HU, Deland JT (1987) Grading the pivot shift. Objective tests with implications for treatment. J Bone Joint Surg Br 69(2):294–299
22. Kuroda R, Hoshino Y, Araki D, Nishizawa Y, Nagamune K, Matsumoto T et al (2012) Quantitative measurement of the pivot shift, reliability, and clinical applications. Knee Surg Sports Traumatol Arthrosc 20(4):686–691
23. Kuroda R, Hoshino Y, Kubo S, Araki D, Oka S, Nagamune K et al (2012) Similarities and differences of diagnostic manual tests for anterior cruciate ligament insufficiency: a global survey and kinematics assessment. Am J Sports Med 40(1):91–99
24. Labbe DR, de Guise JA, Mezghani N, Godbout V, Grimard G, Baillargeon D et al (2010) Feature selection using a principal component analysis of the kinematics of the pivot shift phenomenon. J Biomech 43(16):3080–3084
25. Lane CG, Warren R, Pearle AD (2008) The pivot shift. J Am Acad Orthop Surg 16(12):679–688
26. Lane CG, Warren RF, Stanford FC, Kendoff D, Pearle AD (2008) In vivo analysis of the pivot shift phenomenon during computer navigated ACL reconstruction. Knee Surg Sports Traumatol Arthrosc 16(5):487–492
27. Lopomo N, Signorelli C, Bonanzinga T, Marcheggiani MuICCoIi GM, Visani A, Zaffagnini S (2012) Quantitative assessment of pivot-shift using inertial sensors. Knee Surg Sports Traumatol Arthrosc 20(4):713–717
28. Lopomo N, Zaffagnini S, Bignozzi S, Visani A, MarCASci M (2010) Pivot-shift test: analysis and quantification of knee laxity parameters using a navigation system. J Orthop Res 28(2):164–169
29. Lopomo N, Zaffagnini S, Signorelli C, Bignozzi S, Giordano G, Marcheggiani MuICCoIi GM et al (2012) An original clinical methodology for non-invasive assessment of pivot-shift test. Comput Methods Biomech Biomed Engin 15(12): 1323–1328
30. Losee RE, Johnson TR, Southwick WO (1978) Anterior subluxation of the lateral tibial plateau. A diagnostic test and operative repair. J Bone Joint Surg Am 60(8):1015–1030
31. Maeyama A, Hoshino Y, Debandi A, Kato Y, Saeki K, Asai S et al (2011) Evaluation of rotational instability in the anterior cruciate ligament deficient knee using triaxial accelerometer: a biomechanical model in porcine knees. Knee Surg Sports Traumatol Arthrosc 19(8):1233–1238
32. Muller B, Hofbauer M, Rahnemai-Azar AA, Wolf M, Araki D, Hoshino Y et al (2015) Development of computer tablet software for clinical quantification of lateral knee compartment translation during the pivot shift test. Comput Methods Biomech Biomed Engin 9:1–12
33. Musahl V, Hoshino Y, Ahldén M, Araujo P, Irrgang JJ, Zaffagnini S et al (2012) The pivot shift: a global user guide. Knee Surg Sports Traumatol Arthrosc 20(4):724–731
34. Nishimoto K, Kuroda R, Mizuno K, Hoshino Y, Nagamune K, Kubo S et al (2009) Analysis of the graft bending angle at the femoral tunnel aperture in anatomic double bundle anterior cruciate ligament reconstruction: a comparison of the transtibial and the far anteromedial portal technique. Knee Surg Sports Traumatol Arthrosc 17(3):270–276
35. Noyes FR, Grood ES, Cummings JF, Wroble RR (1991) An analysis of the pivot shift phenomenon. The knee motions and subluxations induced by different examiners. Am J Sports Med 19(2):148–155
36. Pearle AD, Kendoff D, Musahl V, Warren RF (2009) The pivot-shift phenomenon during computer-assisted anterior cruciate ligament reconstruction. J Bone Joint Surg Am 91(Suppl 1):115–118

Use of Inertial Sensors for Quantifying the Pivot Shift Maneuver

25

Per Henrik Borgstrom, Edward Cheung, Keith L. Markolf, David R. McAllister, William J. Kaiser, and Frank A. Petrigliano

Contents

P.H. Borgstrom (✉)
Wireless Health Institute, University of California at Los Angeles, Los Angeles, CA, USA
e-mail: henrikborgstrom@gmail.com

E. Cheung • F.A. Petrigliano • K.L. Markolf
D.R. McAllister
Department of Orthopedic Surgery, University of California at Los Angeles, Los Angeles, CA, USA
e-mail: echeung@mednet.ucla.edu; fpetrigliano@mednet.ucla.edu; dmcallister@mednet.ucla.edu; kmarkolf@mednet.ucla.edu

W.J. Kaiser
Wireless Health Institute, University of California at Los Angeles, Los Angeles, CA, USA
e-mail: kaiser@ee.ucla.edu

25.1 Introduction

The anterior cruciate ligament (ACL) is a primary stabilizer of the knee, accounting for 85 % of the total restraint to anterior tibial translation [6]. Injury to the ACL occurs frequently, comprising 40–50 % of all ligamentous knee injuries [9]. While imaging remains the gold standard in evaluating ACL state, the pivot shift, originally described by Galway, Beaupre, and MacIntosh in 1972 [7], has been shown to be the most specific physical exam maneuver, diagnosing ACL rupture and rotatory instability with up to 98 % specificity [2, 4, 18, 23]. Furthermore, the pivot shift grade has been shown to be associated with patient outcome after ACL reconstruction [12, 13, 17]. However, the subjective nature of this exam and the grading system used to assign a pivot shift score are well-recognized limitations of this test. The clinical grading system is highly dependent on subtle differences in testing technique and perceptions of the examining physician. It has historically been graded using a subjective 0–3 classification [8] with 0 being negative, 1 a glide, 2 a clunk, and 3 a gross clunk. Due to the subjectivity of the pivot shift grading scale, objective quantification of rotational instability with convenient instrumentation could enable the development of a more reliable and reproducible grading system. Such a system would be advantageous for preoperative diagnostic testing, would provide an objective non-biased pivot shift grade, and would be

V. Musahl et al. (eds.), *Rotatory Knee Instability*, DOI 10.1007/978-3-319-32070-0_25

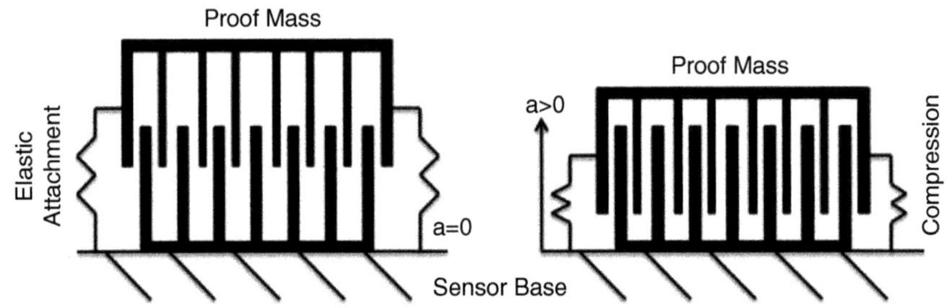

Fig. 25.1 A schematic representation of one type of MEMS accelerometer. The accelerometer consists of a conductive comb rigidly attached to the sensor base and a second comb-shaped proof mass attached via elastic struts. At the left, with the sensor undergoing zero acceleration, the two combs interdigitate only slightly, resulting in a small area of interaction. This yields a low capacitance. At the right, as the sensor undergoes upward acceleration, the inertia of the proof mass causes the elastic struts to compress, yielding increased overlapping between the combs and increased capacitance. Capacitance is measured and converted to acceleration via a linear constant

useful in controlled longitudinal studies. At present, this goal remains elusive. The ideal system for this clinical application is noninvasive, accurate, easily implemented, and low cost. Inertial sensors fulfill many of these criteria and for this reason are currently being utilized for a variety of biomedical applications. This chapter reviews the current application of inertial sensors towards quantification of the pivot shift and describes the current limitations that this technology must overcome prior to widespread clinical use.

25.2 Review of Inertial Sensor Technology

During the previous decade, novel sensor technologies have emerged that may help advance the goal of noninvasively quantifying rotational instability of the knee. Microelectromechanical systems (MEMS) inertial sensors, specifically accelerometers, gyroscopes, and magnetometers, have evolved into low-cost, low-power devices sufficiently small to be embedded into handheld or body-mounted packages. For example, most modern smartphone devices and gaming controllers employ integrated 9 degrees of freedom (9-DOF) sensors that leverage triaxial accelerometers, gyroscopes, and magnetometers. Recent instantiations of such integrated sensors have footprints of $3 \times 3 \times 1$ mm with power consumption on the order of 10 mW and are often combined with sophisticated on-board sensor fusion and signal processing algorithms [10].

25.2.1 MEMS Accelerometer Overview

Accelerometers are used to measure linear acceleration as well as the gravity vector. Conceptually, the modern MEMS accelerometer is a relatively simple device. A typical accelerometer is shown in Fig. 25.1. Whereas one accelerometer measures acceleration only along a single-axis, modern MEMS technology enables three such structures to be manufactured orthogonally, thereby providing triaxial accelerometer measurements.

25.2.2 MEMS Gyroscope Overview

A gyroscope is a device that measures the rate of rotation about an axis. In modern MEMS devices, a vibrating mass is excited to oscillate within a plane. Due to this oscillation, the mass, in accordance with the Coriolis effect, resists rotation with a force that is proportional to the rate of rotation. This force is subsequently measured using a transducer, thereby providing a measure of rotational velocity. This principle of operation is somewhat similar to that of the accelerometer shown in Fig. 25.1, except that the acceleration that induces the change in capacitance is Coriolis acceleration rather than linear acceleration. As with accelerometers, three single-axis devices can be integrated orthogonally in one package to provide measurements of rotations about three axes.

25.2.3 AHRS: Sensor Fusion Systems

In the case of instrumenting the pivot shift, it is desirable to have information regarding leg kinematics during the maneuver. However, neither gyroscopes nor accelerometers enable this directly, as they measure rotational rate and linear acceleration, respectively, not absolute sensor orientation. Integration of the rotational rates measured by the gyroscope yields an approximation of sensor orientation, but it is susceptible to long-term drift due to accumulation of small errors in the integral. On the other hand, the accelerometer can be used to measure the gravity vector and thereby compute the roll and pitch of the device. However, the accelerometer measures the sum of the gravity vector and any acceleration, so an estimate of orientation based solely on this measurement is subject to large noise when the sensor is not static.

To provide a responsive and stable estimate of orientation, gyroscope and accelerometer data are combined to form an attitude and heading reference system (AHRS), in which the long-term stable behavior of the accelerometer is combined with the superior high-frequency properties of the gyroscope. AHRSs have been well studied and characterized, and a number of commonly used methods exist [25].

It should be noted that an AHRS based solely on accelerometer and gyroscope data is not able to generate long-term stable estimates of orientation about the vertical axis, as the accelerometer provides no such information. Thus, drift about this axis accumulates due to integration of the gyroscope signal. A magnetometer is often used as an electronic compass to remedy this long-term drift. However, the pivot shift maneuver occurs rapidly, and accumulation of long-term drift is therefore not a concern in this scenario.

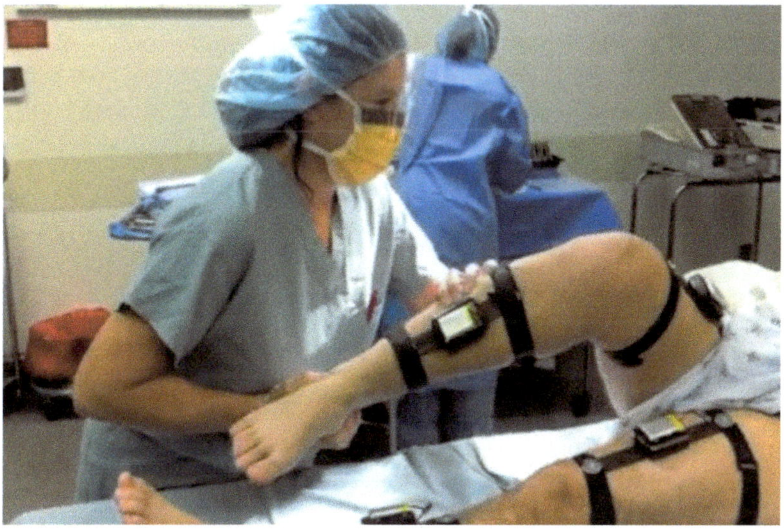

Fig. 25.2 A pivot shift maneuver being performed on an anesthetized subject with triaxial accelerometers and gyroscopes attached along the tibia and femur of each leg. This placement was used to enable computation of knee kinematics as well as to capture the dynamics and accelerations caused by the maneuver. Other trials have placed sensors differently, and there is no consensus on optimal placement

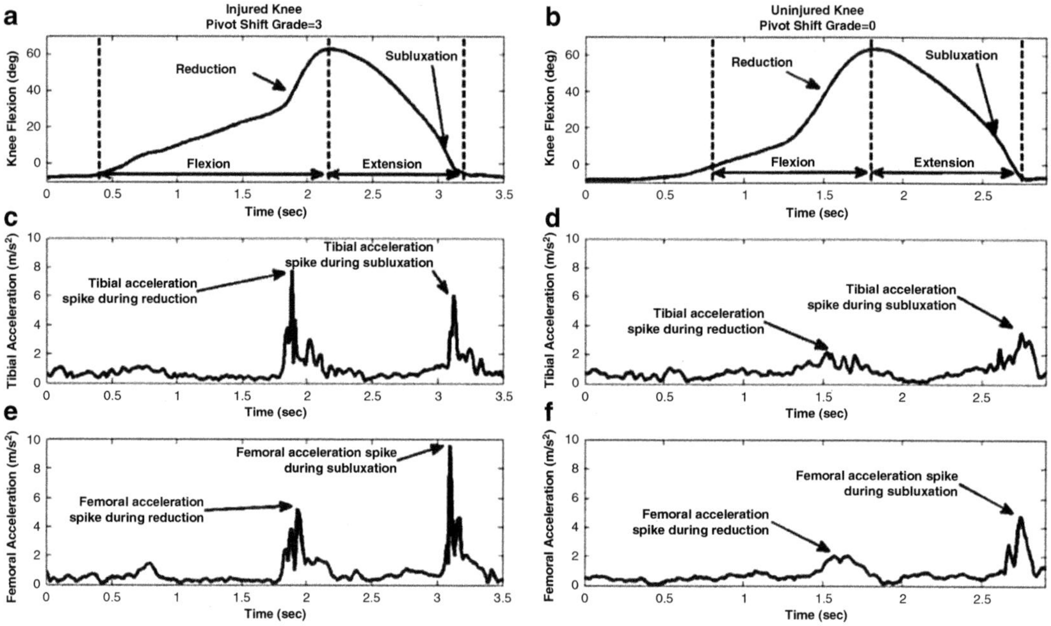

Fig. 25.3 Sample tracings for a patient's injured knee with a grade 3 pivot shown at left (**a**, **c**, **e**) and the uninjured knee shown at right (**b**, **d**, **f**). The two upper plots (**a**, **b**) show flexion angle, while the middle plots (**c**, **d**) show resultant accelerations for femoral sensors, and the lower plots (**e**, **f**) show resultant accelerations for tibial sensors. The large spikes in acceleration shown in (**c**, **e**) are characteristic of a gross pivot shift in an ACL-deficient knee, whereas the smaller and less defined peaks shown in (**d**, **f**) are indicative of an ACL-intact knee

25.3 Inertial Sensors and the Pivot Shift

There is some disagreement in the literature regarding optimal lower extremity placement of inertial sensors in measuring the pivot shift. Some groups have chosen to mount sensors along the tibia [3, 19], and some have placed sensors along both the tibia and femur [1, 5, 14–16]. One example configuration is shown in Fig. 25.2. In this experiment, the subject is equipped with triaxial accelerometers and gyroscopes mounted along both the tibia and femur.

The acceleration metrics or features computed from the raw data also vary. Some papers consider maximum or minimum acceleration values, others consider the range, and some consider the derivative of this measurement, known as jerk. However, the data collected and visualized in all studies is remarkably similar in many ways, regardless of sensor location or subsequent feature extraction; in accelerometer data, pivot shift reduction events appear as spikes or peaks, and the magnitude of these spikes is shown to correlate with ACL state.

Accelerometer waveforms from two example pivot shifts are shown in Fig. 25.3. Here, accelerometer data has been high-pass-filtered to remove the gravity vector, and the norm of the triaxial acceleration vector has been computed and plotted against time. The entire pivot shift maneuver is shown, including both the flexion and extension phase, and data from the femoral and tibial sensors is provided.

> **Fact Box 1**
> Advances in MEMS technology have provided researchers with new, unprecedented means of instrumenting the pivot shift maneuver. Accelerometer measurements during pivot shifts show peaks in acceleration during reduction and subluxation events.

The difference between injured and contralateral knees is seldom as exaggerated as in these plots. In particular, the difference between two knees with pivot shift grades differing by only one grade may be very slight or unnoticeable. Therein lies the primary difficulty in using accelerometer data to determine ACL state and assign a specific pivot shift grade.

Fact Box 2

(1) Accelerations measured during pivot shift maneuvers correlate with rotational instability of the knee, (2) diagnosis of ACL state based purely on accelerometer data is not likely to provide sufficient accuracy for clinical use, and (3) combination of accelerometer and gyroscope data using advanced classification techniques may provide accurate diagnosis of ACL state, although appropriate training of classification models represents a potential difficulty.

25.4 Review of the Current Literature

The availability of low-power, low-cost, and accurate inertial sensors combined with wireless transmission or on-board storage of data enables development of sensor devices appropriate and convenient for clinical use. Since 2010, ascertaining the value of such devices in instrumenting the pivot shift maneuver has emerged as an important research objective. Several groups have contributed significantly, and the overall conclusions of this research are fairly consistent:

Lopomo et al. were among the first to evaluate the use of MEMS accelerometers in the diagnosis of ACL injury [19]. In this study, the authors instrumented 66 patients undergoing ACL reconstruction and examined both knees under anesthesia. The injured and contralateral limbs underwent pivot shift maneuvers and the resulting accelerations were measured by a triaxial accelerometer between Gerdy's tubercle and the anterior tibial tubercle. In this study, the acceleration maximum, minimum, and range were found with strong significance to be larger in ACL injured knees than in the contralateral side. This finding was the first step in validating the use of accelerometers to instrument the pivot shift maneuver.

Further investigation and validation were provided in two subsequent studies [1], wherein the authors compared electromagnetic (EM) position sensors attached to the bone of cadaveric specimens, tissue-mounted EM sensors, and externally mounted accelerometers. The bone-mounted EM sensors were used to determine the actual movement of the tibia and femur in quantifying the pivot shift. Twelve expert surgeons performed pivot shift maneuvers on the knee and graded the pivot shift. The authors considered acceleration measured by each sensor system during reduction in the pivot shift event. The group found that clinical pivot shift grade strongly correlated with the maximal acceleration as measured by both externally mounted accelerometers and bone-mounted electromagnetic sensors. Thus, this study was able to demonstrate correlation between clinical pivot shift grade and accelerometer measurements in a cadaver.

Berruto et al. provided further evidence of the applicability of accelerometer measurements in evaluation of ACL state [3]. One hundred ACL-deficient patients were instrumented with accelerometers prior to surgery, and pivot shift maneuvers were performed on both knees. Additionally, 30 patients were measured at a minimum of 6 months postoperatively. In the preoperative trials, significant differences were found between the maximum accelerations measured in injured and normal knees. In the 30 subjects measured postoperatively, no such difference was found. The authors also consider the problem of correlating clinical pivot shift grade with accelerometer measurements and propose a set of reference values for each clinical grade. Importantly, this study required that the pivot shift be performed in a manner different from that in which it is performed in typical clinical settings, with a slow approach and more careful control of force applied to the femur being considered more suitable for measurement by accelerometers. Initially, examiners struggled to perform this test reliably regardless of experience level. With practice, all examiners learned to perform the maneuver reliably, with experienced surgeons adapting more quickly than less experienced residents and students.

In these critical early evaluations of the use of inertial sensor technology, researchers arrived at the consistent conclusion that accelerations measured using externally mounted inertial sensors correlated with ACL state. Larger overall accelerations were observed in injured knees, and the differences were statistically significant. Further, correlations were found between measured accelerations and clinical pivot shift grades. Additionally, the small form factor, low power, and low cost of such devices made their use in the clinical setting straightforward. However, little mention is made in these studies of the accuracy of ACL diagnosis and pivot shift grading based on accelerometer measurements.

Labbe et al. made a significant step in the direction of ACL diagnosis based on inertial sensing [16]. In this study, 13 ACL-deficient subjects were instrumented with sensor packages containing accelerometers and magnetometers. The magnetometers were used to remove the gravity vector from accelerometer measurements, and these corrected measurements were subsequently correlated with clinical pivot shift grade. It was found that the measured femoral acceleration in these subjects did in fact correlate with pivot shift grade. Statistical significance was found between low clinical grades (0, 1) and higher clinical grades (2, 3). However, no such difference was found between 0 and 1 nor between 2 and 3. Thus, while the study presents promising data specifically in the authors ability to correlate pivot shift grade with inertial sensor measurements, it simultaneously reveals a major shortcoming associated with use of inertial sensors for evaluation of ACL state: if straightforward acceleration metrics are considered, diagnostic accuracy of ACL state is not likely to achieve resolution or accuracy on par with the traditional pivot shift examination. Careful analysis of plots and tables from prior studies indicates similar results, although, without access to raw data, such analysis is only approximate and is not presented here.

Fact Box 3

Increased tibial and femoral acceleration as measured by inertial sensors during a pivot shift maneuver has been shown to correlate with ACL injury in a number of studies. ACL-deficient knees undergo significantly larger accelerations, and pivot shift grade also correlates significantly with measured acceleration.

However, Labbe et al. had already applied more advanced statistical methods with much success using data from EM position sensors, and this methodology bore promise in use with inertial sensor systems. In [14], a method called principle component analysis (PCA) was used to analyze the kinematics of a pivot shift maneuver. PCA is a statistical tool that computes data features that correlate most strongly with an outcome [11]. For example, one might hypothetically suggest that three axes of measured acceleration correlate with pivot shift grade. Further, through careful analysis, one might determine that the anterior axis correlated most strongly, the lateral axis slightly less strongly, and the distal axis least so. Application of PCA to this scenario would yield that the metric most consistent with pivot shift grade is a weighted sum of the three accelerations wherein anterior acceleration is weighted more heavily than lateral, which is weighted more heavily than distal. In this way, PCA is able to rank proposed features in what is roughly speaking their order of usefulness. When PCA was applied to the pivot shift maneuver in [14], a number of data features were found to be valuable, including a large number of acceleration metrics, tibial rotation, and a number of translational distances. Thus, the kinematics and dynamics of the pivot shift appear to be quite complex, and the single-variable analysis that had been previously applied to inertial sensors is not likely to fully capture the phenomenon.

In a subsequent investigation [15], Labbe et al. used a sophisticated classification approach known as support vector machine (SVM) [24] to assign pivot shift grades based on data from EM sensors. The SVM approach here leveraged the optimal feature set computed through PCA and achieved promising results, with 66 % of computed grades matching the clinically determined value and 96 % falling within + −1 grade.

Borgstrom et al. applied computational methods similar to those in [14, 15] to diagnose ACL state and compute pivot shift grades based on inertial sensor data [5]. Thirty-two subjects with unilateral injuries and 29 subjects with two intact ACLs were instrumented with inertial sensors along the femur and tibia of each leg. Pivot shifts were performed preoperatively under anesthesia on each leg. AHRS methods were used to compute knee kinematics during the pivot shift. PCA and SVM methods were used to detect ACL tears with 97 % accuracy and assign pivot shift grades with 77 % accuracy, with 98 % within ± 1 grade. The rate of convergence of statistical methods such as SVM was also considered. In this case, it was found that data from roughly 20 subjects examined by a surgeon were required to train SVM methods before they became reliable and 38 were required for accuracy of diagnosis of ACL tears to reach 90 %. This study did not extend to awake subjects, and only one surgeon was considered, so further work remains to evaluate whether these methods can in fact replace or serve a complementary role to the traditional pivot shift grade. A summary of the primary results presented in literature is provided in Table 25.1.

Fact Box 4

Single-variable analysis of acceleration is not likely to provide sufficiently accurate results to replace or complement the traditional pivot shift grade. Use of advanced statistical methods and classification algorithms has enabled accurate diagnosis via inertial sensor data in one study, but further work is necessary to verify such approaches.

25.5 Conclusions and Future Directions

Instrumentation of the pivot shift using inertial sensors appears promising at this time. Improvements in technology have enabled approaches to making the pivot shift more objective. Correlations have been demonstrated between ACL injury and accelerometer measurement, and subsequent studies have shown that pivot shift grades also correlate with such measurements. Finally, the application of advanced statistical approaches and classification algorithms has achieved accurate diagnosis of ACL state based on inertial sensor data. However, a large amount of research and validation will be required to further support this early work. First, one of the primary difficulties in performing the pivot shift is

Table 25.1 Summary of results presented in literature

	N	Subject State	Sensors used	Primary results
Lopomo et al. [19]	66	Anesthetized	Accelerometer	Increased accelerations in injured knees
Araujo et al. [1]	1	Cadaveric	Accelerometer Electromagnetic	PS grade correlates with measured acceleration
Berruto et al. [3]	100	Awake	Accelerometer	PS grade correlates with accelerations. Increased acceleration in injured knees
Labbe et al. [16]	13	Awake	Accelerometer Magnetometer	PS grade correlates with accelerations but 0 similar to 1, 2 similar to 3
Labbe et al. [14]	70	Awake	Electromagnetic	Large number of parameters found to be important in PS grade
Labbe et al. [15]	56	Awake	Electromagnetic	Accurate diagnosis of PS grade (66 %, 96 % within 1 grade)
Borgstrom et al. [5]	61	Anesthetized	Accelerometer Gyroscope	Accurate diagnosis of PS grade (77 %, 98 % within 1 grade)

PS pivot shift

the tendency of some subjects to "guard" against the shift by tensing the surrounding musculature. This undeniably affects the resulting data, but little has been done to quantify these effects nor to mitigate them in quantifying ACL state.

Further, there are a large number of ways to perform the pivot shift maneuver, some of which add internal rotation to the tibia [20, 22], external rotation, and/or a varying degree of valgus stress [21]. Statistical diagnostic tools leveraging PCA and SVM or other similar methods would need to be trained for each pivot shift method or possibly even for each individual surgeon. It is likely that the forces applied to the knee differ among examiners, yet the effect of these forces on accelerometry measurements has not been well described. Some pivot shift methods may be more or less suitable to the accelerometer approach.

Finally, while the 0–3 pivot shift grade approach is widely accepted and has been shown to correlate with patient outcomes, the rough granularity and inter-physician variability of this approach are well known and are among the primary motivators in the development of new diagnostic technology. However, all studies correlating inertial sensor data with ACL state with diagnostic resolution greater than ruptured or intact rely on the pivot shift grade as ground truth; the new technology is being compared against an old method whose flaws it seeks to remedy. Thus, once inertial sensor instrumentation of the pivot shift has advanced sufficiently, research must be undertaken to correlate these measurements directly with patient outcome without the clinical pivot shift grade as an intermediate variable.

In our clinical practice, we currently use accelerometry as research tool to evaluate the effect of pivot shift characteristics on reconstructive outcomes. In general, we have not adapted the technology to determine a treatment algorithm; however we anticipate that this would be the ultimate goal of this approach. In this framework, those patients with a "high-grade" pivot shift as determined by accelerometry may be a candidate for the addition of extra-articular augmentation or the like. Further work is needed to determine the accelerometry values that define an "at-risk" population of patients.

Fact Box 5

The use of inertial sensors to instrument the pivot shift is currently being investigated as a means to quantify the pivot shift. Correlations between such measurements and ACL state have been demonstrated. Accurate diagnosis of ACL state based on these measurements is likely to require advanced statistical methods. Even with the application of such methods, much work remains to evaluate the new technology clinically for a diverse set of physicians and subjects.

References

1. Araujo PH, Ahlden M, Hoshino Y, Muller B, Moloney G, Fu FH, Musahl V (2012) Comparison of three non-invasive quantitative measurement systems for the pivot shift test. Knee Surg Sports Traumatol Arthrosc 20(4):692–697
2. Benjaminse A, Gokeler A, van der Schans CP (2006) Clinical diagnosis of an anterior cruciate ligament rupture: a meta-analysis. J Orthop Phys Ther 36(5): 267–288
3. Berruto M, Uboldi F, Gala L, Marelli B, Albisetti W (2013) Is triaxial accelerometer reliable in the evaluation and grading of knee pivot shift phenomenon? Knee Surg Sports Traumatol Arthrosc 21(4):981–985
4. Bignozzi S, Zaffagnini S, Lopomo N, Fu FH, Irrgang JJ, Marcacci M (2010) Clinical relevance of static and dynamic tests after anatomical double-bundle ACL reconstruction. Knee Surg Sports Traumatol Arthrosc 18(1):37–42
5. Borgstrom PH, Markolf KL, Wang Y, Xu X, Yang PR, Joshi NB, Yeranosian MG, Petrigliano FA, Hame SL, Kaiser WJ, McAllister DR (2015) Use of inertial sensors to predict pivot-shift grade and diagnose an ACL injury during preoperative testing. Am J Sports Med 43(4):857–864. doi:10.1177/0363546514565090, Epub 2015 Jan 22
6. Butler DL, Noyes FR, Grood ES (1980) Ligamentous restraints to anterior-posterior drawer in the human knee. A biomechanical study. J Bone Joint Surg Am 62(2):259–270
7. Galway RD, Beaupre A, Macintosh DL (1972) Pivot shift: a clinical sign of symptomatic anterior cruciate insufficiency. J Bone Joint Surg Br 54:763–764
8. Hefti F, Muller W, Jakob RP (1993) Staubli HU evaluation of knee ligament injuries with the IKDC form. Knee Surg Sports Traumatol Arthrosc 1:226–234. 13

9. Hirschman HP, Danial D, Miyasaka K (1990) The fate of unoperated knee ligament injuries. In: Daniel D (ed) Knee ligaments structure function. Injury and repair. Raven, New York, pp 481–503
10. Invensense MPU 9250 Datasheet. http://www.invensense.com/products/motion-tracking/9-axis/mpu-9250/. Accessed 31 July 2015
11. Joliffe IT (2002) Principal component analysis. Springer series in statistics. 2nd edn. Springer-Verlag, New York
12. Jonsson H, Riklund-Ahlström K, Lind J (2004) Positive pivot shift after ACL reconstruction predicts later osteoarthrosis: 63 patients followed 5–9 years after surgery. Acta Orthop Scand 75(5):594–599
13. Kocher MS, Steadman JR, Briggs KK et al (2004) Relationships between objective assessment of ligament stability and subjective assessment of symptoms and function after anterior cruciate ligament reconstruction. Am J Sports Med 32:629–634
14. Labbe D, de Guise J, Mezghani N, Godbout V, Grimard G, Baillargeon D, Lavigne P, Fernandes J, Ranger P, Hagemeister N (2010) Feature selection using a principal component analysis of the kinematics of the pivot shift phenomenon. J Biomech 43: 3080–3084
15. Labbe D, de Guise J, Mezghani N, Godbout V, Grimard G, Baillargeon D, Lavigne P, Fernandes J, Ranger P, Hagemeister N (2011) Objective grading of the pivot shift phenomenon using a support vector machine approach. J Biomech 44:1–5
16. Labbe D, Li D, Grimard G, de Guise J, Hagemeister N (2015) Quantitative pivot shift assessment using combined inertial and magnetic sensing. Knee Surg Sports Traumatol Arthrosc 23(8):2330–2338
17. Leitze Z, Losee RE, Jokl P, Johnson TR, Feagin JA (2005) Implications of the pivot shift in the ACL-deficient knee. Clin Orthop Relat Res 436:229–236
18. Lopomo N, Zaffagnini S, Bignozzi S, Visani A, Marcacci M (2010) Pivot-shift test: analysis and quantification of knee laxity parameters using a navigation system. J Orthop Res
19. Lopomo N, Zaffagnini S, Signorelli C, Bignozzi S, Giordano G, Marcheggiani Muccioli GM, Visani A (2012) An original clinical methodology for non-invasive assessment of pivot-shift test. Comput Methods Biomech Biomed Engin 15(12):1323–1328
20. Losee RE (1983) Concepts of the pivot shift. Clin Orthop Relat Res 172:45–51
21. Musahl V, Hoshino Y, Ahlden M et al (2012) The pivot shift: a global user guide. Knee Surg Sports Traumatol Arthrosc 20(4):724–731
22. Petermann J, Trus P, Kunneke M, Gotzen L (1996) The pivot-shift test in relation to hip position and lower leg rotation. A clinical analysis. Unfallchirurg 99(3):191–195
23. Prins M (2006) The Lachman test is the most sensitive and the pivot shift the most specific test for the diagnosis of ACL rupture. Aust J Physiother 52(1):66
24. Suykens JA, Vandenwalle J (1999) Least squares support vector machine classifiers. Neural Proc Letters 9(3):293–300
25. Zhu R, Sun D, Zhou Z, Wang D (2007) A linear fusion algorithm for attitude determination using low cost MEMS-based sensors. Measurement 40(3): 322–328

Part V

Surgery for Rotatory Knee Instability

The MacIntosh Procedure 26

Vehniah K. Tjong and Daniel B. Whelan

Contents

26.1 Introduction

Like many pioneers in surgery, Dr. D.L. MacIntosh developed his lateral reconstruction for the anterior cruciate ligament deficient-knee out of necessity. During his tenure as the orthopedic surgeon for varsity athletes at the University of Toronto in the late 1960s, most of his colleagues were focused on addressing meniscal pathology alone, which did nothing to improve symptoms of recurrent instability. Aside from intra-articular pathology, much attention at the time was focused on the concept of medial and anterolateral rotatory instability of the knee [9, 13]. Only in 1972 was Dr. MacIntosh able to reproduce the mechanism of an ACL injury by a physical exam maneuver that is now widely known as the "pivot shift test" [4]. This clinical examination produces an anterior subluxation of the lateral tibial plateau under the lateral femoral condyle when the limb is supported in full extension with a valgus force applied. Subsequent reduction is felt as the knee reaches 30–50° of flexion. Anatomically, the iliotibial band shifts from having extensor function anterior to the flexion-extension axis when the knee is subluxed to a flexor function posterior to the axis when the knee is reduced [4].

His desire to understand the biomechanics contributing to ACL ruptures in his athletes naturally led to the development of a method to prevent recurrent instability after injury. Dr. John Cameron, one of Dr. MacIntosh's best known fellows, describes how Dr. MacIntosh spoke of the need to "tether the tibia" to avoid the anteromedial to posterolateral displacement of the tibia on the femur [1]. Thus, the MacIntosh anterior cruciate ligament reconstruction was born.

26.1.1 The Evolution of Macintosh Procedure [1]

There have been three well-known iterations of the ACL reconstruction procedure established

V.K. Tjong • D.B. Whelan (✉)
Division of Orthopaedic Surgery,
University of Toronto, Toronto, ON, Canada
e-mail: WhelanD@smh.ca

V. Musahl et al. (eds.), *Rotatory Knee Instability*, DOI 10.1007/978-3-319-32070-0_26

by MacIntosh. All had as their common goal the elimination of the pivot shift phenomenon with or without an anatomic facsimile of the ligament itself. Thus they have often been categorized as "non-anatomic" procedures following the advent of modern intra-articular ACL reconstructive techniques. The MacIntosh I, first outlined in the late 1960s, is an extra-articular reconstruction using the iliotibial band (ITB). The middle third slip of the IT band is detached proximally and transferred deep to the lateral collateral ligament (LCL) and through a subperiosteal window or the lateral intramuscular septum only to be secured back onto the ITB origin (Fig. 26.1). In 1979, Ellison used this concept but modified with a bone block from Gerdy's tubercle rerouted deep to the proximal LCL and securing the iliotibial band anterior to its original insertion [3]. Both of these laterally based reconstructions stabilized rotational control; however in a series of 52 knees, there was residual anterior-posterior laxity in all patients using only this lateral-based technique [10]. The MacIntosh I has provided the foundation for current techniques in anterolateral ligament reconstruction and for similar reasons was found to be more appropriate as an adjunct to eliminate lateral-sided pivot shift since it did not address anterior-posterior laxity [6, 10].

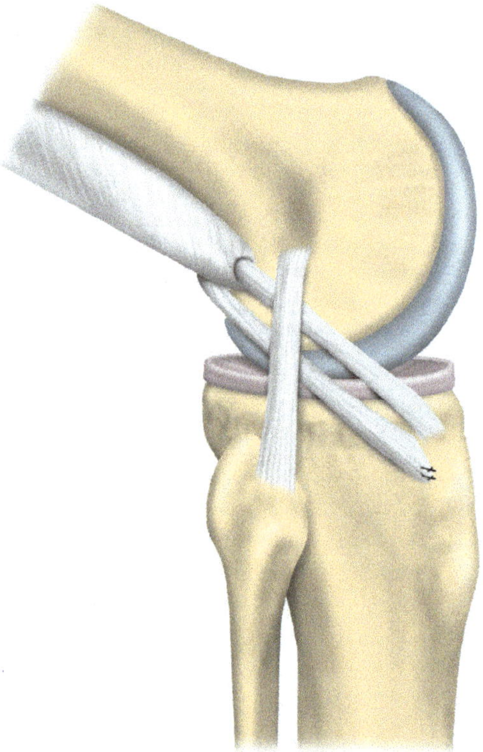

Fig. 26.1 MacIntosh I, lateral extra-articular ligament reconstruction where the iliotibial band graft is passed through the lateral collateral ligament and intermuscular septum and sutured back onto its insertion

Around 1975, MacIntosh refined his original operation with the addition of an intra-articular portion to address the residual A-P laxity noted in some of his previous patients. This became known as the MacIntosh II or lateral substitution over-the-top (LSOT) procedure, which is the technique for which he is most known and described in detail in the section below. The difference in this second iteration includes an intra-articular component where the ITB is passed over the top of the lateral femoral condyle and through a trans-osseous tibial tunnel (Fig. 26.2a, b). This method improved the anterior-posterior laxity experienced by MacI patients, and where his previous patients may have needed screw fixation, MacIntosh described a fixation-free method in his LSOTs by using sutures to secure the reconstruction. It was also noted that patients with concomitant LCL laxity also benefitted from the LSOT as the extra-articular portion of the ITB is weaved through the LCL and ultimately tightened after tensioning.

For acute ACL ruptures where a repair was historically performed, MacIntosh developed a third variation of his procedure called the quadriceps-patellar tendon over the top (QPOT) otherwise known as the MacIntosh III. This method involved using the middle third of the patellar tendon, left attached distally, and extended around the periosteum of the patella and through to the middle third of the quadriceps tendon. This graft was then passed over the top of the lateral femoral condyle as an augment to the acutely ruptured ACL, which was also stitched, passed, and fixated on the lateral femur. Since primary ACL repairs were not performed then, the MacIntosh III procedure consequently grew out of favor (Fig. 26.3).

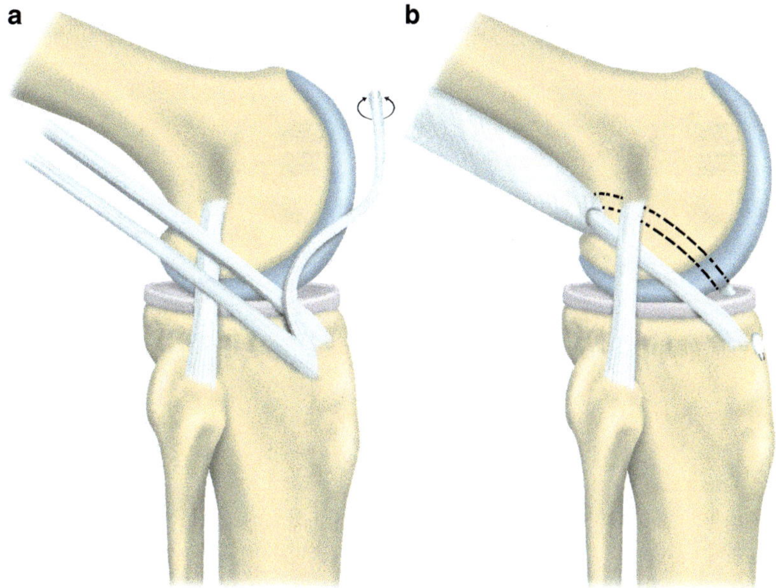

Fig. 26.2 (**a**, **b**) MacIntosh II, iliotibial band graft is passed over the top of the lateral femoral condyle and secured through a tibial tunnel

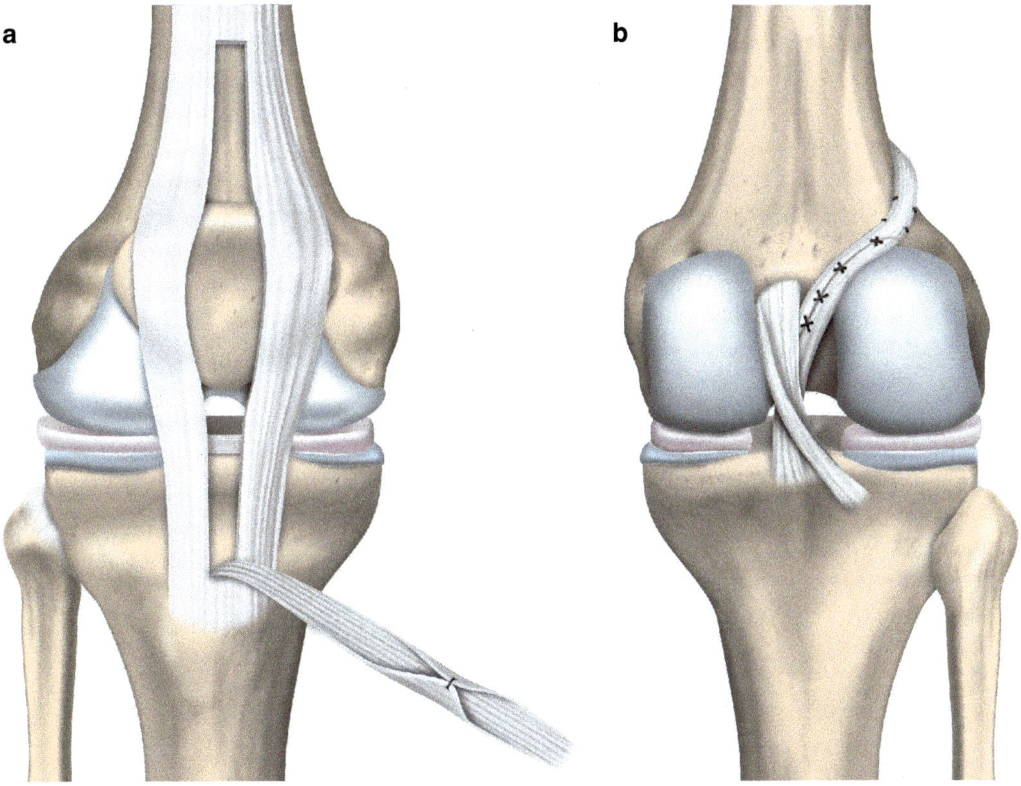

Fig. 26.3 (**a**, **b**) MacIntosh III, quadriceps-patellar tendon over-the-top (QPOT) method usually as an adjunct to an anterior cruciate ligament repair

26.2 Lateral Substitution Over-the-Top Procedure (LSOT) [1, 11]

When it was first described, the indications for the LSOT procedure were focused on individuals with recurrent, symptomatic anterior cruciate ligament instability. The procedure was felt to be ideal for high-demand, contact athletes, athletes who could not wear a brace following injury, and individuals with connective tissue disease and occasionally for failed primary ACL repairs. At present it is occasionally considered in revision cases for patients who have failed anatomic intra-articular ACL reconstructions (in which case it may be used as an augment or a stand-alone procedure) or patients with open growth plates. Surgical goals include a stable, functional, pain-free knee with the restoration of full range of motion and ability to return to sport without the use of a brace if intended.

26.2.1 Surgical Technique for the LSOT or MacIntosh II

Positioning

- Patient is positioned supine with an ipsilateral bump underneath the operative limb.
- An examination under general anesthesia is performed to demonstrate the presence of a positive pivot shift test.
- A high tourniquet is placed, inflated, and leg rested on a footplate.

Initial Incision

- Medial parapatellar arthrotomy is carried out to inspect the knee joint and visualize ACL. Meniscal repair/debridement is done at this time.

ITB Graft Harvest

- With the knee in 90° of flexion, a direct lateral incision is extended approximately 6 cm from distal aspect of the lateral femoral condyle to expose the iliotibial band.
  - The middle third of the iliotibial band approximately 6 cm proximal to its insertion site is harvested while leaving it attached distally on Gerdy's tubercle (Fig. 26.4). It should measure approximately 3 cm wide distally and 5 cm wide proximally.
  - The proximal end of the graft is then tubularized with a whipstitch by using a 0-sized, non-absorbable suture and reflected distally (Fig. 26.5).

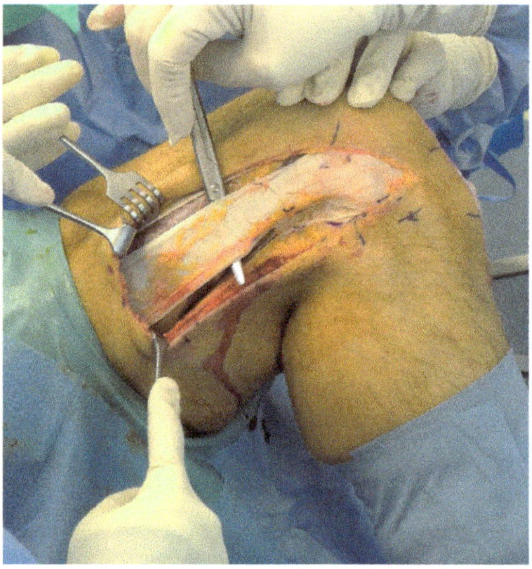

Figs. 26.4 Iliotibial band graft harvest and detachment proximally

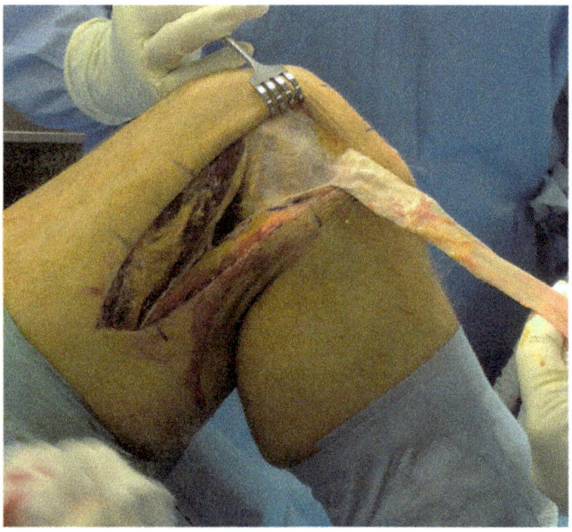

Fig. 26.5 Passage through lateral collateral ligament is developed and marked with Kelly

Tunnel Placement

- The femoral origin of the LCL is isolated and a subperiosteal tunnel from posterior to the femoral origin of the LCL to anterior to the lateral intermuscular septum is created using a curved Kelly (Fig. 26.6).
- A second subperiosteal tunnel is made from posterior to the intermuscular septum into the posterior "over-the-top" area on the femoral condyle (Fig. 26.7).
- The graft is then passed deep to the LCL and through both subperiosteal tunnels into the "over-the-top" region of the intercondylar notch.

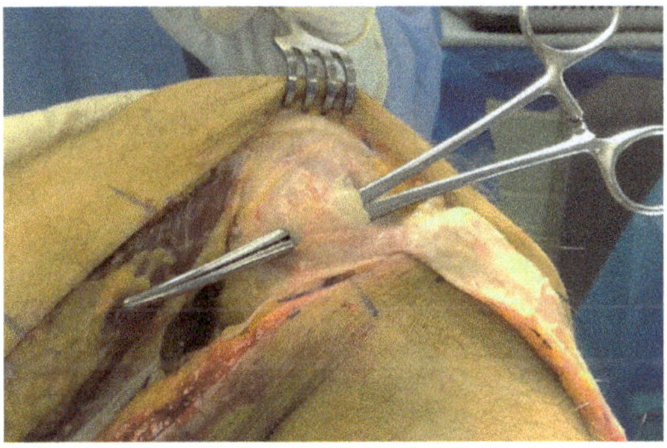

Fig. 26.6 Passage through lateral collateral ligament is developed and marked with Kelly

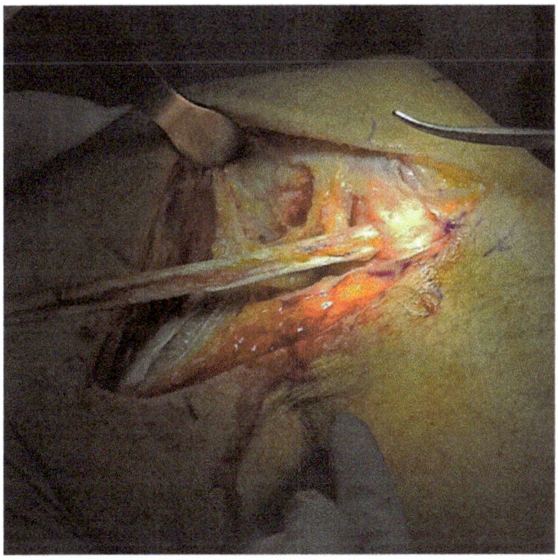

Fig. 26.7 Iliotibial band graft is passed through the lateral collateral ligament tunnel while preparing to pass through intermuscular septum

Tibial Preparation

- A quarter-inch drill hole was made using the 60° guide starting medial to the patellar tendon insertion and exiting slightly posterior to the anterior tibial spine. This is overdrilled with a cannulated 3/8 in. drill bit.

Graft Passage and Tensioning

- With the knee flexed at 90°, a curved Kelly is passed through the intercondylar notch and posterolateral capsule into the over-the-top space where the graft was passed through the notch posteriorly and then through the tibial tunnel from posterior to anterior (Fig. 26.8).
- The graft is tensioned at 70° of flexion with the tibia in external rotation and with a posteriorly directed force. It is then sutured to the femoral origin of the LCL. After emerging from the tibial tunnel, the distal end of the graft is passed deep to the patellar tendon and sutured beyond Gerdy's tubercle onto itself (Figs. 26.9 and 26.10).

Closure

- A drain is placed posterolaterally and the knee lavaged with saline after which a 2-layer close takes place.
- Sterile gauze dressing and Jones bandage are applied.
- A hinged knee brace is applied and locked at 70° of flexion with the tibia in external rotation to decrease tension on the lateral side.

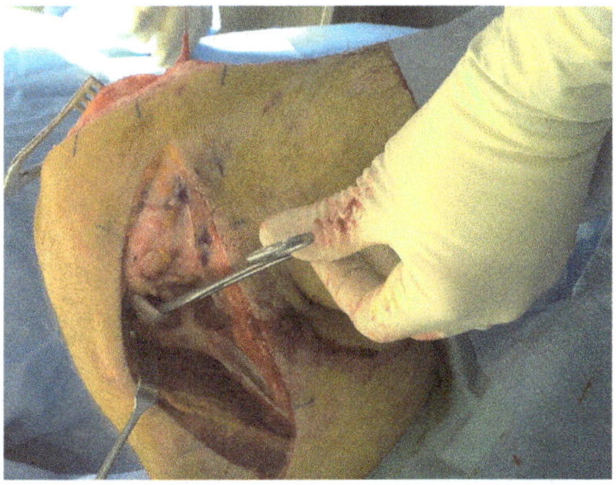

Fig. 26.8 Graft is passed from over-the-top passage through to the notch

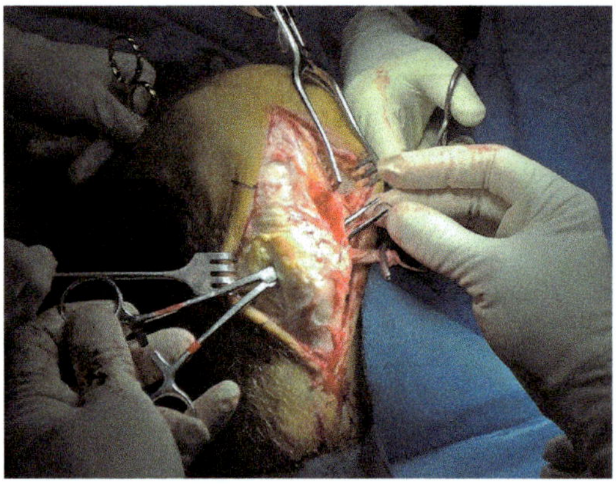

Fig. 26.9 Plane developed for iliotibial band graft to traverse deep to the patellar tendon

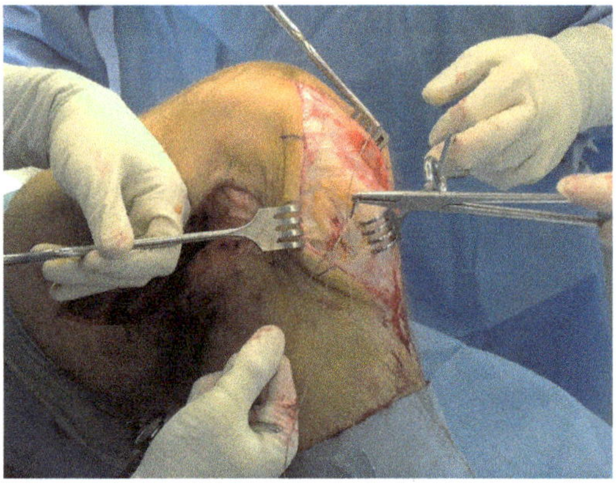

Fig. 26.10 Secure reconstruction back onto its insertion at Gerdy's tubercle

26.3 Discussion

The MacIntosh procedure has gone through several iterations over decades and, in turn, has found itself on the forefront of the discussion around rotational instability of the knee. Its application and efficacy as an adjunct to the intra-articular ACL reconstruction are being studied at length.

Researchers from Italy studied the pivot shift phenomenon in vivo to determine the effect of intra-articular and extra-articular ACL reconstruction. They measured both the maximum anterior tibial translation (ATT) and the axial tibial rotation (ATR). Results highlight that extra-articular reconstruction had minimal effect compared to intra-articular reconstruction in reducing anterior translation of the tibia, whereas tibial rotatory instability was significantly decreased by the use of lateral tenodesis as previously reported [12].

Early results from Ireland and Trickey suggested that after a 2-year follow-up, there was significant improvement in clinical and functional stability after an extra-articular MacIntosh procedure. Seventy-four percent of patients had returned to some form of sporting activity, while 84 % of patients presented with a negative pivot shift test [7]. Furthermore, Dempsey and Tregonning reviewed 25 patients with combined extra- and intra-articular MacIntosh ACL reconstructions or the MacIntosh II as well as 22 patients with isolated extra-articular ACL reconstructions or the MacIntosh I. After 9 years, there were no subjective symptoms of instability with 62 % of knees having good to excellent Lysholm scores and 83 % remaining active in sport. They also found that the addition of the intra-articular component made no significant difference in subjective outcome or long-term function [2].

Decades later, Johnston et al. reported on a retrospective cohort of 84 knees who had undergone the MacIntosh LSOT procedure whose results were similar to the previously published literature (i.e., 61 % of patients with good to excellent Lysholm scores, negative pivot shift in 88 % of knees). They concluded that the LSOT could be a viable substitute for arthroscopically assisted ACL reconstruction for those whose scar cosmesis is not a priority [8].

Most recently, there have been several studies investigating the use of the extra-articular MacIntosh procedure in combination with a more modern intra-articular ACL reconstruction technique using hamstring as a method to reduce rotational instability seen with the latter. Vadala et al. found no significant difference in KT-1000 measurements and Lachman testing between patients who had the combined procedure versus the MacIntosh in isolation. There was, however, a significant residual pivot shift in the group who did not have the extra-articular reconstruction [15]. This supports the concept that the MacIntosh procedure may significantly reduce rotational laxity of the knee following ACL injury. Sonnery-Cottet et al. has reported preliminary data on outcomes of this combined ACL reconstruction and anterolateral ligament reconstruction, which is described as the MacIntosh I. Their indications to apply this combined method include the presence of a Segond fracture, chronic ACL lesion, grade 3 pivot shift, high level of sport participation and pivoting sports, and a radiographic lateral femoral notch sign. After an average follow-up of 2 years, the Lysholm, Tegner, objective and subjective IKDC scores, as well as the pivot shift exam had improved although 10% of knees in their study had persistent pivot shift postoperatively [14]. Long-term results are not yet available, and the effect on posttraumatic OA is also not yet known.

Conclusions

Just as a pendulum returns to its equilibrium once displaced, the original application and theory behind the MacIntosh procedure have swung back into the forefront of orthopedic surgery. Interest in comparing biomechanical and clinical outcomes of ACL reconstruction with or without the augmentation using a lateral extra-articular tenodesis has continued to grow with promising preliminary results. One international, multicenter, randomized control trial is currently underway comparing isolated anatomic ACL reconstruction with an identical procedure augmented with a Macintosh II construct. This study will undoubtedly provide further information on graft failure, function, strength, range of motion, and quality of life when utilizing an extra-articular augment [5].

With recent anatomic advances in the definition and function of the anterolateral ligament of the knee, the Macintosh procedure has regained popularity. The optimal indication for an extra-articular augmentation with primary ACL reconstruction is as yet unknown; however it is likely to be most useful in patients with a chronic Segond-type lesion (i.e., lateral capsular injury, bony, or otherwise) and patients with generalized ligamentous laxity or in revision situations with excess rotational laxity. In the pediatric population it provides an option to impart some stability with less risk of physeal injury. Further research will help to clarify its specific role in primary ACL injury and the longer-term consequences on return to function and the development of arthritis post reconstruction.

Fact Box

- Pivot shift test mimics axial tibial rotatory instability.
- Lateral tenodesis or the MacIntosh procedure has been shown to effectively reduce the pivot shift phenomenon.
- The MacIntosh procedure as an augment or revision to intra-articular ACL reconstruction may effectively address both pivot shifting and anterior translation in patients who experience symptoms of both.
- The extra-articular portion of the original MacIntosh I likely mimics the function of the anterolateral ligament (ALL) and is similar to ALL reconstruction techniques currently described with minor modifications.

References

1. Cameron J (2015) Personal Interview on the history and development of the MacIntosh ACL Reconstruction. V. Tjong, Toronto
2. Dempsey SM, Tregonning RJ (1993) Nine-year follow-up results of two methods of MacIntosh anterior cruciate ligament reconstructions. Clin Orthop Relat Res (294):216–222
3. Ellison AE (1979) Distal iliotibial-band transfer for anterolateral rotatory instability of the knee. J Bone Joint Surg Am 61(3):330–337
4. Galway H et al (1972) Pivot shift: a clinical sign of symptomatic anterior cruciate insufficiency. J Bone Joint Surg Br 54R:763
5. Getgood A (2013 – ongoing) Multicenter randomized clinical trial comparing anterior cruciate ligament reconstruction with and without lateral extra-articular tenodesis in individuals who are at high risk of graft failure. University of Western Ontario, Canada. ClinicalTrials.gov Identifier: NCT02018354
6. Hewison CE et al (2015) Lateral extra-articular tenodesis reduces rotational laxity when combined with anterior cruciate ligament reconstruction: a systematic review of the literature. Arthroscopy 31(10):2022–2034. doi: 10.1016/j.arthro.2015.04.089. Epub 2015 Jun 24.
7. Ireland J, Trickey EL (1980) Macintosh tenodesis for anterolateral instability of the knee. J Bone Joint Surg Br 62(3):340–345
8. Johnston DR et al (2003) Long-term outcome of MacIntosh reconstruction of chronic anterior cruciate ligament insufficiency using fascia lata. J Orthop Sci 8(6):789–795

9. Kennedy JC (1963) Complete dislocation of the knee joint. J Bone Joint Surg Am 45:889–904
10. Kennedy JC et al (1978) Anterolateral rotatory instability of the knee joint. An early analysis of the Ellison procedure. J Bone Joint Surg Am 60(8): 1031–1039
11. MacIntosh D, Darby T (1976) Lateral substitution reconstruction. J Bone Joint Surg Br 58:142
12. Monaco E et al (2014) Extra-articular ACL reconstruction and pivot shift: in vivo dynamic evaluation with navigation. Am J Sports Med 42(7):1669–1674
13. Slocum DB, Larson RL (1968) Pes anserinus transplantation. A surgical procedure for control of rotatory instability of the knee. J Bone Joint Surg Am 50(2):226–242
14. Sonnery-Cottet B et al (2015) Outcome of a combined anterior cruciate ligament and anterolateral ligament reconstruction technique with a minimum 2-year follow-up. Am J Sports Med 43(7):1598–1605
15. Vadalà AP et al (2013) An extra-articular procedure improves the clinical outcome in anterior cruciate ligament reconstruction with hamstrings in female athletes. Int Orthop 37(2):187–192

Surgery for Rotatory Knee Instability: Experience from the Hughston Clinic

27

Champ L. Baker III and Champ L. Baker Jr.

Contents

C.L. Baker III, MD (✉) • C.L. Baker Jr., MD
The Hughston Clinic, Columbus, GA, USA
e-mail: champbaker3@gmail.com

27.1 Introduction

In 1949 Dr Jack Hughston established his orthopedic practice in Columbus, GA. He was an anatomist, a keen observer and recorder of his findings, and a believer in the documentation of long-term follow-up of his results. In the 1950s he began to document the pathological anatomy he observed at surgery and to correlate these findings with his clinical examinations of patients with acute and chronic knee injuries. Over time, Dr Hughston developed a classification system for knee ligament instabilities [5, 6]. He believed that a thorough knowledge of knee anatomy was the key to performing successful surgical repair. This knowledge and his classification system allow the clinician to diagnose tears of specific ligaments and other capsular structures accurately during a ligamentous examination of an injured knee.

The Hughston classification of knee ligament instabilities is based upon the rotational motion of the knee about the central axis of the posterior cruciate ligament (PCL). While not the true mechanical axis, it does provide a reference point. All rotatory instabilities are then defined as subluxations about the axis of the intact PCL and may be present singly or combined. If the PCL is injured, the instability is designated as straight or existing in one plane. The rotatory knee instabilities include three types: anteromedial, anterolateral, and posterolateral. Posteromedial rotatory instability, by contrast, is impossible because

V. Musahl et al. (eds.), *Rotatory Knee Instability*, DOI 10.1007/978-3-319-32070-0_27

when the tibia is internally rotated on the femur, the intact PCL prevents posteromedial rotatory displacement.

27.2 Anteromedial Rotatory Instability

Anteromedial rotatory instability (AMRI) is defined as an anterior subluxation of the medial tibial plateau on the medial femoral condyle resulting from a tear of the medial compartment ligaments. Clinical signs of AMRI include either a positive abduction stress test at 30° of flexion or a positive anterior drawer test with the tibia in slight external rotation or both. When positive, each test demonstrates the anteromedial subluxation of the tibia. An associated tear of the anterior cruciate ligament (ACL) will usually increase the displacement observed in the anterior drawer test. The degree of instability demonstrated during stress testing is graded based on the separation of the joint surfaces. A mild (1+) instability indicates separation of five millimeters or less; a moderate (2+) instability indicates separation between five and ten millimeters; and a severe (3+) instability indicates separation greater than ten millimeters [5]. When performing the anterior drawer in flexion and the tibia in external rotation, tears of the meniscofemoral portion of the mid-third capsular ligament will usually allow an anteromedial subluxation of no more than 1+; however, tears of the meniscotibial portion of the mid-third capsular ligament will result in an AMRI of 2+ or 3+. With an intact meniscotibial ligament, the medial meniscus remains stabilized to the tibia, buttressing the posterior femoral condyle. When this ligament tears, the meniscus becomes mobile, and its stabilizing function is lost, producing the AMRI observed at the anterior drawer test in external rotation.

The tibial collateral ligament lies over the mid-third capsular ligament, which is divided into its meniscofemoral and meniscotibial portions. Hughston and Eilers [8] have described the posterior oblique ligament (POL) anatomy and its importance in repairing the medial structures. The POL attaches to the adductor tubercle and has three arms: superficial, tibial, and capsular. The superficial arm is a thin, fibrous structure that passes over the anterior arm of the semimembranosus to attach distally to the pes anserine fascia. The main tibial arm passes beneath the anterior arm of the semimembranosus and inserts on the proximal medial tibia close to the articular margin with firm attachments to the medial meniscus. The capsular arm of the POL blends with the posterior capsule and oblique popliteal ligament as it arises from the semimembranosus. The capsular arm of the semimembranosus aponeuroses is continuous with the POL anteriorly and the oblique popliteal ligament posteriorly. Contraction of the semimembranosus tenses the POL and the oblique popliteal ligaments and has a dynamic and static stabilizing effect on the meniscus through their firm attachments. The medial meniscus may thus be thought of as the terminal structure in the semimembranosus muscle-ligament-meniscus unit (Fig. 27.1).

The pathological anatomy of the torn medial compartment ligaments can take on a variety of manifestations. Specific injury sites were documented in 170 cases of acute, isolated AMRI requiring operative repair [4]. Notable findings included injury to the tibial attachment of the tibial collateral ligament in 54 % of cases, while in 57 % of cases, the meniscofemoral ligament was torn commonly hidden beneath the intact femoral attachment of the tibial collateral ligament. Additionally, injury to the POL was localized to the femoral attachment in 35 % of knees, to midsubstance in 39 % of knees, and to the tibial attachment in 43 % of cases. For operative repair a medial hockey stick incision is made from the medial aspect of the tibia extending proximally along the medial border of the patellar tendon to the level of the inferior pole and then curving proximally 5–8 cm at a level between the joint space and medial epicondyle. The incision is carried deep to the superficial fascia, and a posterior flap is raised, including the sartorius aponeurosis. The saddle is then palpated between the medial epicondyle and adductor tubercle. The tibial collateral ligament attaches to the medial epicondyle, and the POL attaches to

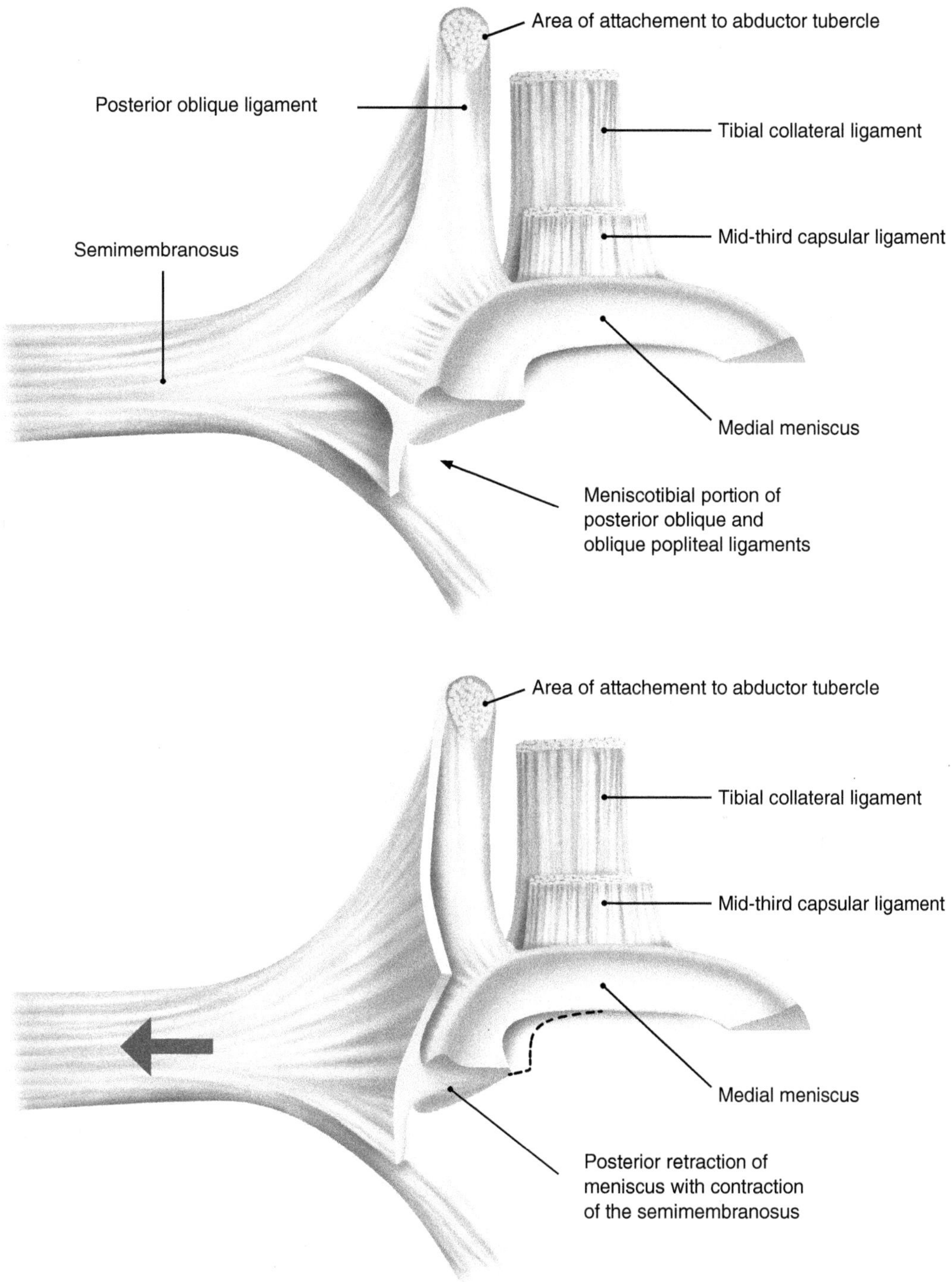

Fig. 27.1 This shows the insertion of the capsular arm of the semimembranosus into the POL and thusly the posterior third of the medial meniscus. Contraction of the semimembranosus creates stability during knee flexion and during cutting and twisting by maintaining the medial meniscus posteriorly

the adductor tubercle. A soft area may be palpated between the posterior border of the tibial collateral ligament and POL. A posteromedial arthrotomy incision is made beginning at the epicondylar area extending distally and anteriorly paralleling the posterior border of the tibial collateral ligament. Retraction of the posteromedial arthrotomy incision anteriorly and posteriorly exposes the mid-third capsular ligaments, the POL, and their attachments to the meniscus. The attachment sites and the substance of the tibial collateral ligament, mid-third capsular ligament, POL, meniscus, oblique popliteal ligament, and semimembranosus are then examined systematically with particular attention to the continuity of the semimembranosus-posterior oblique-medial meniscus complex. Repair of the injured structures then proceeds. The hip is kept in abduction and external rotation with the knee flexed approximately 60°. This flexion angle is maintained during the repair. A bolster or towel is placed under the anterolateral aspect of the foot to internally rotate the tibia and reduce the joint. If torn, the medial meniscus is repaired first to the capsule followed by repair of the meniscofemoral and meniscotibial portions of the mid-third capsular ligament. Next, the tibial collateral ligament, if torn from its attachment sites, is repaired with the use of suture anchors. Historically only periosteal sutures were available. When there is either an avulsion of the POL from the adductor tubercle or an interstitial tear of the ligament, proper tension is restored by advancing the ligament proximally and superiorly to the periosteum of the medial epicondylar and adductor tubercle region. Once tension is restored to the POL, it is advanced onto the previously stabilized mid-third capsular and tibial collateral ligaments with mattress sutures. If the capsular arm of the semimembranosus appears lax, it is then advanced to the POL (Fig. 27.2). Historically after surgery the knee is immobilized in a plaster cast in 60° of flexion for 6 weeks with touchdown weight-bearing restrictions. Over the next several months, the patient gradually regains muscular strength and extension and can discontinue crutches once the knee nears full extension. Quadriceps strengthening is emphasized. Currently at the Hughston Clinic, patients with 3+ AMRI managed operatively are treated with the same repair technique as described by Dr Hughston. After surgery the patient is placed in a hinged knee brace and allowed full range of motion immediately but with protected non-weight-bearing restrictions for 6 weeks followed by progressive therapy.

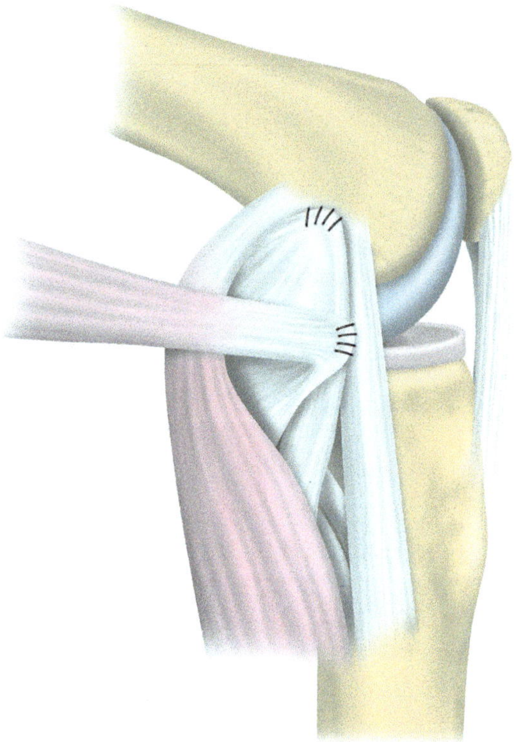

Fig. 27.2 Tension has been restored to the POL by advancement proximally and anteriorly onto the femur and by further advancement with mattress sutures onto the tibial collateral ligament. The capsular arm of the semimembranosus may also be advanced onto the POL if persistent laxity is noted

Several reports have documented the surgical treatment of acute AMRI [3, 7, 8]. In one of his last reports, Dr Hughston presented his long-term results of repair of the medial ligaments in 41 knees with an average of 22 years of follow-up [3]. In 24 patients, the knees had an associated tear of the ACL that was either debrided (17), repaired (6), or augmented (1). At follow-up there was no difference in recurrent instability, meniscal injury, or radiographic degenerative changes in those patients with a torn ACL at the time of operation versus those with an intact ligament. As Dr Hughston had concluded in an earlier report, "it is not the absence of an isolated tear of an anterior cruciate ligament that leads to an anterior cruciate-deficient knee, but rather the presence of an additional ligament lesion that was not perceived either clinically or at operation" [7]. Thirty-eight patients continued to participate in physical fitness and recreational athletics at final follow-up. There were three failures (7 %): two from technical difficulty and one from unrecognized associated anterolateral rotatory instability. Dr Hughston's long-term results of repair with the use of periosteal sutures and primary direct repair in comparison to modern use of implants and ACL graft reconstructions are remarkable.

Fact Box 1
Restoration of the semimembranosus-POL-medial meniscus unit eliminates the AMRI, stabilizes the knee, and protects against future meniscal tearing and degeneration.

27.3 Anterolateral Rotatory Instability

Anterolateral rotatory instability (ALRI) is defined as an anterior subluxation of the lateral tibial plateau on the lateral femoral condyle. Dr Hughston believed that this form of instability could be most accurately demonstrated by a positive jerk test and also by a positive anterior drawer test in neutral rotation. The adduction stress test at 30° is either normal or mildly positive. Dr Hughston described the jerk test as follows: "With the patient supine, the examiner supports the lower extremity, flexing the hip to about 45° and the knee to 90° and internally rotating the tibia. If the right knee is being examined, grasp the foot with the right hand and internally rotate the tibia while the left hand is placed over the proximal end of the tibia and fibula and used to exert a valgus stress. If the test is positive, subluxation of the lateral femorotibial articulation becomes maximum at about 30° of flexion, and then, as the knee extends further, spontaneous relocation occurs. The relocation takes the form of a sudden change in the relative velocities of the tibia and the femur. That is, there is a sudden change in the rate of acceleration of the two surfaces which, in engineering terminology, is called a jerk" [6]. Essentially the jerk test is equivalent to the pivot shift test with the former demonstrating the anterolateral rotatory instability in going from knee flexion to extension and the latter with the knee progressing from knee extension into knee flexion. Dr Hughston believed that a positive pivot shift jerk test could only be elicited in the presence of tears of the lateral capsular or iliotibial tract ligaments or both [4]. He believed that an associated tear of the ACL accentuated the anterolateral rotatory instability but did not cause it.

The mid-third lateral capsular ligament attaches proximally to the femoral lateral epicondyle and distally to the lateral tibial joint margin. Recent research has focused upon the anterolateral ligament (ALL) as a distinct anatomic structure and responsible for anterolateral instability. We believe Dr Hughston's descriptions of the mid-third lateral capsular ligament to be consistent to those reported of the ALL. The iliotibial tract may be divided into aponeurotic, superficial, middle, deep, and capsulo-osseous layers [13]. The deep layer fibers begin at the termination of the lateral intermuscular septum approximately 6 cm proximal to the lateral epicondyle. The layer extends laterally in the coronal plane and curves distally following the lateral femoral condyle to blend with the superficial layer in the sagittal plane. The deep layer strengthens and thickens the superficial layer, while the capsulo-osseous layer functions as a medial retaining wall for the deep layer. It is formed proximally by fascia overlying the plantaris and lateral gastrocnemius, and it extends distally, attaching posterior to the fibula and anterior to the lateral tibial tuberosity. Together the deep and capsulo-osseous layers augment the superficial layer to function as an anterolateral ligament of the knee [13].

In 66 operative cases of acute ALRI, the pathological anatomy was recorded with the following findings: the ACL was torn in all cases, and in 56 cases, the mid-third lateral capsular ligament was torn, and the iliotibial tract was torn either in the superficial (27 knees) or deep (54 knees) fibers or both [4]. Although the ACL is commonly torn in cases with ALRI, Dr Hughston did not believe that isolated injury of this ligament was responsible for ALRI. He believed that injuries to the lateral capsular ligament and iliotibial tract were responsible. In an unpublished review of 228 consecutive cases of chronic ACL tears seen over a 5-year period, only 35 (15 %) were associated with ALRI or combined ALRI and AMRI [6]. Operative management for acute and chronic ALRI included an extra-articular repair of the torn ligamentous and capsular structures. A lateral hockey stick incision is made in line with the iliotibial band extending distally between the tibial tuberosity and Gerdy's tubercle. A large posterior flap is mobilized in the plane between the superficial and deep fascia. The iliotibial band is incised longitudinally just posterior to the intermuscular septum proximally and continuing distally toward the lateral tibial tubercle. Retraction of the iliotibial band both anteriorly and posteriorly exposes the deep iliotibial tract and septum proximally and the lateral capsular ligament distally. A lateral arthrotomy incision is made anterior to the popliteus and paralleling its course to the level of the lateral meniscus. The incision is then changed to a vertical incision and progressed distally to the tibia to protect the arcuate ligament reflection that forms the anterior border of the popliteal recess. Abnormalities may be noted in the mid-third capsular ligament including transverse tears, avulsions from the tibia with or without associated bone, or most commonly interstitial tears with associated laxity. Retractors are placed and the lateral meniscus is inspected for peripheral or body tears. At this point peripheral tears of the meniscus are repaired with suture, and body tears are resected. Posterior inspection includes evaluation of the short head of the biceps and its attachment to the posterolateral capsule. The superficial and deep components of the iliotibial tract and the lateral intermuscular septum attachments to the lateral femoral condyle are inspected for hemorrhage and injury. This completes the surgical approach and identification of the pathological anatomy. As Dr Hughston has stated, the next step is "to restore the tissues, the ligaments, and their muscular attachments back to their natural places, with the proper tension and continuity" [4]. If avulsed the mid-third lateral capsular ligament is repaired back to the tibia with periosteal sutures or, if the tear is interstitial, advanced anteriorly and distally in a pants-over-vest fashion with mattress sutures. If torn the short head of the biceps is then reattached to the posterolateral capsule. Next, the posterior portion of the iliotibial tract is sutured to the intermuscular septum at its attachment to the lateral femoral condyle (Fig. 27.3). The posterior portion of the long head of the biceps insertion may be released and advanced distally to the iliotibial tract just proximal to Gerdy's tubercle to restore tension to this musculotendinous unit.

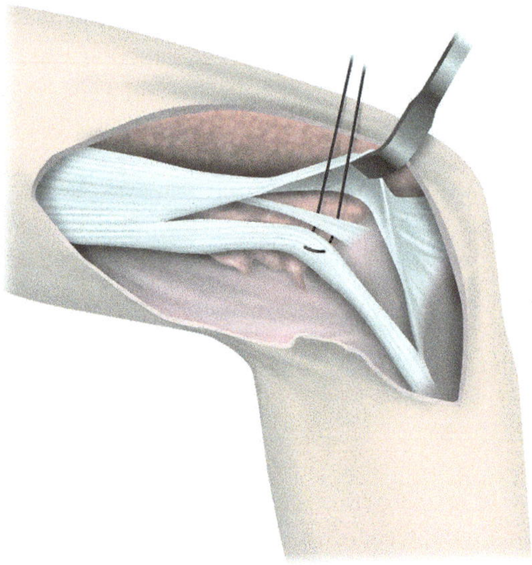

Fig. 27.3 The posterior portion of the iliotibial tract is reconstructed to the lateral intermuscular septum at its point of attachment to the lateral femoral condyle with mattress sutures. In the distal aspect of the iliotibial incision, one may see the closure and advancement of the mid-third lateral capsular ligament (In this illustration the closure and advancement of the lateral capsular ligament has been omitted)

Historically after surgery for ALRI, the knee is immobilized at 70° of flexion in a plaster cast for 6 weeks. Crutch ambulation continues for up to 3 months after surgery with slowly progressive weight bearing as the patient regains knee exten-

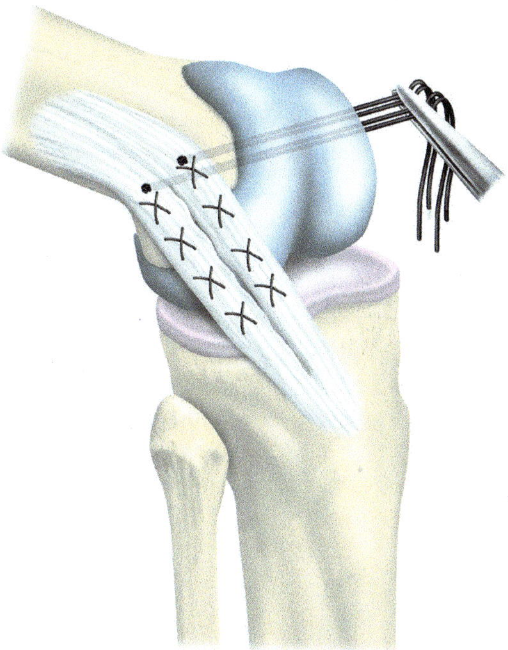

Fig. 27.4 The Andrews extra-articular reconstruction for ALRI. Sutures are tied medially over a bone bridge after passage through drill holes lateral to medial

sion and muscular strength. Full extension may not be achieved until after 6 months of rehabilitation. Patients may expect good stability and function with return to activities at a year after surgery.

Andrews et al. from the Hughston Clinic detailed their experience with a lateral extra-articular iliotibial tract tenodesis in the treatment of 31 knees with acute and chronic ALRI at a minimum of 2 years of follow-up [1]. The injured ACL was repaired in 16 knees, while in 15 knees, no repair was performed with no differences in outcomes at follow-up. Overall 94 % of patients achieved a good or excellent subjective and objective result. Twenty-one patients were able to return to pre-injury level of sport performance, 9 were able to return to sport with decreased performance, and only one was unable to return. The authors noted that the success of the technique is directly related to the minimization or elimination of the rotational instability noted clinically by the jerk test [1]. During the procedure the posterior portion of the distal iliotibial tract is tenodesed to the prepared lateral femoral metaphysis. Two parallel rows of Bunnell sutures are created through the iliotibial tract and then passed through the femur and tied to each other medially over a bone bridge. Fixation points laterally are at the distal insertion of the intermuscular septum on the linea aspera just anterior to the posterior femoral cortex and secondly 1 cm anterior and 0.5 cm distally to the first (Fig. 27.4).

Currently at the Hughston Clinic, ALRI is managed operatively with anatomic ACL reconstruction. Consideration for anterolateral repair/reconstruction is reserved for cases with combined acute posterolateral rotatory instability in which a lateral approach will be undertaken or in revision cases with persistent positive jerk tests. Rehabilitation currently for ALRI is similar to standard ACL reconstruction rehabilitation with immediate full weight bearing and range of motion.

As with other rotatory instabilities, ALRI may coexist with other types including AMRI and posterolateral rotatory instability (PLRI). Success requires identification of all pathology and treatment of associated rotatory instability. Dr Hughston stated "the value and success of the reconstruction depend on re-establishing the anatomy and thereby restoring the dynamic input to the extra-articular ligaments" [4]. Indeed anatomic repair performed with precise technique and combined with appropriate therapy and rehabilitation produces predictably good results.

Fact Box 2

An ACL tear alone does not cause ALRI. ALRI is caused by an injury to either the iliotibial tract or mid-third lateral capsular ligament or both.

27.4 Posterolateral Rotatory Instability

PLRI is a posterior and external rotatory subluxation of the lateral tibial plateau on the lateral femoral condyle. This manifests clinically with either a positive posterolateral drawer test [10], a positive external rotation recurvatum test [5, 6,

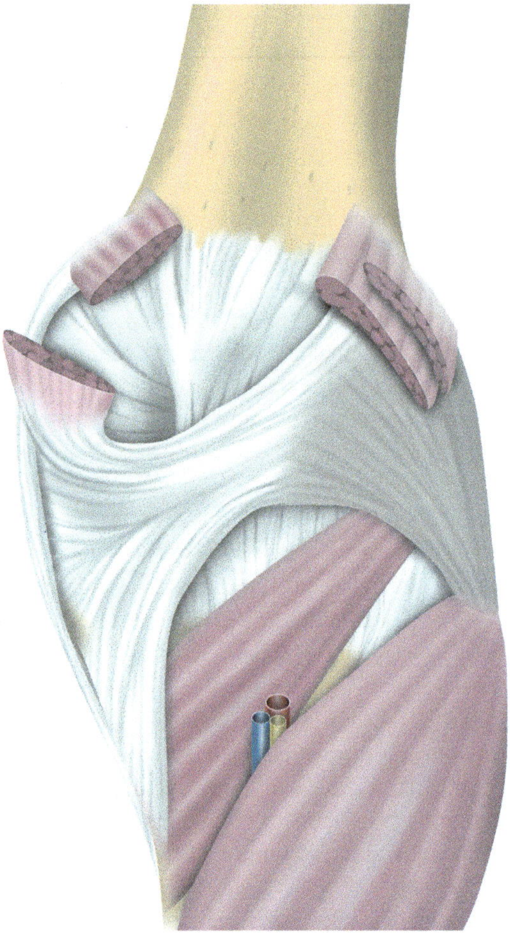

Fig. 27.5 A posterior view of the knee demonstrating the *shaded area* as the arcuate ligament as described by Dr Hughston (where is the shaded area in the illustration?)

10], or both. The posterolateral drawer test is a posterior drawer test performed with the tibia unconstrained and the ankle and foot free to rotate. When the test is positive, the tibial tuberosity rotates externally and appears to sink, losing its prominence. In the external rotation recurvatum test, the examiner grasps the great toe of the injured extremity and lifts up the leg of the supine patient. When positive the tibial tuberosity rotates externally and produces an apparent tibia vara and a degree of recurvatum greater than the uninvolved side. The adduction stress test at 30° is typically mildly to severely positive depending upon the extent of the injury to the fibular collateral ligament. The posterior drawer test in neutral rotation is negative, indicating an intact PCL.

PLRI is produced by an injury to what Dr Hughston termed the arcuate complex, consisting of the arcuate ligament, the fibular collateral ligament, and the popliteus tendon and its aponeurosis. The use of the term arcuate ligament has created confusion in the literature regarding the posterolateral corner anatomy of the knee. It was considered by Dr Hughston to have an attachment to the posterior femur immediately proximal to the articular surface of the lateral femoral condyle. It blended with the oblique popliteal ligament, fascia from the popliteus, and other fascial layers to form distal attachments to the meniscus, tibia, and fibula (Fig. 27.5). In later anatomic dissections from the Hughston Clinic, the arcuate ligament was noted to be comprised of not a single ligament but of several structures giving an arched or arcuate appearance [12]. Further studies at Hughston have demonstrated posterolateral corner injuries often involve injury to multiple different anatomic structures that can account for the clinical differences seen in stability testing [11].

More so than any other rotatory instability, PLRI is often seen as a combined instability with either AMRI or ALRI. Isolated PLRI is much less common. Review of the operative findings in 19 cases of isolated acute PLRI demonstrates injury to the fibular collateral ligament in 12 knees, injury to the popliteus in nine knees, injury to the short head of the biceps in three knees and the long head in six knees, and injury to the tibial portion of the arcuate ligament in nine, mid-third portion in four, and femoral portion of the arcuate ligament in seven [4]. The surgical approach for operative management for acute PLRI is similar to that for acute ALRI. The peroneal nerve is located and protected. The iliotibial band is split just posterior to the intermuscular septum and extended distally to the midpoint of the lateral tibial tubercle. The mid-third lateral capsular ligament is incised as described previously. During the intra-articular inspection, the lateral meniscus and arcuate ligament are probed. The

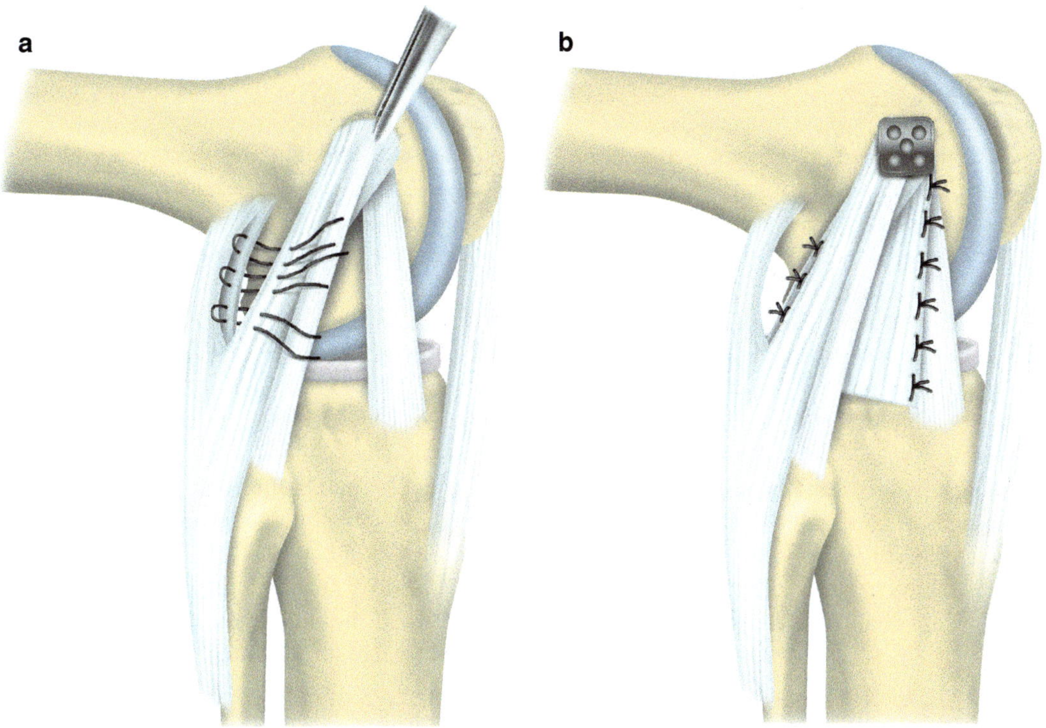

Fig. 27.6 (**a**) Procedure for chronic PLRI. The femoral attachments of the lateral gastrocnemius, fibular collateral ligament, and popliteus are released in an osteotomy. Sutures are passed in the arcuate ligament posteriorly prior to osteotomy fixation. (**b**) The osteotomized portion of bone is fixated to the femur with a staple after advancement. The arcuate ligament sutures are tied. The lateral capsular incision is closed with the distal portion advanced as much as possible

lateral gastrocnemius is then retracted to expose the posterior arcuate. The tibial and fibular attachments of the arcuate ligament are exposed with retraction of the biceps femoris. Primary repair of all injured structures then proceeds. If detached from the femur, tibia, or fibula, the arcuate ligament is sutured back with periosteal sutures or through drill holes. Interstitial or transverse tears are repaired in a pants-over-vest fashion. Tendon avulsions of the gastrocnemius, biceps, and popliteus are similarly directly repaired to their points of normal attachment. In Dr Hughston's approach, postoperatively the knee is placed in a long leg cast at 70° of flexion and neutral rotation with the incorporation of a pelvic band to prevent adduction stress on the lateral compartment. The cast is removed at 6 weeks postoperatively and exchanged for a hinged brace. Active extension exercises are also begun. Partial weight bearing begins when the knee lacks 20° of full extension. The brace is brought gradually into full extension and weight bearing increased to full.

In 1983 Baker et al. [2] reported on Dr Hughston's results in 13 knees with acute PLRI with an average follow-up of over 5 years. One or more components of the arcuate ligament complex were injured in all knees. No patient required later reconstruction for chronic instability. Eighty-five percent of patients returned to athletics at their pre-injury level. Seventy-seven percent achieved a good objective result at follow-up, and 85 % were rated good subjectively. Over the same time frame as this study, over 140 patients were treated for chronic PLRI emphasizing the need for appropriate diagnosis and treatment at the time of injury [9]. Patients with chronic PLRI were treated operatively with an anterior and distal advancement en masse of the arcuate complex on the femur (Figs. 27.6a, b). At follow-up of 2–13 years, 96 knees were evaluated after repair for chronic PLRI. Interestingly 71 of these patients had undergone a combined total of 112 prior operations before referral without addressing the primary pathology. At follow-up 85 % percent achieved a good objective result, and 78 % were rated good subjectively.

Currently at the Hughston Clinic, cases of acute PLRI managed operatively are treated with an approach similar to Dr Hughston's. Injured structures are directly repaired back to their attachment sites. The advent of suture anchors has certainly improved the security of the repair. With midsubstance injuries, or in those cases in which a secure direct repair is not possible, a posterolateral corner reconstruction is performed with the use of allograft tissue.

Fact Box 3
AMRI, ALRI, and PLRI can and do exist in combination and all must be addressed appropriately for a successful outcome.

Conclusion

Dr Hughston's focus on the knee was centered upon both the functional anatomy and the pathological anatomy resulting from the various patterns of injury. His teachings of knowledge of the mechanism of injury, correlation of the clinical examination with the injured structures seen at surgery, and repair of the anatomy with close follow-up of patients with documentation have provided a classification system for management of the acute knee ligament injuries. His definitions of anteromedial (AMRI), anterolateral (ALRI), and posterolateral (PLRI) rotatory instability provide a framework for communication and a foundation for future research. The vast majority of his practice was prior to the successful introduction of ACL reconstruction techniques; however, his surgical techniques appropriately addressed the rotational instabilities identified at clinical examination. Certainly his long-term follow-up studies remain as a testament to his philosophy. As he eloquently stated "no machines or ancillary aids should ever supersede a complete history and physical examination, clinical experience, and good common sense" [4]. Today at the clinic that bears his name, we adhere to his teachings of anatomy and diagnosis of knee rotatory instabilities. Anatomic repair is attempted for acute AMRI and PLRI as taught by Dr Hughston. If direct repair is not possible, graft reconstruction is undertaken. Although Dr Hughston addressed ALRI with repair of the injured lateral capsule and iliotibial tract, we currently reconstruct the ACL to correct the rotational instability and reserve extra-articular repair/reconstruction for revision cases with persistent rotatory instability.

References

1. Andrews JR, Sanders RA, Morin B (1985) Surgical treatment of anterolateral rotatory instability: a follow-up study. Am J Sports Med 13:112–119
2. Baker CL Jr, Norwood LA, Hughston JC (1983) Acute posterolateral rotatory instability of the knee. J Bone Joint Surg Am 65:614–618
3. Hughston JC (1994) The importance of the posterior oblique ligament in repairs of the medial ligaments in knees with and without an associated rupture of the anterior cruciate ligament. Results of long-term follow-up. J Bone Joint Surg Am 76: 1328–1344
4. Hughston JC (1993) Knee ligaments: injury and repair. Hughston Sports Medicine Foundation, Columbus
5. Hughston JC, Andrews JR, Cross MJ, Moschi A (1976) Classification of knee ligament instabilities. Part I: the medial compartment and cruciate ligaments. J Bone Joint Surg Am 58:159–172
6. Hughston JC, Andrews JR, Cross MJ, Moschi A (1976) Classification of knee ligament instabilities. Part II: the lateral compartment. J Bone Joint Surg Am 58:173–179

7. Hughston JC, Barrett GR (1983) Acute anteromedial rotatory instability: long term results of surgical repair. J Bone Joint Surg Am 65:145–153
8. Hughston JC, Eilers AF (1973) The role of the posterior oblique ligament in repairs of acute medial (collateral) ligament tears of the knee. J Bone Joint Surg Am 55:923–940
9. Hughston JC, Jacobson KE (1985) Chronic posterolateral rotatory instability of the knee. J Bone Joint Surg Am 67:351–359
10. Hughston JC, Norwood LA (1980) The posterolateral drawer test and external rotational recurvatum test for posterolateral rotatory instability of the knee. Clin Orthop Relat Res 147:82–87
11. Laprade RF, Terry GC (1997) Injuries to the posterolateral aspect of the knee: association of anatomic injury patterns with clinical instability. Am J Sports Med 25:433–438
12. Terry GC, Laprade RF (1996) The posterolateral aspect of the knee: anatomy and surgical approach. Am J Sports Med 24:732–739
13. Terry GC, Hughston JC, Norwood LA (1986) The anatomy of the iliopatellar band and iliotibial tract. Am J Sports Med 14:39–45

"Over the Top" Single-Bundle ACL Reconstruction with Extra-articular Plasty

28

Stefano Zaffagnini, Tommaso Roberti Di Sarsina, Alberto Grassi, Giulio Maria Marcheggiani Muccioli, Federico Raggi, Tommaso Bonanzinga, Cecilia Signorelli, and Maurilio Marcacci

Contents

S. Zaffagnini (✉) • T.R. Di Sarsina • A. Grassi
G.M. Marcheggiani Muccioli • F. Raggi
T. Bonanzinga • C. Signorelli • M. Marcacci
Clinica Ortopedica e Traumatologica II, Laboratorio di Biomeccanica ed Innovazione Tecnologica, Istituto Ortopedico Rizzoli, Via di Barbiano, 1/10, Bologna 40136, Italy
e-mail: stefano.zaffagnini@biomec.ior.it

28.1 Introduction

Instability can be defined as a ligamentous knee injury resulting in a shift from the primary load-bearing areas to a different location, resulting in overloading of part of the articular cartilage, with a change in both static and dynamic loading with increased stress through the articular cartilage.

The anterior cruciate ligament (ACL) is the most commonly injured knee ligament and it is a primary constraint to anteroposterior joint translation, and isolated lesions are uncommon. Frequently, other ligamentous structures or the menisci are affected, leading to further compromise of joint stability.

However, there is a lack of evidence that ACL reconstruction or meniscus repair prevents the development of osteoarthritis in the long term. There is evidence of radiographic osteoarthritic changes in 50–80% of injured knees even after adequate ACL reconstruction [28]. This can be due to a persistent excessive tibial rotation during demanding activity.

A combined damage of the ACL and the posterolateral structures has been associated with rotational laxity that leads to a severe positive pivot-shift test [6, 30, 36]. Other authors have also recorded possible evidence of damage to these structures along with ACL tears with the presence of the Segond fracture that results from avulsion of the iliotibilial band (ITB) or the

V. Musahl et al. (eds.), *Rotatory Knee Instability*, DOI 10.1007/978-3-319-32070-0_28

"anterior oblique band" of the lateral collateral ligament (LCL) [8]. Further evidence of the gross instability after ACL and lateral structures damage is the lateral tibial subluxation and the subsequent "bone bruising" observed on magnetic resonance imaging [14, 42]. As Dodds and Amis have recently published, these posterolateral structures may not have been yet directly identified, but likely act as secondary restraints to the pivot-shift test, supplementing the primary restraint role of the ACL in anteroposterior laxity, with emphasis on rotatory laxity and internal rotation [2, 15]. The persistence of this rotatory laxity has been reported even after cases of uneventful ACL reconstruction, suggesting that a single-bundle intra-articular reconstruction may not be sufficient to completely restore rotational knee stability in certain patients [1, 3, 35, 43].

28.2 Quantifying the Pivot Shift

Quantification of the pivot-shift phenomenon can be considered one of the major issues facing the orthopedists involved in ACL surgery, both in diagnosis and to assess results after surgery. Recent reviews have highlighted the importance, in present-day clinical practice, of quantifying the pivot-shift maneuver during the assessment of ACL injuries [22] and also underlining the different technologies that have been developed to this end [29, 45, 46].

A noninvasive accelerometer-based method to quantify the pivot shift has been described and validated, which resulted in reliable and high intra-tester repeatability in a controlled setup. This quantification instigates the debate on the additional structures damaged, other than the intra-articular component, and the need to control especially the rotation after ACL reconstruction that gave rise to the strategy to combine intra-articular ACL reconstruction with extra-articular plasty [48]. The main arguments of the supporters of this procedure are: (1) the previously mentioned evidence of the additional structures being damaged in ACL tears favors that there are additional structures required to be addressed in ACL reconstruction, (2) there is the strong association of the posterolateral structures in controlling internal tibial rotation, and (3) the lateral extra-articular plasty is far from the center of the knee rotation and provides a greater lever arm for controlling pivot-shift test and internal rotation than the intra-articular reconstruction [15, 34]. The rationale behind extra-articular plasty is therefore to create a restraint in internal tibial rotation.

Authors who favor the supplementary extra-articular plasty to standard ACL reconstruction record reduced pivot-shift test results and lateral tibial translation [13, 31, 32, 47], but the introduction of evidence-based inclusion criteria for any similar technique as a primary or a revision option is difficult and remains sporadic and empirically based [13, 15, 34]. In the current authors' practice, indications for extra-articular plasty and supplementing the primary intra-articular ACL reconstruction are:

1. Challenging primary cases where gross pivot-shift test is recorded or increased BMI is combined with high-level sports activities
2. Chronic cases of ACL laxity
3. Revision cases of ACL reconstruction, especially cases where patellar tendon (PT) has been used or incorrectly placed
4. Patients with joint hyperlaxity and knee recurvatum

28.3 Surgical Techniques

28.3.1 Arthroscopic Setting

With the patient in the supine position on the operating table, a pneumatic tourniquet is placed as high as possible around the proximal part of the thigh. A support is placed laterally at the upper level of the knee to stress the joint during arthroscopic evaluation. Usually a medial suprapatellar portal is used for the water inflow, an anterolateral viewing portal, and an anteromedial working portal. After confirmation of ACL lesion, the tibial insertion area and the intercondylar notch are prepared. Any soft tissue in the posterior part of the roof that can obstruct the "over-the-top" position must be carefully removed as well.

28.3.2 Graft Harvesting

With the patient's leg in a figure-4 position, the pes anserinus is located by following the hamstring tendons distally to their attachment on the anteromedial tibia. A 3 cm transverse incision is made over the pes anserinus (2 cm distal and 1 cm medial to the tibial tubercle).

Subcutaneous tissue is then dissected and the fascia is incised parallel to the orientation of the pes tendons (Fig. 28.1a). When the gracilis and the semitendinosus have been identified, a meticulous dissection of both tendons from their fascial attachments is performed in order to prevent premature cutting of the tendons when advancing the tendon stripper. Both tendons are harvested using a blunt tendon stripper (Acufex, Microsurgical, Mansfield, MA), with knee in more than 90° flexion to facilitate the detachment of the tendon. The tibial insertion of both tendons is preserved to maintain their neurovascular supply (Fig. 28.1b). In order to gain an additional 1 or 2 two cm in length, the distal attachment of the semitendinosus to the adjacent gracilis tendon could be dissected, and then the tendons are sutured together with three nonabsorbable Flexidene No. 2 stitches (Laboratory Bruneau, Boulogne Billancourt, France), obtaining a graft of 24–28 cm in length.

28.3.3 Tibial Tunnel Preparation

Preparation of the tibial tunnel is performed under arthroscopic visualization by inserting a guide pin on the medial aspect of the tibia through the graft harvesting incision (Fig. 28.2), directed to the medial posterior part of the ACL tibial insertion. After reaming the tibial tunnel according to ligament diameter (usually 8–9 mm), a looped wire passer is inserted from the tibial tunnel into the notch and is brought out from the anteromedial portal under arthroscopic visualization. The edges of the osseous tunnel should be accurately smoothened with a motorized shaver.

28.3.4 Over-the-Top Position

With the knee positioned at 90° flexion and the foot externally rotated, a 3–5 cm longitudinal incision is made directly above the lateral femoral epicondyle (Fig. 28.3). The posterior third of the iliotibial band is divided and is retracted anteriorly. The lateral aspect of the thigh is dissected using electrocautery and scissors, in order to reach the lateral intermuscular septum, which separates the vastus lateralis muscle (above) from the lateral head of the gastrocnemius muscle (below). When the lateral intermuscular septum

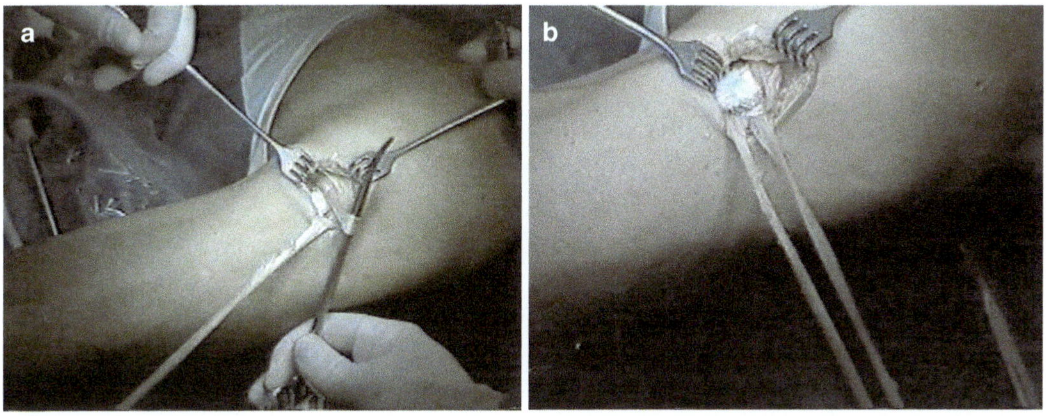

Fig. 28.1 After skin incision over pes anserinus and dissection of subcutaneous tissue, the fascial incision is made parallel to the orientation of the pes tendons (**a**). Both tendons are harvested using a blunt tendon stripper maintaining firm tension on the tendon distally and with knee in more than 90° flexion. The harvested tendons are sutured together using nonabsorbable stitches at the free end. The gracilis and semitendinosus tendons are harvested maintaining the tibial insertion intact (**b**)

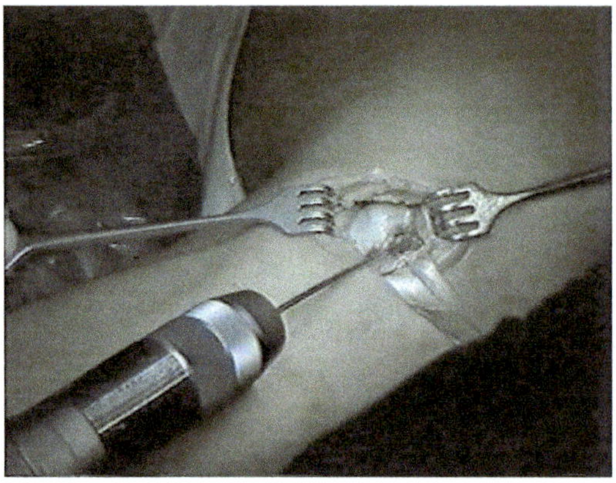

Fig. 28.2 The tibial tunnel is prepared under arthroscopic visualization inserting a guide pin on the medial aspect of the tibia through the graft harvesting incision. The guide pin is directed to the medial posterior part of the ACL tibial insertion. The wire loop is inserted from the tibial tunnel into the notch, grasped with a clamp, and brought out the anteromedial portal

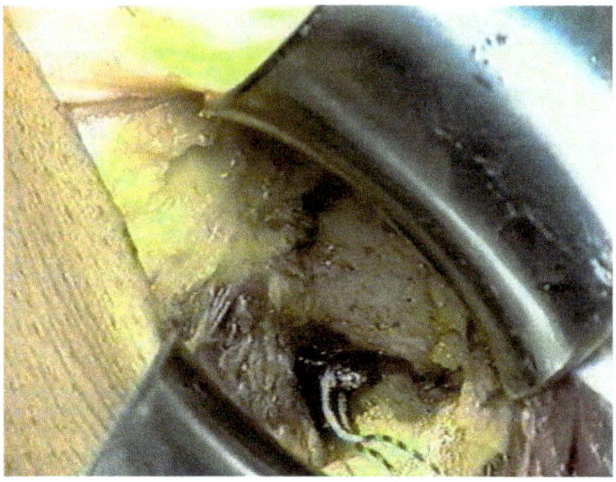

Fig. 28.4 A clamp is inserted in the anteromedial portal and directed to the notch; with a finger in the lateral side of the femur just posterior to the intermuscular septum, it is possible to palpate the tip of the clamp against the posterior part of the capsule in the over the top position. The clamp is pushed through the thin posterior layer of knee capsule, reaching the posterior space previously prepared

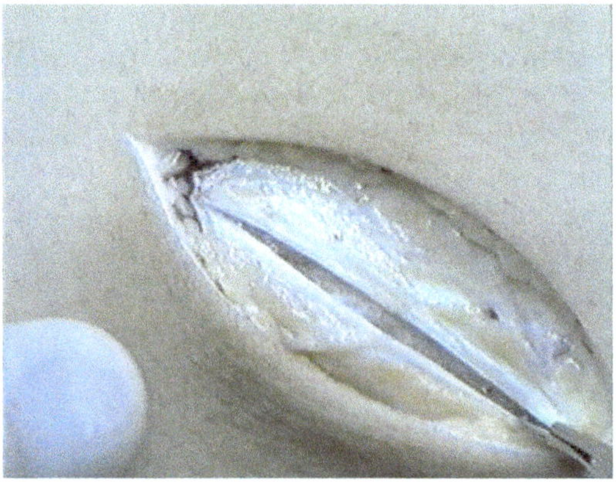

Fig. 28.3 The 3–5 cm incision to reach the over-the-top position is performed longitudinally just above the lateral femoral condyle, with the knee positioned at 90° of flexion and the foot externally rotated

has been clearly identified, it is possible to reach the posterior aspect of the joint capsule by passing over this structure. If this is not possible, the septum can be divided. It is possible to determine the correct placement of the "over-the-top" position and to protect the posterior structures during the next step, by palpating the posterior tubercle of the lateral femoral condyle with a finger. A curved Kelly clamp is passed from the anteromedial portal into the notch, and its tip is placed as far proximally possible against the posterior part of the capsule. After palpating the tip of the clamp from the lateral side of the femur just posterior to the intermuscular septum, it is pushed through the thin posterior layer of knee capsule, reaching the posterior space previously prepared. A suture loop is then placed into the tip of the clamp (Fig. 28.4), pulled anteriorly through the anteromedial portal, and placed into the wire loop previously inserted in the portal. Pulling the wire from the tibial side brings the suture loop at the bottom of the tibial tunnel and out from the tibial incision.

28.3.5 Graft Placement and Fixation

The suture is tied on the free end of the graft and pulled through the knee joint. The graft is retrieved from the lateral incision (Fig. 28.5). A groove is made in the lateral aspect of the femur just proximally to the start of the lateral condyle, allowing the anteriorization of the grafts and the achievement of a more isometric position. Once the graft is placed in the correct position, it is tensioned and the knee cycled through a full range of motion several times to check its stability. Then, the graft can be secured to the lateral femoral

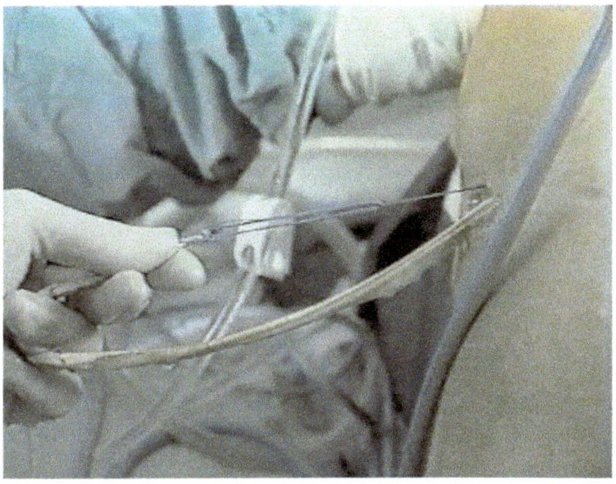

Fig. 28.5 The suture that exits from the tibial tunnel is tied on the free end of the graft. Pulling the suture, the graft passes through the tibial tunnel and in the knee joint. At the end the graft is retrieved from the lateral incision

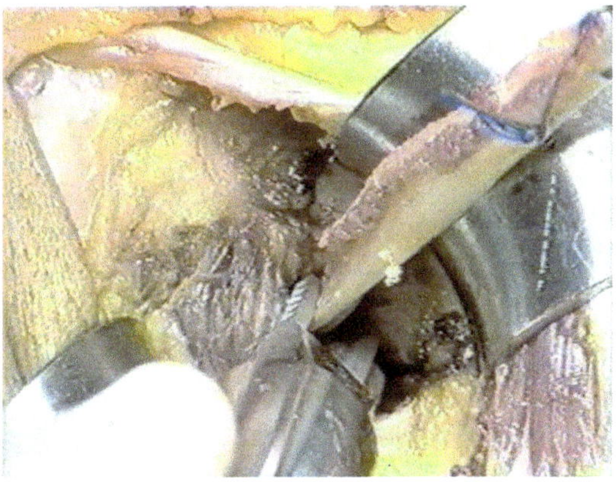

Fig. 28.6 The graft is tensioned with the knee at 90° of flexion and secured with two metal staples on the lateral femoral cortex. Putting under tension the remaining part of the graft, it is possible to check whether or not it is long enough to reach Gerdy's tubercle in the anterolateral aspect of the tibia

cortex into the groove with two metal staples (Fig. 28.6) while maintaining the knee at about 90° of flexion and the foot externally rotated. Putting under tension the remaining part of the graft makes it possible to evaluate its length and whether or not it is long enough to reach Gerdy's tubercle (GT) in the anterolateral aspect of the tibia. If this condition is satisfied, a 1–2 cm skin and fascia incision is performed just below the GT. Then, a small Kelly clamp is passed under the fascia from this incision to the lateral femoral condyle (Fig. 28.7a), where the sutures at the end of the graft are placed in the tip of the clamp and pulled down, emerging from the GT incision. The graft is tensioned and the knee is cycled again to check the isometry of the lateral tenodesis and the freedom of flexion-extension. Another metallic staple is then used to fix the graft below GT to the lateral aspect of the tibia (Fig. 28.7b). An intra-articular drain is threaded through the superomedial portal, and additional drains are inserted in each wound. The iliotibial tract defect is closed, taking care to prevent lateral tilt and patellar compression, while the medial fascia over the pes anserinus is not closed, in order to prevent compartment syndrome

28.4 Rehabilitation Protocol

28.4.1 First Post-Op Phase (Weeks 1–4)

Started the day after surgery:

- Passive range of motion (ROM) restoration, both in flexion and in extension, with continuous passive mobilization (CPM), therapist assisted. CPM must be two times a day and it starts from a ROM between 10° and 30° of flexion, gradually increased according to patient restraint (5–10° per day), in order to reach a ROM between 0° and 110° at 3 weeks.
- Pain and swelling reduction with cryotherapy.
- Muscle atrophy restoration with isometric exercise, without knee articulation load.

From week 2:

- Quadriceps electrostimulation
- After stitches removal, passive patellar mobilization both horizontally and vertically
- 1 week after stitch removal, hydrokinesotherapy
- Restoration of ambulation autonomy

In the first days after surgery, no weight bearing is allowed and it is then progressive to become partial at the end of week 2. From week 3, there is abandon of one crutch (on the operated side)

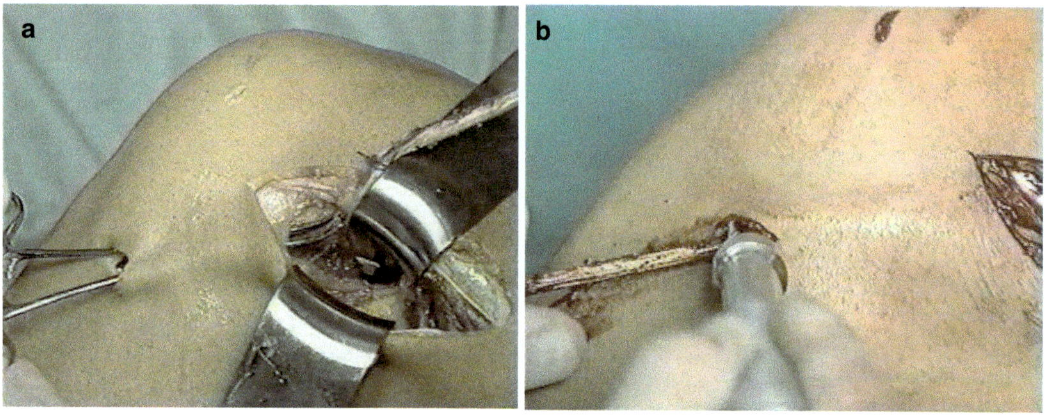

Fig. 28.7 A 1–2 cm skin and fascia incision is performed just below Gerdy's tubercle. A small Kelly clamp is passed below the fascia, to the lateral femoral condyle (**a**). The sutures at the end of the graft are placed in the tip of the clamp and pulled distally. At the end of this maneuver, the graft emerges from the Gerdy's tubercle incision where it can be secured with a metal staple (**b**)

and then the second to regain full weight bearing and autonomy.

28.4.2 Second Phase (Weeks 5–8)

Achievement of the following objectives:

- Operated knee with no swelling
- Complete ROM restoration
- Correct ambulation
- Muscular trophism restoration and strengthening

This can be obtained with:

- Flexion exercises from supine, prone, or sitting position
- Isometric exercises and concentric exercises against resistance with limited articular excursion
- Stationary bicycle
- Proprioceptive exercises in closed kinetic chain, and with balance boards
- Freestyle swimming (avoid frog-style)
- Hydro-kinesotherapy
- Muscular elongation exercises
- Running on treadmill at progressive speed, exercise duration
- Running backwards, in circles, in 8 shapes, and with direction changes

28.4.3 Third Phase (Weeks 9–12)

- Complete muscular strength restoration equal to the healthy limb, through machine-assisted exercises avoiding last 30° of extension, stationary bike, closed kinetic chain exercises until 90° of flexion, and balance boards (improving instability)
- Complete regaining of daily activities (driving, working activity)
- Return to sport-specific training with inferior-to-normal intensity and speed

28.4.4 Fourth Phase (Weeks 13–20)

- Neuromuscular improvement with proprioceptive exercises
- Running and coordination restoration (field in line running, then soft running uphill, in circles, and 8 shape running)

28.4.5 Fifth Phase (Weeks 21–24)

- In this phase the athlete starts restoration of sport-specific gestures, improving strain tolerance and resistance (aerobic exercises, running with sharp turning, direction changes) and gradual return to sport. We recommend return to sport not prior to 6 months after surgery.

28.5 Discussion

The extra-articular plasty was initially performed without concomitant intra-articular ACL reconstruction. The early results were not promising mostly because of the failure to restore anteroposterior stability and the postoperative presence of lateral femorotibial degenerative changes [9, 30, 38, 40, 41]. The main reasons why the interest on these techniques has weakened over 20 years were that the evolution of all-arthroscopic ACL reconstruction was favored over these more invasive and less cosmetic techniques, the absence of concomitant intra-articular ACL reconstruction, the donor-site morbidity, and the long rehabilitation protocols that included a 2-month period of knee immobilization [15].

When extra-articular plasty was combined with intra-articular ACL reconstruction, the results were more encouraging. One hundred and forty-eight patients have been treated with 11.5 years follow-up using open intra-articular ACL reconstruction with patellar tendon and extra-articular plasty with the Lemaire technique [26], and it has been recorded that 89 % scored "satisfied" or "very satisfied" in a subjective score [12]. Using the same technique, 251 cases of chronic ACL laxity have been treated and it has been recorded that 83 % had "good" or "excellent" functional results [11]. In another study, no significant differences between intra-articular ACL reconstruction and additional extra-articular plasty have been found, but it has been recorded that extra-articular plasty reduced the feeling of "giving way" [23]. Similarly, two other studies found significant increase of stability when extra-articular plasty was added to ACL reconstruction [27, 37].

The rationale behind this combined intra- and extra-articular ACL reconstructions with gracilis and semitendinosus tendons is to combine into one operation the advantages of both methods (Table 28.1).

Table 28.1 Principles at the basis of intra- and extra-articular procedures

1. To increase the tensile strength of the reconstruction using two grafts
2. To protect the intra-articular reconstruction from excessive loads, especially in the rehabilitation period
3. To better control rotation laterally, especially in some complex cases as revision ACL surgery
4. To leave the extensor apparatus of the knee undisturbed

The presence of the extra-articular lateral augmentation protects the graft reducing the load applied to the intraarticular portion of the graft. An in vitro analysis has shown that the extra-articular plasty, when used in combination with intra-articular reconstruction, reduces the stress on the graft by approximately 43 % [20]. Other researchers showed by navigation in their "in vivo" study that the addition of an extra-articular tenodesis to single-bundle ACL reconstruction may be effective in controlling coupled tibial translation during the Lachman test and in reducing anteroposterior laxity at 90° of flexion [4].

The site of femoral fixation is the key step to obtain a good extra-articular plasty. This point corresponds to the optimal isometric position, as defined by Krackow et al. [25] and Draganich et al. [16, 17–19]. A study performed in 1992 concluded that the role of extra-articular procedures in the final outcome is limited [39]. Although we acknowledge that most of ACL injuries can be solved by an isolated intra-articular reconstruction, we do believe that the importance of extra-articular augmentation should be reconsidered [40].

Successful results were published in a study where the authors used an intra-articular reconstruction with doubled hamstrings graft and an extra-articular reconstruction by a modification of the MacIntosh procedure for ACL revision cases [21]. Marcacci et al. reported the long-term results of their non-anatomic over-the-top ACL reconstruction combined with lateral tenodesis using hamstrings graft [33]. The authors recommended the technique for primary ACL reconstruction since they recorded that 90 % of 54 consecutive cases scored "good" or "excellent" results in IKDC after an average of 11 years [33]. In another study, the same non-anatomic over-the-top technique using allograft tendons has been utilized, for multiple-revision ACL reconstruction, reporting "good" or "excellent" results in 83 % of patients and 92 % with "normal" to "nearly normal" pivot-shift test [5]. Also, the results of ACL revision with additional lateral plasty have been reported, showing better results in terms of stability and failure rate compared to isolated intra-articular reconstruction [44].

Apart from the graft choice and its versatile course until its usual final insertion in the lateral femoral condyle, most of these authors agree that the critical point for the success of the extra-articular plasty is the point of femoral fixation [15, 34]. This has been defined to be located slightly posteriorly and proximally to the femoral insertion of the LCL [7, 16, 25]. Colombet published a technique where navigation was used in order to facilitate the identification of this femoral insertion point [10]. Although the over-the-top position does not allow an exact anatomic reconstruction, it has been shown in a prospective study there are no significant clinical differences between patients who underwent hamstring ACL reconstruction using the "over-the-top" technique and patients who had femoral graft placement through femoral condylar tunnel [24]. The first technique is highly reproducible and eliminates the risk of surgical error associated with placement of the femoral tunnel (especially for not experienced knee surgeons). Moreover this extra-articular procedure does not damage any lateral structures commonly used in other extra-articular augmentation procedures (like the iliotibial band). Another benefit of this technique is the need of only three titanium staples for graft fixation, which results in a reduction of surgical costs. This fast and cheap technique is also a simple solution for revision cases, eliminating the issues of management of femoral tunnel malposition, presence of intra-articular hardware, or tunnel enlargement. As previously showed by Zaffagnini et al. [45] in a prospective randomized fashion, a simple intra-articular procedure combined with an extra-articular augmentation may achieve better results in maintaining rotational control with less risk of technical error and better clinical results than a single-bundle ACL reconstruction (either PT or hamstring). More recently, the same group compared double-bundle ACL reconstruction versus single-bundle ACL reconstruction with extra-articular plasty and recorded that the latter resulted in better control of static knee laxity, reduced mediolateral instability in early flexion, and reduced rotatory instability at 90° of flexion [47].

Conclusion

The highly satisfactory results obtained over the time with the above-reported techniques show that a combination of intra- and extra-articular procedures for ACL reconstruction is a valid surgical option in the ACL-deficient knee given that the appropriate indications are followed. More recent literature demonstrated in vitro and in vivo the efficacy of the extra-articular plasty in limiting rotatory knee instability as a result of ACL lesion and in improving final clinical results. ACL ruptures need to be well documented and need an objective preoperative laxity evaluation to properly identify which knee necessitates an extraarticular reconstruction combined with intrarticular ACL reconstruction. More insight on the anatomical and biomechanical features of anterolateral compartment will allow a more anatomical reconstruction. The long-term effect of these new procedures still needs a long-term clinical evaluation.

References

1. Acquitter Y, Hulet C, Locker B et al (2003) Patellar tendon-bone autograft reconstruction of the anterior cruciate ligament for advanced-stage chronic anterior laxity: is an extra-articular plasty necessary? A prospective randomized study of 100 patients with five year follow-up. Rev Chir Orthop Reparatrice Appar Mot 89(5):413–422
2. Amis AA, Scammell BE (1993) Biomechanics of intra-articular and extra-articular reconstruction of the anterior cruciate ligament. J Bone Joint Surg Br 75(5):812–817
3. Andrews JR, Sanders RA, Morin B (1985) Surgical treatment of anterolateral instability: a follow-up study. Am J Sports Med 13:112–119
4. Bignozzi S, Zaffagnini S, Lopomo N et al (2009) Does a lateral plasty control coupled translation during antero-posterior stress in single-bundle ACL reconstruction? An in vivo study. Knee Surg Sports Traumatol Arthrosc 17(1):65–70

5. Buda R, Ruffilli A, Di Caprio F (2013) Allograft salvage procedure in multiple-revision anterior cruciate ligament reconstruction. Am J Sports Med 41(2): 402–410
6. Bull AMJ, Amis AA (1998) The pivot-shift phenomenon: a clinical and biomechanical perspective. Knee 5(5):141–158
7. Bylski-Austrow DI, Grood ES, Hefzy MS et al (1990) Anterior cruciate ligament replacements: a mechanical study of femoral attachment location, flexion angle at tensioning, and initial tension. J Orthop Res 8(4):522–531
8. Campos JC, Chung CB, Lektrakul N et al (2001) Pathogenesis of the Segond fracture: anatomic and MR imaging evidence of an iliotibial tract or anterior oblique band avulsion. Radiology 219(2):381–386
9. Christel P, Djian P (2002) Anterio-lateral extra-articular tenodesis of the knee using a short strip of fascia lata. Rev Chir Orthop Reparatrice Appar Mot 88(5):508–513
10. Colombet PD (2011) Navigated intra-articular ACL reconstruction with additional extra-articular tenodesis using the same hamstring graft. Knee Surg Sports Traumatol Arthrosc 19(3):384–389
11. Dejour H, Walch G, Neyret P et al (1988) Results of surgically treated chronic anterior laxities. Apropos of 251 cases reviewed with a minimum follow-up of 3 years. Rev Chir Orthop Reparatrice Appar Mot 74(7): 622–636
12. Dejour H, Dejour D, Ait Si Selmi T (1999) Chronic anterior laxity of the knee treated with free patellar graft and extra-articular lateral plasty: 10-year follow-up of 148 cases. Rev Chir Orthop Reparatrice Appar Mot 85(8):777–789
13. Dejour D, Vasconcelos W, Bonin N et al (2013) Comparative study between mono-bundle bone-patellar tendon-bone, double-bundle hamstring and mono-bundle bone-patellar tendon-bone combined with a modified Lemaire extra-articular procedure in anterior cruciate ligament reconstruction. Int Orthop 37:193–199
14. Delzell PB, Schils JP, Recht MP (1996) Subtle fractures about the knee: innocuous-appearing yet indicative of significant internal derangement. AJR Am J Roentgenol 167(3):699–703
15. Dodds AL, Gupte CM, Neyret P et al (2011) Extra-articular techniques in anterior cruciate ligament reconstruction: a literature review. J Bone Joint Surg Br 93(11):1440–1448
16. Draganich LF, Reider B, Ling M, Samuelson M (1990) An in vitro study of an intraarticular and extraarticular reconstruction in the anterior cruciate ligament deficient knee. Am J Sports Med 18:262–266
17. Draganich LF, Hsieh YF, Reider B (1995) Iliotibial band tenodesis: a new strategy for attachment. Am J Sports Med 23(2):186–195
18. Duthon VB, Magnussen RA, Servien E et al (2013) ACL reconstruction and extra-articular tenodesis. Clin Sports Med 32(1):141–153
19. Ellison AE (1979) Distal iliotibial-band transfer for anterolateral rotatory instability of the knee. J Bone Joint Surg Am 61(3):330–337
20. Engebretsen L, Lew WD, Lewis JL et al (1990) The effect of an iliotibial tenodesis on intraarticular graft forces and knee joint motion. Am J Sports Med 18(2): 169–176
21. Ferretti A, Conteduca F, Monaco E et al (2006) Revision anterior cruciate ligament reconstruction with doubled semitendinosus and gracilis tendons and lateral extra-articular reconstruction. J Bone Joint Surg Am 88(11):2373–2379
22. Giraud B, Besse JL, Cladiere F et al (2006) Intra-articular reconstruction of the anterior cruciate ligament with and without extra-articular supplementation by quadricipital tendon plasty: seven-year follow-up. Rev Chir Orthop Reparatrice Appar Mot 92(8): 788–797
23. Jensen JE, Slocum DB, Larson RL et al (1983) Reconstruction procedures for anterior cruciate ligament insufficiency: a computer analysis of clinical results. Am J Sports Med 11(4):240–248
24. Karlson JA, Steiner ME, Brown CH, Johnston J (1994) Anterior cruciate ligament reconstruction using gracilis and semitendinosus tendons. Comparison of through-the-condyle and over-the-top graft placements. Am J Sports Med 22:659–666
25. Krackow KA, Brooks RL (1983) Optimization of knee ligament position for lateral extraarticular reconstruction. Am J Sports Med 11(5):293–302
26. Lemaire M (1975) Chronic knee instability. Technics and results of ligament plasty in sports injuries. J Chir (Paris) 110(4):281–294
27. Lerat JL, Chotel F, Besse JL et al (1998) The results after 10–16 years of the treatment of chronic anterior laxity of the knee using reconstruction of the anterior cruciate ligament with a patellar tendon graft combined with an external extra-articular reconstruction. Rev Chir Orthop Reparatrice Appar Mot 84(8): 712–727
28. Lohmander LS, Ostenberg A, Englund M, Roos H (2004) High prevalence of knee osteoarthritis, pain, and functional limitations in female soccer players twelve years after anterior cruciate ligament injury. Arthritis Rheum 50:3145–3152
29. Lopomo N, Zaffagnini S, Amis AA (2013) Quantifying the pivot shift test: a systematic review. Knee Surg Sports Traumatol Arthrosc 21:767–783
30. Losee RE, Johnson TR, Southwick WO (1978) Anterior subluxation of the lateral tibial plateau. A diagnostic test and operative repair. J Bone Joint Surg Am 60(8):1015–1030
31. Macintosh DL, Darby JA (1976) Lateral substitution reconstruction. Proceedings of the Canadian Orthopaedic Association. J Bone Joint Surg Br 58:142
32. Marcacci M, Zaffagnini S, Iacono F et al (1998) Arthroscopic intra- and extra-articular anterior cruciate ligament reconstruction with gracilis and semitendinosus tendons. Knee Surg Sports Traumatol Arthrosc 6(2):68–75

33. Marcacci M, Zaffagnini S, Giordano G et al (2009) Anterior cruciate ligament reconstruction associated with extra-articular tenodesis: a prospective clinical and radiographic evaluation with 10- to 13-year follow-up. Am J Sports Med 37(4):707–714
34. Marcacci M, Zaffagnini S, Marcheggiani Muccioli GM et al (2011) Arthroscopic intra- and extra-articular anterior cruciate ligament reconstruction with gracilis and semitendinosus tendons: a review. Curr Rev Musculoskelet Med 4(2):73–77
35. Monaco E, Labianca L, Conteduca F et al (2007) Double bundle or single bundle plus extraarticular tenodesis in ACL reconstruction? A CAOS study. Knee Surg Sports Traumatol Arthrosc 15(10):1168–1174
36. Norwood LA Jr, Andrews JR, Meisterling RC et al (1979) Acute anterolateral rotatory instability of the knee. J Bone Joint Surg Am 61(5):704–709
37. Noyes FR, Barber SD (1991) The effect of an extra-articular procedure on allograft reconstructions for chronic ruptures of the anterior cruciate ligament. J Bone Joint Surg Am 73(6):882–892
38. O'Brien SJ, Warren RF, Pavlov H et al (1991) Reconstruction of the chronically insufficient anterior cruciate ligament with the central third of the patellar ligament. J Bone Joint Surg Am 73(2):278–286
39. Pearl AJ, Bergfeld JA (eds) (1992) Extraarticular reconstruction in the anterior cruciate ligament deficient knee. Human Kinetics Books, Champaign
40. Roth JH, Kennedy JC, Lockstadt H et al (1987) Intra-articular reconstruction of the anterior cruciate ligament with and without extra-articular supplementation by transfer of the biceps femoris tendon. J Bone Joint Surg Am 69(2):275–278
41. Strum GM, Fox JM, Ferkel RD et al (1989) Intraarticular versus intraarticular and extraarticular reconstruction for chronic anterior cruciate ligament instability. Clin Orthop Relat Res 245:188–198
42. Tashiro Y, Okazaki K, Miura H et al (2009) Quantitative assessment of rotatory instability after anterior cruciate ligament reconstruction. Am J Sports Med 37(5):909–916
43. Tashman S, Collon D, Anderson K et al (2004) Abnormal rotational knee motion during running after anterior cruciate ligament reconstruction. Am J Sports Med 32(4):975–983
44. Trojani C, Beaufils P, Burdin G (2012) Revision ACL reconstruction: influence of a lateral tenodesis. Knee Surg Sports Traumatol Arthrosc 20(8):1565–1570
45. Zaffagnini S, Marcacci M, Lo Presti M et al (2006) Prospective and randomized evaluation of ACL reconstruction with three techniques: a clinical and radiographic evaluation at 5 years follow-up. Knee Surg Sports Traumatol Arthrosc 14(11):1060–1069
46. Zaffagnini S, Marcheggiani Muccioli GM, Lopomo N et al (2012) Can the pivot-shift be eliminated by anatomic double-bundle anterior cruciate ligament reconstruction? Knee Surg Sports Traumatol Arthrosc 20:743–751
47. Zaffagnini S, Signorelli C, Lopomo N et al (2012) Anatomic double-bundle and over-the-top single-bundle with additional extra-articular tenodesis: an in vivo quantitative assessment of knee laxity in two different ACL reconstructions. Knee Surg Sports Traumatol Arthrosc 20(1):153–159
48. Zaffagnini S, Lopomo N, Signorelli C, Marcheggiani Muccioli GM, Bonanzinga T, Grassi A, Raggi F, Visani A, Marcacci M (2014) Inertial sensors to quantify the pivot shift test in the treatment of anterior cruciate ligament injury. Joints 2(3):124–129

ACL and Extra-articular Tenodesis

29

Benjamin V. Herman, Timothy D. Lording, and Alan Getgood

Contents

29.1 Introduction

Anterior cruciate ligament reconstruction (ACLR) is one of the most common orthopedic surgical procedures performed. With modern arthroscopic techniques, good patient-reported outcomes have been typically reported. However, return to high-level sport has been reported as low as 63 % at 2 years [1]. One contributing reason could be the inability of the conventional ACLR to reliably restore normal tibial rotational kinematics.

Various methods of lateral extra-articular tenodesis (LET) were introduced over 40 years ago. These methods were developed as the biomechanical understanding of anterior cruciate ligament (ACL) injury improved, specifically the lack of anterolateral rotational stability in an ACL-deficient knee. Concerns with the resultant biomechanics, specifically of over-constraint and outcomes of LET procedures of the past, along with improvements in intra-articular ACLR techniques led to a departure from the LET procedure in isolation. Due to the aforementioned concerns with current ACLR outcomes, there is a renewed interest in performing LET as an adjunct procedure.

B.V. Herman, MD, FRCSC • A. Getgood, MPhil, MD, FRCS (Tr & Orth) (✉)
Department of Surgery, Fowler Kennedy Sport Medicine Clinic, Western University, London, ON N6A 3K7, Canada
e-mail: bherman@ualberta.ca; alan.getgood@uwo.ca

T.D. Lording, MBBS, FRACS
Melbourne Orthopaedic Group, Department of Orthopaedic Surgery, The Alfred Hospital, Melbourne, VIC, Australia
e-mail: tlording@iinet.net.au

V. Musahl et al. (eds.), *Rotatory Knee Instability*, DOI 10.1007/978-3-319-32070-0_29

29.2 Anatomical and Biomechanical Rationale for the Lateral Extra-articular Tenodesis

29.2.1 Anatomy

The ACL is a primary restraint to anterior translation and contributes to the restraint of internal tibial rotation and varus/valgus laxity. It has been described as being comprised of two bundles, each having a different kinematic role – the anteromedial and posterolateral bundles are taut in flexion and extension, respectively. The noncontact mechanism of injury involves a combination of forces, but has been described as similar to those forces involved in the pivot shift test – an axial load on the lateral compartment with a valgus force as the knee moves from flexion to extension [2]. This mechanism results in the pathognomonic bone bruising of the posterior aspect of the lateral tibial plateau and anterolateral lateral femoral condyle that is seen on magnetic resonance imaging.

The mechanism of injury in an "isolated" ACL rupture often results in additional injuries to soft tissue structures including the lateral capsuloligamentous structures, among several others. Recent anatomical studies have identified the anterolateral ligament (ALL) (Fig. 29.1) as a discrete lateral structure that acts as a secondary stabilizer to internal tibial rotation [3–6]. There have been several studies in the past that have implicated various structures on the lateral side of the knee and identified them as having an important role in restraining anterolateral rotational laxity [3, 5, 7–10]. The pathognomonic Segond fracture was originally hypothesized to be an avulsion of the middle third of the lateral capsular ligament [11]. Norwood et al. [12] identified the lateral capsular ligament and/or iliotibial band injuries in 32 of 36 knees with acute anterolateral rotatory instability. It would seem that many of the structures identified in previous studies may be synonymous with the ALL, and it is now with modern techniques in imaging and histology that investigators are able to more accurately characterize this structure [6]. A recent study has confirmed the ALL to be associated with the Segond fracture [13].

It should be noted that the ALL is not the only structure that has an effect on rotational control. Posterior root tears of the lateral meniscus and meniscocapsular separations of the medial meniscus both impact the degree of rotational laxity in an ACL-deficient knee [14–16]. The iliotibial band (ITB) has also been shown to have an impact on the control of anterolateral rotation since it attaches to Gerdy's tubercle. In particular, recent research would suggest that the capsulo-osseous layer of the ITB, attaching proximally from the posterior Kaplan fibers on the distal femur to distally on the posterior aspect of Gerdy's tubercle [17], is a major contributor to anterolateral rotational control. We can therefore surmise that anterolateral rotational control is provided by a combination of intra- and extra-articular structures, with the ACL, lateral meniscus, ITB, and ALL working in unison. Furthermore, ACL injury may therefore result in a combination of injuries to these important structures. It is important, therefore, to look for peripheral injuries in addition to the ACL and address these as appropriate.

29.2.2 Biomechanics and Results of ACLR

The conventional intra-articular ACLR is typically successful at reducing anterior tibial translation and less so at controlling rotational stability. Recent advancements in ACLR techniques have aimed to restore normal knee kinematics, with varying degrees of success. Double-bundle ACLR techniques have increased the complexity of the surgery, and although biomechanical studies suggest the additional posterolateral bundle helps control rotational laxity [18, 19], clinical studies have not shown any significant benefit over traditional single-bundle techniques [20]. The anatomic single-bundle ACLR is the most recent technique development. This places the femoral tunnel within the ACL footprint and results in a lower graft position with a more oblique angle than previous single-bundle techniques [21]. Theoretically, increased graft obliquity should provide a biomechanical advantage for control-

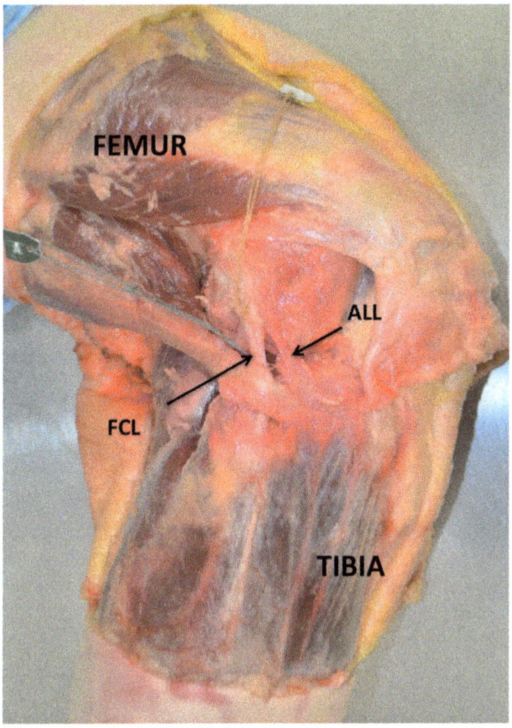

Fig. 29.1 Gross anatomy of the anterolateral aspect of the knee. The ALL is highlighted. Reprinted with permission from the American Journal of Sports Medicine

ling tibial rotation [22]. There is a growing body of literature supporting the improved rotational control and patient-reported outcomes of a more oblique graft position [23–26] and, furthermore, an anatomic single-bundle ACLR [27–29].

However, the clinical outcomes of current ACLR techniques have shown some concerning issues. The rate of reinjury in patients under the age of 20 may be as high as 20% [30–33], with many studies reporting a high incidence of persistent rotational laxity as measured by the pivot shift test. It is known that a positive pivot shift test correlates with decreased patient satisfaction and increased functional instability [23, 34, 35], with a growing body of literature emerging that shows current ACLR techniques are not effective at reducing rotational laxity [32]. Furthermore, rates of return to sport to a pre-injury level may be as low as 63%, while return to competitive sport is even lower at 44% [1]. Lastly, the incidence and severity of post-operative posttraumatic osteoarthritis (PTOA) seem to be higher in ACLR knees compared to the uninjured side [36]; however, direct causation is unclear. A positive pivot shift may be predictive of abnormal articular cartilage contact stress and the subsequent development of increased wear [37]; however, the molecular events that occur at the time of injury are most likely to be the primary factor in PTOA development [38, 39].

Although current ACLR techniques do have good patient-reported outcomes [36], it is evident that there is a lack of consistent restoration of rotational control, and clinical issues remain. Many authors hypothesize that these clinical issues may be mitigated by addressing the rotational laxity.

29.2.3 Biomechanics of LET

LET techniques were developed to recreate the anterolateral capsular structures to address the laxity present in an ACL-deficient knee [40], prior to the development of intra-articular ACLR procedures. Theoretically, it is thought that an extra-articular reconstruction has a biomechanical advantage over an intra-articular reconstruction with regard to anterolateral rotational control. The longer lever arm exerted by the peripherally based extra-articular reconstruction would theoretically be more able to resist torque. Ellison [41] described the ACL as "the hub of the wheel" and suggested that "it is easier to control rotation of a wheel at its rim than at its hub."

The LET has also been shown to protect the ACL graft. As previously mentioned, the obliquity of the graft is increased in the anatomic ACLR technique. This may expose the graft to higher than normal forces since it should theoretically resist more rotational torques [27]. This could lead to graft failure due to stretching or rupture. In a cadaver model, an LET has been shown to decrease the stress on an ACL graft by 43% [42]. A cadaver model has also shown a load-sharing relationship between an intra-articular ACLR and an LET during both anterior translation and internal rotation [43]. Similar benefits have been seen in an in vivo model. At the time of surgery, LET added to a single-bundle ACLR was shown to significantly reduce tibial internal rotation compared to a single-bundle

ACLR alone or a double-bundle ACLR [44]. Zaffagnini et al. [45] also showed patients had improved restraint to internal tibial rotation at 90° flexion in addition to improved varus-valgus laxity in full extension.

The biomechanics and reconstruction of the lateral side of the knee has been more rigorously investigated in recent years. The renewed interest in the ALL resulted in the development of an anatomic ALL reconstruction with the goal of restoring rotational stability. Biomechanical testing has shown that the ALL does play a role in controlling anterolateral rotatory laxity; however, its clinical effect may be small. In a recent study by Spencer et al. [46], sectioning the ALL in a cadaveric ACL-deficient knee resulted in a significant increase in internal rotation during a simulated pivot shift maneuver, though the increase was only 2° and may not prove to be clinically significant. Furthermore, reconstruction of the ALL using the previously described technique did not restore the kinematics of the native ALL intact state. However, when an LET was performed utilizing a strip of the ITB and routing it under the fibular collateral ligament (FCL) attaching it to the distal femoral metaphysis (modified Lemaire technique), this resulted in a significant reduction in anterior translation and internal rotation in the ACL-deficient state. This study showed that the LET was superior to the anatomic ALL reconstruction, which may be in part due to issues with the position of the femoral attachment and tensioning of the latter structure.

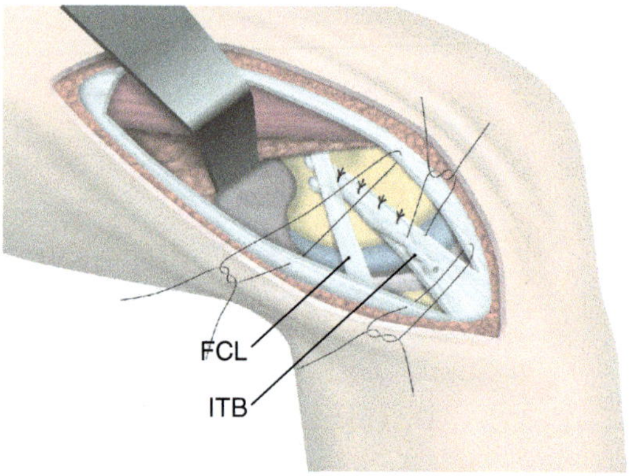

Fig. 29.2 The Lemaire procedure. A) and B) show the original description by Lemaire, utilizing a strip of IT band left attached on Gerdy's and passed through a bone tunnel proximal and deep to the FCL origin on the femur; C) shows the modification by Neyret et al., where a gracilis graft is pulled through the bone block of a bone-patella tendon-bone ACL graft which is introduced into the knee from outside in. The gracilis graft is then fixed to Gerdy's Tubercle via a bone tunnel

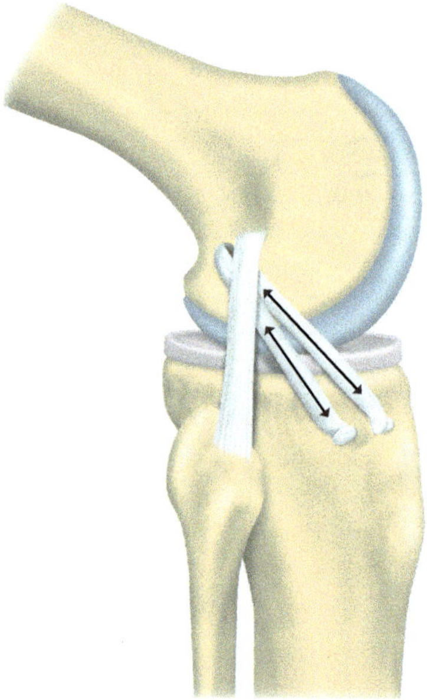

Fig. 29.3 The Losee procedure

29.3 Clinical Results of the LET

29.3.1 Isolated LET Procedures

Several methods for LET procedures have been developed, and initially, these procedures were done in isolation without addressing the ACL (Figs. 29.2, 29.3, 29.4, and 29.5). The original Lemaire technique was described in 1967 and used an 18 cm × 1 cm strip of IT band [47]. It was left attached at Gerdy's tubercle, passed under the fibular collateral ligament (FCL), and secured in a bone tunnel proximal to the FCL femoral insertion. The graft was then passed back distally and secured in a second tunnel at Gerdy's tubercle. Losee described passing the IT band from anterior to posterior through a femoral tunnel, around the arcuate complex, under the FCL,

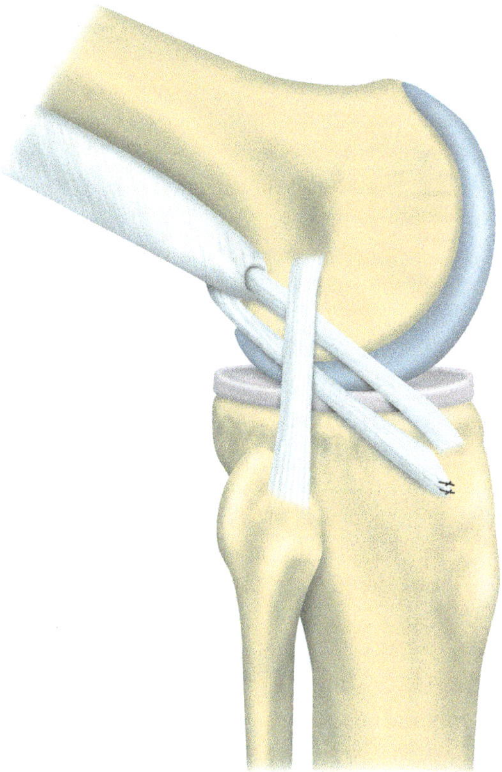

Fig. 29.4 The Ellison procedure

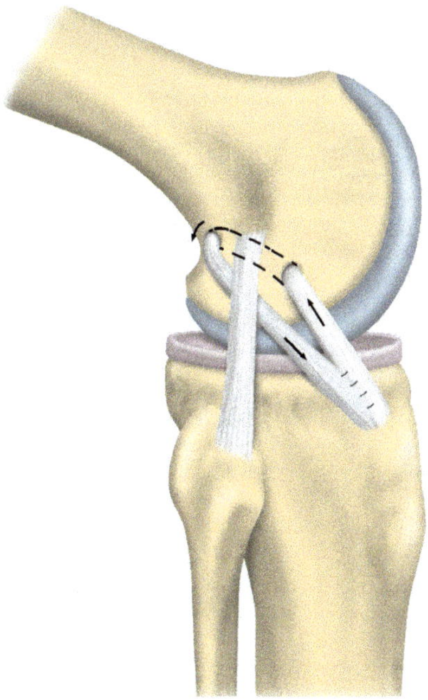

Fig. 29.5 The MacIntosh procedure

and attaching it to Gerdy's tubercle with a staple [48]. The Ellison procedure, described in 1979, harvested an IT band graft from Gerdy's tubercle with a bone plug and passed it under the proximal aspect of the FCL before stapling the bone plug anterior to Gerdy's tubercle [49]. The MacIntosh procedure was described in 1980 and was similar to the Lemaire procedure [50]. The graft was passed on the femoral side through a subperiosteal tunnel posterior to the FCL origin and looped behind the lateral intermuscular septum before being passed distally again. A modification of the MacIntosh procedure looped the IT band graft around the lateral femoral condyle and intra-articular through a tunnel in the tibia (MacIntosh 2). Another MacIntosh iteration took a strip of the quadriceps-patellar tendon dissected off the anterior patella, left it attached distally, passed the graft through the notch, and secured it to the lateral aspect of the femur [51]. The Andrews "mini-reconstruction" was published in 1983 and split the IT band longitudinally before tenodesing part of it to the lateral femur [52].

29.3.2 Results of Isolated LET Procedures

Results for the various isolated LET procedures have been generally poor. Patient satisfaction in terms of good to excellent results has been reported at rates of as low as 57–63 % for the Ellison procedure [53, 54] and 52 % for the Lemaire procedure [55]. Return to previous level of sport was seen in less than half of patients with a MacIntosh procedure despite a negative pivot shift in 84 % of patients [50]. Objective testing of the pivot shift in isolated LET procedures usually found a positive result more often than not [53, 55]. Andrews (1983) was able to report 94 % objectively acceptable and 91 % subjectively acceptable results with his technique [52]. Unfortunately, given the body of results of other isolated procedure studies, these results are looked upon with hesitation since they came from an era of nonvalidated scoring systems [56].

In addition to the poor clinical outcomes, there were other concerns that led to the abandonment of the isolated LET. The nonanatomic nature of LET procedures was thought to result in poor knee kinematics. Several studies have shown over-constraint in the form of abnormal resting tibial position in external rotation [42, 57–59]. However, this is likely a result of tensioning the LET graft in excessive external rotation [60]. There was also concern about this over-constraint possibly predisposing patients to osteoarthritis (OA) of the lateral compartment. However, the evidence supporting this relationship is underwhelming [57].

29.3.3 Combined LET Procedures

As arthroscopic ACLR techniques improved and became the gold standard, surgeons experimented with the LET as an adjunctive procedure. Some surgeons employed the MacIntosh or Lemaire procedure to compliment intra-articular graft reconstruction [61–65]. Marcacci developed a technique in 1992 that used hamstring grafts to reconstruct both the ACL and lateral reconstruction [66]. After passing the ACL portion of the graft, it is then brought through the "over the top" position, passed deep to the IT band and over the FCL down to Gerdy's tubercle where it is secured. Colombet employed a similar technique, but instead of the "over the top" position, the graft was passed through a femoral tunnel from the anteromedial bundle of the ACL to a point 1 cm proximal and posterior to the "femoral lateral tubercle" [67].

29.3.4 Results of Combined LET Procedures

Results for combined intra-articular ACLR and LET procedures have been more promising. A meta-analysis of 29 articles revealed a statistically significant reduction in the pivot shift in favor of a combination ACLR+LET compared to ACLR alone [68]. No significant difference was seen in anterior translation as measured by KT1000/2000 arthrometry or in International Knee Documentation Committee scores. The meta-analysis also highlights the amount of heterogeneity in the studies as several factors were different including type of ACL graft (bone-patellar tendon-bone (BTB) vs hamstring tendon (HT)) and method of LET. Overconstraint has not been shown in cadaver studies [43], and similarly, clinical studies have failed to show an increased risk of lateral compartment OA – even with the LET graft tensioned with tibial external rotation [69, 70].

29.4 The Fowler Kennedy Approach

29.4.1 Indications

The current practice at our institution is to perform an isolated ACLR in most primary cases with either a BTB or HT autograft. The addition of an LET procedure is considered in the setting of a revision ACLR where no other significant pathology needs to be addressed (i.e., posterolateral corner, medial collateral ligament reconstruction, meniscus transplantation, etc.) and particularly if allograft is being used. This is supported in a study by Trojani et al. [71] where a negative pivot shift was found in 80 % of revision patients receiving an LET augment compared to 63 % in ACLR alone. There are no clear indications for LET in the primary setting. However, consideration is given to patients who present with a combination of specific (see Fact Box 29.1) risk factors, in which case the senior author (AG) may recommend the additional procedure due to perceived increased risk of graft failure.

Fact Box 1: Risk Factors to Consider for Addition of LET

- Grade 2 or 3 pivot shift (high-grade rotational laxity)
- Young age <25 years
- Generalized ligamentous laxity
- Genu recurvatum >10°
- Returning to pivoting sport (i.e., soccer, basketball)

Others have proposed an individualized treatment algorithm for treating ACL ruptures based on the constellation of concomitant injuries [72]. Musahl suggests consideration of LET in a patient with a grade 2 or 3 pivot shift test in the absence of a meniscus or collateral ligament injury. In these cases, permanent capsular strain, generalized ligamentous laxity, or underlying morphologic abnormalities may be the cause for the abnormal pivot shift. Lerat et al. [73] suggest that patients with differential translation of the lateral side of the knee during the Lachman test (i.e., obvious internal rotation during anterior translation) may benefit from LET. Lording et al. [74] suggest that a significant injury to the medial meniscus may be another indication given the fact its loss increases stress within the ACL graft and negatively affects postoperative knee stability [75, 76].

29.4.2 Surgical Technique (Fig. 29.6)

Following the final tensioning of the ACLR, a modified Lemaire procedure is performed [77, 78]. A 6 cm curvilinear incision is placed just posterior to the lateral femoral epicondyle. The posterior border of the ITB is identified and freed of any fascial attachments to the level of Gerdy's tubercle. An 8 cm long × 1 cm wide strip of ITB is harvested from the posterior half of the ITB, ensuring that the most posterior fibers of the capsulo-osseous layer remain intact. It is left attached distally at Gerdy's tubercle, freed of any deep attachments to vastus lateralis, released proximally, and a #1 Vicryl whip stitch is placed in the free end of the graft. The FCL is then identified. Small capsular incisions are made anterior and posterior to the proximal portion of the ligament, and Metzenbaum scissors are placed deep to the FCL to bluntly dissect out a tract for graft passage. An attempt is made to remain extracapsular while ensuring there is no iatrogenic damage to the popliteus. The ITB graft is then passed beneath the FCL from distal to proximal. The lateral femoral supracondylar area is then cleared of the small fat pad found proximal to the lateral head of the gastrocnemius using electrocautery. The attachment site should be identified just anterior and proximal to the lateral gastrocnemius tendon. The periosteum is cleared using a cob on the metaphyseal flare of the lateral femoral condyle. Care is taken not to damage ACL femoral fixation as the suspensory loop button is often found close to this location. The graft is then held taut but not over-tensioned, with the knee at 60° flexion and the foot in neutral rotation to avoid lateral compartment over-constraint. The graft is secured using a small Richards staple and then folded back distally and sutured to itself using the #1 Vicryl whip stitch. The wound is irrigated, hemostasis is confirmed, and closure is performed in layers. We do not close the posterior aspect of the ITB where the graft was harvested from to avoid over-tightening the lateral patellofemoral joint. Postoperative rehabilitation is the same as for any ACLR and weight bearing, and range of motion is performed as tolerated so long as there is no significant meniscal repair.

Fact Box 2: Technical Pearl
Place the leg in the figure-4 position to place the fibular collateral ligament under tension to help identify it in order to pass the LET graft deep to it.

Fact Box 3: Technical Pearl
Apply minimal tension to the LET graft during fixation and secure it with the knee at 60° of flexion and the foot in neutral rotation to avoid over-constraint.

29.4.3 Future Directions

The role of LET will become more clear as studies more accurately identify those patients who are at an increased risk of failure with an isolated ACLR. Many risk factors are known with regard to graft rupture and ACLR failure. Young age, female sex, use of allograft, concomitant injuries (loss of medial meniscus), and return to high-risk sport involving pivoting or jumping have all been

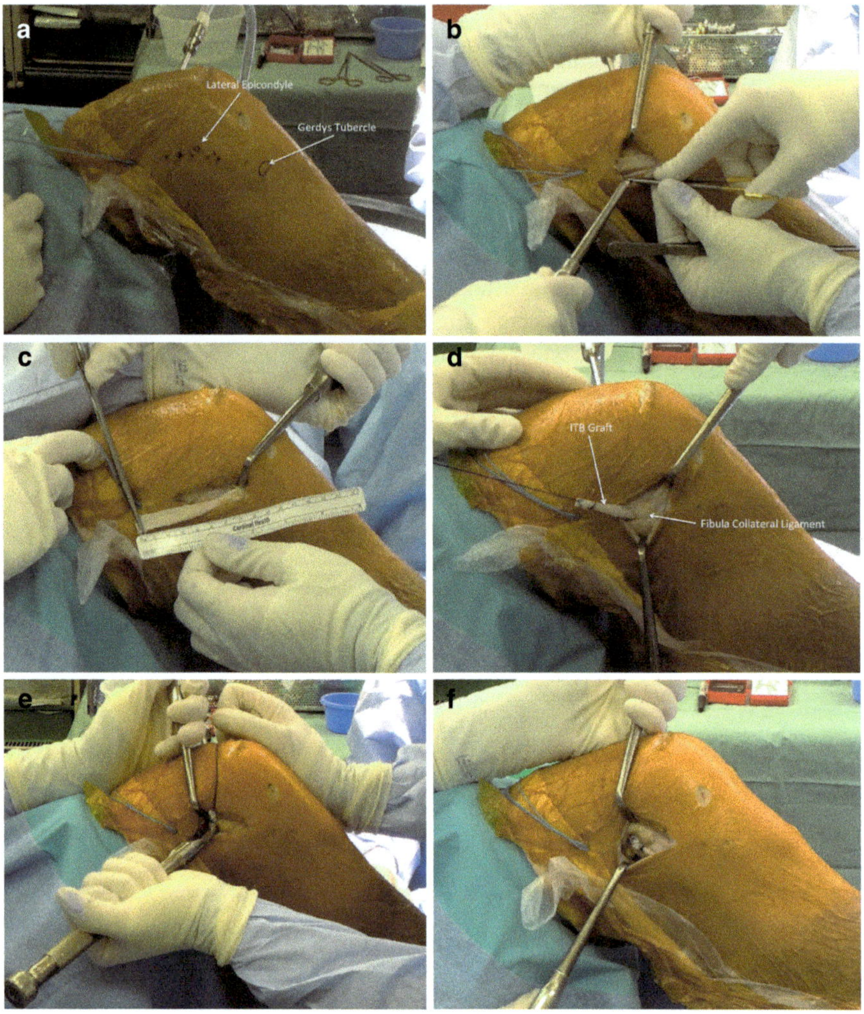

Fig. 29.6 Surgical technique of the Modified Lemaire LET. A) A 6 cm curvilinear incision (dotted line) is placed just posterior to the lateral femoral epicondyle; B & C) An 8cm long x 1cm wide strip of ITB is harvested from the posterior half of the ITB, ensuring that the most posterior fibers of the capsuloosseous layer remain intact; D) The FCL is identified and the ITB graft is then passed beneath the FCL from distal to proximal; E) The attachment site should be identified just anterior and proximal to the lateral gastrocnemius tendon. The graft is fixed with a small Richards staple, held taught but not over tensioned, with the knee at 60 degrees flexion and the foot in neutral rotation to avoid lateral compartment over-constraint; F) The graft is sutured back on itself and the ITB is left open to avoid over tightening the lateral retinaculaum

implicated as possible causes of failure [30, 79–81]. It will take well-designed studies to determine who, if anyone, will benefit most from an adjunctive LET procedure.

Our center is currently leading a multicenter randomized clinical trial aimed at determining if there is a clinical benefit to performing LET in the primary setting in high-risk patients [82]. The STAbiLiTY (Standard ACL Reconstruction vs ACL + Lateral Extra-Articular Tenodesis) study has been enrolling patients at eight centers in Canada and Europe since January 2014 and is aiming to recruit 600 participants. Patients are included if they are under the age of 25 and have any two of the following characteristics: greater than a grade 2 pivot shift, participation in a pivoting sport, or generalized ligamentous laxity. Two-year follow-up will be performed with a primary outcome of graft failure, which is defined as instability requiring revision surgery or a positive pivot shift test.

Fact Box 4

Start using the LET in the revision scenario as this will demonstrate its ability to control anterolateral rotation. Once comfortable with the technique, it may be used in the high-risk primary ACLR such as the young patient with generalized ligamentous laxity, genu recurvatum, and high-grade pivot shift wishing to return to pivoting sport.

Conclusion

Recent research has demonstrated the combined roles of the ACL, lateral meniscus posterior root, ALL, and ITB in controlling anterolateral rotation and the pivot shift. While the ALL has received significant attention, it is likely that the high-grade rotational laxity that results from an ACL injury is a combination of injury to many of these structures. The literature supports the biomechanical benefits of providing an extra-articular restraint to internal tibial rotation. LET is widely accepted in the European orthopedic community and is beginning to be recognized in North America as a useful adjunct to current ACLR techniques in certain patient populations. With modern techniques, it is a low-morbidity procedure with minimal complications. However, more clinical studies are needed to determine the particular patient population that may best benefit from receiving the additional procedure and if this will confer any benefit in the medium to long term.

Acknowledgments We are grateful for research funding for the STAbiLiTY study has been provided through the Multicenter Grant competition from the International Society of Arthroscopy, Knee Surgery, and Orthopedic Sports Medicine (ISAKOS) and the Orthopedic Research and Education Foundation (OREF).

Dr. Getgood also thanks Dr. David Dejour and Dr. Peter Verdonk for demonstrating their respective techniques of lateral extra-articular tenodesis.

References

1. Ardern CL, Webster KE, Taylor NF, Feller JA (2011) Return to sport following anterior cruciate ligament reconstruction surgery: a systematic review and meta-analysis of the state of play. Br J Sports Med 45:596–606
2. Boden BP, Sheehan FT, Torg JS, Hewett TE (2010) Noncontact anterior cruciate ligament injuries: mechanisms and risk factors. J Am Acad Orthop Surg 18:520–527
3. Claes S, Vereecke E, Maes M, Victor J, Verdonk P, Bellemans J (2013) Anatomy of the anterolateral ligament of the knee. J Anat 223:321–328
4. Vieira EL, Vieira EÁ, da Silva R, dos Santos Berlfein PA, Abdalla RJ, Cohen M (2007) An anatomic study of the iliotibial tract. Arthrosc J Arthrosc Relat Surg 23:269–274
5. Vincent JP, Magnussen RA, Gezmez F, Uguen A, Jacobi M, Weppe F et al (2012) The anterolateral ligament of the human knee: An anatomic and histologic study. Knee Surg Sports Traumatol Arthrosc 20:147–152
6. Caterine S, Litchfield R, Johnson M, Chronik B, Getgood A (2014) A cadaveric study of the anterolateral ligament: re-introducing the lateral capsular ligament. Knee Surg Sports Traumatol Arthrosc. [Internet]. [cited 2015 Mar 5];1–10. Available from: http://www.ncbi.nlm.nih.gov/pubmed/24929656
7. Hughston JC, Andrews JR, Cross MJ, Moschi A (1976) Classification of knee ligament instabilities. Part II. The lateral compartment. J Bone Joint Surg. Am. [Internet]. [cited 2014 Nov 17];58:173–179. Available from: http://www.ncbi.nlm.nih.gov/pubmed/1254620
8. Dietz GW, Wilcox DM, Montgomery JB (1986) Segond tibial condyle fracture: lateral capsular ligament avulsion. Radiology [Internet]. [cited 2015 Apr 29];159:467–469. Available from: http://www.ncbi.nlm.nih.gov/pubmed/3961179
9. Goldman AB, Pavlov H, Rubenstein D (1988) The Segond fracture of the proximal tibia: a small avulsion that reflects major ligamentous damage. AJR Am J Roentgenol. [Internet]. [cited 2015 Apr 29];151:1163–1167. Available from: http://www.ncbi.nlm.nih.gov/pubmed/3263770
10. Johnson LL (1979) Lateral capsular ligament complex: anatomical and surgical considerations. Am J Sports Med. [Internet]. [cited 2015 Apr 29];7:156–160. Available from: http://www.ncbi.nlm.nih.gov/pubmed/464170
11. Segond P (1879) Recherches cliniques et experimentales sur les epanchements sanguins du genou par entorse. Progres Medical, Paris

12. Norwood LA, Andrews JR, Meisterling RC, Clancy GL (1979) Acute anterolateral rotatory instability of the knee. J Bone Joint Surg Am 61-A:704–709
13. Claes S, Luyckx T, Vereecke E, Bellemans J (2014) The Segond fracture: a bony injury of the anterolateral ligament of the knee. Arthroscopy [Internet]. [cited 2015 Jul 3];30:1475–1482. Available from: http://www.ncbi.nlm.nih.gov/pubmed/25124480
14. Bhatia S, LaPrade CM, Ellman MB, LaPrade RF (2014) Meniscal root tears: significance, diagnosis, and treatment. Am J Sports Med. [Internet]. [cited 2015 Apr 29];42:3016–3030. Available from: http://www.ncbi.nlm.nih.gov/pubmed/24623276
15. Tanaka M, Vyas D, Moloney G, Bedi A, Pearle AD, Musahl V (2012) What does it take to have a high-grade pivot shift? Knee Surg. Sports Traumatol. Arthrosc. [Internet]. [cited 2015 Mar 5];20:737–742. Available from: http://www.ncbi.nlm.nih.gov/pubmed/22222616
16. Thompson WO, Fu FH (1993) The meniscus in the cruciate-deficient knee. Clin Sports Med. [Internet]. [cited 2015 Apr 29];12:771–796. Available from: http://www.ncbi.nlm.nih.gov/pubmed/8261525
17. Kittl C, El Daou H, Athwayl K, Gupte C, Weiler A, Williams A et al (2015) The role of the anterolateral structures and the ACL in controlling internal rotational knee laxity. ISAKOS Bienn Congr. [Internet]. Lyon; [cited 2015 Jun 15]. Available from: https://www.isakos.com/meetings/2015congress/AbstractView?EventID=8115
18. Zelle BA, Vidal AF, Brucker PU, Fu FH (2007) Double-bundle reconstruction of the anterior cruciate ligament: anatomic and biomechanical rationale. J Am Acad Orthop Surg 15:87–96
19. Yagi M, Wong EK, Kanamori A, Debski RE, Fu FH, Woo SL-Y (2002) Biomechanical analysis of an anatomic anterior cruciate ligament reconstruction. Am J Sports Med 30:660–666
20. Meredick RB, Vance KJ, Appleby D, Lubowitz JH (2008) Outcome of single-bundle versus double-bundle reconstruction of the anterior cruciate ligament: a meta-analysis. Am J Sports Med 36:1414–1421
21. Bedi A, Raphael B, Maderazo A, Pavlov H, Williams RJ (2010) Transtibial versus anteromedial portal drilling for anterior cruciate ligament reconstruction: a cadaveric study of femoral tunnel length and obliquity. Arthrosc J Arthrosc Relat Surg. [Internet]. Elsevier Inc.; 6:342–350. Available from: http://dx.doi.org/10.1016/j.arthro.2009.12.006
22. Markolf KL, Jackson SR, McAllister DR (2010) A comparison of 11 o'clock versus oblique femoral tunnels in the anterior cruciate ligament-reconstructed knee: knee kinematics during a simulated pivot test. Am J Sports Med 38:912–917
23. Lee MC, Seong SC, Lee S, Chang CB, Park YK, Jo H et al (2007) Vertical femoral tunnel placement results in rotational knee laxity after anterior cruciate ligament reconstruction. Arthroscopy [Internet]. [cited 2015 Apr 29];23:771–778. Available from: http://www.ncbi.nlm.nih.gov/pubmed/17637414
24. Loh JC, Fukuda Y, Tsuda E, Steadman RJ, Fu FH, Woo SLY (2003) Knee stability and graft function following anterior cruciate ligament reconstruction: Comparison between 11 o'clock and 10 o'clock femoral tunnel placement. Arthrosc J Arthrosc Relat Surg 19:297–304
25. Scopp JM, Jasper LE, Belkoff SM, Moorman CT (2004) The effect of oblique femoral tunnel placement on rotational constraint of the knee reconstructed using patellar tendon autografts. Arthroscopy [Internet]. [cited 2015 Apr 29];20:294–299. Available from: http://www.ncbi.nlm.nih.gov/pubmed/15007318
26. Jepsen CF, Lundberg-Jensen AK, Faunoe P (2007) Does the position of the femoral tunnel affect the laxity or clinical outcome of the anterior cruciate ligament-reconstructed knee? A clinical, prospective, randomized, double-blind study. Arthroscopy [Internet]. [cited 2015 Apr 29];23:1326–1333. Available from: http://www.ncbi.nlm.nih.gov/pubmed/18063177
27. Kato Y, Ingham SJM, Kramer S, Smolinski P, Saito A, Fu FH (2009) Effect of tunnel position for anatomic single-bundle ACL reconstruction on knee biomechanics in a porcine model. Knee Surg Sports Traumatol Arthrosc 18:2–10
28. Kato Y, Maeyama A, Lertwanich P, Wang JH, Ingham SJM, Kramer S et al (2012) Biomechanical comparison of different graft positions for single-bundle anterior cruciate ligament reconstruction. Knee Surg Sports Traumatol Arthrosc 21:816–823
29. Kondo E, Merican AM, Yasuda K, Amis AA (2011) Biomechanical comparison of anatomic double-bundle, anatomic single-bundle, and nonanatomic single-bundle anterior cruciate ligament reconstructions. Am J Sports Med. [Internet]. [cited 2015 Jun 16];39:279–288. Available from: http://ajs.sagepub.com/content/39/2/279.short
30. Shelbourne K, Gray T, Haro M (2009) Incidence of subsequent injury to either knee within 5 years after anterior cruciate ligament reconstruction with patellar tendon autograft. Am J Sports Med 37:246–251
31. Kaeding CC, Aros B, Pedroza A, Pifel E, Amendola A, Andrish JT et al (2011) Allograft versus autograft anterior cruciate ligament reconstruction: predictors of failure from a MOON prospective longitudinal cohort. Sports Health 3:73–81
32. Mohtadi NG, Chan DS, Dainty KN, Whelan DB (2011) Patellar tendon versus hamstring tendon autograft for anterior cruciate ligament rupture in adults. Cochrane Database Syst Rev. [Internet]. [cited 2015 Apr 29];CD005960. Available from: http://www.ncbi.nlm.nih.gov/pubmed/21901700
33. Magnussen RA, Lawrence JTR, West RL, Toth AP, Taylor DC, Garrett WE (2012) Graft size and patient age are predictors of early revision after anterior cruciate ligament reconstruction with hamstring autograft. Arthroscopy [Internet]. [cited 2015 Apr

29];28:526–531. Available from: http://www.ncbi.nlm.nih.gov/pubmed/22305299
34. Kocher MS, Steadman JR, Briggs K, Zurakowski D, Sterett WI, Hawkins RJ (2002) Determinants of patient satisfaction with outcome after anterior cruciate ligament reconstruction. J Bone Joint Surg Am 84-A:1560–1572
35. Ayeni OR, Chahal M, Tran MN, Sprague S (2012) Pivot shift as an outcome measure for ACL reconstruction: a systematic review. Knee Surg Sports Traumatol Arthrosc. [Internet]. [cited 2015 Apr 29];20:767–777. Available from: http://www.ncbi.nlm.nih.gov/pubmed/22218828
36. Leiter JRS, Gourlay R, McRae S, de Korompay N, MacDonald PB (2014) Long-term follow-up of ACL reconstruction with hamstring autograft. Knee Surg Sports Traumatol Arthrosc. [Internet]. [cited 2015 Apr 29];22:1061–1069. Available from: http://www.ncbi.nlm.nih.gov/pubmed/23595537
37. Jonsson H, Riklund-Ahlström K, Lind J (2004) Positive pivot shift after ACL reconstruction predicts later osteoarthrosis: 63 patients followed 5-9 years after surgery. Acta Orthop Scand 75:594–599
38. Catterall JB, Stabler T V, Flannery CR, Kraus VB (2010) Changes in serum and synovial fluid biomarkers after acute injury (NCT00332254). Arthritis Res Ther. [Internet]. [cited 2015 Jun 24];12:R229. Available from: http://www.pubmedcentral.nih.gov/articlerender.fcgi?artid=3046542&tool=pmcentrez&rendertype=abstract
39. Natoli RM, Scott CC, Athanasiou KA (2008) Temporal effects of impact on articular cartilage cell death, gene expression, matrix biochemistry, and biomechanics. Ann Biomed Eng. [Internet]. [cited 2015 Jun 24];36:780–792. Available from: http://www.ncbi.nlm.nih.gov/pubmed/18299988
40. Schindler OS (2012) Surgery for anterior cruciate ligament deficiency: a historical perspective. Knee Surg Sports Traumatol Arthrosc 20:5–47
41. Ellison A (1978) Anterolateral rotatory instability. In: Funk F Jr (ed) Symposium on the athlete's knee, surgical repair and reconstruction. American Academy of Orthopaedic Surgeons, St. Louis, AAOS, pp 178–193
42. Engebretsen L, Lew WD, Lewis JL, Hunter RE (1990) The effect of an iliotibial tenodesis on intraarticular graft forces and knee joint motion. Am J Sports Med 18:169–176
43. Draganich LF, Reider B, Ling M, Samuelson M (1990) An in vitro study an intraarticular and extraarticular reconstruction in the anterior cruciate ligament deficient knee. Am J Sports Med 18:262–266
44. Monaco E, Labianca L, Conteduca F (2007) De Carli a., Ferretti a. Double bundle or single bundle plus extraarticular tenodesis in ACL reconstruction?: AAA CAOS study. Knee Surg Sports Traumatol Arthrosc 15:1168–1174
45. Zaffagnini S, Signorelli C, Lopomo N, Bonanzinga T, Marcheggiani Muccioli GM, Bignozzi S et al. (2012) Anatomic double-bundle and over-the-top single-bundle with additional extra-articular tenodesis: an in vivo quantitative assessment of knee laxity in two different ACL reconstructions. Knee Surg Sports Traumatol Arthrosc. [Internet]. [cited 2015 Apr 29];20:153–159. Available from: http://www.ncbi.nlm.nih.gov/pubmed/21710111
46. Spencer L, Burkhart TA, Tran MN, Rezansoff AJ, Deo S, Caterine S et al. (2015) Biomechanical Analysis of Simulated Clinical Testing and Reconstruction of the Anterolateral Ligament of the Knee. Am J Sports Med [Internet]. [cited 2015 Jun 24];0363546515589166. Available from: http://ajs.sagepub.com/content/early/2015/06/19/0363546515589166.abstract
47. Lemaire M (1967) Ruptures anciennes du ligament croise anterieur du genou: Requence, Clinique, Traitement. (46 cas). J Chir 93:311–320
48. Losee RE, Johnson TR, Southwick WO (1978) Anterior subluxation of the lateral tibial plateau. A diagnostic test and operative repair. J Bone Joint Surg Am. [Internet]. [cited 2015 Apr 29];60:1015–1030. Available from: http://www.ncbi.nlm.nih.gov/pubmed/721850
49. Ellison AE (1979) Distal iliotibial-band transfer for anterolateral rotatory instability of the knee. J Bone Joint Surg Am 61-A:330–337
50. Ireland J, Trickey E (1980) MacIntosh tenodesis for anterolateral instability of the knee. J Bone Joint Surg Br 62-B:340–345
51. McCulloch PC, Lattermann C, Boland AL, Bach BR (2007) An illustrated history of anterior cruciate ligament surgery. J Knee Surg 20:95–104
52. Andrews JR, Sanders R (1983) A "mini-reconstruction" technique in treating anterolateral rotatory instability (ALRI). Clin Orthop Relat Res 172:93–96
53. Kennedy JC, Stewart R, Walker DM (1978) Anterolateral rotatory instability of the knee joint. J Bone Joint Surg Am 60-A:1031–1039
54. Fox JM, Blazina ME, Del Pizzo W, Ivey FM, Broukhim B (1980) Extra-articular stabilization of the knee joint for anterior instability. Clin Orthop Relat Res 56–61
55. Neyret P, Palomo JR, Donell ST, Dejour H (1994) Extra-articular tenodesis for anterior cruciate ligament rupture in amateur skiers. Br J Sports Med 28:31–34
56. Johnson DS, Smith RB (2001) Outcome measurement in the ACL deficient knee – what's the score? Knee 8:51–57
57. Sydney S, Haynes D, Hungerford D, Gerdes M (1987) The altered kinematic effect of an iliotibial band tenodesis on the anterior cruciate deficient knee. Orthopaedic Research Society, Transaction of Annual Meeting, p. 340
58. Draganich LF, Reider B, Miller PR (1989) An in vitro study of the Muller anterolateral femorotibial ligament tenodesis in the anterior cruciate ligament deficient knee. Am J Sports Med 17:357–362
59. Amis AA, Scammell BE (1993) Biomechanics of intra-articular and extra-articular reconstruction of the anterior cruciate ligament. J Bone Joint Surg Br 75:812–817

60. Anderson AF, Snyder RB, Lipscomb AB (2001) Anterior cruciate ligament reconstruction. A prospective randomized study of three surgical methods. Am J Sports Med 29:272–279
61. Dandy DJ (1995) Some clinical aspects of reconstruction for chronic anterior cruciate ligament deficiency. Ann R Coll Surg Engl 77:290–298
62. Bertoia JT, Urovitz EP, Richards RR, Gross AE (1985) Anterior cruciate reconstruction using the MacIntosh lateral-substitution over-the-top repair. J Bone Joint Surg Am 67-S:1183–1188
63. Zarins B, Rowe CR (1986) Combined anterior cruciate-ligament reconstruction using semitendinosus tendon and iliotibial tract. J Bone Joint Surg Am 68-A:160–177
64. Rackemann S, Robinson A, Dandy DJ (1991) Reconstruction of the anterior cruciate ligament with an intra-articular patellar tendon graft and an extra-articular tenodesis: results after six years. J Bone Joint Surg Br 73-B:368–373
65. Dejour H, Walsh G, Neyret P, Adeleine P (1988) Resultats des laxites chroniques anterieures operees. Rev Chir Orthop 74:622–636
66. Marcacci M, Zaffagnini S, Iacono F, Neri MP, Loreti I, Petitto A (1998) Arthroscopic intra- and extra-articular anterior cruciate ligament reconstruction with gracilis and semitendinosus tendons. Knee Surg Sports Traumatol Arthrosc. [Internet]. [cited 2015 Apr 29];6:68–75. Available from: http://www.ncbi.nlm.nih.gov/pubmed/9604189
67. Colombet PD (2011) Navigated intra-articular ACL reconstruction with additional extra-articular tenodesis using the same hamstring graft. Knee Surg Sports Traumatol Arthrosc 19:384–389
68. Hewison CE, Tran MN, Kaniki N, Remtulla A, Bryant D, Getgood AM (2015) Lateral extra-articular tenodesis reduces rotational laxity when combined with anterior cruciate ligament reconstruction: a systematic review of the literature. Arthroscopy [Internet]. Elsevier; [cited 2015 Jul 25]; Available from: http://www.arthroscopyjournal.org/article/S0749806315003862/fulltext
69. Marcacci M, Zaffagnini S, Giordano G, Iacono F, Presti ML (2009) Anterior cruciate ligament reconstruction associated with extra-articular tenodesis: a prospective clinical and radiographic evaluation with 10- to 13-year follow-up. Am J Sports Med 37:707–714
70. Zaffagnini S, Marcacci M, Lo Presti M, Giordano G, Iacono F, Neri MP (2006) Prospective and randomized evaluation of ACL reconstruction with three techniques: a clinical and radiographic evaluation at 5 years follow-up. Knee Surg Sports Traumatol Arthrosc 14:1060–1069
71. Trojani C, Beaufils P, Burdin G, Bussière C, Chassaing V, Djian P et al (2012) Revision ACL reconstruction: influence of a lateral tenodesis. Knee Surg Sports Traumatol Arthrosc 20:1565–1570
72. Musahl V, Kopf S, Rabuck S, Becker R, van der Merwe W, Zaffagnini S et al (2012) Rotatory knee laxity tests and the pivot shift as tools for ACL treatment algorithm. Knee Surg Sports Traumatol Arthrosc 20:793–800
73. Lerat JL, Moyen BL, Cladière F, Besse JL, Abidi H (2000) Knee instability after injury to the anterior cruciate ligament. Quantification of the Lachman test. J Bone Joint Surg Br 82:42–47
74. Lording TD, Lustig S, Servien E, Neyret P (2014) Lateral reinforcement in anterior cruciate ligament reconstruction. Asia-Pacific J Sport Med Arthrosc Rehabil Technol. [Internet]. 1:3–10. Available from: http://linkinghub.elsevier.com/retrieve/pii/S2214687313000034
75. Papageorgiou CD, Gil JE, Kanamori A, Fenwick JA, Woo SL, Fu FH (2001) The biomechanical interdependence between the anterior cruciate ligament replacement graft and the medial meniscus. Am J Sports Med 29:226–231
76. Trojani C, Sbihi A, Djian P, Potel JF, Hulet C, Jouve F et al (2011) Causes for failure of ACL reconstruction and influence of meniscectomies after revision. Knee Surg Sports Traumatol Arthrosc 19:196–201
77. Christel P, Djian P (2002) Anterio-lateral extra-articular tenodesis of the knee using a short strip of fascia lata. Rev Chir Orthop Reparatrice Appar Mot. [Internet]. [cited 2015 Apr 29];88:508–513. Available from: http://www.ncbi.nlm.nih.gov/pubmed/12399717
78. Getgood A (2014) Lateral Extra-Articular Tenodesis (LET) – indications and technique [Internet]. VuMedi. [cited 2015 Jun 15]. Available from: https://www.vumedi.com/video/lateral-extra-articular-tenodesis-let-indications-and-technique/
79. Salmon L, Russell V, Musgrove T, Pinczewski L, Refshauge K (2005) Incidence and risk factors for graft rupture and contralateral rupture after anterior cruciate ligament reconstruction. Arthroscopy 21:948–957
80. Wright RW, Dunn WR, Amendola A, Andrish JT, Bergfeld J, Kaeding CC et al (2007) Risk of tearing the intact anterior cruciate ligament in the contralateral knee and rupturing the anterior cruciate ligament graft during the first 2 years after anterior cruciate ligament reconstruction: a prospective MOON cohort study. Am J Sports Med. [Internet]. [cited 2015 Mar 9];35:1131–1134. Available from: http://www.ncbi.nlm.nih.gov/pubmed/17452511
81. Brophy R, Schmitz L, Wright RW (2012) Return to play and future ACL injury risk after ACL reconstruction in soccer athletes from the Multicenter Orthopaedic Outcomes Network (MOON) group. Am J Sports Med 40:2517–2522
82. Getgood A (2013) Standard ACL reconstruction vs ACL+lateral extra-articular tenodesis study (STAbiLiTY) [Internet]. ClinicalTrials.gov. [cited 2015 Jun 16]. Available from: https://clinicaltrials.gov/ct2/show/NCT02018354

ACL and Hidden Meniscus Lesions

30

Bertrand Sonnery-Cottet, Benjamin Freychet,
Nicolas Jan, François-Xavier Gunepin,
Romain Seil, and Mathieu Thaunat

Contents

B. Sonnery-Cottet (✉) • B. Freychet
N. Jan • M. Thaunat
Centre Orthopédique Santy, FIFA Medical Center of Excellence, Groupe Ramsay-Générale de Santé, Hôpital privé Jean Mermoz, 24 Avenue Paul Santy, Lyon 69008, France
e-mail: sonnerycottet@aol.com; benjamin.freychet@gmail.com; nicojan.nj@gmail.com; mathieuthaunat@yahoo.fr

F.-X. Gunepin
Service d'orthopédie, Clinique mutualiste de la porte de L'Orient, Rue Robert de la Croix, Lorient 56100, France
e-mail: francois-xavier.gunepin@clinique.mutualite56.fr

R. Seil
Department of Orthopaedic Surgery, Centre Hospitalier de Luxembourg–Clinique d'Eich, Luxembourg City, Luxembourg
e-mail: rseil@yahoo.com

30.1 Introduction

Data from anterior cruciate ligament (ACL) registries demonstrate that ACL tears are associated in 47–61 % with meniscal lesions [1, 17]. The most common intra-articular lesion associated with ACL ruptures involves the posterior horn of medial meniscus (MM) [26]. Specific types of MM lesions, such as meniscosynovial or meniscocapsular tears, cannot be diagnosed arthroscopically from the anterior compartment. These lesions were described in the 1980s by Hamberg [18] and Strobel [36], who called them "ramp" lesions [33]. Increased attention has been paid to this entity over the last few years [3, 9, 23, 32]. It has been shown that they are associated with ACL tears in 9–17 %, and they cannot be recognized on preoperative magnetic resonance imaging (MRI) scans [9, 23, 32]. In order to visualize them properly, the posterior compartment requires inspection. Various methods have been described to improve the visualization of the posteromedial corner of the knee [6, 8, 13, 15, 22, 23, 37]. Furthermore, several techniques and good clinical results have been described for meniscal repairs via an additional

V. Musahl et al. (eds.), *Rotatory Knee Instability*, DOI 10.1007/978-3-319-32070-0_30

posteromedial portal [3, 4, 25, 28]. Among the arthroscopic techniques, the all-inside repair through a standard anterior portal with meniscal suture anchor implants has increased in popularity as a result of its easy application [21]. Despite this, complications have been reported with these devices [35]. Biomechanically, the horizontal sutures of these devices have inferior strength when compared to the vertical sutures [7]. Morgan described the vertical suture of the posterior segment of the MM through a posteromedial portal with a suture hook, but this technique fell out of favor possibly because of its technical challenge [25]. However, a better healing rate for posterior horn MM lesions may be expected with better visualization, allowing for an improved diagnosis and an improved quality of the debridement prior to the repair and the control of a complete closure of the lesion through a posteromedial portal with a simple vertical suture [34].

30.2 Anatomy

Anatomically, the circumferential collagen fibers of the medial meniscal body are prolonged posteriorly to the meniscotibial ligament, which attaches to the subchondral bone of the tibia distal to the joint space. This structure represents a fibrocartilaginous transitional zone, possibly assisting with the progressive stiffness transition between ligamentous and bony tissues. The posterior horn is well attached to the tibia, preventing its posterior displacement during knee motion. Damage to the posterior part, involving the posteromedial corner and/or the posterior meniscotibial ligament, could lead to instability of the posterior horn [24]. One can hypothesize that hidden lesions represent an injury to the meniscotibial ligament (Fig. 30.1) which may be suspected, but not confirmed, from an anterior portal by visualization.

30.3 Diagnostic

30.3.1 Historical Background

Multiple studies have shown a high tear rate of the posterior horn of the MM in ACL-deficient knees. Several of them have also shown that the majority of errors in arthroscopic diagnosis result from the failure to recognize peripheral posterior horn tears of the medial meniscus, which are not adequately visualized from anterior portals [14, 16, 19, 20, 37]. Ireland et al. [19] demonstrated a 5.8 % incidence of failure to diagnose tears of the posterior horn of the MM in a series of 135 knee arthroscopies and emphasized the difficulty in visualizing the posterior third of the MM, as a result of obstruction by the medial femoral condyle. Gillies et al. [14] reported a 14 % and Kimori et al. [20] a 15 % incidence of overlooked MM posterior horn tears at arthroscopy. Bollen et al. [9] recently described a series of meniscocapsular lesions, which could be diagnosed only with a systematic inspection of the posterior compartment. These lesions were associated with ACL injuries and were present in 9.3 % of his prospective series of 183 ACL reconstructions. A combined mild anteromedial rotatory subluxation was suspected in this group. Liu et al. [23] described a prevalence of 16.6 % in a series of 868 consecutive arthroscopic ACL reconstructions. This corresponds exactly to the rate of the lesions we identified through direct visualization and probing of the posteromedial compartment.

> **Fact Box 1**
> Hidden MM lesions are associated with ACL tears in 9–17 % of cases.

30.3.2 Arthroscopy Technique

A systematic arthroscopic exploration of the medial meniscus was performed in three steps with a classic 30° arthroscope [23]:

- Step 1, standard arthroscopic exploration: The presence of a meniscal tear and its pattern was evaluated through standard anterior visualization via an anterolateral portal with meticulous probing of the meniscal tissue (Fig. 30.2a).

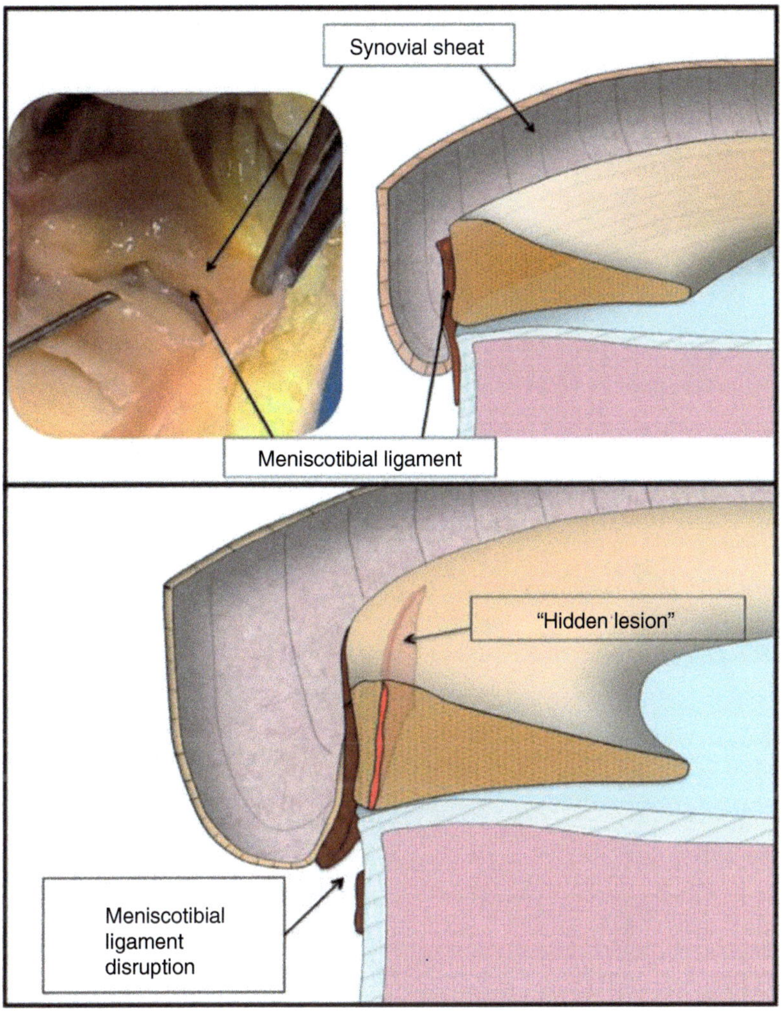

Fig. 30.1 Hidden lesion of the posterior horn of the medial meniscus

- Step 2, posteromedial compartment exploration:
- To gain access to the posteromedial compartment, the arthroscope was introduced through the anterolateral portal deeply into the notch and underneath the posterior cruciate ligament. Sometimes the help of a blunt trocar was necessary if the passage of the camera was difficult. In this position, the optical lens was rotated to allow for a good visualization of the posteromedial compartment and especially the meniscocapsular junction to assess the presence of a ramp lesion. A 70° arthroscope was not required in any of the cases.
- Step 3, posteromedial portal:
- A standard posteromedial portal was created under direct arthroscopic visualization of the posteromedial capsule. The entry point was localized with a needle to find the safe entry point, after which a skin incision and subcutaneous dissection were performed. The portal entry was just above the meniscus, proximal to the medial femoral condyle. The posterior horn of the MM was explored with a needle or a probe to detect an eventual ramp lesion (Fig. 30.2b). The posterior horn could be directly visualized by switching the arthroscope to the posteromedial portal. A minimal debridement of a superficial soft-tissue layer with a motorized shaver could discover the tear. This

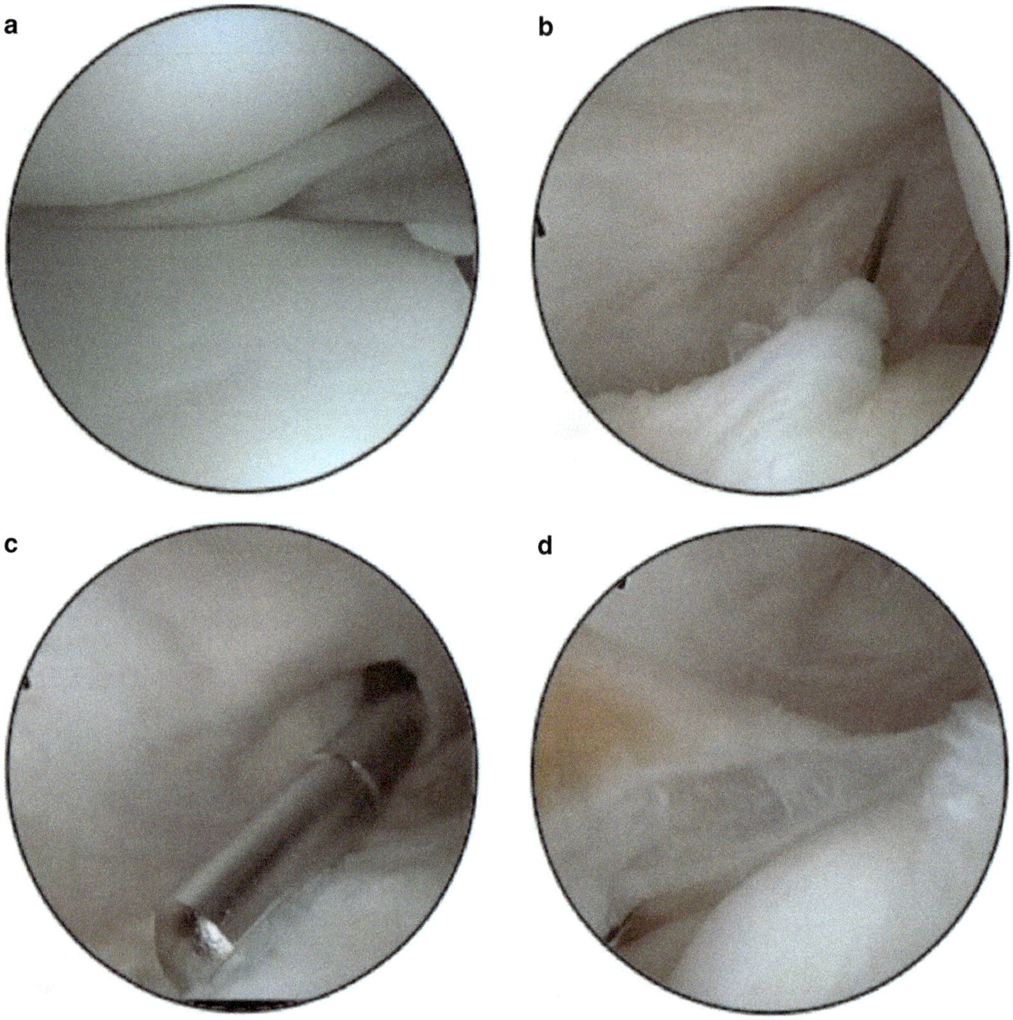

Fig. 30.2 (**a**) Anterior translation of the posterior horn of the medial meniscus during anterior probing, (**b**) visualization of the posterior compartment, and exploration of a superficial layer with a needle, (**c**) after a minimal debridement, (**d**) and discovery of a "hidden" lesion of the medial meniscus

type of lesion was called a "hidden lesion" (Fig. 30.2c, d).

125 meniscus tears were diagnosed using the three arthroscopic steps described above; 75 (60 %) medial meniscal body lesions were diagnosed through standard anterior portal exploration, 29 (23.2 %) ramp lesions were diagnosed at posteromedial compartment exploration, and 21 (16.8 %) were discovered at step 3 by probing the tear through a posteromedial portal and after a minimal debridement of a superficial soft-tissue layer with a motorized shaver [34].

Fact Box 2: Exploration of the MM

- Step 1, standard anterior arthroscopic exploration:
  Discovery of 60 % of the MM lesions
- Step 2, exploration of the posteromedial compartment through the anterolateral portal deeply into the notch and underneath the posterior cruciate ligament:
  Discovery of 23 % of the MM lesions
- Step 3: through a posteromedial portal, a needle or a probe is used to detect a ramp lesion:
  Discovery of 17 % of the MM lesions

30.4 Classification

We propose a classification for medial meniscocapsular tears. Type 1 is ramp lesion behind the meniscotibial ligament with low mobility at probing. Type 2 is a partial superior lesion in front of the meniscotibial ligament with low mobility at probing. Type 3 is a partial inferior lesion (hidden lesion) with high mobility at probing. Type 4 is a complete lesion with very high mobility at probing Type 5 is a double lesion (Fig. 30.3).

30.5 Biomechanical Consequence on ACL-Deficient Knee

Longitudinal tears of the MM posterior horn represent an important, prevalent, and often missed lesion associated with an ACL rupture. For many authors [2, 9, 11] when left untreated, these lesions predispose to increased anterior tibial translation and increased ACL strain and for SR. Bollen, to a mild anteromedial rotatory subluxation. Moreover, these studies demonstrated that repairing these lesions at the time of ACL reconstruction is very important in order to restore knee biomechanics and minimize stress on the ACL graft.

30.6 Treatment

30.6.1 Historical Background

Despite the development of new devices, the failure rate for repairs of MM posterior horn tears remains high [12, 21]. With classic anterior portals, failure to visualize the posterior horn of the MM may result in insufficient debridement of the lesion, while *all-inside suture device* placement may be at risk for becoming a blind procedure. Furthermore, with visualization from anterior portals alone, it is not always possible to be sure that a complete closure of the lesion is achieved. *There is a risk of inadequately positioning the all-inside suture devices between the central and peripheral zone, which leads to inadequate reduction of the tear and potential failure* [38]. Without an excellent view of the lesion, meniscal repair devices may induce different complications, including migration or breakage of the implant [10, 38, 39], leading to iatrogenic cartilage damage [35]. Hence, a better healing rate of posterior horn MM lesions may be expected through better visualization, allowing for an improved diagnosis [29], an improved quality of the debridement prior to the repair, and the control of a complete closure of the lesion [5]. Better visualization also allows the placement of vertical sutures perpendicular to the deep fibers of the menisci, which are biomechanically more adapted. The reduction of the lesion is visualized during the procedure, which is not possible in the all-inside implantation. *The same hooked suture passer can be used to pass multiple sutures throughout the hidden meniscus tear.*

30.6.2 Surgical Technique

During the procedure, the patients are placed supine on the operating table with a tourniquet placed high on the thigh. The knee is placed at 90° of flexion with a foot support to allow for a full range of knee motion. We use a standard high lateral parapatellar portal for the arthroscope and the medial parapatellar portal for the instruments [33]. In case of a dislocated bucket-handle tear, reduction is performed. The possibility of engaging the probe in the posterior segment of the meniscus and of bringing it under the condyle is an indirect sign of lesion and instability criteria. Direct visualization of the posteromedial compartment must always be done in order to diagnose and repair these lesions.

The arthroscope is introduced into the anterolateral portal in the triangle *formed* by the medial condyle, the PCL, and the tibial spines. After the contact with this zone, the arthroscope can pass through the space at the condyle border when applying a valgus force, first in flexion and then in extension. An internal rotation is applied to the tibia to help visualization; this causes the posterior tibial plateau to sublux and a posterior translation of the middle segment. With this maneuver, two-thirds of peripheral lesions from the posterior segment up to the middle segment

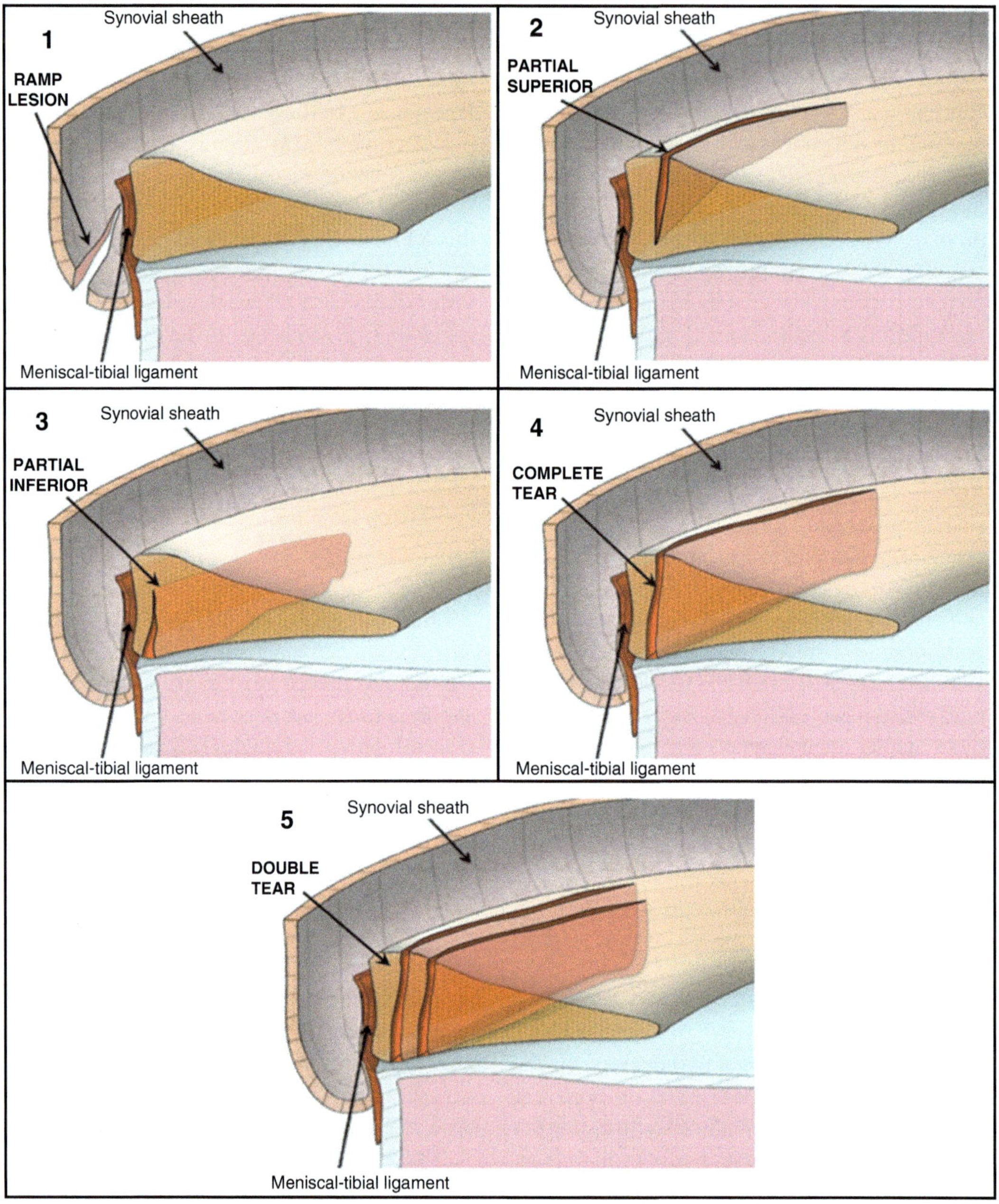

Fig. 30.3 The five typical types of medial meniscocapsular tears

can be seen. In the case of a tear of the posterior segment, a posteromedial approach is performed. Transillumination allows the surgeon to observe the veins and nerves that must be avoided. The point where the needle is introduced is above the hamstring tendons, 1 cm posterior to the medial femorotibial joint line. The knee must be flexed at 90° to avoid the popliteal structures. The needle must be introduced from outside to inside, in the direction to the lesion. The approach is done with a number 11 blade scalpel under arthroscopic control and dissection via the same approach, again under arthroscopic control. The all-inside suture can then be performed (Fig. 30.4).

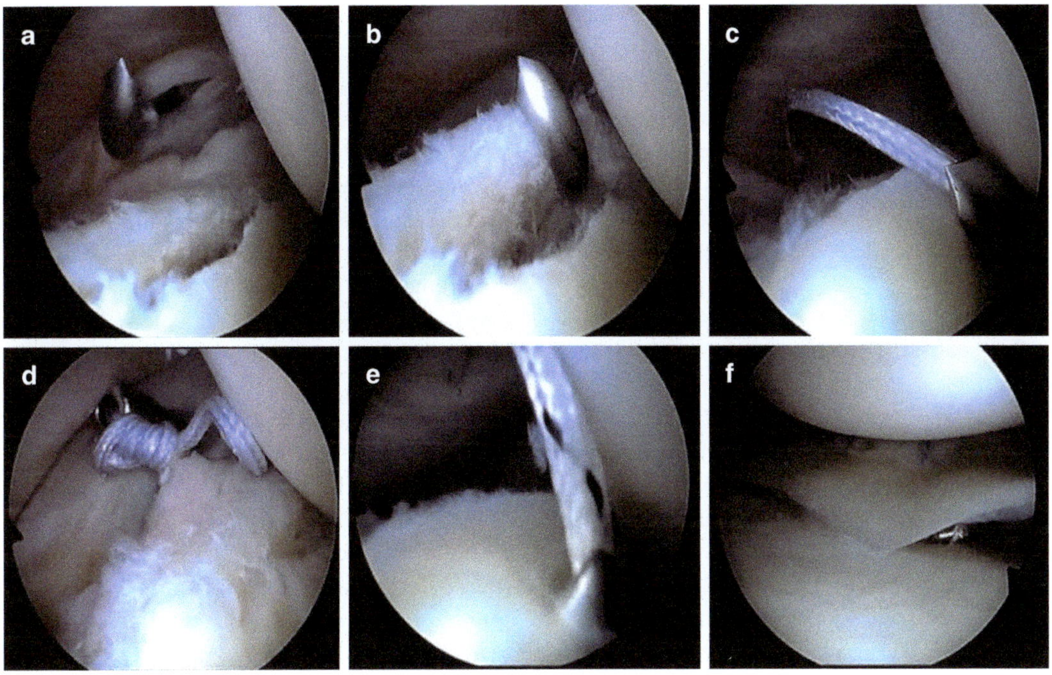

Fig. 30.4 (**a, b**) Suture of the posterior segment of the medial meniscus of the right knee through a posteromedial portal with a suture hook device; (**c**) the sharp tip penetrated the peripheral wall of the medial meniscus from outside to inside; (**d**) next, the suture hook is passed through the center (the inner portion) of the medial meniscus; (**e**) the first knot is tied with a knot pusher; (**f**) a second suture is performed 5 mm more posterior to the first one. The final suture with nonabsorbable suture from the anterior portal

Initially, the lesion is debrided and edges of the tear are trimmed with a shaver. A left-curved hook is used for a right knee and vice versa. The 25° hook loaded with a N° 2 non-resorbable braided composite suture is introduced through the posteromedial portal. The foot is positioned in maximal internal rotation in order to take away the medial condyle from the posterior segment of the meniscus. The suture hook is manipulated by hand so that the sharp tip penetrates the peripheral wall of the medial meniscus from outside to inside. Next, the suture hook is passed through the central (inner) portion of the medial meniscus. The free end of the suture in the posteromedial space is grasped and brought up to posteromedial portal. A sliding knot (fishing knot type) is applied to the most posterior part of the meniscus with the help of a knot pusher and is then cut. This maneuver is repeated as required, depending on the length of the tear (one knot was inserted every 5 mm). Care is taken during this technique to avoid tangling the sutures. Once the posteromedial *part* is finished, the knee is positioned in valgus, near extension, and the suture is tested and repeated if necessary. The posterior suture is completed with a repair through standard anterior portal with a meniscal suture anchor when the tear extends to the pars intermedia and/or by outside-in sutures if the tear extends to the anterior segment of the meniscus. The stability of the suture is then tested with the probe.

Fact Box 3: Tips and Tools for Posteromedial Meniscus Suture

- Internal rotation is applied to the tibia to help visualization of the posterior horn of the MM.
- A 25° hook suture passer loaded with a resorbable n°1 PDS suture.
- To know a sliding knot.

30.6.3 Rehabilitation

Postoperatively, both active and passive ranges of motion are limited to 0–90° in the first 6 weeks. Progression to full weight bearing occurs by postoperative week 3. Jogging is permitted after week 12, pivoting activity at 6 months, and full activity at 9 months for all patients.

30.7 Results

We prospectively evaluated 132 consecutive patients in whom 132 medial menisci underwent a MM repair with a suture hook device loaded with a N° 2 non-resorbable braided composite suture in conjunction with ACL reconstruction. Nine patients (6.8 %) had failure of the meniscal repair with repeat surgical intervention involving resection or revision of the repair. With failure as the end point, the cumulative survival rate of all-inside suture repair of the MM through a posteromedial portal during ACL reconstruction was 93.2 % (95 % CI 0.887–0.974) at the final follow-up, with an *average of 24 months (range, 21–26 months)*.

When the healing rate of this study is compared to those previously reported using this method of suture, an abnormally high rate of recurrent meniscal lesions was found. However, the healing rate at the location of the initial tear was comparable to the rate of 96.4 % reported by Ahn et al. in a recent study with a second-look arthroscopy [4].

The nine recurrent tears showed the following aspect at arthroscopy:

- Two flaps between the intermediate and the posterior portions of the meniscus. The initially sutured lesion was a bucket-handle tear ($n=2$).
- Recurrent ramp lesion ($n=2$).
- New tear located more anteriorly to the initial tear (white/white zone) with the latter being healed ($n=5$) (Fig. 30.5).

The high rate of recurrent tear was explained by newly formed injuries, which were confirmed on the surface of five menisci. It is conceivable that these injuries were attributable to a residual cleft left by the path of the suture lasso and maintained by the use of a strong N° 2 nonabsorbable suture (Fig. 30.6). These clefts on the avascular meniscal substance may remain in situ without healing and would favor the recurrence of a more centrally located lesion in the white/white zone. Therefore, we decided to change our suture from a strong non-resorbable suture to a PDS suture in order to reduce the risk of newly formed injury. From a biomechanical point of view, PDS 0 and PDS 1 sutures are recommended for meniscal sutures to guarantee a high primary stability, small amount of gapping, and fewer partial tissue failure [31] and was used by Ahn et al. [4], and they did not report any newly formed injury in their series of 140 knees which had a second-look arthroscopy at a mean follow-up of 37.7 months after an all-inside suture of the posterior segment of the MM through a posteromedial portal. However, in these five cases, the amount of meniscectomy was decreased when compared with the initial lesion. As advocated by Pujol et al. [30], the meniscus can be partially saved and that a risk of a partial failure should be *accepted* when possible.

30.8 Complications

The disadvantages of the all-inside suture technique through a PM portal are that a second incision is necessary, requiring more operative time. There is also a significant learning curve in placing and tying the sutures. A potential risk for synovial fistula has been reported, but no cases were encountered in the series of the current authors [40]. The main risk of posteromedial access is injury to the saphenous nerve and

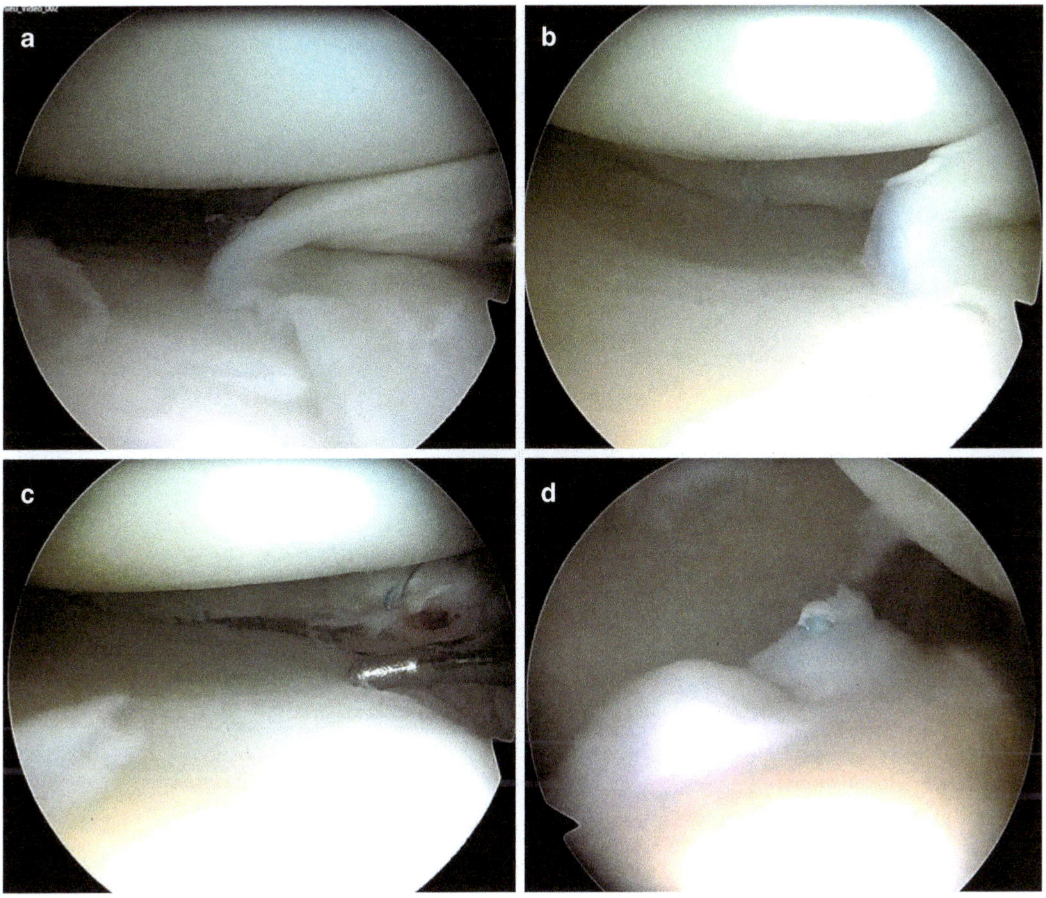

Fig. 30.5 (**a**) Newly formed injury after the medial meniscal repair of the right knee; (**b**) a meniscal flap with an anterior pedicle located in the red/white zone is detached; (**c**) this newly formed injury is identified by a residual nonabsorbable suture material on the meniscus; (**d**) aspect of the medial meniscus after economical subsequent meniscectomy of the unstable flap; the vertical suture from the primary repair is left alone. View of the posterior segment with the scope placed deep in the notch; the original tear site is healed completely

vein. The popliteal artery, common fibular nerve, and tibial nerve are situated more laterally. According to anatomical studies, the portal is located at least 1.5 cm from the saphenous nerve and vein. Morgan describes one case of transient hypoesthesia of the sartorius branch of the saphenous nerve in one series of 70 cases, likely due to an accessory access portal situated too anteriorly [25]. The clinical review of 179 patients who underwent posterior approaches did not show serious complications, but included three cases (1.7 %) of residual hypoesthesia in the saphenous nerve and two cases of puncture of the saphenous vein [27]. The specific technique for passage of the arthroscope through the intercondylar notch is necessary to provide transillumination in order to avoid this complication.

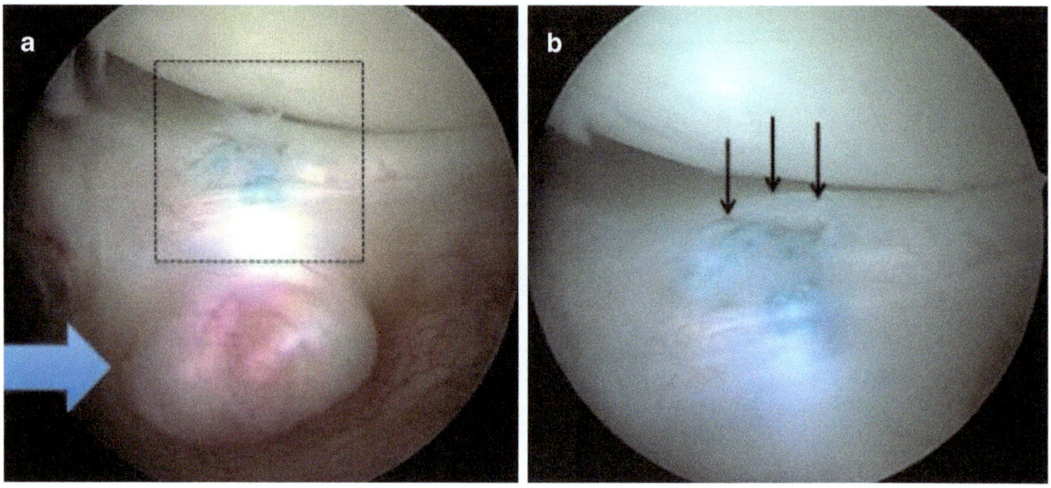

Fig. 30.6 (**a**) Second-look arthroscopy 2 years after posterior view of a MM posterior horn repair with #2 nonabsorbable sutures. The *blue arrow* shows the synovial coverage of the knot. View from posteromedial portal, left knee at 90° of flexion; (**b**) magnification shows the residual cleft (*black arrows*) created by the path of the suture lasso. These clefts may remain in situ and may favor the recurrence of a second meniscus tear. For these reasons the authors changed suture materials from strong nonabsorbable material to resorbable PDS sutures.

Conclusion

Posterior visualization and posteromedial probing of the posterior horn of the MM can provide assistance in discovering a higher rate of lesions that may be easily missed through a standard anterior exploration. In numerous cases, these lesions were "hidden" under a membrane-like tissue and were discovered only after a minimal debridement through a posteromedial portal. This additional portal allows for a better visualization, easier access, and sufficient debridement prior to repair. Repaired medial menisci in ACL-reconstructed knees using a suture hook through a posteromedial portal showed good healing with a low rate of revision at an average of 2-year follow-up. It seems to be a promising technique because it allows the placement of vertically oriented sutures with good tissue approximation. It has been previously demonstrated that repairing these lesions at the time of ACL reconstruction is very important in order to restore knee biomechanics and minimize stress on the ACL graft.

References

1. Ahldén M, Samuelsson K, Sernert N, Forssblad M, Karlsson J, Kartus J (2012) The Swedish National Anterior Cruciate Ligament Register: a report on baseline variables and outcomes of surgery for almost 18,000 patients. Am J Sports Med 40(10): 2230–2235
2. Ahn JH, Bae TS, Kang KS, Kang SY, Lee SH (2011) Longitudinal tear of the medial meniscus posterior horn in the anterior cruciate ligament-deficient knee significantly influences anterior stability. Am J Sports Med 39(10):2187–2193. doi:10.1177/0363546511416597
3. Ahn JH, Kim SH, Yoo JC, Wang JH (2004) All-inside suture technique using two posteromedial portals in a medial meniscus posterior horn tear. Arthroscopy 20:101–108
4. Ahn JH, Lee YS, Yoo JC, Chang MJ, Koh KH, Kim MH (2010) Clinical and second-look arthroscopic evaluation of repaired medial meniscus in anterior cruciate ligament-reconstructed knees. Am J Sports Med 38(3):472–477. doi:10.1177/0363546509348102
5. Ahn JH, Wang JH, Yoo JC (2004) Arthroscopic all-inside suture repair of medial meniscus lesion in anterior cruciate ligament–deficient knees: results of second-look arthroscopies in 39 cases. Arthroscopy 20:936–945

6. Amin KB, Cosgarea AJ, Kaeding CC (1999) The value of intercondylar notch visualization of the posteromedial and posterolateral compartments during knee arthroscopy. Arthroscopy 15:813–817
7. Aşík M, Sener N (2002) Failure strength of repair devices versus meniscus suturing techniques. Knee Surg Sports Traumatol Arthrosc 10(1):25–29
8. Bedi A, Dines J, Dines DM, Kelly BT, O'Brien SJ, Altchek DW, Allen AA (2010) Use of the 70 ° arthroscope for improved visualization with common arthroscopic procedures. Arthroscopy 26:1684–1696. doi:10.1016/j.arthro.2010.04.070
9. Bollen SR (2010) Posteromedial meniscocapsular injury associated with rupture of the anterior cruciate ligament: a previously unrecognized association. J Bone Joint Surg Br 92:222–223. doi:10.1302/0301-620X.92B2.22974
10. Calder SJ, Myers PT (1999) Broken arrow: a complication of meniscal repair. J Arthrosc Relat Surg 15(6):651–652
11. Cory E, James KW, Elifho O, Connor Z, Dale NR, Robert AA (2015) Posteromedial meniscocapsular tear: prevalence, detection sensitivity, biomechanics, and repair technique. In Scientific Exhibit SE81. American Academy of Orthopaedic surgeons. http://aaos2015.conferencespot.org/58906-aaos-1.1965581/cory-edgar-1.1970358
12. Ellermann A, Siebold R, Buelow JU, Sobau C (2002) Clinical evaluation of meniscus repair with a bioabsorbable arrow: a 2- to 3-year follow-up study. Knee Surg Sports Traumatol Arthrosc 10(5):289–293
13. Fakioglu O, Ozsoy MH, Ozdemir HM, Yigit H, Cavusoglu AT, Lobenhoffer P (2013) Percutaneous medial collateral ligament release in arthroscopic medial meniscectomy in tight knees. Knee Surg Sports Traumatol Arthrosc 21(7):1540–1545. doi:10.1007/s00167-012-2128-x
14. Gillies H, Seligson D (1979) Precision in the diagnosis of meniscal lesions: a comparison of clinical evaluation, arthrography, and arthroscopy. J Bone Joint Surg Am 61:343–346
15. Gillquist J, Hagberg G, Oretorp N (1979) Arthroscopic examination of the posteromedial compartment of the knee joint. Int Orthop 3:13–18
16. Gold DL, Schaner PJ, Sapega AA (1995) The posteromedial portal in knee arthroscopy: an analysis of diagnostic and surgical utility. Arthroscopy 11:139–145
17. Granan LP, Inacio MC, Maletis GB, Funahashi TT, Engebretsen L (2012) Intraoperative findings and procedures in culturally and geographically different patient and surgeon populations: an anterior cruciate ligament reconstruction registry comparison between Norway and the USA. Acta Orthop 83:577–582. doi: 10.3109/17453674.2012.741451
18. Hamberg P, Gillquist J, Lysholm J (1983) Suture of new and old peripheral meniscus tears. J Bone Joint Surg Am 65(2):193–197
19. Ireland J, Trickey EL, Stoker DJ (1980) Arthroscopy and arthrography of the knee: a critical review. J Bone Joint Surg Br 62:3–6
20. Kimori K, Suzu F, Yamashita F, Sakakida K, Hirasawa Y (1989) Evaluation of arthrography and arthroscopy for lesions of the posteromedial corner of the knee. Am J Sports Med 17:638–643
21. Kotsovolos ES, Hantes ME, Mastrokalos DS, Lorbach O, Paessler HH (2006) Results of all-inside meniscal repair with the FasT-Fix meniscal repair system. J Arthrosc Relat Surg 22(1):3–9
22. Lewicky RT, Abeshaus MM (1982) Simplified technique for posterior knee arthroscopy. Am J Sports Med 10:22–23
23. Liu X, Feng H, Zhang H, Hong L, Wang XS, Zhang J (2011) Arthroscopic prevalence of ramp lesion in 868 patients with anterior cruciate ligament injury. Am J Sports Med 39:832–837. doi:10.1177/0363546510388933
24. Mariani PP (2011) Posterior horn instability of the medial meniscus a sign of posterior meniscotibial ligament insufficiency. Knee Surg Sports Traumatol Arthrosc 19:1148–1153. doi:10.1007/s00167-011-1424-1
25. Morgan CD (1991) The "all-inside" meniscus repair. Arthroscopy 7:120–125
26. Noyes FR, Chen RC, Barber-Westin SD, Potter HG (2011) Greater than 10-year results of red-white longitudinal meniscal repairs in patients 20 years of age or younger. Am J Sports Med 39:1008–1017. doi:10.1177/0363546510392014
27. Ogilvie-Harris DJ, Weisleder L (1995) Arthroscopic synovectomy of the knee: is it helpful? J Arthrosc Relat Surg 11(1):91–95
28. Park IS, Kim SJ (2006) New meniscus repair technique for peripheral tears near the posterior tibial attachment of the posterior horn of the medial meniscus. Arthoscopy 22:908.e1–908.e4
29. Peltier A, Lording TD, Lustig S, Servien E, Maubisson L, Neyret P (2015) Posteromedial meniscal tears may be missed during anterior cruciate ligament reconstruction. Arthroscopy 31(4):691–698. doi:10.1016/j.arthro.2014.12.003
30. Pujol N, Barbier O, Boisrenoult P, Beaufils P (2011) Amount of meniscal resection after failed meniscal repair. Am J Sports Med 39(8):1648–1652. doi:10.1177/0363546511402661
31. Seil R, Rupp S, Jurecka C, Rein R, Kohn D (2001) Effect of various suture strength factors on behavior of meniscus sutures in cyclic loading conditions. Unfallchirurg 104(5):392–398
32. Seil R, VanGiffen N, Pape D (2009) Thirty years of arthroscopic meniscal suture: what's left to be done? Orthop Traumatol Surg Res 95:S85–S96. doi:10.1016/j.otsr.2009.09.004
33. Sonnery-Cottet B, Archbold P, Zayni R, Thaunat M, Bortolletto J, Fayard JM, Chambat P (2011) High

lateral portal for sparing the infrapatellar fat-pad during ACL reconstruction. Orthop Traumatol Surg Res 97:870–873. doi:10.1016/j.otsr.2011.08.007
34. Sonnery-cottet B, Conteduca J, Thaunat M, Gunepin FX, Seil R (2014) Hidden lesions of the posterior horn of the medial meniscus: a systematic arthroscopic exploration of the concealed portion of the knee. Am J Sports Med 42(4):921–926. doi:10.1177/0363546514522394
35. Sonnery-Cottet B, Mortati R, Gadea F, Thaunat M, Moyere F, Chouteau J (2013) Osteolysis of the tibial plateau after meniscal repair with hybrid suture anchor. Knee Surg Sports Traumatol Arthrosc 21(9):2137–2140. doi:10.1007/s00167-012-2296-8
36. Strobel MJ (1988) Menisci. In: Fett HM, Flechtner P (eds) Manual of arthroscopic surgery. Springer, New York, pp 171–178
37. Tolin BS, Sapega AA (1993) Arthroscopic visual field mapping at the periphery of the medial meniscus: a comparison of different portal approaches. Arthroscopy 9:265–271
38. Walgrave S, Claes S, Bellemans J (2013) High incidence of intraoperative anchorage failure in FasT-fix all inside meniscal suturing device. Acta Orthop Belg 79(6):689–693
39. Wilmes P, Lorbach O, Brogard P, Seil R (2008) Complications with all-inside devices used in reconstructive meniscal surgery. Orthopade 37:1088–1089, 1091–1095, 1097–1098. doi:10.1007/s00132-008-1307-4
40. Yiannakopoulos CK (2007) Diagnosis and treatment of postarthroscopic synovial knee fistulae: a report of four cases and review of the literature. J Knee Surg 20(1):34–38

Double-Bundle Anterior Cruciate Ligament Reconstruction

31

Sebastián Irarrázaval, Jonathan N. Watson, Marcio Albers, Daniel Guenther, and Freddie H. Fu

Contents

S. Irarrázaval, MD • J.N. Watson, MD • M. Albers, MD
D. Guenther, MD • F.H. Fu, MD (✉)
Department of Orthopaedic Surgery, University of Pittsburgh Medical Center, Kaufman Building Suite 1011, 3471 Fifth Avenue, Pittsburgh, PA 15213, USA
e-mail: ffu@upmc.edu

31.1 Introduction

ACL ruptures are one of the most common sports injuries, affecting approximately 30 out of every 100,000 people each year in the United States [16]. This injury can result in both acute and chronic problems, including recurrent knee instability, meniscal tears, articular cartilage degeneration, and subsequent osteoarthritis (OA) [4, 39, 42]. The ACL does not have an intrinsic capacity to heal, and as such, surgical reconstruction is therefore the standard treatment in active patients [6, 13]. The objective of ACL reconstruction is to reestablish knee function as closely as possible to the native knee and prevent future meniscal and chondral damage, which can lead to degenerative changes [7, 8, 23].

Traditionally, ACL reconstruction has focused on one portion of the ACL, the anteromedial (AM) bundle, and relied on the transtibial technique. This approach typically results in nonanatomic tunnel placement. Accordingly, studies have demonstrated persistent laxity and abnormal knee kinematics with functional testing after this reconstruction [11, 12, 56]. In addition, several studies have shown that up to 50 % of patients develop radiological signs of OA within 12 years after this procedure [34, 37].

In an attempt to restore knee laxity and function and improve clinical outcomes, anatomic

V. Musahl et al. (eds.), *Rotatory Knee Instability*, DOI 10.1007/978-3-319-32070-0_31

double-bundle (DB) ACL reconstruction was developed, recreating both bundles to potentially optimize and restore normal knee kinematics [14, 15, 59].

The objective of this chapter is to describe the anatomic ACL reconstruction concept and determine, following an evidence-based approach, whether DB reconstruction restores knee rotatory laxity closer to normal than nonanatomic SB ACL reconstruction.

Fact Box 1

Transtibial ACL reconstruction: surgical technique in which the femoral tunnel is drilled through the tibial tunnel. It can be used for single- or double-bundle ACL reconstruction.

Anteromedial portal ACL reconstruction: surgical technique in which the femoral tunnel is drilled inside out through an accessory anteromedial portal, allowing to more accurately reach the femoral insertion site compared to the transtibial technique. It can be used for single- or double-bundle ACL reconstruction.

Two-incision ACL reconstruction: surgical technique in which the femoral tunnel is drilled outside-in through a mini-open incision on the lateral side of the distal femur, also allowing to more accurately reach the femoral insertion site compared to the transtibial procedure. It can be used for single- or double-bundle ACL reconstruction.

Anatomic ACL reconstruction concept: restoration of the ACL to its native dimensions, collagen orientation, and insertion sites. It's a concept that can be applied to different surgical techniques including SB reconstruction, DB reconstruction, augmentation, and ACL revision surgery.

Individualized ACL reconstruction: part of the anatomic ACL reconstruction concept, in which the surgical technique (DB or SB) and graft size are chosen depending on preoperative (MRI) and intraoperative measurements of the patient's native ACL and bony anatomy.

31.2 Anatomy and Biomechanics of the Native ACL

The anatomy of the ACL consists of two functional bundles, the AM and the posterolateral (PL) bundles. The bundles are covered by a thin membrane and are separated by a distinct septum containing vascular-derived stem cells [40] (Fig. 31.1).

Biomechanically, the AM and PL bundles function together to provide stability throughout knee range of motion. The AM bundle length stays constant during knee range of motion, showing maximum tension between 45° and 60° of knee flexion. The PL bundle has maximum tension in full extension, with decreasing tension during knee flexion. The orientation of the bundles changes throughout the arc of motion. In extension, the bundles are parallel, while in flexion they become crossed in the coronal, sagittal, and axial planes, twisting around each other [9]. The AM bundle is primarily responsible for stabilization of the knee in the AP direction, whereas the PL bundle primarily stabilizes knee rotation [65] (Fig. 31.2).

The AM and PL bundles have differing exposures to in situ forces. The forces experienced by each bundle are complementary in nature, with the AM bundle experiencing a majority of the load across all flexion angles, with the PL seeing greater loads at lower flexion angles, more specifically 0–30° [62].

Knowledge of the biomechanical relationship of the two bundles is important when it comes to anatomic ACL reconstruction. If the AM and PL bundles are anatomically restored, the graft should experience the same forces as the native ACL. If the graft is placed in a nonanatomic position, it will see lower than normal forces [27, 65].

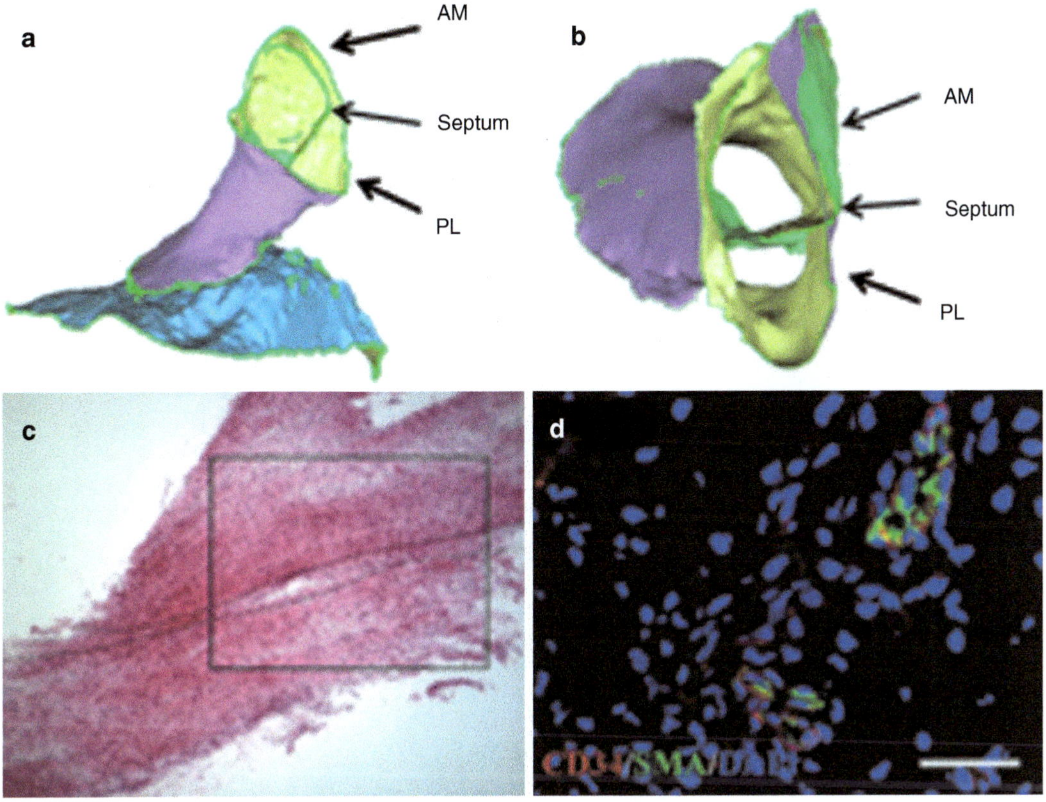

Fig. 31.1 ACL bundles and septum. (**a**, **b**) 3D laser scan of the ACL showing anteromedial (*AM*) and posterolateral (*PL*) bundle morphology and the septum between them (Reprinted with permission from Fu et al. [15]). (**c**) Histologic cut of fetal ACL, which shows the septum dividing the AM and PL bundles (*dotted lines*). (**d**) In the septum region, CD34 (+) and CD146 (+) (*both red*) were located surrounding smooth muscle actin (*SMA*) (*green*) arterioles. Scale bar: 50 mm (Reprinted with permission from Matsumoto et al. [40])

> **Fact Box 2: Anatomy and Biomechanics of the ACL**
> 1. The ACL is composed of AM and PL bundles.
> 2. The primary function of the AM bundle is to restrain AP translation. The primary function of the PL bundle is to resist rotatory translation.
> 3. The majority of load experienced by the AM bundle occurs during knee flexion, while the PL bundle experiences the most loading during extension.

While this may decrease risk of graft failure, these forces can be distributed throughout the joint, increasing the contact pressures on the cartilage, potentially predisposing the joint to abnormal kinematics and the development of early OA [10].

31.3 Anatomic ACL Reconstruction

Anatomy is the basis of orthopedic surgery and the approach to ACL reconstruction is governed by this principle as well. The concept of anatomic ACL reconstruction is based on four fundamental principles: (1) restoration of the two functional bundles of the ACL, (2) restoration of the native

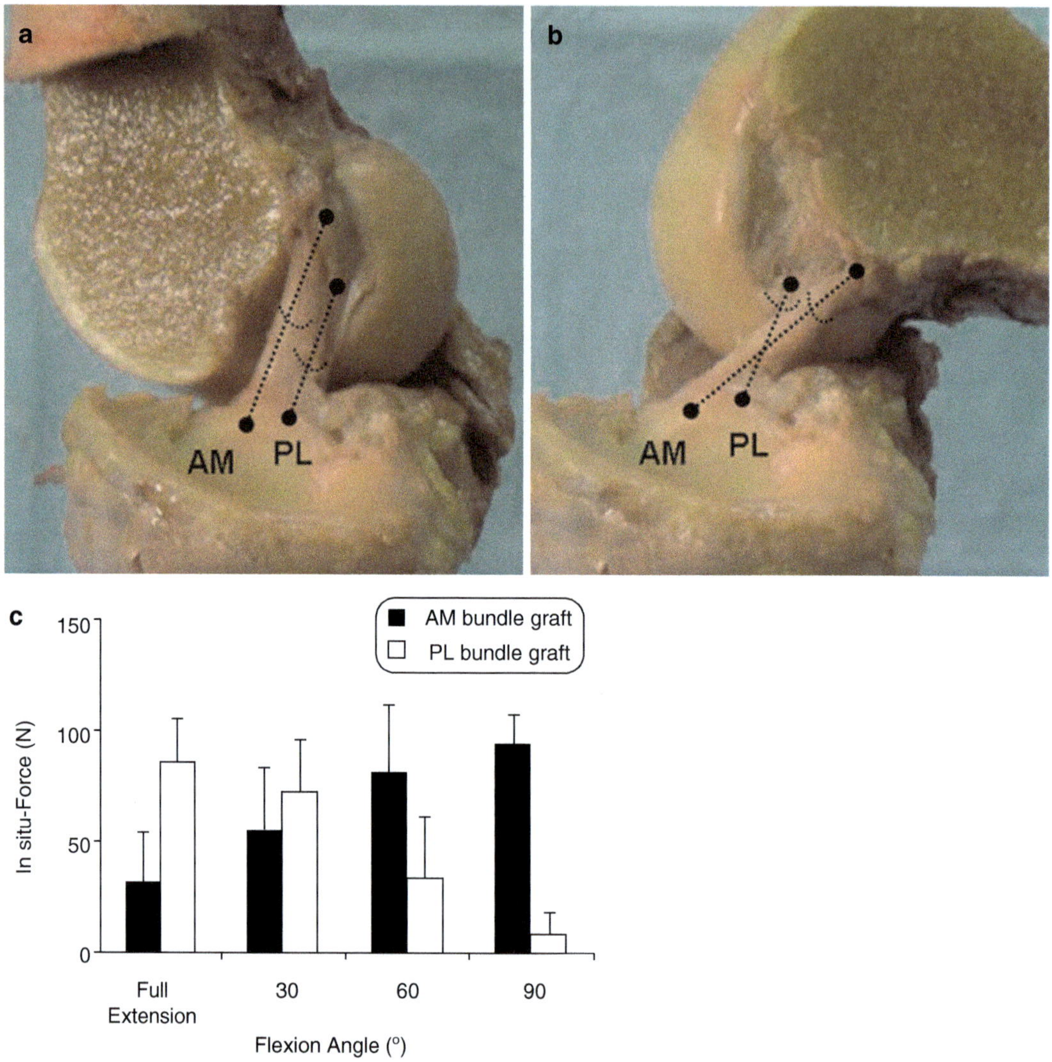

Fig. 31.2 Synergistic function of two bundles. (**a**) Knee in extension shows both femoral insertions oriented vertically and the bundles are parallel. (**b**) Knee in 90° of flexion shows both femoral insertions oriented horizontally and the bundles are crossed (Reprinted with permission from Chhabra et al. [9]). (**c**) In situ force in anteromedial (*AM*) and posterolateral (*PL*) bundle grafts for the anatomic ACL reconstruction in response to a 134 N anterior tibial load. The magnitude of the in situ force in the AM bundle increases with higher flexion angles, whereas the in situ force in the PL bundle increases with higher extension angles (Reprinted with permission from Yagi et al. [65])

insertion sites of the ACL by placing the tunnels in their true anatomic positions, (3) correct tensioning of each bundle, and (4) individualization of surgery for each patient, where tunnel diameter and graft size are dictated by native insertion sites.

Anatomic ACL reconstruction aims to restore the ACL to its native dimensions, collagen orientation, and insertion sites. This concept can be applied to SB and DB reconstruction, augmentation, and revision surgery [15] (Fig. 31.3).

Fact Box 3: Anatomic ACL Reconstruction

1. Anatomic ACL reconstruction is used to restore the ACL to its native insertion sites, collagen fibers, and orientation.
2. Anatomic reconstruction can be performed in both SB and DB ACL reconstruction techniques.

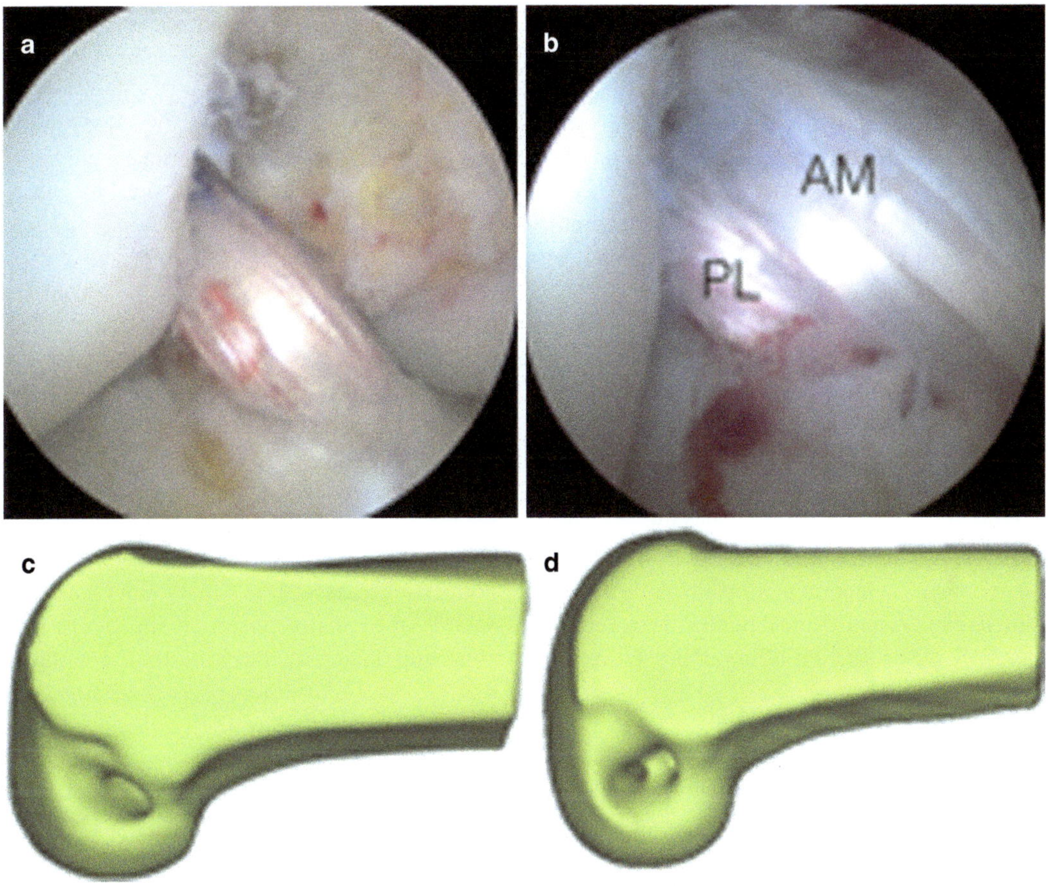

Fig. 31.3 Anatomic ACL reconstruction concept aims for the restoration of the ACL to its native dimensions, collagen orientation, and insertion sites. This concept can be applied to different surgical techniques including SB reconstruction and DB reconstruction. (**a**, **b**) Intraoperative pictures of SB and DB reconstruction, respectively. (**c**, **d**) Postoperative 3D CT of SB and DB reconstruction, respectively (*AM* anteromedial bundle, *PL* posterolateral bundle)

31.4 Biomechanics

Biomechanical studies have shown that DB reconstruction restores knee kinematics better than transtibial SB reconstruction, leading to less rotational laxity, increased tibiofemoral contact area, and lower contact pressures [44, 61, 65, 66, 71]. Woo et al. [61] reported in a controlled laboratory study that transtibial SB reconstruction was inadequate for resisting rotational loads. Their findings suggested that improved reconstruction techniques that could accurately restore the anatomy of the ACL were needed. In a biomechanical study, Yagi et al. [65] reported that the normalized in situ force with a combined rotatory load at 30° of flexion was significantly higher with DB reconstruction (91 % ± 35 % of intact knee) than SB reconstruction (66 % ± 40 %) ($p < 0.05$). This means that DB reconstruction restored the in situ forces of the knee closer to the intact knee compared with SB reconstruction, when a combined rotatory load was applied.

In another cadaveric study, Yamamoto et al. [66] compared femoral tunnel placement close to the PL insertion versus anatomic reconstruction and found that lateral tunnel placement could restore rotatory and anterior knee laxity similar to anatomic reconstruction, but only when the knee was near extension. Considering that most of normal knee activities are in flexion, this study also suggests that to reproduce the function of the ACL, both bundles should be reconstructed. In the same line, in an in vivo controlled laboratory study, Kopf et al. [32] evaluated kinematic tests with a computer navigation system. The authors showed that isolated PL bundle reconstruction improves laxity in an ACL-deficient knee and that the addition of AM bundle reconstruction further improves laxity. Tests that were evaluated were the Lachman, anterior drawer, and varus-valgus stress at 30° of knee flexion. Musahl et al. [46] performed a biomechanical study with a surgical navigation system and mechanized pivot-shift test, comparing transtibial SB, AM single-bundle, and DB techniques. They reported that DB reconstruction offers improved restoration of anterior and rotational laxity compared to SB reconstructions.

The above-noted anatomic and biomechanical studies have facilitated an interest in clinical studies of both DB reconstruction and anatomic ACL reconstruction techniques.

Fact Box 4: Biomechanics

1. DB reconstruction restores knee kinematics better than SB reconstruction.
2. DB reconstruction restores the in situ forces of the knee better than SB reconstruction.

31.5 Influence of Double-Bundle ACL Reconstruction on Clinical Outcomes

Several prospective level I or II clinical studies have reported superior results of anatomic DB reconstruction compared with SB reconstruction [2, 3, 6, 22, 23, 25, 26, 28, 29, 33, 41, 45, 53, 64, 65, 68, 69]. On the other hand, other studies have shown no difference between DB and SB reconstruction in terms of improvement in laxity or function [1, 48, 50, 55]. However, for several of the abovementioned studies, it remains unclear whether both the DB and SB reconstructions performed in these studies were anatomic or not.

In many studies that compare SB reconstruction with anatomic DB reconstruction, the femoral tunnels are drilled utilizing a transtibial method, in both SB reconstructions and the AM bundle in DB reconstructions [2, 3, 6, 23, 25, 26, 28, 29, 41, 45, 53, 59, 60, 64, 68, 69]. Discrepancy between tunnel position and the native ACL insertion site is common when the femoral tunnel is drilled in a transtibial fashion. Some studies have shown that tunnel placement outside of the native insertion site can result in abnormal knee kinematics, limited range of motion, supraphysiologic graft tension, and, ultimately, graft failure [5, 17, 18, 31, 52, 54, 59, 70].

Park et al. [48] evaluated DB reconstruction versus transtibial SB reconstruction and revealed no differences in laxity or patient satisfaction. However, they used the clockface method to drill the femoral tunnels for DB reconstruction, which can often lead to malalignment and nonanatomic positioning because of the three-dimensional nature of the intercondylar notch [19, 31, 52].

In a level 1 study comparing 40 patients with SB and DB reconstructions, Sastre et al. [50] placed the femoral tunnels more horizontally in both groups and found no significant differences between SB and DB techniques. The authors concluded that placing the femoral tunnel in a more horizontal position in the SB group produced similar rotatory and AP laxity to that obtained with the DB technique in patients with low functional demands. However, they drilled the femoral AM tunnel of DB reconstruction using a transtibial technique and they included a limited number of patients.

Yasuda et al. [67] performed a prospective, comparative, study on anatomic DB, nonanatomic

DB, and transtibial SB in 72 patients total. Their results showed that anatomic DB was significantly better than SB based on AP and rotation laxity restoration, using KT-2000 and pivot-shift test, respectively ($p<0.05$). There were no significant differences between the anatomic and nonanatomic DB groups. They also found no significant differences between the 3 groups in terms of International Knee Documentation Committee (IKDC) evaluation, range of motion, and muscle torque. This emphasizes that in terms of AP and rotational laxity, DB reconstruction (anatomic or nonanatomic) is superior to SB reconstruction.

In a randomized clinical trial, Hussein et al. [21] compared conventional nonanatomic SB, anatomic SB, and anatomic DB reconstruction. AP laxity was measured with KT-1000 and rotatory laxity was tested with pivot shift. Anatomic SB resulted in superior restoration of AP and rotational laxity compared to transtibial SB reconstruction. Average side-to-side difference for anterior tibial translation was 1.6 mm versus 2.0 mm, respectively ($p=0.002$), and negative pivot shift was 66.7 % versus 41.7 % ($p=0.003$). Additionally, anatomic DB reconstruction was superior to anatomic SB reconstruction. Average side-to-side difference for anterior tibial translation was 1.2 mm versus 1.6 mm, respectively ($p=0.002$), and negative pivot shift was 93.1 % versus 66.7 % ($p<0.001$). This high-quality study confirmed not only the improved results with DB reconstruction but also the relevance of anatomic reconstruction in SB and DB techniques, with focus on restoring the native ACL insertions.

Another study from Hussein et al. [20] aimed to compare the results of SB and DB reconstruction, using an anatomic and individualized approach. According to this approach, depending on intraoperative measurements of the ACL insertion site, patients were selected for either anatomic SB or DB reconstruction. There were no significant differences between the groups in terms of Lysholm score (93.9 vs 93.5), subjective IKDC (93.3 vs 93.1), anterior tibial translation (1.5 vs 1.6 mm side-to-side difference), and pivot shift (92 % vs 90 % with negative pivot-shift examination). This study implies that anatomic DB reconstruction is not superior to anatomic SB reconstruction, when an individualized anatomic ACL reconstruction technique is used. This individualized approach not only considers the anatomic ACL reconstruction concept but also the restoration of the native insertion sites according to their sizes.

Fact Box 5: Influence of Double-Bundle Reconstruction on Clinical Outcomes

1. Several studies have shown no difference in outcomes between SB and DB reconstructions; however many of the techniques used were not standardized.
2. An anatomic or individualized approach to ACL reconstruction has been shown to have excellent outcomes, whether performed using an SB or DB technique.

31.6 Meta-analysis of Double-Bundle ACL Reconstruction

On the basis of the evolution of clinical studies comparing SB and DB reconstruction, multiple authors have conducted systematic reviews and meta-analyses comparing both types of reconstruction [12, 30, 35, 36, 38, 41, 57, 58, 63, 73]. Recently, the nine available overlapping meta-analyses of SB versus DB reconstruction were evaluated, in an attempt to reconcile conclusions from both techniques [38]. Three of the meta-analyses included level I evidence only [30, 35, 41], and six included level I and level II evidence [12, 36, 57, 58, 63, 73].

	Li et al. [36]	Desai et al. [12]	Zhu et al. [73]	Kongtharvonskul et al. [30]	Li et al. [35]	Xu et al. [63]	Tiamklang et al. [57]	Van Eck et al. [58]	Meredick et al. [41]
Clinical indices: Lysholm Subjective IKDC Tegner	+	–	±	±	±	+	+	±	–
Knee stability: Pivot shift Instrumented laxity	+	+	+	+	+	+	+	+	+
Knee stability: Navigated AP laxity IKDC stability Lachman Anterior drawer	±	±	±	±	±	±	+	±	–
Range of motion and strength	–	±	–	–	+	–	±	±	–
Subjective outcomes: Return to pre-injury activity level	–	–	–	–	–	–	+	–	–
Complications	±	±	±	±	±	–	+	±	–

Using quality assessment tools for meta-analyses [24, 43, 47, 49], the current highest level of evidence suggests that DB reconstruction provides improved postoperative knee laxity compared with SB reconstruction. This was evaluated using mainly KT arthrometer, Lachman, and anterior drawer tests for AP translation and the pivot-shift test for rotational laxity.

Nevertheless this difference between DB and SB clinical results should be interpreted cautiously. Although DB showed statistically significant better results using a KT arthrometer, this difference may have questionable clinical significance because its magnitude ranged from 0.56 to 0.74 mm. Also, the differences for the clinical tests (Lachman, anterior drawer, and pivot shift) were heterogeneous between studies. This can be explained by the subjectivity in grading, interexaminer variability, and dependence on patient cooperation for these tests.

The other clinical outcomes and risk of graft failure were not found to be significantly different between DB and SB in this systematic review of overlapping meta-analysis.

Of the nine studies included in this review, only three had the highest level of evidence, without major flaws with their methodology [36, 57, 58].

The first of these studies was a meta-analysis from Tiamklang et al. [57] which reported no significant differences between DB and SB reconstructions in subjective IKDC score, Tegner activity score, Lysholm score, adverse effects, and complications, including graft failure (1.8 % vs 2.4 %). However, they found significant differences favoring DB reconstruction in terms of return to pre-injury level of activity (91 % vs 82 %), long-term follow-up IKDC (normal 94 % vs 90 %), knee laxity measured with KT-1000 arthrometry (mean difference –0.74 mm), and rotational knee laxity tested by the pivot-shift test (normal or nearly normal: 98 % vs 92 %). There were also significant differences in favor of DB reconstruction for secondary meniscal injury (3.8 % vs 6.7 %).

In a meta-analysis, Van Eck et al. [58] showed DB reconstruction to be superior than SB reconstruction for anterior and rotational laxity (KT arthrometer testing, Lachman testing, IKDC grading, and pivot-shift testing). However there

Study	Number of studies/ patients analyzed	Outcomes in favor of DB ACL-R	Outcomes in favor of SB ACL-R	Outcomes without differences between DB and SB ACL-R
Tiamklang et al. [57]	17/1433	Return to play IKDC grade KT-1000 Pivot shift	None	IKDC score Tegner score Lysholm score Complications
Van Eck et al. [58]	12/1127	KT-1000 Pivot shift Lachman IKDC grade	None	Flexion Extension Lysholm Complications
Li et al [36]	19/1686	Pivot shift IKDC grade KT-1000	None	IKDC score KT-1000 Lysholm Tegner Complications

were no differences in range of motion, Lysholm scores, or complications when compared with SB reconstruction. Considering knee rotational laxity, the pivot-shift test results favored DB reconstruction with a relative risk (RR) of 0.31 (95 % CI 0.16–0.61) for the randomized studies. This indicates that in comparison with DB ACL reconstruction, DB reconstruction reduces the risk of a positive pivot-shift test by 69 %.

Li et al. [36] showed in a meta-analysis that DB reconstruction patients had improved pivot-shift test, KT grading, and IKDC grading, but showed no differences in terms of functional outcomes when compared with SB reconstruction (IKDC score, KT arthrometer testing, Lysholm score, Tegner score, and complication rate). The analysis across all studies showed a significant difference in pivot shift, with an odds ratio (OR) of 0.27 (95 % CI 0.20–0.36) favoring DB reconstruction, indicating that this technique reduces the risk of a positive pivot-shift test by 73 % [72].

Recently, clinical practice guidelines for management of ACL injuries were published according to the results of a systematic review of the current scientific and clinical information [51]. This review confirmed the similarity between the clinical outcomes of SB and DB techniques. Considering "high strength" studies with consistent findings, the authors state that in patients undergoing ACL reconstruction, the surgeon should use either the SB or DB technique, because the measured outcomes are similar [51].

One possible limitation of the studies that compare SB and DB reconstruction is the lack of statistical power. Small clinical effects may not be statistically significant in studies with small sample sizes. Also, much of the available studies comparing SB and DB reconstruction consist of relatively short-term follow-up, such that a significant difference that only manifests itself in long-term follow-up would be missed in this analysis. Another limitation is related to the heterogeneity among the included studies, specifically in terms of combined analysis of anatomic and nonanatomic ACL reconstruction techniques, which may yield different outcomes in terms of restoration of rotational laxity [28].

Fact Box 6: Meta-analysis of Double-Bundle ACL Reconstructions

1. There have been 3 high-quality meta-analyses comparing SB and DB ACL reconstruction, with all of them showing improved rotational laxity compared to SB reconstruction.
2. Improved clinical outcomes have not been shown in these studies; however rates of secondary meniscal injury and return to play were improved in 1/3 of the analyses.
3. Most updated clinical guidelines strongly recommend that for ACL reconstruction, the SB or DB technique can be used, considering the similarity of measured clinical outcomes.

Conclusions

Anatomic ACL reconstruction aims to restore the ACL to its native dimensions, collagen orientation, and insertion sites, focusing on providing the patient with the best potential for a successful outcome.

The best evidence from the highest quality meta-analyses suggests that anatomic DB reconstruction yields superior restoration of knee laxity (based on KT arthrometry and pivot-shift testing) when compared with transtibial SB reconstruction.

The modest improvement in some clinical tests like KT arthrometry afforded by DB reconstruction needs to be further examined in both laboratory and long-term clinical cohort studies.

These future studies should determine the best treatment for ACL reconstruction, in which the ultimate goal is the improvement of patients' clinical outcomes and prevention of secondary degenerative changes of the knee.

References

1. Adachi N, Ochi M, Uchio Y, Iwasa J, Kuriwaka M, Ito Y (2004) Reconstruction of the anterior cruciate ligament. Single- versus double-bundle multistranded hamstring tendons. J Bone Joint Surg Br 86:515–520
2. Aglietti P, Giron F, Cuomo P, Losco M, Mondanelli N (2007) Single-and double-incision double-bundle ACL reconstruction. Clin Orthop Relat Res 454:108–113
3. Aglietti P, Giron F, Losco M, Cuomo P, Ciardullo A, Mondanelli N (2010) Comparison between single-and double-bundle anterior cruciate ligament reconstruction: a prospective, randomized, single-blinded clinical trial. Am J Sports Med 38:25–34
4. Ajuied A, Wong F, Smith C, Norris M, Earnshaw P, Back D, Davies A (2014) Anterior cruciate ligament injury and radiologic progression of knee osteoarthritis: a systematic review and meta-analysis. Am J Sports Med 42:2242–2252
5. Allen CR, Giffin JR, Harner CD (2003) Revision anterior cruciate ligament reconstruction. Orthop Clin North Am 34:79–98
6. Bach BR, Levy ME, Bojchuk J, Tradonsky S, Bush-Joseph CA, Khan NH (1998) Single-incision endoscopic anterior cruciate ligament reconstruction using patellar tendon autograft. Minimum two-year follow-up evaluation. Am J Sports Med 26:30–40
7. Beynnon BD, Johnson RJ, Abate JA, Fleming BC, Nichols CE (2005) Treatment of anterior cruciate ligament injuries, part 2. Am J Sports Med 33:1751–1767
8. Beynnon BD, Johnson RJ, Abate JA, Fleming BC, Nichols CE (2005) Treatment of anterior cruciate ligament injuries, part I. Am J Sports Med 33:1579–1602
9. Chhabra A, Starman JS, Ferretti M, Vidal AF, Zantop T, Fu FH (2006) Anatomic, radiographic, biomechanical, and kinematic evaluation of the anterior cruciate ligament and its two functional bundles. J Bone Joint Surg 88(Suppl 4):2–10
10. Chu CR, Williams AA, West RV, Qian Y, Fu FH, Do BH, Bruno S (2014) Quantitative magnetic resonance imaging UTE-T2* mapping of cartilage and meniscus healing after anatomic anterior cruciate ligament reconstruction. Am J Sports Med 42:1847–1856
11. Debandi A, Maeyama A, Hoshino Y, Asai S, Goto B, Smolinski P, Fu FH (2013) The effect of tunnel placement on rotational stability after ACL reconstruction: evaluation with use of triaxial accelerometry in a porcine model. Knee Surg Sports Traumatol Arthrosc 21:589–595
12. Desai N, Bjornsson H, Musahl V, Bhandari M, Petzold M, Fu FH, Samuelsson K (2014) Anatomic single- versus double-bundle ACL reconstruction: a meta-analysis. Knee Surg Sports Traumatol Arthrosc 22(5):1009–1023. doi:10.1007/s00167-013-2811-6
13. Duthon VB, Barea C, Abrassart S, Fasel JH, Fritschy D, Ménétrey J (2006) Anatomy of the anterior cruciate ligament. Knee Surg Sports Traumatol Arthrosc 14:204–213
14. Fu FH, van Eck CF, Tashman S, Irrgang JJ, Moreland MS (2014) Anatomic anterior cruciate ligament reconstruction: a changing paradigm. Knee Surg Sports Traumatol Arthrosc. doi:10.1007/s00167-014-3209-9
15. Fu FH, van Eck CF, Tashman S, Irrgang JJ, Moreland MS (2015) Anatomic anterior cruciate ligament reconstruction: a changing paradigm. Knee Surg Sports Traumatol Arthrosc 23:640–648
16. Gianotti SM, Marshall SW, Hume PA, Bunt L (2009) Incidence of anterior cruciate ligament injury and other knee ligament injuries: a national population-based study. J Sci Med Sport 12(6):622–627
17. Harner CD, Giffin JR, Dunteman RC, Annunziata CC, Friedman MJ (2001) Evaluation and treatment of recurrent instability after anterior cruciate ligament reconstruction. Instr Course Lect 50:463–474
18. Heming JF, Rand J, Steiner ME (2007) Anatomical limitations of transtibial drilling in anterior cruciate ligament reconstruction. Am J Sports Med 35(10):1708–1715
19. Hensler D, Illingworth KD, Fu FH (2010) Principle considerations in anatomic ACL reconstruction. Arthroscopy 26:1414–1415
20. Hussein M, van Eck CF, Cretnik A, Dinevski D, Fu FH (2012) Individualized anterior cruciate ligament surgery: a prospective study comparing anatomic single- and double-bundle reconstruction. Am J Sports Med 40:1781–1788
21. Hussein M, van Eck CF, Cretnik A, Dinevski D, Fu FH (2012) Prospective randomized clinical evaluation

of conventional single-bundle, anatomic single-bundle, and anatomic double-bundle anterior cruciate ligament reconstruction: 281 cases with 3- to 5-year follow-up. Am J Sports Med 40:512–520
22. Ibrahim SAR, Hamido F, Al Misfer AK, Mahgoob A, Ghafar SA, Alhran H (2009) Anterior cruciate ligament reconstruction using autologous hamstring double bundle graft compared with single bundle procedures. J Bone Joint Surg Br 91:1310–1315
23. Jacobsen K (1977) Osteoarthrosis following insufficiency of the cruciate ligaments in man. A clinical study. Acta Orthop Scand 48:520–526
24. Jadad AR, Cook DJ, Browman GP (1997) A guide to interpreting discordant systematic reviews. Can Med Assoc J 156:1411–1416
25. Järvelä T (2007) Double-bundle versus single-bundle anterior cruciate ligament reconstruction: a prospective, randomize clinical study. Knee Surg Sports Traumatol Arthrosc 15:500–507, Springer-Verlag
26. Järvelä T, Moisala A-S, Sihvonen R, Järvelä S, Kannus P, Järvinen M (2008) Double-bundle anterior cruciate ligament reconstruction using hamstring autografts and bioabsorbable interference screw fixation: prospective, randomized, clinical study with 2-year results. Am J Sports Med 36:290–297
27. Kato Y, Maeyama A, Lertwanich P, Wang JH, Ingham SJM, Kramer S, Martins CQA, Smolinski P, Fu FH (2013) Biomechanical comparison of different graft positions for single-bundle anterior cruciate ligament reconstruction. Knee Surg Sports Traumatol Arthrosc 21:816–823
28. Kondo E, Merican AM, Yasuda K, Amis AA (2011) Biomechanical comparison of anatomic double-bundle, anatomic single-bundle, and nonanatomic single-bundle anterior cruciate ligament reconstructions. Am J Sports Med 39:279–288
29. Kondo E, Yasuda K, Azuma H, Tanabe Y, Yagi T (2008) Prospective clinical comparisons of anatomic double-bundle versus single-bundle anterior cruciate ligament reconstruction procedures in 328 consecutive patients. Am J Sports Med 36:1675–1687
30. Kongtharvonskul J, Attia J, Thamakaison S, Kijkunasathian C, Woratanarat P, Thakkinstian A (2013) Clinical outcomes of double- vs single-bundle anterior cruciate ligament reconstruction: a systematic review of randomized control trials. Scand J Med Sci Sports 23:1–14
31. Kopf S, Forsythe B, Wong AK, Tashman S, Anderst W, Irrgang JJ, Fu FH (2010) Nonanatomic tunnel position in traditional transtibial single-bundle anterior cruciate ligament reconstruction evaluated by three-dimensional computed tomography. J Bone Joint Surg Am 92:1427–1431
32. Kopf S, Musahl V, Bignozzi S, Irrgang JJ, Zaffagnini S, Fu FH (2014) In vivo kinematic evaluation of anatomic double-bundle anterior cruciate ligament reconstruction. Am J Sports Med 42:2172–2177
33. Kopf S, Pombo MW, Szczodry M, Irrgang JJ, Fu FH (2011) Size variability of the human anterior cruciate ligament insertion sites. Am J Sports Med 39:108–113
34. Li RT, Lorenz S, Xu Y, Harner CD, Fu FH, Irrgang JJ (2011) Predictors of radiographic knee osteoarthritis after anterior cruciate ligament reconstruction. Am J Sports Med 39:2595–2603. American Orthopaedic Society for Sports Medicine
35. Li X, Xu C-p, J-q S, Jiang N, Yu B (2013) Single-bundle versus double-bundle anterior cruciate ligament reconstruction: an up-to-date meta-analysis. Int Orthop 37:213–226
36. Li YL, Ning GZ, Wu Q, Wu QL, Li Y, Hao Y, Feng SQ (2014) Single-bundle or double-bundle for anterior cruciate ligament reconstruction: a meta-analysis. Knee 21:28–37
37. Lohmander LS, Ostenberg A, Englund M, Roos H (2004) High prevalence of knee osteoarthritis, pain, and functional limitations in female soccer players twelve years after anterior cruciate ligament injury. Arthritis Rheum 50:3145–3152. Wiley Subscription Services, Inc., A Wiley Company
38. Mascarenhas R, Cvetanovich GL, Sayegh ET, Verma NN, Cole BJ, Bush-Joseph C, Bach BR Jr (2015) Does double-bundle anterior cruciate ligament reconstruction improve postoperative knee stability compared with single-bundle techniques? A systematic review of overlapping meta-analyses. Arthroscopy 31:1185–1196
39. Mascarenhas R, Tranovich M, Karpie JC, Irrgang JJ, Fu FH, Harner CD (2010) Patellar tendon anterior cruciate ligament reconstruction in the high-demand patient: evaluation of autograft versus allograft reconstruction. Arthroscopy 26:S58–S66
40. Matsumoto T, Ingham SM, Mifune Y, Osawa A, Logar A, Usas A, Kuroda R, Kurosaka M, Fu FH, Huard J (2012) Isolation and characterization of human anterior cruciate ligament-derived vascular stem cells. Stem Cells Dev 21:859–872
41. Meredick RB, Vance KJ, Appleby D, Lubowitz JH (2008) Outcome of single-bundle versus double-bundle reconstruction of the anterior cruciate ligament: a meta-analysis. Am J Sports Med 36:1414–21
42. Meuffels DE, Favejee MM, Vissers MM, Heijboer MP, Reijman M, Verhaar JAN (2009) Ten year follow-up study comparing conservative versus operative treatment of anterior cruciate ligament ruptures. A matched-pair analysis of high level athletes. Br J Sports Med 43:347–351
43. Moher D, Cook DJ, Eastwood S, Olkin I, Rennie D, Stroup DF (1999) Improving the quality of reports of meta-analyses of randomised controlled trials: the QUOROM statement. Quality of reporting of meta-analyses. Lancet 354:1896–1900
44. Morimoto Y, Ferretti M, Ekdahl M, Smolinski P, Fu FH (2009) Tibiofemoral joint contact area and pressure after single- and double-bundle anterior cruciate ligament reconstruction. Arthroscopy 25:62–69
45. Muneta T, Koga H, Mochizuki T, Ju Y-J, Hara K, Nimura A, Yagishita K, Sekiya I (2007) A prospective randomized study of 4-strand semitendinosus tendon anterior cruciate ligament reconstruction comparing single-bundle and double-bundle techniques. Arthroscopy 23:618–628

46. Musahl V, Voos JE, O'Loughlin PF, Choi D, Stueber V, Kendoff D, Pearle AD (2010) Comparing stability of different single- and double-bundle anterior cruciate ligament reconstruction techniques: a cadaveric study using navigation. Arthroscopy 26:S41–8
47. Oxman AD, Guyatt GH (1991) Validation of an index of the quality of review articles. J Clin Epidemiol 44:1271–1278
48. Park S-J, Jung YB, Jung H-J, Jung H-J, Shin HK, Kim E, Song K-S, Kim G-S, Cheon H-Y, Kim S (2010) Outcome of arthroscopic single-bundle versus double-bundle reconstruction of the anterior cruciate ligament: a preliminary 2-year prospective study. Arthroscopy 26:630–636
49. Poolman RW, Abouali JAK, Conter HJ, Bhandari M (2007) Overlapping systematic reviews of anterior cruciate ligament reconstruction comparing hamstring autograft with bone-patellar tendon-bone autograft: why are they different? J Bone Joint Surg 89:1542–1552
50. Sastre S, Popescu D, Núñez M, Pomes J, Tomas X, Peidro L (2010) Double-bundle versus single-bundle ACL reconstruction using the horizontal femoral position: a prospective, randomized study. Knee Surg Sports Traumatol Arthrosc 18:32–36
51. Shea KG, Carey JL, Richmond J, Sandmeier R, Pitts RT, Polousky JD, Chu C, Shultz SJ, Ellen M, Smith A, LaBella CR, Anderson AF, Musahl V, Meyer GD, Jevsevar D, Bozic KJ, Shaffer W, Cummins D, Murray JN, Patel N, Shores P, Woznica A, Martinez Y, Gross L, Sevarino K, American Academy of Orthopaedic Surgeons (2015) The American Academy of Orthopaedic Surgeons evidence-based guideline on management of anterior cruciate ligament injuries. J Bone Joint Surg Am 97(8):672–674
52. Shen W, Forsythe B, Ingham SM, Honkamp NJ, Fu FH (2008) Application of the anatomic double-bundle reconstruction concept to revision and augmentation anterior cruciate ligament surgeries. J Bone Joint Surg Am 90(Suppl 4):20–34
53. Siebold R, Dehler C, Ellert T (2008) Prospective randomized comparison of double-bundle versus single-bundle anterior cruciate ligament reconstruction. Arthroscopy 24:137–145
54. Steiner ME, Battaglia TC, Heming JF, Rand JD, Festa A, Baria M (2009) Independent drilling outperforms conventional transtibial drilling in anterior cruciate ligament reconstruction. Am J Sports Med 37:1912–1919. American Orthopaedic Society for Sports Medicine
55. Streich NA, Friedrich K, Gotterbarm T, Schmitt H (2008) Reconstruction of the ACL with a semitendinosus tendon graft: a prospective randomized single blinded comparison of double-bundle versus single-bundle technique in male athletes. Knee Surg Sports Traumatol Arthrosc 16:232–238
56. Tashman S, Collon D, Anderson K, Kolowich P, Anderst W (2004) Abnormal rotational knee motion during running after anterior cruciate ligament reconstruction. Am J Sports Med 32(4):975–983
57. Tiamklang T, Sumanont S, Foocharoen T, Laopaiboon M (2012) Double-bundle versus single-bundle reconstruction for anterior cruciate ligament rupture in adults. Cochrane Database Syst Rev. (11):CD008413. John Wiley & Sons, Ltd
58. van Eck CF, Kopf S, Irrgang JJ, Blankevoort L, Bhandari M, Fu FH, Poolman RW (2012) Single-bundle versus double-bundle reconstruction for anterior cruciate ligament rupture: a meta-analysis – does anatomy matter? Arthroscopy 28:405–424
59. van Eck CF, Lesniak BP, Schreiber VM, Fu FH (2010) Anatomic single- and double-bundle anterior cruciate ligament reconstruction flowchart. Arthroscopy 26(2):258–268. doi:10.1016/j.arthro.2009.07.027
60. van Eck CF, Schreiber VM, Mejia HA, Samuelsson K, van Dijk CN, Karlsson J, Fu FH (2010) "Anatomic" anterior cruciate ligament reconstruction: a systematic review of surgical techniques and reporting of surgical data. Arthroscopy 26:S2–S12
61. Woo SLY, Kanamori A, Zeminski J, Yagi M, Papageorgiou C, Fu FH (2002) The effectiveness of reconstruction of the anterior cruciate ligament with hamstrings and patellar tendon. A cadaveric study comparing anterior tibial and rotational loads. J Bone Joint Surg 84-A:907–914
62. Wu J-L, Seon J-K, Gadikota HR, Hosseini A, Sutton KM, Gill TJ, Li G (2010) In situ forces in the anteromedial and posterolateral bundles of the anterior cruciate ligament under simulated functional loading conditions. Am J Sports Med 38:558–563. American Orthopaedic Society for Sports Medicine
63. Xu M, Gao S, Zeng C, Han R, Sun J, Li H, Xiong Y, Lei G (2013) Outcomes of anterior cruciate ligament reconstruction using single-bundle versus double-bundle technique: meta-analysis of 19 randomized controlled trials. Arthroscopy 29:357–365
64. Yagi M, Kuroda R, Nagamune K, Yoshiya S, Kurosaka M (2007) Double-bundle ACL reconstruction can improve rotational stability. Clin Orthop Relat Res 454:100–107
65. Yagi M, Wong EK, Kanamori A, Debski RE, Fu FH, Woo SLY (2002) Biomechanical analysis of an anatomic anterior cruciate ligament reconstruction. Am J Sports Med 30:660–666
66. Yamamoto Y, Hsu W-H, Woo SLY, Van Scyoc AH, Takakura Y, Debski RE (2004) Knee stability and graft function after anterior cruciate ligament reconstruction: a comparison of a lateral and an anatomical femoral tunnel placement. Am J Sports Med 32:1825–1832
67. Yasuda K, Kondo E, Ichiyama H, Tanabe Y, Tohyama H (2006) Clinical evaluation of anatomic double-bundle anterior cruciate ligament reconstruction procedure using hamstring tendon grafts: comparisons among 3 different procedures. Arthroscopy 22:240–251
68. Yasuda K, Tanabe Y, Kondo E, Kitamura N, Tohyama H (2010) Anatomic double-bundle anterior cruciate ligament reconstruction. Arthroscopy 26:S21–S34
69. Zaffagnini S, Bruni D, Marcheggiani Muccioli GM, Bonanzinga T, Lopomo N, Bignozzi S, Marcacci M

(2011) Single-bundle patellar tendon versus non-anatomical double-bundle hamstrings ACL reconstruction: a prospective randomized study at 8-year minimum follow-up. Knee Surg Sports Traumatol Arthrosc 19:390–397
70. Zantop T, Diermann N, Schumacher T, Schanz S, Fu FH, Petersen W (2008) Anatomical and nonanatomical double-bundle anterior cruciate ligament reconstruction: importance of femoral tunnel location on knee kinematics. Am J Sports Med 36:678–685. American Orthopaedic Society for Sports Medicine
71. Zelle BA, Vidal AF, Brucker PU, Fu FH (2007) Double-bundle reconstruction of the anterior cruciate ligament: anatomic and biomechanical rationale. J Am Acad Orthop Surg 15:87–96
72. Zhang J, Yu KF (1998) What's the relative risk? A method of correcting the odds ratio in cohort studies of common outcomes. JAMA 280:1690–1691
73. Zhu Y, Tang R-K, Zhao P, Zhu S-S, Li Y-G, Li J-B (2013) Double-bundle reconstruction results in superior clinical outcome than single-bundle reconstruction. Knee Surg Sports Traumatol Arthrosc 21:1085–1096

ACL and Posterolateral Instability

32

Guan-yang Song, Yue Li, and Hua Feng

Contents

32.1 Introduction

Management of the patient with combined ligamentous knee instability can be a challenging problem. Several studies have suggested that posterolateral knee instability accompanies anterior cruciate ligament (ACL) injury in 10–15 % of patients [28, 35, 43]. This combined injury pattern is an entity that the orthopedic surgeon must be able to recognize and appropriately address. In recent years, biomechanical studies have demonstrated that function of the posterolateral corner (PLC) interacts with the ACL. These in vitro studies have shown that deficiency of the posterolateral structures significantly increases the varus load on the ACL graft, thereby resulting in an increased risk for ACL graft failure [27]. Therefore, in the combined injury setting, the consequence of missing a PLC lesion may affect the outcome of ACL reconstruction. However, a consensus on the treatment of combined ACL and PLC injuries is still lacking. The purpose of this chapter is to discuss the current state of combined anterior and posterolateral instability.

G.-y. Song • Y. Li • H. Feng (✉)
Sports Medicine Service, Beijing Jishuitan Hospital, No. 31 Xinjiekou East Street, Xi Cheng District, Beijing 100035, China
e-mail: fenghua20080617@126.com

32.2 Pathophysiology/Biomechanics

The ACL is the primary restraint to anterior tibial translation and at 30° of knee flexion is responsible for 82–89 % of the restraint of an anterior applied load [6]. Others have shown that in the setting of ACL deficiency, there is a "coupled" increase in internal tibial rotation [1, 15]. This "coupled" function of the ligament as a secondary restraint against rotational loads occurs as a

V. Musahl et al. (eds.), *Rotatory Knee Instability*, DOI 10.1007/978-3-319-32070-0_32

result of the axis of rotation of the tibial plateau being close to the ACL [30].

The primary restraints to rotational control appear to be the more peripheral ligamentous structures of the knee, predominantly the PLC [48]. The most important structures, from a clinical perspective with regard to stability, are the lateral collateral ligament (LCL), the popliteus tendon (Pop-T), and the popliteofibular ligament (PFL) [4, 22] (Fact Box 1). Biomechanical studies, in which these structures were selectively sectioned, have demonstrated that they are important in resisting primary varus and external tibial rotation, as well as coupled external tibial rotation [36, 39].

Some authors examined the biomechanical properties of the knee ligamentous structures by focusing on combined ACL/PLC injuries. Wroble et al. [46] noted in a cadaveric study that there was an increase in primary anterior translation, primary varus, and external tibial rotation with sectioning of both the ACL and PLC. Moreover, LaPrade et al. [27] demonstrated the significance of the combined ACL/PLC injury pattern in a cadaveric study that examined the forces upon the ACL graft in the setting of PLC deficiency. In this study, they reconstructed the ACL of eight fresh-frozen cadaveric knees with central one-third bone-patellar tendon-bone autografts and then assessed the forces imparted upon the ACL graft prior to and after sequentially sectioning the PLC. They found that the graft force was significantly higher after LCL transection with varus loading at both 0° and 30° of knee flexion. This increase in graft force was continued with further sequential sectioning of the Pop-T and the PFL, leading the authors to conclude that untreated PLC injuries might contribute to clinical ACL graft failure by allowing higher forces to stress the graft [27].

Fact Box 1 Main stabilizers of posterolateral corner and their respective biomechanical functions

Main stabilizers	Biomechanical functions
Lateral collateral ligament	Primary stabilizer to lateral joint opening with the knee in extension
Popliteus tendon	Important role in restraining posterolateral motion of the knee
Popliteofibular ligament	Important in limiting excessive external rotation of the knee joints

32.3 Clinical Evaluation

A proper diagnosis is the foundation upon which an appropriate and successful treatment protocol is developed in the patient with combined ACL/PLC injuries. It is essential to perform a complete clinical workup consisting of obtaining a careful history, performing a thorough physical examination, and obtaining appropriate imaging studies. Moreover, there are certain findings that can be noted at the time of diagnostic arthroscopy (Fact Box 2).

32.3.1 History and Physical Examination

The clinical diagnosis of the combined ACL/PLC injury should begin with obtaining the history of injury. Several authors have reported that the application of a varus force in the hyperextended knee is the most common injury mechanism of the PLC [5, 19]. This knee position stresses not only the PLC but also the ACL. Ross et al. [38] reported that in their cohort of 13 patients who sustained combined ACL/PLC injuries, all occurred via a hyperextension and varus mechanism. Therefore, patient-directed questions should assess the mechanism of injury (with higher suspicion for a varus-hyperextension force), whether or not there were the sensation of a "pop," presence and timing of associated swelling, and any subsequent feelings of instability (typically at full extension).

The physical examination should begin with a thorough neurovascular exam. The incidence of peroneal nerve injury in the setting of a PLC injury has been reported to be 12–16% [5, 19]. Serial examinations should be done to ensure an occlusive vascular lesion is not developing on a delayed basis, and the utilization of the ankle-brachial index (ABI) may be useful in determining a need for further evaluation and intervention. An ABI

Fact Box 2 Key points of clinical evaluations

History	Imaging studies
Common injury mechanism: blow to anteromedial tibia causing excessive knee hyperextension, external tibial rotation, and lateral joint opening	AP, lateral, and full standing radiographs (with mechanical axis)
The ACL injury often occurs with PLC injuries	Telos stress radiographs (anterior displacement and lateral joint opening)
	MRI (especially for T2-weighted coronal oblique views)
Physical examinations	**Diagnostic arthroscopy**
Neurovascular exam (peroneal nerve and ABI)	Confirmation of cruciate status
Gait (severe hyperextension stance phase)	Lateral compartment "drive-through" test with varus stress at 30° of knee flexion (>1 cm is indicative of a grade III PLC injury)
Lachman and pivot-shift test	"Lateral gutter drive-through" test (effective in identifying the acute femoral "peel-off" lesions and chronic cases with posterolateral instability)
Varus stress test at both 0° and 30° of knee flexion	
Posterolateral drawer test	
External rotation recurvatum test	
Dial test in either supine or prone position	

Abbreviations: *ACL* anterior cruciate ligament, *PLC* posterolateral corner, *ABI* ankle-brachial index, *AP* anterior-posterior, *MRI* magnetic resonance imaging

<0.9 should alert the physician to an increased likelihood of significant arterial injury [32].

The physical examination should continue with an assessment of the patient's standing alignment. Any varus malalignment should be identified and further evaluated with a long-standing hip-to-ankle anterior-posterior (AP) radiograph. The surgeon should also evaluate the patient's gait pattern, specifically checking for a varus thrust. These findings are clinically important as they may be indicators of concomitant PLC injury, as described by Noyes et al. in the "double and triple varus" knees [34]. Since ligamentous reconstruction in the setting of baseline varus malalignment has an increased risk of PLC graft failure, some of these patients may benefit from a high tibial osteotomy in addition to ligament reconstruction [27, 34].

Important tests to assess the integrity of the ACL include the Lachman and pivot-shift tests. The PLC should be examined in every patient with a suspected ACL injury. Varus instability at 30° of knee flexion suggests an LCL injury (Fig. 32.1). Maneuvers such as the posterolateral drawer test and the external rotation recurvatum test can be useful in establishing a diagnosis of PLC injury [17]. The posterolateral drawer test is performed with the hip flexed 45° and the knee flexed 80° and at 10–15° of external tibial rotation [16]. In the setting of PLC deficiency, the lateral tibial plateau externally rotates around the PCL, and there is relative posterior translation with a

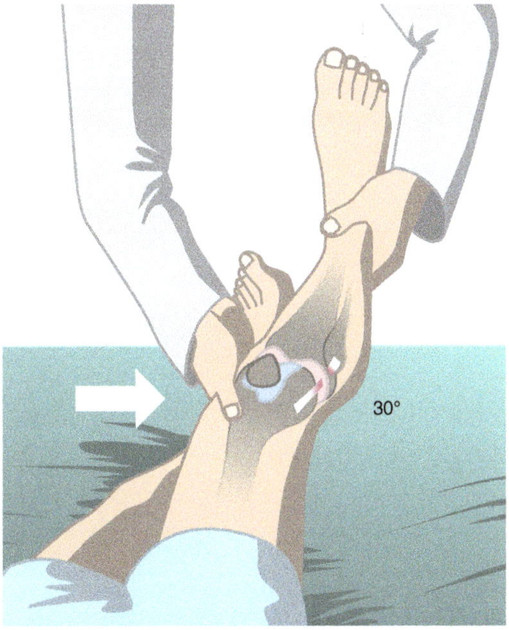

Fig. 32.1 Diagram of varus stress test performed at 30° of knee flexion

posteriorly directed force. The external rotation recurvatum test assesses the PLC in extension and is performed by grasping the great toes of both feet and elevating the legs off the bed [16]. Careful observation will reveal a relative tibia vara and hyperextension of the lateral knee in the patient with PLC injury. Finally, the dial test, which has been described in either the supine or prone position with the leg hanging off the bed, may also be beneficial in diagnosing a PLC injury [3]. If there is asymmetric tibial external rotation of 10° or more in 30° of knee flexion, this is suggestive of a PLC injury (Fig. 32.2; Fact Box 3).

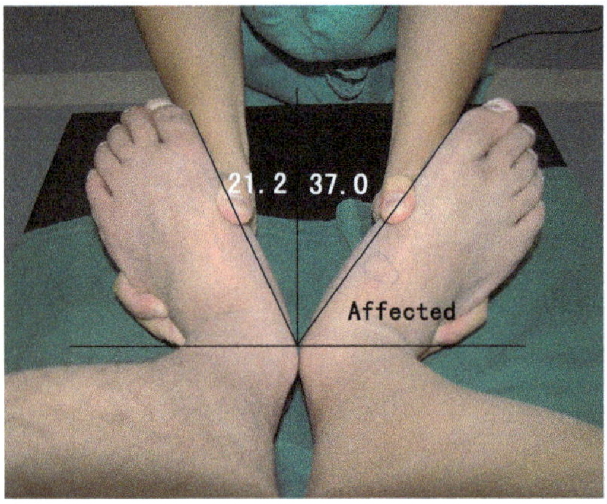

Fig. 32.2 Dial test performed at 30° of knee flexion showed that the external tibial rotation of the affected side was 15.8° greater than that on the contralateral normal side, indicating posterolateral instability

Fact Box 3 Key physical examinations to diagnose combined ACL/PLC injuries

For ACL injury	For PLC injury
Lachman test	Neurovascular exam (peroneal nerve and ABI)
Pivot-shift test	Gait (severe hyperextension stance phase)
Instrumental tests (KT-1000/KT-2000)	Varus stress test at both 0° and 30° of knee flexion
	Posterolateral drawer test
	External rotation recurvatum test
	Dial test in either supine or prone position

Abbreviations: *ACL* anterior cruciate ligament, *PLC* posterolateral corner, *ABI* ankle-brachial index

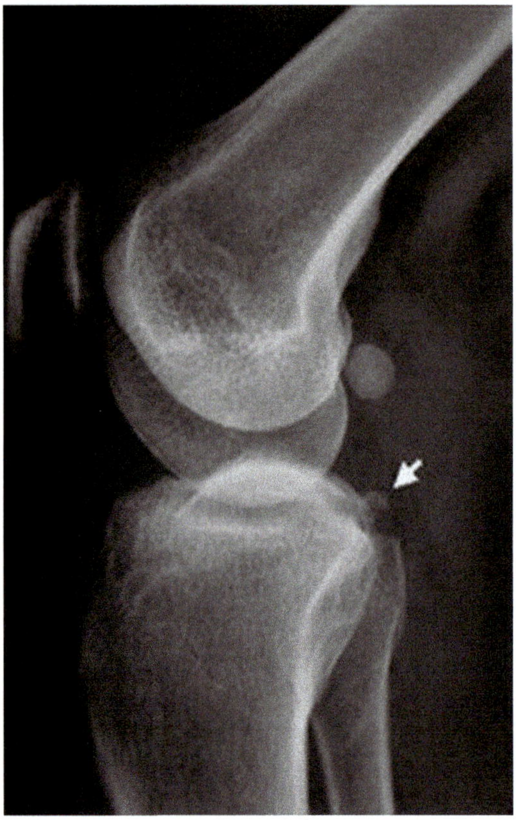

Fig. 32.3 A 45-year-old man sustained an anteromedial strike on the left tibia during a traffic accident. The radiograph showed an avulsed bone fragment (*white arrow*) off the fibular head

32.3.2 Imaging Studies

Plain radiographs of the knee should be obtained not only to assess for the presence of any periarticular or intra-articular fractures but also to evaluate for certain secondary findings that can be seen in the setting of a ligamentous knee injury. A small avulsion fragment off of the fibular head, termed the arcuate sign, may be noted and is indicative of injury to the PLC (Fig. 32.3) [20]. There may also be an avulsion fracture of the lateral tibial plateau, termed the Segond fracture, which is due to the pull of the lateral capsule and may be seen with an ACL injury [12].

Stress radiography is a widely used diagnostic tool that provides objective quantification of knee ligamentous instability. Its applications include diagnosing acute and chronic injuries, comparing instability preoperatively and postoperatively, and monitoring stability in nonoperatively treated patients [18]. Side-to-side differences in the amount of anterior displacement and varus gapping increase suspicion of a functional deficit in combined ACL/PLC injuries (Fig. 32.4). Compared with physical examination, stress radiographs provide a quantifiable and retrievable record of instability.

Magnetic resonance imaging (MRI) is useful to assess the extent of injury and facilitate preoperative planning. It has been reported to be 92.3 % sensitive in identifying acute tears of the ACL in the multi-ligamentous injured knee [13]. It is excellent in identifying injuries of the PLC as well, especially to the LCL or Pop-T; it is reported to be less accurate (53–68 %) in assessing the PFL [47]. LaPrade et al. [25] have recommended obtaining T2-weighted coronal oblique views to assist in identifying injuries to the PLC.

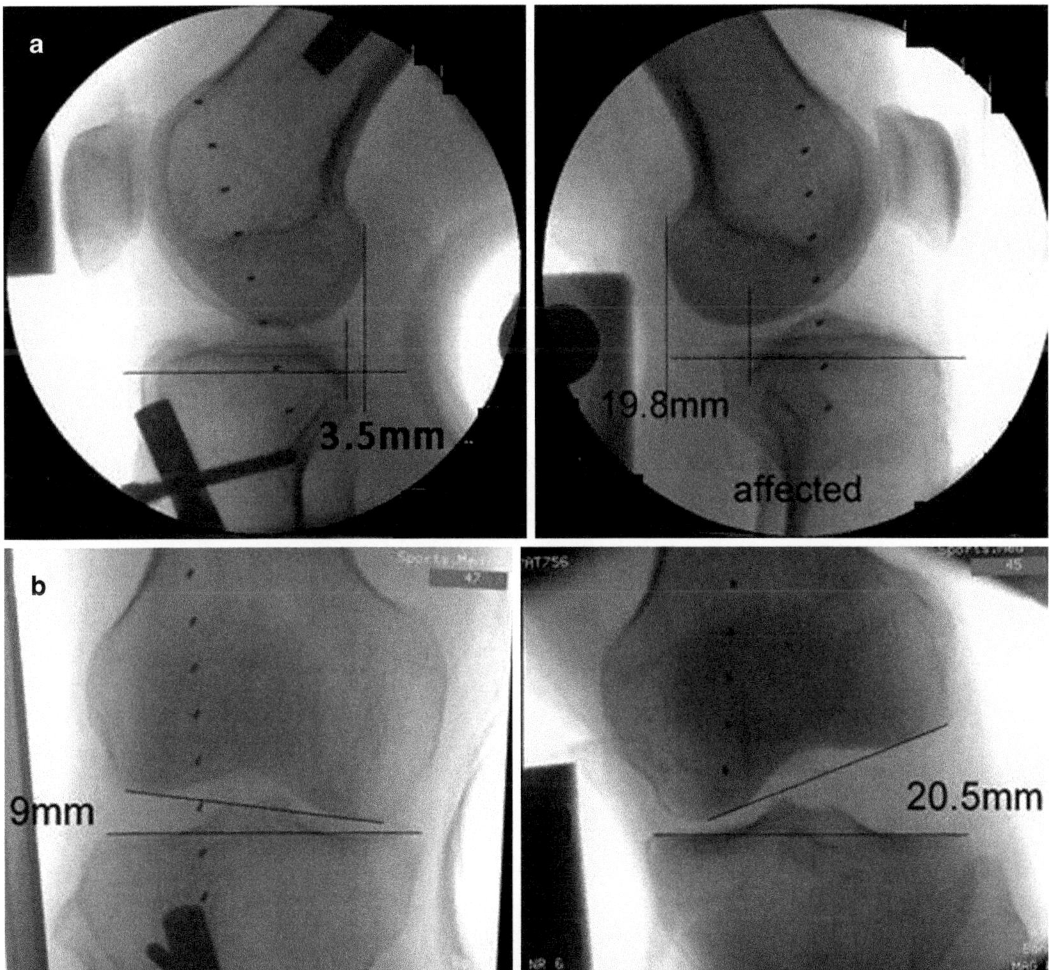

Fig. 32.4 The Telos stress radiography performed on a patient suspected with multi-ligamentous injuries. The side-to-side differences of (**a**) anterior tibial displacement and (**b**) lateral joint opening were 16.3 mm and 11.5 mm, respectively, indicating a combined ACL/PLC injury

32.3.3 Diagnostic Arthroscopy

Diagnostic arthroscopy is becoming increasingly important to investigate the patient undergoing routine ACL reconstruction with no clear preoperative suspicion of PLC injury so that a concomitant PLC injury is not missed. The Pop-T can be easily visualized from the lateral compartment. LaPrade et al. [24] described an arthroscopic "drive-through" sign of the knee where opening of the lateral compartment greater than 1 cm with varus stress at 30° of knee flexion was indicative of a grade III PLC injury.

We recently described a "lateral gutter drive-through" (LGDT) sign, where the arthroscope may be placed deep into the posterolateral compartment via the lateral gutter due to an increased interval between the lateral femoral condyle and the Pop-T at 30° of knee flexion seen in PLC injury. In the case of acute proximal avulsion of the Pop-T from the femur, the bare femoral insertion area, with ecchymosis, scar tissue, and hematoma, can generally be found in the lateral gutter (Fig. 32.5). It was reported that the LGDT sign was effective in identifying the acute femoral "peel-off" lesions, in which the femoral avulsions of the Pop-T and LCL were commonly encountered [8–11]. Moreover, the LGDT sign proved to be useful in diagnosing chronic cases with posterolateral instability, with both the sensitivity and the specificity reaching above 90 % [41].

32.4 Nonoperative Management

Important factors to consider for nonoperative management include the patient's activity level, comorbidities, and the overall nature of the injury. Nonoperative management may be appropriate for the older, sedentary patient with a milder injury pattern who wishes to "cope" via the use of a brace and physical therapy. However, recent evidence does suggest that nonoperative management of combined ACL/PLC injuries may lead to an increased risk of osteoarthritis [31]. Moreover, as discussed earlier, if an associated PLC injury is not addressed in conjunction with an ACL reconstruction, the ACL graft is at an increased risk for early failure [27].

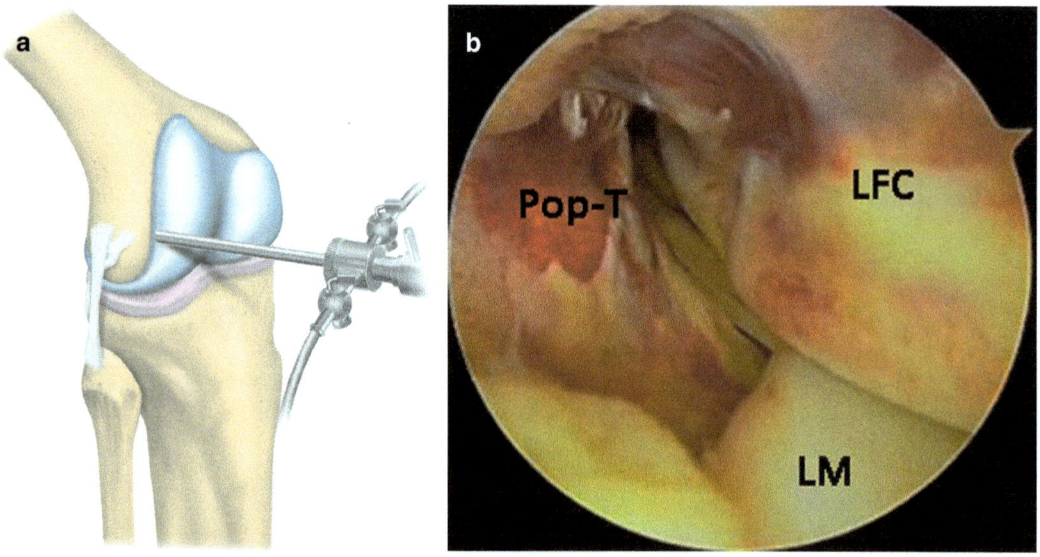

Fig. 32.5 (**a**) Diagram of the "lateral gutter drive-through" test. In those patients with acute proximal avulsion of the popliteus tendon (*Pop-T*) of the femur, the arthroscope can be inserted deeply into the posterolateral compartment through the interval between the Pop-T and the lateral femoral condyle. (**b**) The arthroscopic view from the anterolateral portal shows the interval between the Pop-T and the lateral femoral condyle. The bare femoral insertion area with ecchymosis also can be found in the lateral gutter, which is an indirect sign of an acute femoral "peel-off" lesion (*LFC* lateral femoral condyle, *LM* lateral meniscus)

32.5 Surgical Indications and Contraindications

In the clinical practice of the current authors, surgical intervention is favored in patients who sustain a combined ACL/PLC injury. While these injuries in isolation may be treated successfully by nonoperative management, together they often produce significant instability that remains symptomatic for the patient. Indications for surgery include any active patient involved in pivoting, cutting, or deceleration activities. The authors advocate surgery in young patients and those with concomitant meniscal and/or cartilage pathology, mechanical symptoms, or loss of motion. Any patient that fails from nonoperative management and has continued instability should undergo surgical interventions. Relative contraindications to surgery include morbid obesity, advanced age, limited pre-injury function, extensive scar tissue, circulation dysfunction after previous vascular surgery of the involved lower extremity, knee extension deficit >10°, deep vein thrombosis (DVT), or patients with significant medical contraindications to surgery. However, these patients should be managed with initial immobilization, aggressive rehabilitation, and functional bracing (Fact Box 4).

Fact Box 4 Key points for surgical indications and contraindications

Indications	Contraindications
Active patient involved in pivoting, cutting, or deceleration activities	Morbid obesity (BMI > 30)
Young patients	Advanced aged, sedentary patient with low level of daily activities
Concomitant meniscal and/or cartilage pathologies with mechanical symptoms or loss of motion	Limited pre-injury function (prior joint infection, uncorrected severe varus malalignment, advanced joint arthritis)
Failed nonoperative management with continued instability	Anticipated to be noncompliant with nonoperative management
	Extensive scar tissue
	Knee extension deficit >10°
	Deep vein thrombosis (DVT)
	Circulation dysfunction after previous vascular surgery of the involved lower extremity
	Significant medical contraindications to surgery

Abbreviations: *BMI* body mass index

32.6 Surgical Management

Treatment algorithms are often based on whether the injury is acute or chronic [29, 33]. While there is general consensus in the literature that surgical interventions of the PLC should be performed if the ACL is reconstructed to reduce the risk of early graft failure, some surgeons advocate repair, whereas others prefer reconstruction by a variety of techniques, which will be discussed below.

32.6.1 Acute Combined ACL/PLC Injuries

Initial treatment of the acute combined ACL/PLC injured knee should consist of immobilization, modalities to reduce soft tissue swelling and intra-articular effusion, and therapy to maximize preoperative range of motion. It is the author's preference to delay surgery for 5–7 days. During this time, a complete preoperative workup, as described above, should be performed and an operative plan should be made.

Debate remains on whether to repair or reconstruct the PLC injury in acute combined ACL/PLC injuries. Some authors recommend acute repair of PLC injuries if the quality of the torn structures is adequate to facilitate a repair [38]. Shelbourne et al. [40] reported excellent clinical outcomes in a cohort of 7 patients treated with acute repairs of PLC injuries at a mean follow-up of 5 years. Three injury patterns for an acute femoral "peel-off" lesion were recently described [10]. Type I and II lesions were both femoral bony avulsions without any mid-substance or

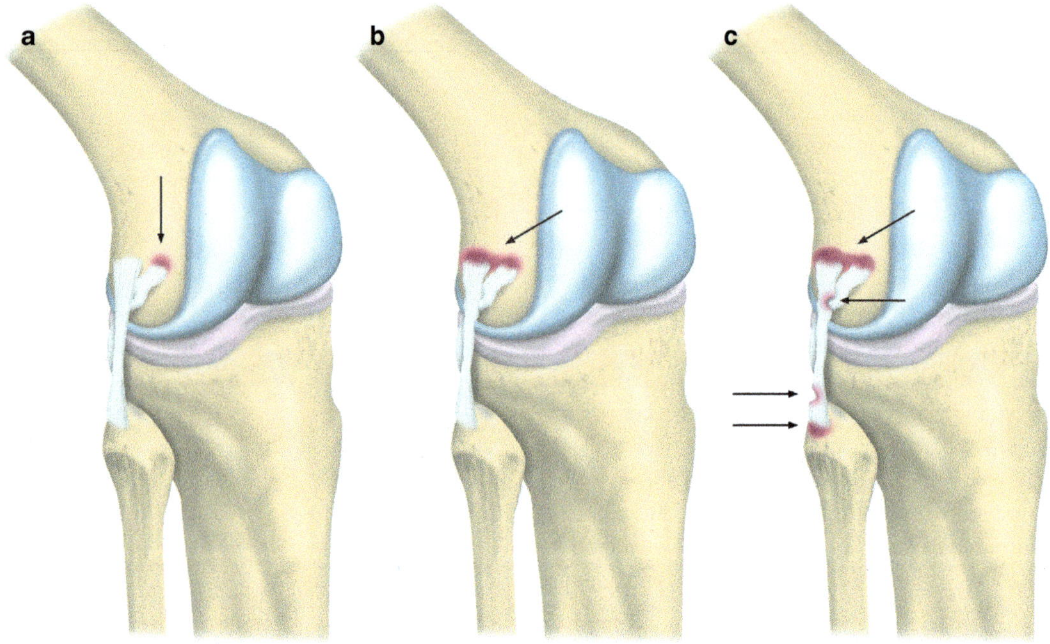

Fig. 32.6 The femoral "peel-off" lesions were typically categorized into three types: (**a**) type I, isolated popliteus tendon (Pop-T) tear (the Pop-T is torn from the femoral insertion site) (*black arrow*); (**b**) type II, combined Pop-T and lateral collateral ligament (LCL) tear (the Pop-T and LCL are torn from the femoral insertion site) (*black arrows*); and (**c**) type III, complex tear (both the Pop-T and the LCL are torn from the femoral insertion site with complex mid-substance injuries) (*black arrows*)

fibular injury to the PLC structures (Fig. 32.6). Acute PLC repair was performed in these patients using strong metal fixation devices and the early clinical outcomes were promising.

However, even in the acute setting, the PLC tissues are often inadequate, especially with mid-substance ruptures. Reconstruction of the PLC can follow either anatomic or nonanatomic principles, and there are proponents of both methods.

As it has been shown that the PFL plays an important role in the posterolateral stability of the knee, current techniques emphasize its reconstruction in addition to the LCL [44]. Veltri and Warren [45] described reconstructing the Pop-T and PFL with a split patellar tendon or Achilles tendon graft, in which the bone plug was fixed in the common femoral tunnel and the two limbs were passed through tunnels in the proximal tibia and fibula. They then addressed the LCL independently. Stannard et al. [42] described what they termed a "modified two-tailed" technique, where a tibialis allograft tendon was tensioned through transtibial and transfibular tunnels and fixed on a single isometric point on the lateral femoral condyle with a spiked washer and screw. Unlike Veltri's technique, this reconstructs the Pop-T, PFL, and LCL simultaneously.

Many surgeons advocate eliminating the tibial tunnel and utilizing only a transfibular tunnel. In this regard, a recent biomechanical study showed that the transfibular tunnel was as equally effective as the dual tibial/fibular tunnels at restoring external rotation and varus stability [37]. Not only is this technically easier, but it also reduces the overall volume of tibial tunnel, which is especially pertinent in the reconstruction of the multi-ligamentous injured knee where there may already be multiple tibial tunnels for ACL/PCL grafts. Others have shown that reconstruction of the PLC with a single sling through a fibular tunnel has better rotational stability, less morbidity, and less operative time when compared to a tibial tunnel [21].

Anatomic reconstruction of the PLC, which involves the placement of two femoral tunnels to replicate both the insertion point of the LCL on the lateral femoral condyle and the Pop-T anterior and distal to it, has been shown by several authors to yield excellent results [23, 26]. One study by

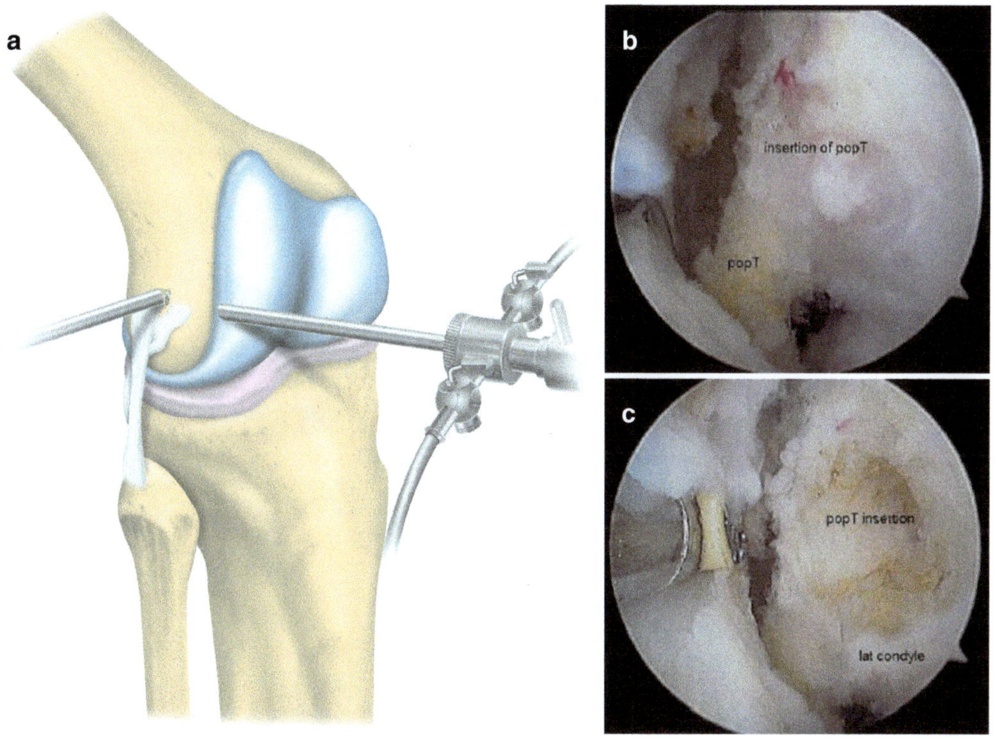

Fig. 32.7 (**a**) Diagram of the preparation of the arthroscopic portals for all-arthroscopic popliteus tendon (*Pop-T*) reconstruction on a right knee; (**b**) arthroscopic view from the lateral portal shows the Pop-T insertion after debridement of covered synovium; (**c**) the femoral insertion of the Pop-T, which is marked by an electrocautery device. (*lat* lateral)

Ho et al. [14] showed improved knee kinematics with better rotational stability and resistance to posterior translation in anatomic PLC reconstructions with two femoral tunnels, compared to a nonanatomic single femoral tunnel technique.

Senior Author's Preferred Technique In the combined ACL/PLC injured knee, graft selection becomes very important. The choice of the senior author is to reconstruct the ACL in a single-bundle manner with autogenous bone-patellar tendon-bone (B-PT-B) in young high-level individuals. In older patients, the patient is offered all of the graft options, but semitendinosus and gracilis tendon autografts are typically recommended. In order to minimize donor site morbidity from the harvesting of multiple grafts, allografts are utilized in all patients for PLC reconstruction since it is easily available and robust.

The authors tend to determine their PLC reconstruction protocols based on the classification system introduced by Fanelli et al. [7]. In cases where increased external tibial rotation is the only presenting finding or when combined with minimal varus laxity (Fanelli type A and type B), the surgical techniques to reconstruct the popliteus complex (including the Pop-T and/or the PFL) can restore normal external tibial rotational stability [49–51]. Motivated by this, an all-arthroscopic Pop-T reconstruction technique was developed [8] and will be presented below.

Under general or spinal anesthesia, the patient is placed in a supine position. The affected limb is placed in a foot and leg support providing 90° of knee flexion and 45° of hip flexion. A 5-mm-diameter anterior tibialis allograft is prepared, and No. 2 Ethibond suture (Ethicon, Somerville, NJ) is used to whipstitch suture each end of the graft. From the standard anterolateral portal, the femoral portion of the Pop-T is visualized through the lateral compartment and lateral gutter. The accessory superolateral portal (close to the femoral insertion area of the native Pop-T) is established with a spinal needle through an outside-in technique. Electrocautery is used to mark the central point of the femoral footprint (Fig. 32.7). An eyelet guide pin is drilled into the center of the footprint, and a 6-mm-diameter socket (approximately 25 mm in depth) is then created over the guide pin.

With 90° of knee flexion, the posteromedial, posterolateral, and transseptal arthroscopic portals are established. The arthroscope is introduced from the posteromedial portal and passed through the transseptal portal to reach the posterolateral compartment. The posterolateral capsule of the knee joint is carefully separated from the synovial edge of the posterior horn of the lateral meniscus with a motorized shaver (3.5 mm in diameter) inserted from the posterolateral portal until the popliteus musculotendinous junction is identified (Fact Box 5). An ACL tibial guide is then brought in through the posterolateral portal, advanced, and targeted to the popliteus musculotendinous junction area on the posterior tibia. A Kirschner wire is passed from the anterior tibial cortex to the posterior aspect of the lateral tibial plateau (Fig. 32.8).

Fact Box 5 Key points for all-arthroscopic popliteus tendon reconstruction

To obtain complete visualization of the musculotendinous junction, the most central portion of the posterior horn of the lateral meniscus is detached from the posterior capsule and meniscal aponeurosis of the popliteus for more than 10 mm downward from the articular surface
As bony landmark, the shallow groove in the posterolateral aspect of the lateral tibial plateau makes the location of the popliteus tunnel
To improve visualization of the popliteus femoral portion, a switching rod sometimes can be introduced from the superolateral portal and passed into lateral gutter to act as a "lift-up hanger." The lateral capsule and skin are lifted up, affording the arthroscopic surgeon a larger space for viewing and instrumental manipulation

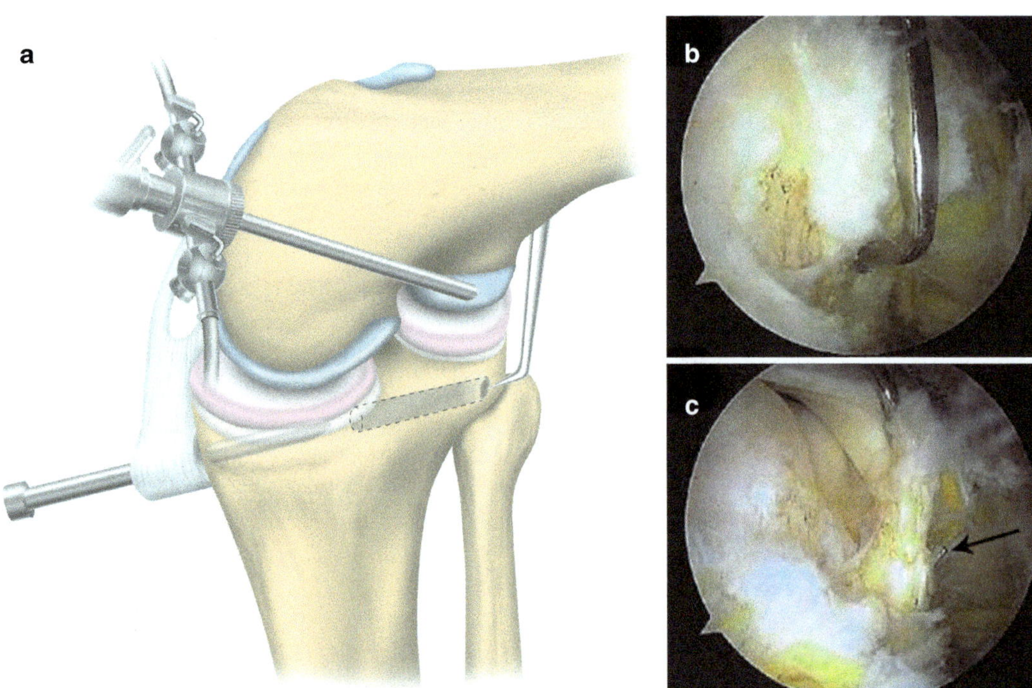

Fig. 32.8 (**a**) Assisted by the transseptal portal, the surgeon introduced the anterior cruciate ligament tibial guide from the posterolateral portal and positioned it to the popliteus musculotendinous junction of the posterior tibia; (**b**) arthroscopic view and positioning of the tibial guide; (**c**) relationship of guide pin (*black arrow*) and groove of popliteus tendon on posterior tibia

Once positioned, a tunnel is made with a cannulated reamer usually 6 mm in diameter. The graft is then pulled through the tibial tunnel and into the femoral socket under the guidance of the passing suture.

Fixation of the ACL is completed before the Pop-T is reconstructed. The surgeon completes the Pop-T reconstruction by pulling on the passing suture and tensioning the graft from the medial side of the knee. Then the graft is fixed into the femoral socket with a bioabsorbable screw (usually 1 size larger than the tunnel diameter). The tibial fixation is then completed with another bioabsorbable interference screw (again 1 size larger than the tunnel diameter), while the knee is held at 30° of flexion with neutral tibial rotation (Fig. 32.9).

In cases where increased external tibial rotation is combined with significant varus laxity (Fanelli type C), an additional LCL reconstruction is indicated. The current authors tend to use B-PT-B allograft to reconstruct the LCL. Initially, both the femoral and fibular tunnels are drilled at the anatomic attachment sites. Then the distal bone portion of the graft is gently tapped into the fibular tunnel and fixed with two small-fragment cortical screws engaging both fibular cortices. Finally, the proximal bone of the graft is advanced into the femoral tunnel and fixed with a soft tissue interference screw at 30° of knee flexion with neutral tibial rotation (Fig. 32.10).

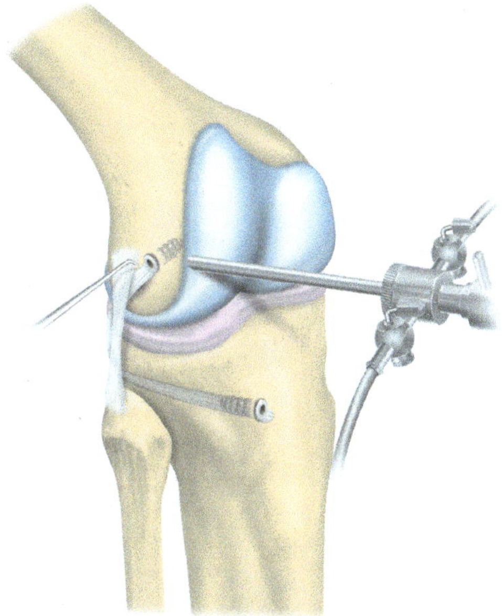

Fig. 32.9 Diagram of the reconstructed popliteus tendon shows the graft and tunnel positions on tibial and femoral sides

32.6.2 Chronic Combined ACL/PLC Injuries

It is not uncommon for patients to present to the surgeon's office with a combined ACL/PLC injury in a delayed manner. They may be chronic injuries that were either initially unrecognized or those that failed from a trial of nonoperative management. In this setting, patents may present with significant swelling and reduced motion and require crutches for ambulation. As with the acutely injured knee, any patient should undergo a vigorous course of therapy to regain range of motion and resume a fairly normal gait prior to considering surgical intervention. Reconstruction of the stiff, swollen knee predisposes the patient to the postoperative complication of significant motion loss.

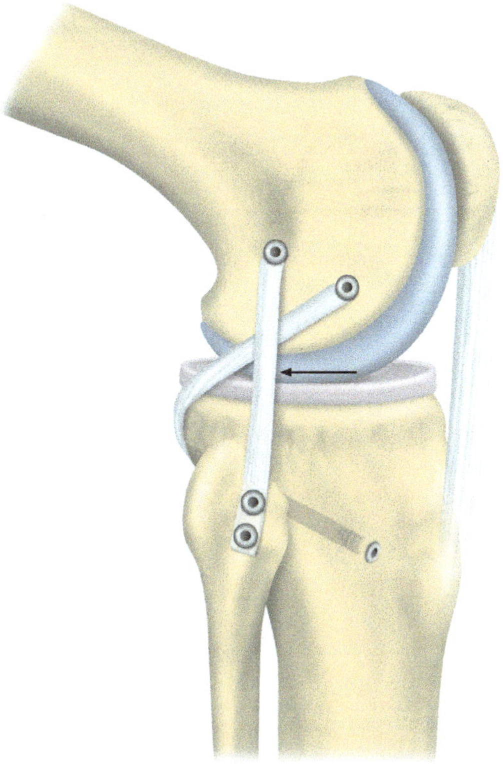

Fig. 32.10 Diagram of combined lateral collateral ligament (*black arrow*) and popliteus tendon reconstruction for Fanelli type C injury

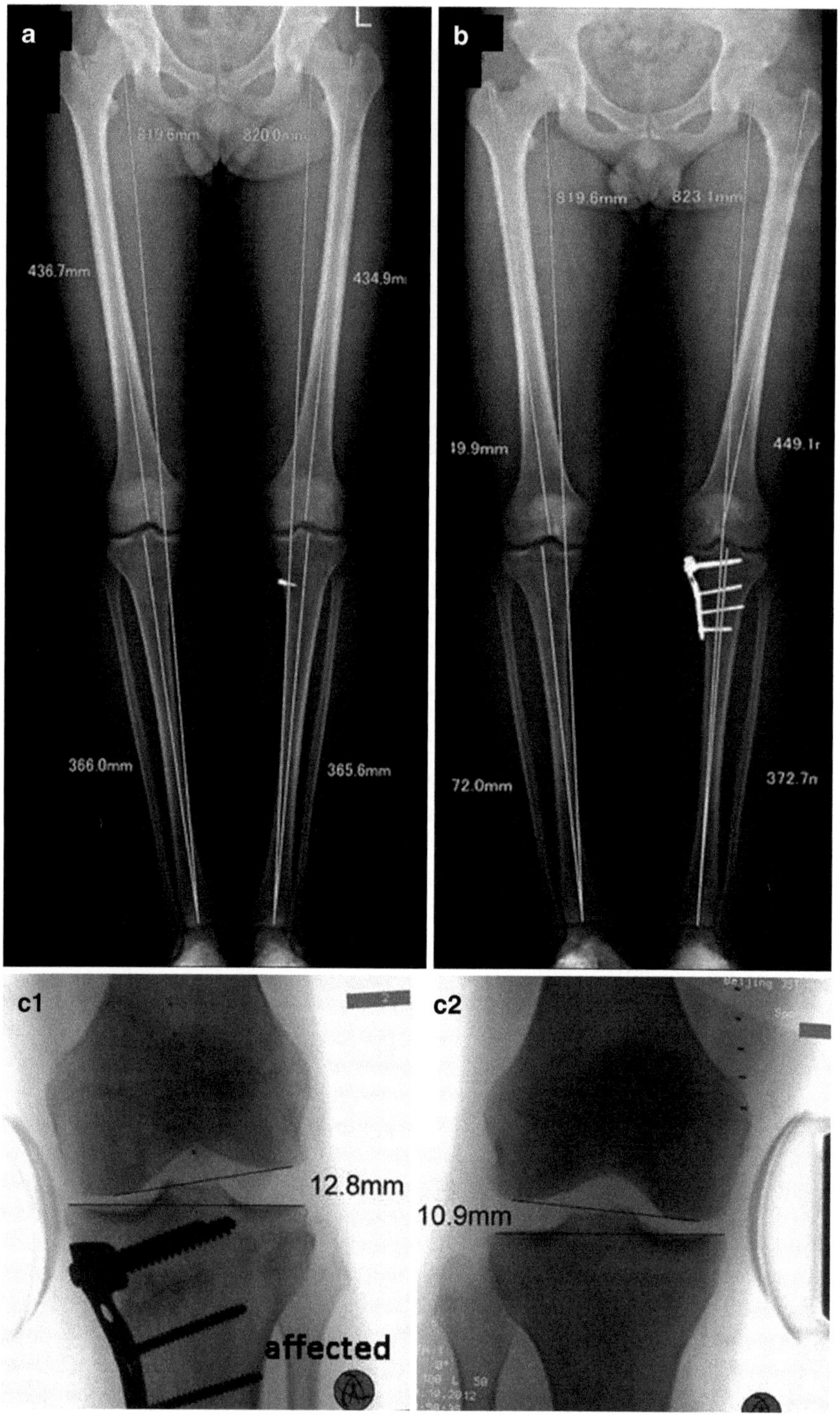

Fig. 32.11 A 24-year-old man presented 5 months after failure of an anterior cruciate ligament (ACL) hamstring autograft reconstruction. Physical examination revealed a grade II pivot shift, 7 mm of increased anterior displacement on KT-1000 testing. (**a**) Full standing radiographs showed a varus deformity of the affected lower extremity. The patient was treated with a staged procedure of a corrective opening wedge high tibial osteotomy (HTO), followed 6 months later with a bone-patellar tendon-bone autograft revision ACL reconstruction. At a 24-month follow-up evaluation, (**b**) full standing radiographs showed that the varus deformity was corrected. (**c**) The side-to-side difference of lateral joint opening was 1.9 mm. The pivot-shift test was negative. The patient had returned to work and light recreational sports without problems

Chronic injuries are associated with poor tissue quality; thus reconstruction of the PLC is indicated, and there is no role for a primary repair. In the chronically unstable knee, surgical intervention is warranted, and we follow the same technical guidelines as those described above for the acute injury. It must be emphasized that it is extremely important in the chronic injured knee to thoroughly evaluate the alignment of the whole extremity, as it is not uncommon for the patient to have a double or triple varus knee from long-standing instability [34]. These patients may benefit from an opening wedge high tibial osteotomy to complement the ligament reconstructions (Fig. 32.11).

32.7 Postoperative Complications

Potential complications from the surgical management of combined ACL/PLC injuries include would infection, hematoma, loss of motion, failure of reconstruction with recurrent pain and/or instability, and hardware irritation. The peroneal nerve can also be injured during the operative approach or reconstruction; the surgeon must be alert and careful with dissection [2].

Conclusions

There are several key points when approaching a patient with combined ACL/PLC injury:

1. In the setting of an ACL injury, it is important not to miss a concomitant PLC injury or varus malalignment as these can lead to early graft failure of the reconstructed ACL.
2. Diligent physical examination and appropriate imaging studies are prerequisites of an accurate diagnosis of combined ACL/PLC injury.
3. A thorough neurovascular examination is critical in preventing catastrophic consequences.
4. Clinical outcomes of "anatomic" PLC reconstruction techniques are promising in controlling both varus and external rotational instability.
5. The assessment of lower limb alignment and role of high tibial osteotomy cannot be understated.
6. The senior author's preferred treatment algorithm of combined ACL/PLC injury is provided (Fig. 32.12).

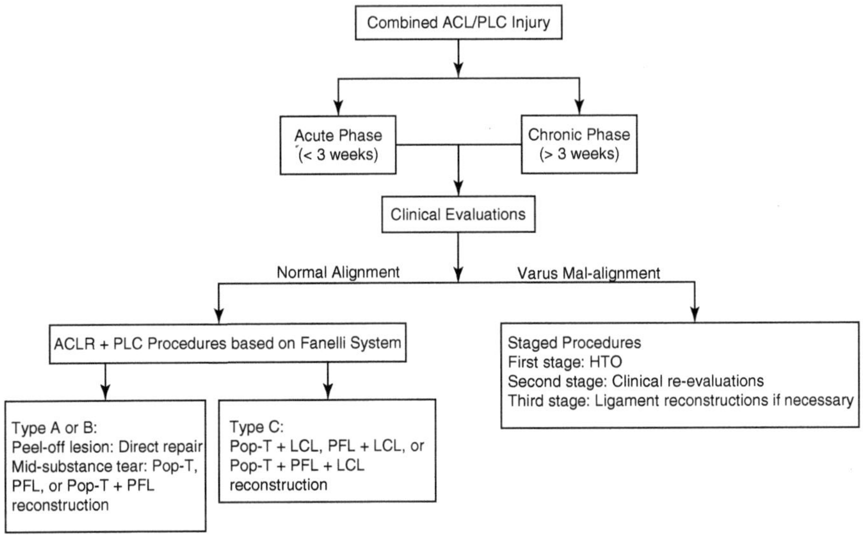

Fig. 32.12 Suggested treatment algorithm of combined ACL/PLC injury (*ACL* anterior cruciate ligament, *PLC* posterolateral corner, *ACLR* anterior cruciate ligament reconstruction, *Pop-T* popliteus tendon, *PFL* popliteofibular ligament, *LCL* lateral collateral ligament, *HTO* high tibial osteotomy)

References

1. Amis AA, Scammell BE (1993) Biomechanics of intra-articular and extra-articular reconstruction of the anterior cruciate ligament. J Bone Joint Surg Br 75(5):812–817
2. Bottomley N, Williams A, Birch R, Noorani A, Lewis A, Lavelle J (2005) Displacement of the common peroneal nerve in posterolateral corner injuries of the knee. J Bone Joint Surg Br 87(9):1225–1226
3. Cooper JM, McAndrews PT, LaPrade RF (2006) Posterolateral corner injuries of the knee: anatomy, diagnosis, and treatment. Sports Med Arthrosc 14(4): 213–220
4. Covey DC (2001) Injuries of the posterolateral corner of the knee. J Bone Joint Surg Am 83-A(1):106–118
5. DeLee JC, Riley MB, Jr Rockwood CA (1983) Acute posterolateral rotatory instability of the knee. Am J Sports Med 11(4):199–207
6. Dienst M, Burks RT, Greis PE (2002) Anatomy and biomechanics of the anterior cruciate ligament. Orthop Clin North Am 33(4):605–620
7. Fanelli GC, Edson CJ (2004) Combined posterior cruciate ligament-posterolateral reconstructions with Achilles tendon allograft and biceps femoris tendon tenodesis: 2- to 10-year follow-up. Arthroscopy 20 (4):339–345
8. Feng H, Hong L, Geng XS, Zhang H, Wang XS, Zhang J (2009) Posterolateral sling reconstruction of the popliteus tendon: an all-arthroscopic technique. Arthroscopy 25(7):800–805
9. Feng H, Song GY, Shen JW, Zhang H, Wang MY (2014) The "lateral gutter drive-through" sign revisited: a cadaveric study exploring its real mechanism based on the individual posterolateral structure of knee joints. Arch Orthop Trauma Surg 134(12): 1745–1751
10. Feng H, Zhang H, Hong L, Wang XS, Cheng KB, Zhang J (2011) Femoral peel-off lesions in acute posterolateral corner injuries: incidence, classification, and clinical characteristics. Arthroscopy 27(7): 951–958
11. Feng H, Zhang H, Hong L, Wang XS, Zhang J (2009) The "lateral gutter drive-through" sign: an arthroscopic indicator of acute femoral avulsion of the popliteus tendon in knee joints. Arthroscopy 25(12):1496–1499
12. Goldman AB, Pavlov H, Rubenstein D (1988) The Segond fracture of the proximal tibia: a small avulsion that reflects major ligamentous damage. AJR Am J Roentgenol 151(6):1163–1167
13. Halinen J, Koivikko M, Lindahl J, Hirvensalo E (2009) The efficacy of magnetic resonance imaging in acute multi-ligament injuries. Int Orthop 33(6):1733–1738
14. Ho EP, Lam MH, Chung MM, Fong DT, Law BK, Yung PS, Chan WY, Chan KM (2011) Comparison of 2 surgical techniques for reconstructing posterolateral corner of the knee: a cadaveric study evaluated by navigation system. Arthroscopy 27(1):89–96
15. Hughston JC, Andrews JR, Cross MJ, Moschi A (1976) Classification of knee ligament instabilities. Part I. The medial compartment and cruciate ligaments. J Bone Joint Surg Am 58(2):159–172
16. Hughston JC, Andrews JR, Cross MJ, Moschi A (1976) Classification of knee ligament instabilities. Part II. The lateral compartment. J Bone Joint Surg Am 58(2):173–179
17. Hughston JC, Jr Norwood LA (1980) The posterolateral drawer test and external rotational recurvatum test for posterolateral rotatory instability of the knee. Clin Orthop Relat Res 147:82–87
18. James EW, Williams BT, LaPrade RF (2014) Stress radiography for the diagnosis of knee ligament injuries: a systematic review. Clin Orthop Relat Res 472(9):2644–2657
19. Jr Baker CL, Norwood LA, Hughston JC (1983) Acute posterolateral rotatory instability of the knee. J Bone Joint Surg Am 65(5):614–618
20. Juhng SK, Lee JK, Choi SS, Yoon KH, Roh BS, Won JJ (2002) MR evaluation of the "arcuate" sign of posterolateral knee instability. AJR Am J Roentgenol 178(3):583–588
21. Jung YB, Jung HJ, Kim SJ, Park SJ, Song KS, Lee YS, Lee SH (2008) Posterolateral corner reconstruction for posterolateral rotatory instability combined with posterior cruciate ligament injuries: comparison between fibular tunnel and tibial tunnel techniques. Knee Surg Sports Traumatol Arthrosc 16(3):239–248
22. Kanamori A, Sakane M, Zeminski J, Rudy TW, Woo SL (2000) In-situ force in the medial and lateral structures of intact and ACL-deficient knees. J Orthop Sci 5(6):567–571
23. Kim JG, Ha JG, Lee YS, Yang SJ, Jung JE, Oh SJ (2009) Posterolateral corner anatomy and its anatomical reconstruction with single fibula and double femoral sling method: anatomical study and surgical technique. Arch Orthop Trauma Surg 129(3):381–385
24. LaPrade RF (1997) Arthroscopic evaluation of the lateral compartment of knees with grade 3 posterolateral knee complex injuries. Am J Sports Med 25(5):596–602
25. LaPrade RF, Gilbert TJ, Bollom TS, Wentorf F, Chaljub G (2000) The magnetic resonance imaging appearance of individual structures of the posterolateral knee. A prospective study of normal knees and knees with surgically verified grade III injuries. Am J Sports Med 28(2):191–199
26. LaPrade RF, Johansen S, Wentorf FA, Engebretsen L, Esterberg JL, Tso A (2004) An analysis of an anatomical posterolateral knee reconstruction: an in vitro biomechanical study and development of a surgical technique. Am J Sports Med 32(6):1405–1414
27. LaPrade RF, Resig S, Wentorf F, Lewis JL (1999) The effects of grade III posterolateral knee complex injuries on anterior cruciate ligament graft force. A biomechanical analysis. Am J Sports Med 27(4): 469–475

28. Lee SH, Jung YB, Jung HJ, Song KS, Ko YB (2010) Combined reconstruction for posterolateral rotatory instability with anterior cruciate ligament injuries of the knee. Knee Surg Sports Traumatol Arthrosc 18(9): 1219–1225
29. Levy BA, Dajani KA, Morgan JA, Shah JP, Dahm DL, Stuart MJ (2010) Repair versus reconstruction of the fibular collateral ligament and posterolateral corner in the multiligament-injured knee. Am J Sports Med 38(4):804–809
30. Lipke JM, Janecki CJ, Nelson CL, McLeod P, Thompson C, Thompson J, Haynes DW (1981) The role of incompetence of the anterior cruciate and lateral ligaments in anterolateral and anteromedial instability. A biomechanical study of cadaver knees. J Bone Joint Surg Am 63(6):954–960
31. Mihelic R, Jurdana H, Jotanovic Z, Madjarevic T, Tudor A (2011) Long-term results of anterior cruciate ligament reconstruction: a comparison with non-operative treatment with a follow-up of 17–20 years. Int Orthop 35(7):1093–1097
32. Mills WJ, Barei DP, McNair P (2004) The value of the ankle-brachial index for diagnosing arterial injury after knee dislocation: a prospective study. J Trauma 56(6):1261–1265
33. Noyes FR, Barber-Westin SD (2007) Posterolateral knee reconstruction with an anatomical bone-patellar tendon-bone reconstruction of the fibular collateral ligament. Am J Sports Med 35(2):259–273
34. Noyes FR, Barber-Westin SD, Hewett TE (2000) High tibial osteotomy and ligament reconstruction for varus angulated anterior cruciate ligament-deficient knees. Am J Sports Med 28(3):282–296
35. O'Brien SJ, Warren RF, Pavlov H, Panariello R, Wickiewicz TL (1991) Reconstruction of the chronically insufficient anterior cruciate ligament with the central third of the patellar ligament. J Bone Joint Surg Am 73(2):278–286
36. Pasque C, Noyes FR, Gibbons M, Levy M, Grood E (2003) The role of the popliteofibular ligament and the tendon of popliteus in providing stability in the human knee. J Bone Joint Surg Br 85(2):292–298
37. Rauh PB, Jr Clancy WG, Jasper LE, Curl LA, Belkoff S, Moorman CR (2010) Biomechanical evaluation of two reconstruction techniques for posterolateral instability of the knee. J Bone Joint Surg Br 92(10):1460–1465
38. Ross G, DeConciliis GP, Choi K, Scheller AD (2004) Evaluation and treatment of acute posterolateral corner/anterior cruciate ligament injuries of the knee. J Bone Joint Surg Am 86-A(Suppl 2):2–7
39. Shahane SA, Ibbotson C, Strachan R, Bickerstaff DR (1999) The popliteofibular ligament. An anatomical study of the posterolateral corner of the knee. J Bone Joint Surg Br 81(4):636–642
40. Shelbourne KD, Haro MS, Gray T (2007) Knee dislocation with lateral side injury: results of an en masse surgical repair technique of the lateral side. Am J Sports Med 35(7):1105–1116
41. Shen J, Zhang H, Lv Y, Hong L, Wang X, Zhang J, Feng H (2013) Validity of a novel arthroscopic test to diagnose posterolateral rotational instability of the knee joint: the lateral gutter drive-through test. Arthroscopy 29(4):695–700
42. Stannard JP, Brown SL, Robinson JT, Jr McGwin G, Volgas DA (2005) Reconstruction of the posterolateral corner of the knee. Arthroscopy 21(9):1051–1059
43. Staubli HU, Birrer S (1990) The popliteus tendon and its fascicles at the popliteal hiatus: gross anatomy and functional arthroscopic evaluation with and without anterior cruciate ligament deficiency. Arthroscopy 6(3):209–220
44. Veltri DM, Deng XH, Torzilli PA, Maynard MJ, Warren RF (1996) The role of the popliteofibular ligament in stability of the human knee. A biomechanical study. Am J Sports Med 24(1):19–27
45. Veltri DM, Warren RF (1994) Operative treatment of posterolateral instability of the knee. Clin Sports Med 13(3):615–627
46. Wroble RR, Grood ES, Cummings JS, Henderson JM, Noyes FR (1993) The role of the lateral extraarticular restraints in the anterior cruciate ligament-deficient knee. Am J Sports Med 21(2):257–262
47. Yu JS, Salonen DC, Hodler J, Haghighi P, Trudell D, Resnick D (1996) Posterolateral aspect of the knee: improved MR imaging with a coronal oblique technique. Radiology 198(1):199–204
48. Zantop T, Schumacher T, Diermann N, Schanz S, Raschke MJ, Petersen W (2007) Anterolateral rotational knee instability: role of posterolateral structures. Winner of the AGA-DonJoy Award 2006. Arch Orthop Trauma Surg 127(9):743–752
49. Zhang H, Hong L, Wang XS, Zhang J, Geng XS, Liu X, Feng H (2010) Single-bundle posterior cruciate ligament reconstruction and mini-open popliteofibular ligament reconstruction in knees with severe posterior and posterolateral rotation instability: clinical results of minimum 2-year follow-up. Arthroscopy 26(4):508–514
50. Zhang H, Hong L, Wang XS, Zhang J, Liu X, Feng H (2011) All-arthroscopic repair of arcuate avulsion fracture with suture anchor. Arthroscopy 27(5):728–734
51. Zhang H, Zhang J, Liu X, Shen JW, Hong L, Wang XS, Feng H (2013) In vitro comparison of popliteus tendon and popliteofibular ligament reconstruction in an external rotation injury model of the knee: a cadaveric study evaluated by a navigation system. Am J Sports Med 41(9):2136–2142

Part VI

Functional Rehabilitation and Return to Sport

Criterion-Based Approach for Returning to Sport After ACL Reconstruction

33

Rick Joreitz, Andrew Lynch, Christopher Harner, Freddie H. Fu, and James J. Irrgang

Contents

R. Joreitz, PT, DPT, SCS, ATC • A. Lynch, PT, PhD
C. Harner, MD • F. H. Fu, MD, DSc
J.J. Irrgang, PT, PhD, ATC, FAPTA (✉)
Pittsburgh, PA, USA
e-mail: irrgangjj@upmc.edu

Anterior cruciate ligament (ACL) reconstruction rehabilitation protocols for the acute postsurgical phase are prevalent. Protocols to guide rehabilitation through the return-to-sport progressions and phases are not as widely available. The purpose of this clinical review is to present the protocol developed at the University of Pittsburgh Medical Center (UMPC) Center for Sports Medicine for the late phases of rehabilitation and return-to-sport progress after ACL reconstruction with references to the literature.

A comprehensive literature search was performed to identify return-to-sport criteria and risk factors for reinjury and revision. The results of that literature search were used to create an evidence-based, criterion-based progression for return to sports that emphasizes injury prevention and mastery of basic sports and athletic skills.

A progression which emphasizes mastery of a hierarchy of functional tasks is presented with criterion to progress between phases including running, agility drills, jumping, hopping/cutting/pivoting, and return to participation in practice which was created with consideration for mitigating injury risk factors that is presented. A complete protocol is presented to guide rehabilitation for return to practice and return to full sports participation phases. Further research is needed to justify a protracted rehabilitation phase that emphasizes mastery of lower-level functional rehabilitation tasks before progression to more demanding tasks. Long-term follow-up with outcomes defined as return to pre-injury

V. Musahl et al. (eds.), *Rotatory Knee Instability*, DOI 10.1007/978-3-319-32070-0_33

levels of sport participation without reinjury must be completed to determine the effectiveness of this protocol. The return-to-play progression presented here has been developed to be specific to the individual with consideration for the best available evidence for healing and function after ACL reconstruction.

33.1 Introduction

Return to sports and avoiding knee joint instability associated with reinjury are key measures of success after anterior cruciate ligament (ACL) reconstruction [18]. The guidelines presented here for the later phases of rehabilitation address factors known to limit success and lead to reinjury – neuromuscular control in basic and advanced sport-specific movements and quadriceps strength. The purpose of this chapter is to aid clinicians in understanding the necessities of late-phase rehabilitation to promote safe and effective return to sports with respect to maximizing performance and mitigating the risk factors for reinjury using criterion-based guidelines.

The clinical decision-making process for return to sport emphasizes a highly structured set of objective tests with associated criteria for progression between phases which is recommended but has not been commonly reported in the literature [4, 31].

The program outlined here serves two purposes. The primary purpose is to provide structure to the rehabilitation process after resolution of early postoperative impairments with a criterion-based progression for resumption of sports activities and participation. During the first 4–6 weeks after surgery, the patient and physical therapist have specific goals for range of motion and criteria for discharge of crutches and postoperative brace, with numerous protocols available in the literature [1, 21, 33]. There are fewer protocols for the return-to-sport phase and a lack of clear goals and standards for progression for the physical therapist and patient. The principles remain the same during the beginning and end of the rehabilitation process, but the exercises are chosen to resolve each individual's impairments as well as prepare them for their specific sport and position. Strategies for prevention of ACL injury are included throughout the program with a focus on balance and proprioception, motor control, agility, and plyometric training [8, 14, 15, 19, 20, 29]. The second purpose is to make this protocol generalizable to all clinical settings and to all individuals. The tests and measures described in this chapter can be applied with minimal specialized equipment and to all individuals regardless of surgical procedure. Specific attention is paid to concomitant procedures and each individual's presentation when making decisions to progress through the protocol.

Individuals progress through this rehabilitation program in five phases. The first phase begins immediately after surgery and is centered on regaining range of motion, strength, patella mobility, flexibility, and normalizing gait. Phases 2 through 5 encompass progressive return to running, agility training, jumping, hopping, and cutting and assume clearance from the surgeon for running and agreement with the criteria established for advancement to subsequent stages. The objective tests and criteria to progress between phases focus on three areas to determine whether or not individuals are ready to attempt more demanding activities [1] mastery of the current phase [2], neuromuscular control, and [3] quadriceps strength (see Table 33.1). Phases 2 through 5 involve working with a physical therapist to initiate new activities. Independent practice is encouraged when the individual demonstrates the ability to safely complete the exercises.

33.2 Assessment of Mastery

Individuals must demonstrate mastery of the rehabilitation goals of the current phase before progressing to the next phase (i.e., individuals must demonstrate the ability to run 2 miles without gait deviations or signs of inflammation before being cleared to perform low-level agility tasks). Mastery is typically assessed through observation of the highest level of performance allowed in the progression. Failure to master the tasks of an individual phase is mediated with

Table 33.1 Criteria to advance to each new phase

Criteria to enter phase 2 – running:		
Phase 1 mastery	Symmetrical range of motion, minimal knee joint effusion (trace or less) Maximal treadmill walking ×15 min without deviations[a]	
Neuromuscular control	Step and hold	30 repetitions without deviation[a]
	Single-leg squats	Ten repetitions to 45° of knee flexion without deviation[a]
	Y-balance test[b]	≥90 % composite score
Quadriceps strength	Strength battery	Leg press ≥ 80 % 1-RM LSI[d] (90–0°)
		Leg extension ≥ 80 % 1-RM LSI[d] (90–45°)
	Or	
	Isometric dynamometry	≥80 % Limb symmetry index
Criteria to enter phase 3 – low-level agility drills:		
Phase 2 mastery	Run 2 miles continuously without pain, swelling, warmth, or gait deviations	
Neuromuscular control	Single-leg squats[c]	Ten repetitions to > 45° of knee flexion without deviation[a] and 75 % LSI
	Y-balance test[b]	≥100 % composite score
Quadriceps strength	Strength battery	Leg press ≥ 85 % 1-RM LSI[d] (90–0°)
		Leg extension ≥ 85 % 1-RM LSI[d] (90–0°)
	Or	
	Isometric dynamometry	≥85 % Limb symmetry index
Criteria to enter phase 4 – double-leg jumping:		
Phase 3 mastery	No compensation patterns with deceleration during phase 3 agility drills performed at full speed	
Neuromuscular control	Single-leg squats[c]	ten repetitions to 60° of knee flexion without deviation[a] and 85 % LSI
Quadriceps strength	Strength battery	Leg press ≥ 90 % 1-RM LSI[d] (90–0°)
		Leg extension ≥ 90 % 1-RM LSI[d] (90–0°)
	Or	
	Isometric dynamometry	≥90 % Limb symmetry index
Criteria to enter phase 5 – single-leg hopping and cutting:		
Phase 4 mastery	No deviations when initiating and landing jumps	
Neuromuscular control	Single-leg squats[c]	Ten repetitions to 60° of knee flexion without deviation[a] and 85 % LSI
Quadriceps strength	Strength battery	Leg press ≥ 90 % 1-RM LSI[d] (90–0°)
		Leg extension ≥ 90 % 1-RM LSI[d] (90–0°)
	Or	
	Isometric dynamometry	≥90 % Limb symmetry index

[a]Deviations include loss of balance, excessive motion outside of the sagittal plane, abnormal trunk movement, contralateral pelvic drop, femoral internal rotation, and medial collapse of the knees

[b]Y-balance test composite score: $\frac{\text{anterior reach} + \text{posteromedial reach} + \text{posterolateral reach}}{3 \times \text{limb length}} * 100\ \%$

[c]Single-limb squat limb symmetry index: $\frac{\text{External load during involved limb single} - \text{leg squat}}{\text{External load during uninvolved limb single} - \text{leg squat}} * 100\ \%$

[d]1-RM LSI: $\frac{\text{Involved limb 1} - \text{RM}}{\text{Uninvolved limb 1} - \text{RM}} * 100\ \%$

focused practice and instruction in proper technique. The inclusion of activity mastery as a prerequisite for advancement to the next phase ensures that individuals take time to practice each skill and incorporate good movement patterns during dynamic tasks even if their strength and neuromuscular control would allow them to progress in multiple phases (i.e., when being tested for phase 2 – running – individuals must demonstrate they can run 2 miles continuously without increased inflammation before progressing to agility drills, regardless whether they can demonstrate greater than 85 % strength and a Y-balance test greater than 100 % of leg length).

33.3 Strength Measurement

Quadriceps strength should be measured as precisely and accurately as possible within the clinical setting due to its importance in the recovery of function and its propensity to be under-rehabilitated. When available, isometric or isokinetic dynamometry should be used, as it isolates the quadriceps and provides reliable measures of strength without compensation. In our clinic, quadriceps and hamstring strength are measured with a maximum volitional isometric contraction for five seconds on an electromechanical dynamometer. To reduce the risk of patellar fractures [26], isometric strength testing with a dynamometer is delayed until 4 or 5 months post-op, and the knee is positioned at 60° of knee flexion to reduce bending forces across the patella.

In cases where dynamometry is not available, a 1-repetition maximum (1-RM) on a knee extension machine [3, 23] or leg press machine [23] can been used to assess strength. For the 1-RM leg press, the individual is positioned on the leg press with the hip and knee being tested flexed to 90°. The heel is in contact with the platform, and the ball of the foot is off the edge (Fig. 33.1: leg press) to limit compensation with the gastrocnemius-soleus complex. The contralateral leg cannot assist in initiating the lift and cannot be on the floor or on the platform. For the 1-RM leg extension, the individual is positioned in 90° hip and knee flexion with the resistance pad placed proximally to the malleoli. The individual is instructed to extend their knee as smoothly as possible to 45° of knee flexion (early phases of rehabilitation) or full knee extension (after 5 months post-op) against the weight. Both the unilateral leg press and the unilateral leg extension should be included in the postoperative protocol for quadriceps strengthening, thus making the individual familiar with the exercises. At the 4- or 5-month time

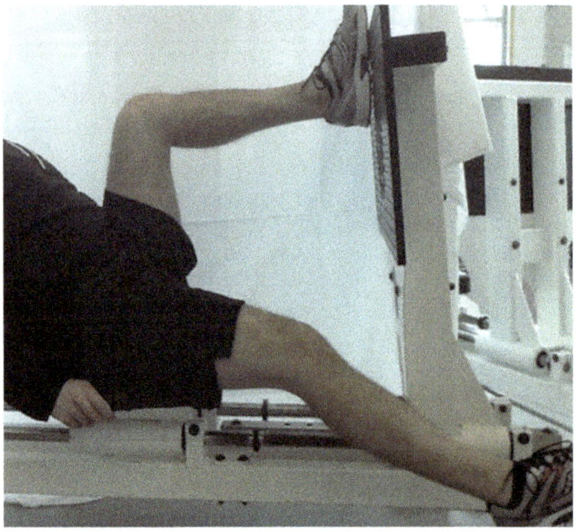

Fig. 33.1 Foot positioning for leg press 1-repetition maximum testing. The ball of the foot is moved up to limit the ability of the gastrocnemius and soleus to contribute to raising the weight

frame when strength testing occurs, there should be no limitations on the range of motion for either weight bearing or non-weight bearing exercise.

The limb symmetry index is calculated as the 1-repetition maximum load of the involved limb divided by the 1-repetition maximum load of the uninvolved limb expressed as a percentage. Neither the leg press 1-RM test nor the leg extension 1-RM test has been validated to measure limb symmetry compared to isometric dynamometry. While both tests can measure the strength of the lower extremity, the leg extension test is preferred by the authors as it better isolates the quadriceps. The leg press can be used as a general measure of lower extremity strength; however, there is the possibility of significant compensation with the gluteal muscles and the triceps surae. When available, isokinetic or isometric dynamometry should be utilized. At the transition to each new phase, strength tests must be repeated to ensure that strength has been maintained and not regressed.

33.4 Neuromuscular Control

Movement patterns and stability are tested with three basic tests, with progressively more stringent criteria to advance to the next phase. The

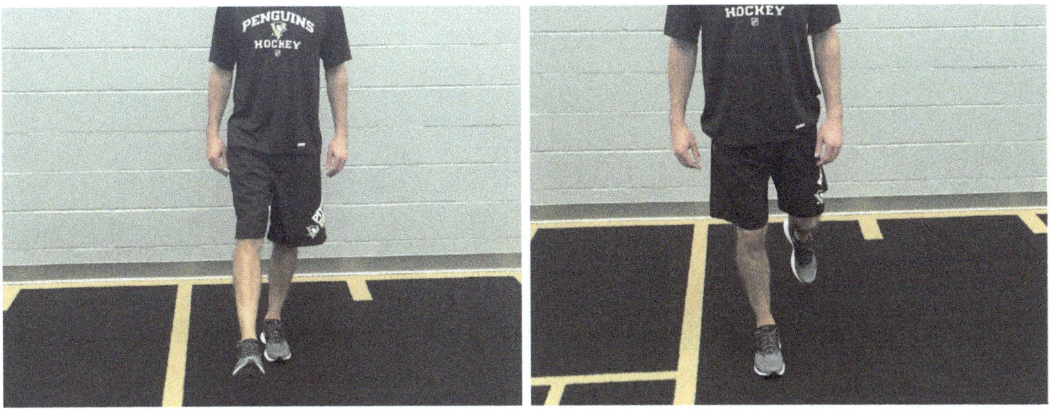

Fig. 33.2 Step and hold. Patients must perform 30 step and holds without loss of balance or excessive motion outside of the sagittal plane

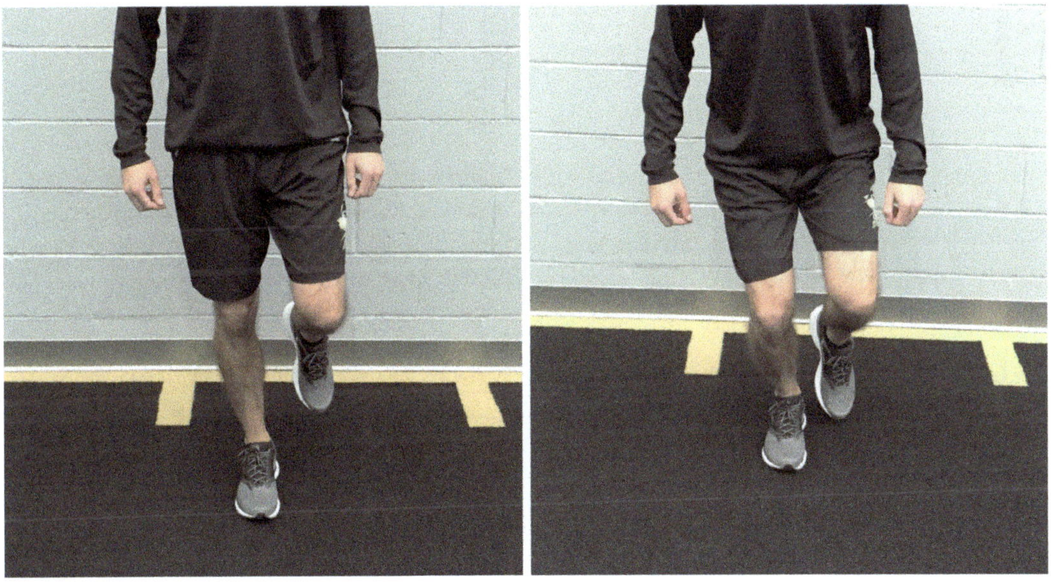

Fig. 33.3 Single-leg squat. Patients must perform ten consecutive single-leg squats to 45° of knee flexion without loss of balance, abnormal trunk movement, Trendelenburg sign, femoral IR, or the knee deviating medially causing the tibial tuberosity to cross an imaginary vertical line over the medial border of the foot

step and hold is a low-level approximation of running to screen for abnormal mechanics and pain. The individual steps from the uninjured limb onto the injured limb, at least the distance of the individual's normal stride length. The individual is cued to imagine they are stepping over a puddle of water and to land with a heel-toe gait pattern to simulate walking and progressing the distance to prepare for running without excessive stiffening or excessive knee flexion (Fig. 33.2: step and hold). The single-leg squat is performed to the appropriate prescribed angle of knee flexion for ten repetitions to screen for deviations (Fig. 33.3: single-leg squat). Deviations are operationally defined as the use of compensatory patterns including loss of balance, contralateral hip drop, excessive femoral abduction or adduction, excessive femoral internal rotation (IR), or abnormal trunk movement. Progression to phases 3, 4, and 5 requires the individual to complete the single-leg squat with additional weight to increase the challenge. The limb symmetry index

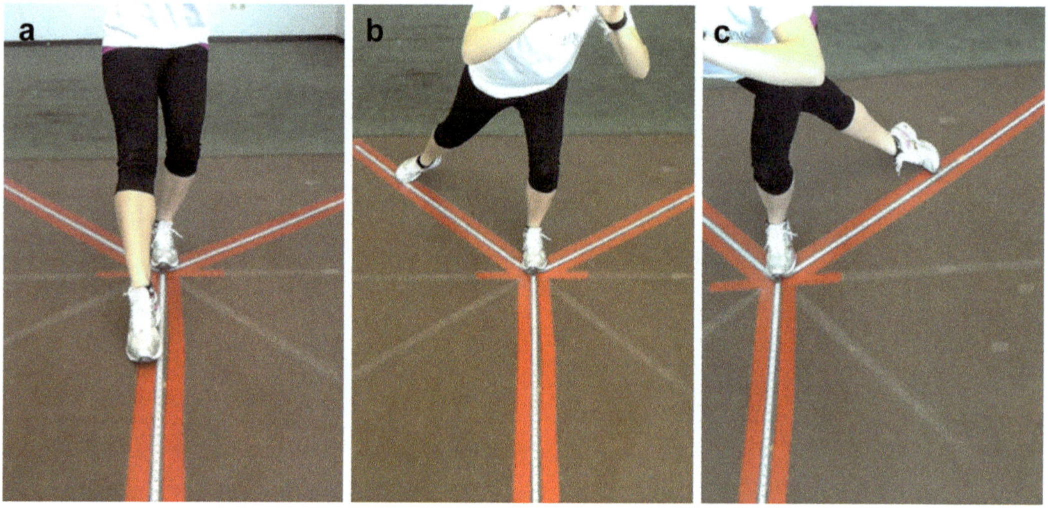

Fig. 33.4 Y-balance test. The individual stands with the toe of the testing foot at the center of the Y and reaches as far along each point as possible without transferring weight to the reach limb. (**a**) Anterior reach on the right leg; (**b**) posteromedial reach on the right leg; (**c**) posterolateral reach on the right leg

for the single-leg squat is expressed as the ratio of external weight tolerated during the involved single-leg squat compared to the external weight tolerated during the uninvolved single-leg squat (body weight is excluded).

$$\text{LSI} = \text{Weight held on involved} / \text{weight held on uninvolved}$$

The Y-balance test is a measure of stability between limbs [11]. The individual stands with their toe at the center of a "Y" made of tape on the floor. The stem of the Y faces forward, with the two arms at 135° clockwise and counterclockwise. The individual reaches as far along each point as possible with the opposite leg while not shifting any weight to the limb that is reaching (Fig. 33.4: Y-balance test). Two practice trials and two measured trials are completed. The distance is measured from the center of the Y in centimeters, with the maximum reach in each direction used for comparison. Reach distances are normalized to leg length measured from the inferior aspect of the anterior superior iliac spine to the most prominent aspect of the lateral malleolus. Comparisons are made for each reach distance and a composite reach distance with progressively strict criteria to progress between phases. The Y-balance test correlates with future injury risk and provides an inter-limb comparison of limits of stability [27].

$$\text{Y balance composite score} = \frac{(\text{Anterior reach} + \text{posteromedial reach} + \text{posterolateral reach})}{(3 \times \text{limb length})}$$

33.5 The UPMC Center for Sports Medicine Functional Training and Return-to-Sport Rehabilitation Protocol

The following sections outline the various phases of the functional training and return-to-sport program. The functional testing criteria and forms can be found in Tables 33.1 and 33.2.

33.5.1 Phase 2: Running

The return to running allows individuals a controlled environment to begin dynamically loading their reconstructed limb. The functional testing to determine readiness to begin running typically occurs between 4 and 5 months after surgery, depending on surgeon preference and surgical factors (graft, concomitant procedures). This

Table 33.2 Post-op ACL reconstruction return-to-sport test

Hop tests	Involved limb performance	Uninvolved limb performance	Limb symmetry index (≥90 % to pass)
Single-leg forward hop			
Single-leg triple hop			
Single-leg triple crossover			
Timed 6-m single leg			
Single-leg vertical hop			
Single broad jump, single-leg landing			
Triple broad jump, single-leg landing			
Single-leg lateral hop			
Single-leg medial hop			
Single-leg medial rotating hop			
Single-leg lateral rotating hop			
Functional runs	**Patient performance**	**Recommended range for males**	**Recommended range for females**
10-yard lower extremity functional test[a]		**18–22 s**	**20–24 s**
Trial 1			
Trial 2			
10-yard pro-agility run[b]		**4.5–6.0 s**	**5.2–6.5 s**
Toward injured limb			
Toward uninjured limb			

[a]Lower extremity functional test
Sprint/backpedal, shuffle, carioca, and sprint
Must perform at perceived full speed and not display hesitation or compensation strategies when decelerating
[b]10-yard pro-agility test
Must perform at perceived full speed and not display hesitation or compensation strategies when decelerating
Criteria to return to practice
MD clearance.
Pass return-to-sport test with ≥90 % results for each test.
Criteria to return to competition
MD clearance.
Tolerate full practice sessions with opposition and contact (if applicable) performed at 100 % effort without any increased pain, increased effusion, warmth, or episodes of giving way.

conservative time frame for beginning running is based on the best available data for healing time frames and is later than has been previously suggested. Mastery of phase 1 is assessed with a measurement of range of motion, effusion, and gait in a demanding scenario. Individuals must have range of motion symmetrical to the uninvolved limb and a trace or less effusion. Gait is assessed during a maximal treadmill walk for 15 min at speed short of jogging (individual still demonstrates a double-support phase) with a physical therapist observing the patient to assess for gait deviations including decreased stride length, contralateral pelvic drop, femoral internal rotation, and medial collapse of the knees. This is tested first to induce fatigue for the other tests. The neuromuscular control tests include 30 step and holds and 10 consecutive single-leg squats on the involved leg to at least 45° of knee flexion without compensatory patterns. The individual must also demonstrate a Y-balance test composite score of at least 90 %. Finally, the individual must demonstrate 80 % quadriceps strength symmetry on an isometric dynamometer or by means of both a 1-RM leg press and a 1-RM leg extension. If individuals do not pass any of the five tests, treatment continues with a focus on the remaining deficits.

Fact Box 1: Criteria to Start Jogging at 4–6 Months Post-op

- No abnormal gait patterns while walking as fast as they can on the treadmill for 15 min
- 30 step and holds without loss of balance or excessive motion outside of the sagittal plane
- Ten consecutive single-leg squats to 45° of knee flexion without loss of balance, abnormal trunk movement, Trendelenburg sign, femoral IR, or the knee deviating medially causing the tibial tuberosity to cross an imaginary vertical line over the medial border of the foot
- ≥80 % 1-repetition maximum (1-RM) on the leg press (90–0°)
- ≥80 % 1-repetition maximum (1-RM) on the knee extension machine (90–45°)
- ≥90 % composite score on Y-balance test

When the individual passes these tests without pain, increased effusion, or signs and symptoms of inflammation, they will be directed to the surgeon for final clearance to begin a jogging progression. Alternating periods of walking and jogging are implemented with progressive increases in distance (see example in Adams 2012 [1]). The authors advocate a distance-based progression over a time-based progression to more accurately control the load experienced by the knee joint. The individual should complete at least three sessions of running on a treadmill under the supervision of their physical therapist to monitor for compensatory patterns. When an appropriate gait pattern is consistently observed, the individual can complete the running progression independently. When the individual can run 2 miles consecutively without increased inflammation, testing for progression to phase 3 can occur.

33.5.2 Phase 3: Basic Agility Drills

Fact Box 2: Criteria to Start Agility Training

- ≥85 % 1-RM on the leg press (90–0°).
- ≥85 % 1-RM on the knee extension machine (90–0°) or Biodex testing if available.
- Ten consecutive single-leg squats >45° of knee flexion without loss of balance, abnormal trunk movement, Trendelenburg sign, femoral IR, or the knee deviating medially causing the tibial tuberosity to cross an imaginary vertical line over the medial border of the foot while holding ≥ 75 % extra weight compared to the other side

(dumbbells, weight vest, etc.). Body weight is not part of the equation.
- 100 % composite score on Y-balance test.
- Be able to run 2 miles continuously without pain, swelling, warmth, or gait deviations.

To demonstrate mastery of phase 2, the individual must run 2 miles continuously without any complaints of pain, without signs or symptoms of inflammation, and without gait deviations. Neuromuscular control is tested with ten consecutive weighted single-leg squats to 45° of knee flexion without aberrant movements with a limb symmetry index of at least 75 % and a Y-balance test with a composite score of at least 100 %. Individuals must also demonstrate an 85 % LSI on 1-RM leg extension and 1-RM leg press.

Basic agility drills include forward/backward shuttle running, side shuffling, carioca (lateral shuffling while crossing your trail leg over the lead leg), and "quick feet" drills using a ladder or hurdles in forward and lateral directions. Deceleration with hip and knee flexion to absorb the load for direction changes is emphasized when running and preparing to change directions. Effort begins at approximately 50 % speed and continues at that level until the individual can complete the drills without hesitation or compensation during deceleration to change directions. The individual should initially perform the agility progression under the supervision of their physical therapist or athletic trainer to monitor movement patterns. When the individual demonstrates acceptable performance and reports full confidence decelerating on the involved leg, they can complete the progression independently, with weekly to biweekly monitoring from their physical therapist.

33.5.3 Stage 4: Double-Limb Jumping

To demonstrate mastery of low-level agility drills, the individual must complete forward/backward shuffling, side shuffling, carioca, and ladder drills at full speed without compensation patterns. Individuals must also demonstrate neuromuscular control by performing ten consecutive weighted single-leg squats to at least 60° of knee flexion with a limb symmetry index of at least 85 % and demonstrate an improved quadriceps strength symmetry of a 90 % LSI.

Fact Box 3: Criteria to Start Jumping

- ≥90 % 1-RM on the leg press (90–0°).
- ≥90 % 1-RM on the knee extension machine (90–0°) or Biodex testing if available.
- Ten consecutive single-leg squats to 60° of knee flexion without loss of balance, abnormal trunk movement, Trendelenburg sign, femoral IR, or the knee deviating medially causing the tibial tuberosity to cross an imaginary vertical line over the medial border of the foot while holding ≥ 85 % extra weight compared to the other side (dumbbells, weight vest, etc.). Body weight is not part of the equation.
- No compensation patterns with deceleration during agility drills performed at near 100 % effort.

The individual begins with forward jumps and jumps onto a box. Cues are given to emphasize avoiding dynamic valgus, to exaggerate hip and knee flexion, and equally distribute weight on both extremities when loading into the jump and landing [8, 14, 19, 25]. When the individual demonstrates good form with forward jumps, they will progress with lateral jumps and rotational jumps. When the individual demonstrates good technique for jumping onto a box, they will progress to jumps off of the box. Lastly, the individual will progress from single jumps where they have to reset each time to consecutive rebounding jumps, both from the floor and from the box to the floor. Jumping drills are initiated in the clinic under supervision and progressed in weekly to biweekly follow-ups with independent practice at home.

33.5.4 Phase 5: Single-Limb Hopping and Cutting and Sport-Specific Drills

Fact Box 4: Criteria to Start Hopping and Cutting

- Ten consecutive single-leg squats to 60° without loss of balance, abnormal trunk movement, Trendelenburg sign, femoral IR, or the knee deviating medially causing the tibial tuberosity to cross an imaginary vertical line over the medial border of the foot while holding ≥ 90 % extra weight compared to the other side (dumbbells, weight vest, etc.). Body weight is not part of the equation.
- No display of medial collapse of the knees when loading into or landing from jumps and equal weight distribution when initiating and landing the jumps.

To demonstrate mastery of double-limb jumping, individuals must not display any compensatory patterns with jumping, with particular attention being paid to loading into and out of the jump symmetrically and without medial collapse of the knee. To demonstrate neuromuscular control, individuals must perform ten consecutive weighted single-leg squats to at least 60° of knee flexion with a limb symmetry index of at least 90 % and demonstrate quadriceps strength symmetry of at least 90 % LSI.

Hopping follows the same progression as jumping in phase 4 – single forward hops on the floor and onto a box, progressing to hops out of the sagittal plane and multiple hops. For cutting activities, individuals should first practice running in an "S" pattern or a figure 8, then progress to 45° cuts, and then to sharper angle cuts. Pivoting should begin when the individual is competent with cutting at sharp angles. As with low-level agility drills, confidence and performance dictate the speed of cutting and pivoting drills, and the individual should not progress with high-level cutting and pivoting drills if they demonstrate compensation patterns or express decreased confidence at higher speeds [7]. Individuals should be able to tolerate controlled cutting and pivoting at full speed before practicing unanticipated cutting and sport-specific movements. Once the individual is familiar with all agility, plyometric, and cutting exercises, rehabilitation will solely focus on the specific demands needed to return to sport.

33.5.5 Return to Practice Testing and Return to Sports

Return to practice testing can occur when the individual can run and perform all agility, plyometric, and sport-specific drills without any hesitation, without compensatory patterns, and with no complaints of increased pain or instability or display of any signs or symptoms of inflammation. The return-to-sport test (Table 33.2) includes a strength assessment, functional testing for symmetrical performance, and functional testing for running situations. Individuals must demonstrate a 90 % quadriceps LSI to pass the return-to-sport test. Functional testing follows the strength assessment.

33.6 Objective Functional Symmetry Testing

Unilateral hop tests mimic the demands of sport participation in a controlled setting allowing for assessment of performance and movement quality. As normative data for these tests are sparse [31], the uninjured limb is consistently used as a benchmark for performance of the reconstructed limb [12, 13, 16, 17, 22, 24]. Limb symmetry indexes of 85 % [5], 90 % [12, 13, 16, 17, 22], and even 95–100 % [31, 32] are used to indicate "normal" or symmetrical performance and for clearance to return to sports. However, none of these cutoffs have been determined to accurately predict the ability to safely return to sports after ACLR and are thus based on expert opinion.

The most common testing involves the single hop for distance [4, 10] although recommendations for and the use of functional testing batteries are becoming more prevalent [12, 13, 16, 17,

22, 31, 32]. For clinics without the benefit of electromechanical dynamometry, unilateral hop tests correlate with quadriceps strength [16, 17] and are affected by quadriceps strength [30]. However these relationships are not strong enough to allow for the use of the hop tests to replace isolated testing of quadriceps strength because hop tests at best only account for approximately 50 % of the variation in quadriceps strength. In addition to measuring performance for potential return to sport, early functional testing at the 6-month time frame is predictive of those individuals who will self-report normal knee function at 1-year follow-up [16].

The use of multiple hop tests including maximal hop tests (for distance or height) and exertional hop tests (for time) presents a comprehensive and robust measurement of individual performance [31]. The most frequently used hop test battery involves four tests – the single hop for distance, the triple hop for distance, the triple crossover hop for distance, and the timed six-meter hop [6, 9, 24, 28]. All of the distance hops begin and end in single-limb stance on the limb being tested in a controlled manner, without using excessive balance reactions. The single hop involves one maximal hop. The triple hop involves three consecutive hops for maximum distance. The triple crossover hop includes three consecutive hops where the individual must land outside of two parallel lines spaced 15 cm apart. Individuals must not pause between hops on the triple or crossover hops. Performance is evaluated by normalizing the performance of the involved limb to the uninvolved limb and expressing the ratio as a percentage, termed the limb symmetry index (LSI). The timed six-meter hop requires the individual to hop as quickly as possible down a six-meter course on a single limb in as many or as few hops as needed. The landing is not controlled after the completion of the six-meter course. Because the uninvolved limb is expected to move the individual more rapidly down the line, the uninvolved limb is expressed as a percentage of the involved limb to maintain the convention that scores less than 100 % indicate superior performance of the uninvolved limb.

Functional muscular power is tested with a single-limb vertical hop test. The individual stands next to a wall and jumps as high as possible from one limb, using their preferred countermovement strategy. The landing is uncontrolled, but monitored for compensations. The individual attempts to jump as high as possible, with height measured by either having the individual put a piece of tape on the wall or using a Vertec System (Gill Athletics, Champaign, IL) to measure jump height. Limb performance is expressed as a ratio of the best recorded jump height of three trials on the reconstructed limb compared to the contralateral limb.

Individuals must demonstrate limb symmetry indices of at least 90 % on these five hop tests to pass. An LSI threshold of 90 % is used as opposed to 95 % or 100 % as recommended by the European Sports Rehabilitation Board [31] as these thresholds may be too stringent and prevent returning to practice with symmetry levels that are in normal ranges.

33.7 Novel Functional Symmetry Testing

In addition to previously established hop tests, the authors are implementing additional hop tests to investigate any additional benefits for determining readiness for return to sport and prediction of future injury. The single-legged medial, lateral, and rotating hops are used to challenge stability in the frontal and transverse planes. The medial and lateral hop tests place additional varus and valgus stresses on the knee joint and may provide a perspective on the ability of the individual to control motion under much higher frontal plane loads. Distance is measured as the maximum distance hopped on each limb, and a limb symmetry index is calculated. The rotating hop places a large rotational moment on the knee and should be performed first in a clockwise direction for the right knee and a counterclockwise direction for the left knee as these will less mimic the position of injury. Upon successful completion of those rotating hops, the directions can be reversed as a more challenging test. Performance is measured by using a goniometer to measure the change in angle from the starting position. These tests are not as directly related to competition and performance as the functional hop series; however, they provide an additional standardized method of evaluating movement quality and side-to-side symmetry. The neuromuscular control risk factors of impaired postural stability and frontal and transverse collapse (dynamic valgus) can be observed in these tests to monitor deficits and identify areas for further rehabilitation. The final two tests are a single and triple jump, where the patient must land on one foot. A single and triple broad jump allows for more power development, and we are testing the ability of the involved leg to control that landing. Threshold values of at least 90 % LSI are encouraged for these tests as well.

33.8 General Functional Agility Testing

Agility tests during the course of rehabilitation give clinical insight into gross movement patterns and glaring asymmetries; however, they are not sensitive enough to establish limb asymmetries that are present during unilateral testing [22]. In the final return-to-sport test, individuals complete two functional runs that focus on quickness, confidence when making directional changes, and quality of movement. The lower extremity functional run (Fig. 33.5a) is set up on a 10-yard course marked by two cones. The athlete begins with a 10-yard sprint followed by a 10-yard backpedal, a 10-yard side shuffle in each direction, and a 10-yard carioca in each direction and ends with a final 10-yard sprint. The pro-agility test (Fig. 33.5b) begins with the individual straddling the centerline of a 10-yard course marked by three cones each 5 yards apart. The athlete must sprint five yards and touch the cone, change direction, sprint back 10 yards and touch the cone, change direction, and sprint back through the centerline. The timer begins with the athlete's first movement to either end of the course and ends with the final crossing of the centerline. Suggested cutoff times are available; however, as bilateral functional tests do not differentiate unilateral deficits, these two functional runs are included for the therapist to evaluate movement quality and direction changes.

When individuals demonstrate 90 % limb symmetry and demonstrate good movement quality with agility tests, they return to their physician for final clearance to return to practice. When individuals return to practice, they again follow a progression specific to their sport and timeline. Individuals typically begin practice with unopposed drills with sport-specific movements and general conditioning. When their unopposed performance is sufficient per the discretion of the coach and athletic trainer, individuals can begin controlled contact drills. Lastly, individuals can return to full intra-squad scrimmaging. Individuals return to their physician for full return to competition clearance when they can practice at 100 % effort (with contact if applicable) and have no complaints of pain or signs and symptoms of inflammation.

33.9 Conclusion

This guideline for functional testing and progression has been developed to be patient specific in light of the best available evidence concerning healing of the reconstructed ACL with consideration for both modifiable and nonmodifiable risk factors. The focus is on consistent implementation of functional tests to provide clear goals for the individual and therapists to pursue while eliminating some of the uncertainty that surrounds the return to activity decision. We are currently testing this protocol to determine areas of inconsistency and insufficiency.

33.9.1 Clinical Recommendations with Strength of Recommendation Taxonomy (SORT) Grades

Grade C. A progression through multiple phases of increasing difficulty should be implemented and progressed based on strength, neuromuscular control, and task mastery to improve return to sports after ACL reconstruction.

Grade C. Comprehensive physical testing to identify limb symmetry in strength and performance should be used as the final test to

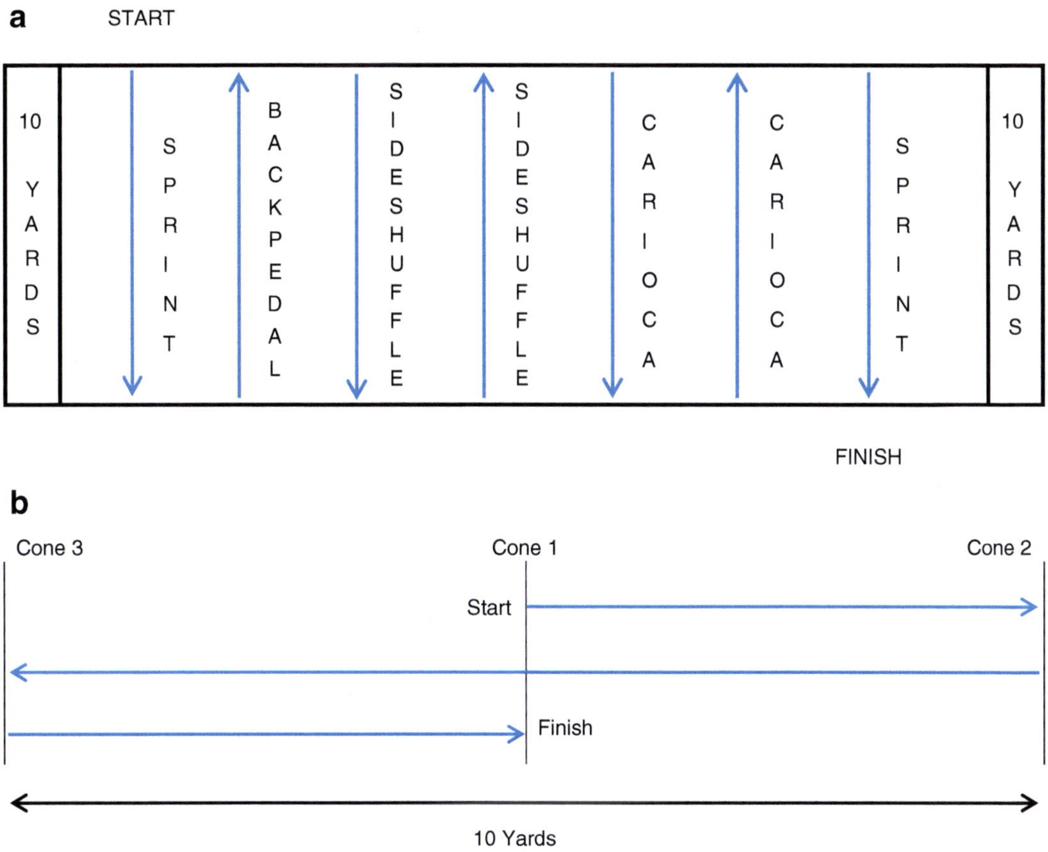

Fig. 33.5 General functional agility runs. (**a**) Lower extremity functional run. Patients will sprint 10 yards and then backpedal to the starting line, side-shuffle 10 yards and back, carioca 10 yards and back, and finally sprint 10 yards to the finish line. To pass this test, patients must run and change direction at full speed without any compensation patterns. (**b**) Pro-agility test. Patients will start facing the tester straddling cone 1. When indicated, they will turn and sprint 5 yards and touch cone 2; then sprint 10 yards and touch cone 3; and finally, sprint 5 yards past cone 1. They will then repeat this test in reverse order (cones 1–3 to 2–1). To pass this test, patients must run and change direction at full speed without any compensation patterns

clear individuals for returning to practice after ACL reconstruction.

Grade C. Assessment of task mastery and movement quality should be included in all assessments to provide a general impression of risk for injury.

References

1. Adams D, Logerstedt D, Hunter-Giordano A, Axe MJ, Snyder-Mackler L (2012) Current concepts for anterior cruciate ligament reconstruction: a criterion-based rehabilitation progression. J Orthop Sports Phys Ther 42(7):601–614
2. Angelozzi M, Madama M, Corsica C et al (2012) Rate of force development as an adjunctive outcome measure for return-to-sport decisions after anterior cruciate ligament reconstruction. J Orthop Sports Phys Ther 42(9):772–780
3. Augustsson J, Thomee R, Karlsson J (2004) Ability of a new hop test to determine functional deficits after anterior cruciate ligament reconstruction. Knee Surg Sports Traumatol Arthrosc 12(5):350–356
4. Barber-Westin SD, Noyes FR (2011) Factors used to determine return to unrestricted sports activities after anterior cruciate ligament reconstruction. Arthroscopy 27(12):1697–1705
5. Barber SD, Noyes FR, Mangine RE, McCloskey JW, Hartman W (1990) Quantitative assessment of functional limitations in normal and anterior cruciate ligament-deficient knees. Clin Orthop Relat Res 255:204–214

6. Cascio BM, Culp L, Cosgarea AJ (2004) Return to play after anterior cruciate ligament reconstruction. Clin Sports Med 23(3):395–408, ix
7. Chmielewski TL, Jones D, Day T, Tillman SM, Lentz TA, George SZ (2008) The association of pain and fear of movement/reinjury with function during anterior cruciate ligament reconstruction rehabilitation. J Orthop Sports Phys Ther 38(12):746–753
8. Di Stasi S, Myer GD, Hewett TE (2013) Neuromuscular training to target deficits associated with second anterior cruciate ligament injury. J Orthop Sports Phys Ther 43(11):777–792, A1–11
9. Fitzgerald GK, Axe MJ, Snyder-Mackler L (2000) Proposed practice guidelines for nonoperative anterior cruciate ligament rehabilitation of physically active individuals. J Orthop Sports Phys Ther 30(4):194–203
10. Frobell RB, Roos HP, Roos EM, Roemer FW, Ranstam J, Lohmander LS (2013) Treatment for acute anterior cruciate ligament tear: five year outcome of randomised trial. BMJ 346:f232 (Clinical research ed)
11. Gribble PA, Hertel J, Plisky P (2012) Using the Star Excursion Balance Test to assess dynamic postural-control deficits and outcomes in lower extremity injury: a literature and systematic review. J Athl Train 47(3):339–351
12. Grindem H, Logerstedt D, Eitzen I et al (2011) Single-legged hop tests as predictors of self-reported knee function in nonoperatively treated individuals with anterior cruciate ligament injury. Am J Sports Med 39(11):2347–2354
13. Hartigan EH, Axe MJ, Snyder-Mackler L (2012) Time line for noncopers to pass return-to-sports criteria after anterior cruciate ligament reconstruction. J Orthop Sports Phys Ther 40(3):141–154
14. Hewett TE, Di Stasi SL, Myer GD (2013) Current concepts for injury prevention in athletes after anterior cruciate ligament reconstruction. Am J Sports Med 41(1):216–224
15. Hewett TE, Myer GD, Ford KR, Paterno MV, Quatman CE (2012) The 2012 ABJS Nicolas Andry Award: the sequence of prevention: a systematic approach to prevent anterior cruciate ligament injury. Clin Orthop Relat Res 470(10):2930–2940
16. Logerstedt D, Grindem H, Lynch A et al (2012) Single-legged hop tests as predictors of self-reported knee function after anterior cruciate ligament reconstruction: the Delaware-Oslo ACL cohort study. Am J Sports Med 40(10):2348–2356
17. Logerstedt D, Lynch A, Axe MJ, Snyder-Mackler L (2013) Symmetry restoration and functional recovery before and after anterior cruciate ligament reconstruction. Knee Surg Sports Traumatol Arthrosc 21(4):859–868
18. Lynch AD, Logerstedt DS, Grindem H et al (2013) Consensus criteria for defining 'successful outcome' after ACL injury and reconstruction: a Delaware-Oslo ACL cohort investigation. Br J Sports Med 23
19. Mandelbaum BR, Silvers HJ, Watanabe DS et al (2005) Effectiveness of a neuromuscular and proprioceptive training program in preventing anterior cruciate ligament injuries in female athletes: 2-year follow-up. Am J Sports Med 33(7):1003–1010
20. Myer GD, Ford KR, Brent JL, Hewett TE (2012) An integrated approach to change the outcome part II: targeted neuromuscular training techniques to reduce identified ACL injury risk factors. J Strength Cond Res 26(8):2272–2292
21. Myer GD, Paterno MV, Ford KR, Quatman CE, Hewett TE (2006) Rehabilitation after anterior cruciate ligament reconstruction: criteria-based progression through the return-to-sport phase. J Orthop Sports Phys Ther 36(6):385–402
22. Myer GD, Schmitt LC, Brent JL et al (2011) Utilization of modified NFL combine testing to identify functional deficits in athletes following ACL reconstruction. J Orthop Sports Phys Ther 41(6):377–387
23. Neeter C, Gustavsson A, Thomee P, Augustsson J, Thomee R, Karlsson J (2006) Development of a strength test battery for evaluating leg muscle power after anterior cruciate ligament injury and reconstruction. Knee Surg Sports Traumatol Arthrosc 14(6): 571–580
24. Noyes FR, Barber SD, Mangine RE (1991) Abnormal lower limb symmetry determined by function hop tests after anterior cruciate ligament rupture. Am J Sports Med 19(5):513–518
25. Paterno MV, Schmitt LC, Ford KR et al (2010) Biomechanical measures during landing and postural stability predict second anterior cruciate ligament injury after anterior cruciate ligament reconstruction and return to sport. Am J Sports Med 38(10): 1968–1978
26. Piva SR, Childs JD, Klucinec BM, Irrgang JJ, Almeida GJ, Fitzgerald GK (2009) Patella fracture during rehabilitation after bone-patellar tendon-bone anterior cruciate ligament reconstruction: 2 case reports. J Orthop Sports Phys Ther 39(4):278–286
27. Plisky PJ, Rauh MJ, Kaminski TW, Underwood FB (2006) Star Excursion Balance Test as a predictor of lower extremity injury in high school basketball players. J Orthop Sports Phys Ther 36(12): 911–919
28. Reid A, Birmingham TB, Stratford PW, Alcock GK, Giffin JR (2007) Hop testing provides a reliable and valid outcome measure during rehabilitation after anterior cruciate ligament reconstruction. Phys Ther 87(3):337–349
29. Risberg MA, Holm I, Myklebust G, Engebretsen L (2007) Neuromuscular training versus strength training during first 6 months after anterior cruciate ligament reconstruction: a randomized clinical trial. Phys Ther 87(6):737–750
30. Schmitt LC, Paterno MV, Hewett TE (2012) The impact of quadriceps femoris strength asymmetry on functional performance at return to sport following anterior cruciate ligament reconstruction. J Orthop Sports Phys Ther 42(9):750–759

31. Thomee R, Kaplan Y, Kvist J et al (2011) Muscle strength and hop performance criteria prior to return to sports after ACL reconstruction. Knee Surg Sports Traumatol Arthrosc 19(11):1798–1805
32. Thomee R, Neeter C, Gustavsson A et al (2012) Variability in leg muscle power and hop performance after anterior cruciate ligament reconstruction. Knee Surg Sports Traumatol Arthrosc 20(6):1143–1151
33. Wilk KE, Reinold MM, Hooks TR (2003) Recent advances in the rehabilitation of isolated and combined anterior cruciate ligament injuries. Orthop Clin North Am 34(1):107–137

Return to Sport following ACL Reconstruction: The Australian Experience

34

Kate E. Webster, Julian A. Feller, and Timothy S. Whitehead

Contents

K.E. Webster, PhD
School of Allied Health, La Trobe University, Melbourne, VIC, Australia

J.A. Feller, MBBS, FRACS
Department of Orthopaedic Surgery, OrthoSport Victoria, Epworth HealthCare, Melbourne, VIC, Australia

School of Allied Health, La Trobe University, Melbourne, VIC, Australia

T.S. Whitehead, MBBS, FRACS (✉)
Department of Orthopaedic Surgery, OrthoSport Victoria, Epworth HealthCare, Melbourne, VIC, Australia
e-mail: tswhitehead@osv.com.au

34.1 Introduction

Return to sport has become an important outcome measure following anterior cruciate ligament (ACL) reconstruction surgery. A group of researchers based in Melbourne, Australia, has been interested in return to sport as an outcome since 2002 and has published widely on the topic [1, 3–8, 14, 18, 19, 31]. This chapter summarises the work of this group and also data from other centres in Australia. Since the authors of the chapter are all members of the Melbourne-based research group, studies emanating from the group are frequently referred to in the first person.

Return to sport following ACL reconstruction has been routinely recorded by the Melbourne researchers since 2002. Initially, the question was whether patients who had been playing high-impact sports prior to injury successfully returned to these sports following their surgery. Anecdotally, we had noted that a number of our patients had not returned to their pre-injury sport when they returned for review at 12 months, and we felt this warranted further exploration. The results of this investigation confirmed our impression and indeed showed a relatively low rate of return to pre-injury sport despite the surgery being apparently otherwise successful [8]. This initial investigation is described in detail in the following section, along with subsequent studies from our group regarding return to sport after primary and revision ACL reconstruction.

V. Musahl et al. (eds.), *Rotatory Knee Instability*, DOI 10.1007/978-3-319-32070-0_34

In order to put our research into context, we also conducted a systematic review of the published literature and performed meta-analyses to determine the rate of return to any kind of sports participation, as well as the rates of return to pre-injury and competitive sports following ACL reconstruction [7]. We evaluated 48 studies that reported on outcomes in 5,770 patients at a mean follow-up of 42 months. Overall, 82 % of patients returned to some kind of sport, but only 63 % were participating in their pre-injury sport at follow-up. When competitive sport was considered, only 44 % were participating at follow-up. These participation rates were in contrast to the finding that around 90 % of patients were rated normal or nearly normal on impairment-based outcomes, such as strength and knee laxity.

This review was updated in 2014 to include a total of 69 studies reporting on 7,556 patients [4]. In the update, 81 % returned to some kind of sport, 65 % returned to their pre-injury sport, and 55 % returned to competitive sport. The larger data set allowed us to explore the influence of key background factors, such as age, gender, and pre-injury sports participation level. Our results showed that being younger, male, and playing at an elite level of sport all favoured a return to pre-injury-level sport. Results in terms of graft type were mixed with hamstring tendon autografts favouring a return to competitive sport at various levels and patellar tendon autografts favouring a return to pre-injury sport, although this discrepancy may reflect definitions and terminology used in different studies. Having a positive psychological response was also shown to be strongly associated with a return to pre-injury sport, and this is another area in which our group has published widely [1, 5, 18, 19, 31].

Fact Box 1

In a 2014 systematic review, the rates of return to some kind of sport and to pre-injury sport following ACL reconstruction were 81 % and 65 %, respectively.

This chapter is in three sections: in the first, we describe in detail the results of the return to sport studies conducted in Melbourne, Australia; in the second, the wider Australian literature is presented; and in the third, the Melbourne work in terms of the psychological impact of returning to sport is discussed.

34.2 The Melbourne Return to Sport Experience

34.2.1 Return to Sport Following Primary ACL Reconstruction

We have conducted a number of studies on return to sport following ACL reconstruction [3–8]. Two studies investigated return to sport at two different time points in patients who had undergone primary ACL reconstruction surgery by a single surgeon. The two patient cohorts were slightly different, but were both active in sport prior to their ACL injury.

The first study [8] involved 503 patients (68 % male, 32 % female, mean age of 26 at the time of surgery) who participated in competitive-level Australian rules football, basketball, netball, or soccer prior to their ACL injury. The four sports represented the most common setting for an ACL injury in the local population, and all are demanding sports from the point of view of ACL injury. The most common two sports played prior to injury were Australian rules football (39 %) and netball (24 %). Eighty-six per cent of patients sustained their ACL injury during an organised league game, 12 % during recreational sport and 2 % in nonsporting activities.

The patient group was derived from a total of 1201 primary ACL reconstructions using autologous hamstring tendons performed by a single surgeon over a 5-year period. Of these patients, 88 % returned for follow-up examination at 12 months. In general, patients were advised that they could resume training for their sport from 6 months postoperatively and return to play at 9–10 months from surgery, providing their recovery had been uncomplicated.

The 12-month follow-up examination included a custom-designed self-report questionnaire, which covered information regarding the main sport played before injury and the level of competition in which the patient was involved when the injury occurred, as well as postoperative sports participation and the patient's plans regarding return to sport. Specifically, the patients were asked whether they had attempted to play their main sport following surgery. The response options were: not at all, training and/or modified competition, or full competition. Patients who had not attempted full competition postoperatively were asked to indicate whether they planned to return to their main sport. The response options for intentions regarding return to sport were: yes, unable to play or have given up sport because of my knee, or have given up sport or not been able to return to sport for reasons other than my knee.

Clinical data collected and used in the analysis included the International Knee Documentation Committee (IKDC) knee evaluation form, single-limb hop for distance, and triple crossover hop.

At the 12-month follow-up, one-third of patients had attempted full competition and one-third had attempted training or modified competition. The remaining third had not attempted to play sport or train. Males were more likely than females to have attempted full competition. There were no differences in terms of attempting full competition between those patients who rated highly on IKDC and those who did not. However, patients with a hop test limb symmetry index of greater than 85 % were more likely to have attempted full competition than those with a limb symmetry index of less than 85 %.

Fact Box 2

In a study of athletes competing in team ball sport prior to their ACL injury, only one-third had returned to pre-injury competitive sport at 12 months following their ACL reconstruction. Another one-third had returned to training or competition at a lower level.

Half of the patients who had not attempted full competition indicated that they were planning to return to sport. Twelve per cent had stopped participating in sport for reasons other than the knee, 13 % had given up sport because of their knee function, and 25 % did not report whether they intended to return to competitive sport.

Given the high number of patients who indicated that they still intended returning to their competition sport, it was concluded that patients may require more than 12 months to make a return to competitive sport after ACL reconstruction. The reasons for this, however, were unclear.

In the second study [3], the patient cohort was derived from the same 1201 patients who had undergone primary hamstring tendon ACL reconstruction by one surgeon over a 5-year period. The inclusion criteria for this study were different from the first study. To be eligible, patients must have had surgery at least 2 years previously, received clearance to return to play from the treating surgeon, attended a routine 12-month follow-up, and been participating in sport at least twice per week before their ACL injury. In other words, this group included patients who were potentially a little less active in sport than the first study (as they were not required to have been participating in competitive sport in order to be included).

Of 533 patients who met the inclusion criteria, 59 % (314) participated in the study. There were more females in this cohort than in the first study – 42 % compared with 32 %. The mean age at review was a little higher – 32.5 compared with 27 – and the mean time from surgery was 40 months. The same four sports were the most commonly played prior to injury. Sixty-three per cent of participants played at a competitive level prior to injury.

Patients completed a custom-designed self-report questionnaire. With regard to sport, they were asked whether they had attempted to play any form of sport since surgery, whether they had attempted to play their pre-injury sport, and whether they had attempted competitive sport. Participants were asked about their sports participation at any time since their surgery, as well as at the time of completing the survey. Those who had not attempted to play any sport since surgery were asked about their future intentions. Patients who indicated they had changed or reduced their level of sports participation, or ceased sport, were asked whether this was because of their operated knee or for other reasons. Patients were also asked a series of questions about knee function and symptoms.

At the time of follow-up, participants generally reported satisfactory knee function with a mean score of 87 out of a maximum of 100. Sixty-six per cent of the patients were participating in sport. Forty-five per cent were playing at their pre-injury level. The rate of return to pre-injury level of sport at final follow-up was significantly influenced by age, with participants older than 32 years being less likely to be participating at that level. Gender was not associated with the rate of return to pre-injury sport. Similarly, return to sport or not at 12 months postoperatively was not associated with longer-term participation rates.

When the rate of return to sport at *any* time since surgery was examined, higher participation rates were noted. Ninety-three per cent had played some kind of sport and 61 % had returned to their pre-injury level of sport. The same association between older age and a lower rate of return to sport was noted. Once again, gender did not appear to be an influential factor. Of those patients who had not attempted sport at their pre-injury level, 56 % indicated that they had changed their sports participation because of the function of their operated knee.

> **Fact Box 3**
> Age plays an important role in return to sport following ACL reconstruction, with older patients less likely to return to their pre-injury sport.

On the basis of these two studies, it appears that a significant proportion of patients make a return to their pre-injury sport beyond the 12-month mark but that there is a significant drop-off in participation by 4 years postoperatively. Age may play an important role. The lower participation rate of older patients may well reflect lifestyle factors.

34.2.2 Return to Sport Following Revision ACL Reconstruction

The Melbourne group has also examined rates of return to sport following revision ACL reconstruction (manuscript under review) [13]. One hundred and nine of 136 (80 %) eligible patients who had undergone their first revision ACL reconstruction over a 4-year period completed a sports activity survey at a mean 5-year follow-up (minimum 3 years).

Overall, there did not appear to be much difference between the rates of return following the revision ACL reconstruction (46 %) and following the primary procedure (50 %), although it should be noted that the rate of return to pre-injury sport after the primary surgery was lower than in the two studies described above. Of the patients who were not able to return to their pre-injury level of sport after primary reconstruction, 33 % improved to the point that they were able to do so after revision. In the majority of cases, this was felt to be due to correction of technical problems or errors in the primary surgery.

Once again, younger patients were more likely to have returned to their pre-injury level of sport, whilst the same rate of return was seen in males and females. Perhaps not surprisingly, those who returned to their pre-injury level of sport also scored higher on the Marx activity, KOOS-QOL, and IKDC subjective scores.

With regard to the status of the knee at the time of revision ACL reconstruction, patients with less than 50% thickness articular cartilage lesions were more likely to have returned to their pre-injury level and had significantly better Marx activity, KOOS-QOL, and IKDC scores at follow-up. The status of the menisci at the time of revision surgery was not associated with rates of return to sport, but patients with an intact medial meniscus had significantly higher KOOS-QOL scores at follow-up.

Overall, it appears that satisfactory rates of return to sport can be achieved following revision ACL reconstruction surgery, particularly if there is little articular cartilage damage and the medial meniscus is intact. An inability to return to sport following primary ACL reconstruction may reflect technical problems at the time of surgery. If these can be corrected at revision surgery, improved outcomes can be expected [30].

34.2.3 Return to Sport in Australian Rules Football

Australian rules football is a code of football unique to Australia. It has a high participation rate, particularly in the southern states. It is a contact and very athletic game, played on a large ground, and the demands on footballers include speed, endurance, jumping ability, and foot and hand skills. Apart from a mouthguard, no protection is worn. The game involves frequent pivoting, cutting, and landing and a player can be tackled from any direction, including from behind. As noted from the above studies, it is a frequent source of ACL injuries. The Melbourne group has looked at return to sport in both professional and nonprofessional Australian rules footballers.

In an unpublished study [14], a comprehensive questionnaire was completed by 78 patients who were a minimum of 2 years following ACL reconstruction by a single surgeon and who played Australian rules prior to injury (nonprofessionally) and indicated a desire to return to play following ACL reconstruction. Sixty-seven per cent of participants had a patellar tendon graft and 23% a hamstring tendon graft. The mean age of participants at follow-up was 29.6 years.

Eighty-eight per cent returned to competition football, with exactly the same rate for both graft types. Five subjects (6%) changed their mind about returning to football following surgery, but all indicated this was for reasons other than their operated knee. Of the other four participants who did not return to football, three indicated this was because of their operated knee. The other participant sustained an ACL rupture in the contralateral knee. Seventy-seven per cent of the players felt that the surgery had successfully enabled them to return to their previous level of football.

In a personal series of 52 primary ACL reconstructions in professional Australian rules footballers who suffered an ACL rupture whilst playing or training at the highest level (Australian Football League), the rate of return to play is even higher. At a minimum of 12 months following primary ACL reconstruction, 49 (94%) returned to play at the same level of competition. Two players retired immediately upon suffering their injury and one player who had a hamstring graft was unable to resume play at the same level due to hamstring graft site problems.

The Melbourne experience has been that the rates of return to pre-injury sport appear to be higher in professional footballers playing at the very elite level than in the more general population of patients undergoing ACL reconstruction.

Illustrations

Australian rules football

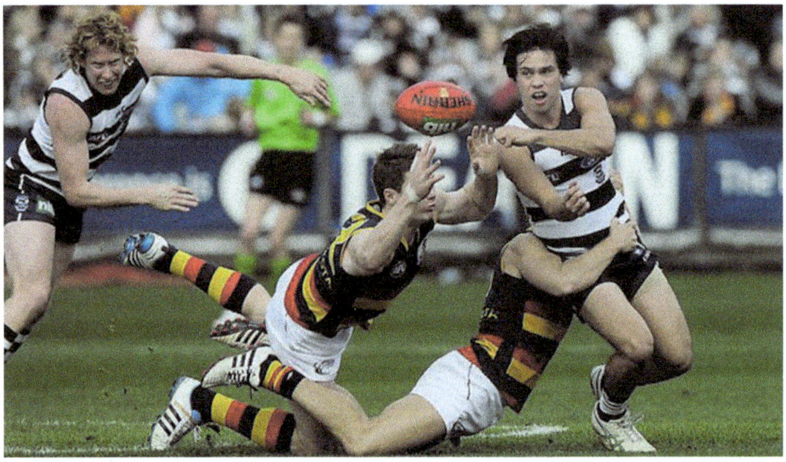

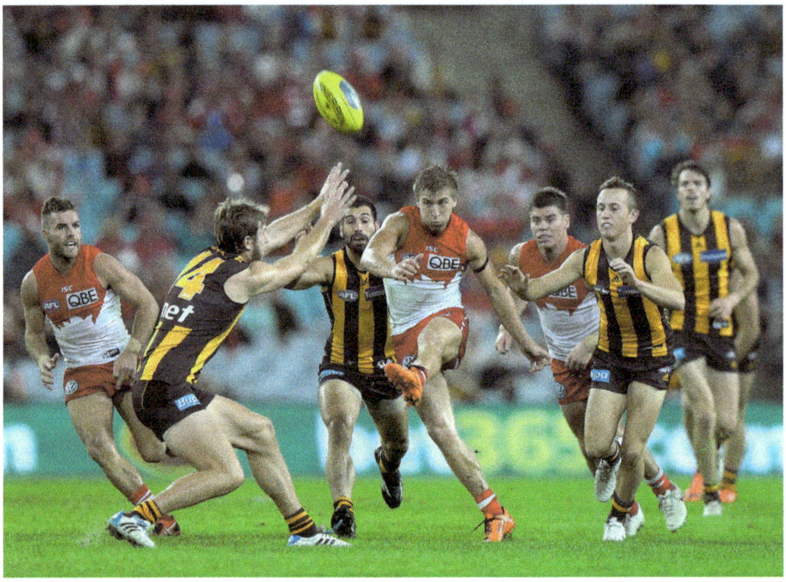

34.3 An Australian Perspective

34.3.1 Return to Sport in Australian Rules Football

Despite the high rate of return to sport in the single-surgeon series, such results have not been universally reported. Liptak and Angel [21] performed a retrospective analysis of 115 elite AFL players who underwent an ACL reconstruction (63 % patellar tendon, 34 % hamstring) between 1990 and 2000. This study examined return to play, reinjury rates, and return to previous playing competency.

Overall, 30 players (26 %) did not return to play AFL football at the elite level, whereas of the remaining 85 players (74 %), 41 (48 %) played less than 1 year following surgery and 44 (52 %) played 1 year or longer. Players were less likely to play if they were older (30 years or older), their dominant knee was injured, or they were of lighter body weight (70–79 kg). Of the

85 players that returned to play, 24 (28 %) had a further ACL injury in either their operated (16 %) or contralateral knee (12 %). The reinjury rates were higher in those who returned to play less than 1 year following surgery. Return to form was analysed by examining match day statistics prior to the ACL injury and comparing them to those at 1, 2, and 3 years following return to play. On average, most players did not return to their pre-injury level of form by 3 years, although young (17–24 years) and older (over 30 years) players demonstrated a greater drop-off in form in the first 12 months.

34.3.2 Return to Sport Following Primary ACL Reconstruction

Although no other Australian studies have examined return to sport and activity as a primary outcome measure, several have reported this as a secondary outcome measure. Most of these studies originate from the same centre and report on the long-term outcomes following an ACL reconstruction [10, 11, 20, 25–27].

Bourke et al. [11] performed a retrospective analysis of 673 patients (89 % follow-up) who had undergone an ACL reconstruction with either a patellar tendon (47 %) or quadrupled hamstring graft (53 %) at a minimum of 15 years following their surgery. There were 241 female (36 %) and 432 male (74 %) patients with a mean age of 29 years at the time of surgery. Interestingly, the rate of return to their pre-injury sporting activity was similar to those of the Melbourne group, with 73 % achieving this at some stage over the 15-year period. Gender did not influence these results. Of those who had not returned to their previous level of activity (180 patients), 71 % attributed this to their operated knee, whereas the remainder reported other reasons. Not surprisingly, activity levels deteriorated over time, with only 51 % patients participating in high-demand sport at the 15-year follow-up. This percentage was significantly higher in males (58 %). Although the type of graft did not influence the within-gender activity rates, significantly fewer female patients with a patellar tendon graft participated in high-demand activities when compared with the other three groups.

The same researchers in a separate study reported the long-term (mean 15-year follow-up) outcomes for 186 patients with an "isolated" ACL rupture who underwent ACL reconstruction using hamstring tendon autograft [10]. Several exclusion criteria were used to define an isolated ACL rupture, including significant chondral damage (any patients with full-thickness lesions were excluded), previous meniscectomy, and excision of more than one-third of either meniscus or significant meniscal root avulsion at the time of surgery. Despite these strict criteria, participation in strenuous sporting activities at 15 years' follow-up was still only 52 %. In a similar study of patients who had a reconstruction using a patellar tendon graft, 62 % were participating in strenuous or very strenuous sport at 15 years [15]. This would appear to suggest that return to activity rates following ACL reconstruction deteriorate over time regardless of the status of the menisci or articular cartilage at the time of surgery.

The influence of graft type on outcomes was further studied by the same group who performed a prospective analysis of 180 patients with an isolated ACL rupture who underwent ACL reconstruction utilising either a hamstring graft ($n=90$, mean age=24 years) or patellar tendon graft ($n=90$, mean age=25 years) [20, 25, 26]. There were no significant demographic differences between the groups. At the 5-year review, the IKDC score (level 1, strenuous activities requiring jumping and pivoting; level 2, moderate activities such as tennis and skiing) was used to ascertain activity levels. Although there was no significant difference between the two groups, activity levels again deteriorated over time. Eighty-four per cent of the hamstring patients and 74 % of the patellar tendon patients participated in level 1 or 2 activities at 2 years, but these percentages dropped to 69 % and 60 %, respectively, at 5 years. The same cohort of patients was studied by Leys et al. [20] who performed a 15-year analysis. The modified IKDC activity score was used for this study, making comparisons of activity levels between time periods difficult. Patients were asked to rate their current activity level as being very strenuous (jumping, pivoting), strenuous (skiing, tennis), moderate (running), light (walking), or unable to perform any of the above activities. Overall, the hamstring group demonstrated significantly higher activity levels, with 77 % participating in either strenuous or very strenuous activities, compared with 62 % of the patellar tendon group. Although the patellar tendon group maintained their activity level over time (5–15 years), the hamstring group surprisingly demonstrated an increased activity level. It is not clear whether this increased activity level was real or a product of the slightly different activity scores used at the two time points. Factors such as specific type, frequency, and intensity of activity were not recorded.

Fact Box 4

Gender does not appear to play a role in return to sport following ACL reconstruction in Australian patient cohorts.

Although the lack of homogeneity of scoring systems, study aims, and design make between-studies comparisons difficult, some conclusions regarding return to sporting activities following ACL reconstruction can be made. At 2 years' follow-up after surgery, at least two-thirds of patients had returned to either their pre-level or a higher level of activity, regardless of graft type. In general, as expected with increasing age, these rates do not increase over time. Gender appears to have little or no influence on the results.

34.4 The Psychological Impact of Returning to Sport

The Anterior Cruciate Ligament-Return to Sport after Injury (ACL-RSI) scale was developed by Webster et al. [31] to specifically investigate the psychological impact of returning to sport after ACL injury. Development started in 2003 in response to there being a paucity of psychological measures specific to sports injury rehabilitation. There was emerging evidence at the time to suggest that returning to sport after an ACL injury had a significant psychological impact on some athletes. The scale was operationally defined as measuring psychological readiness to return to sport, and this section will summarise its development and ability to predict return to sports outcomes.

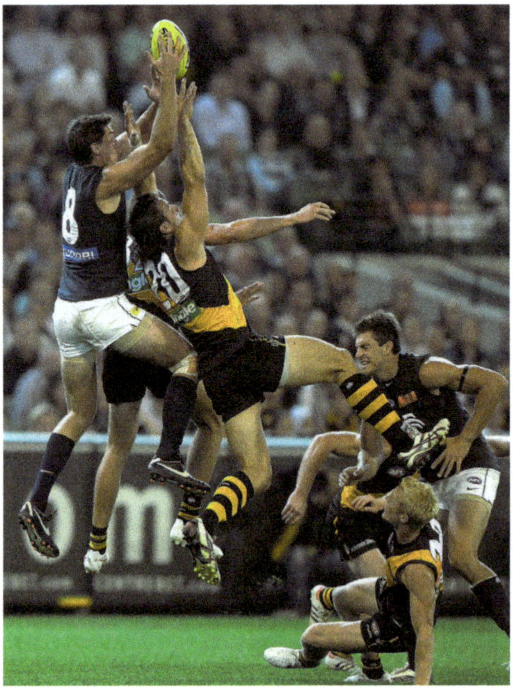

Netball

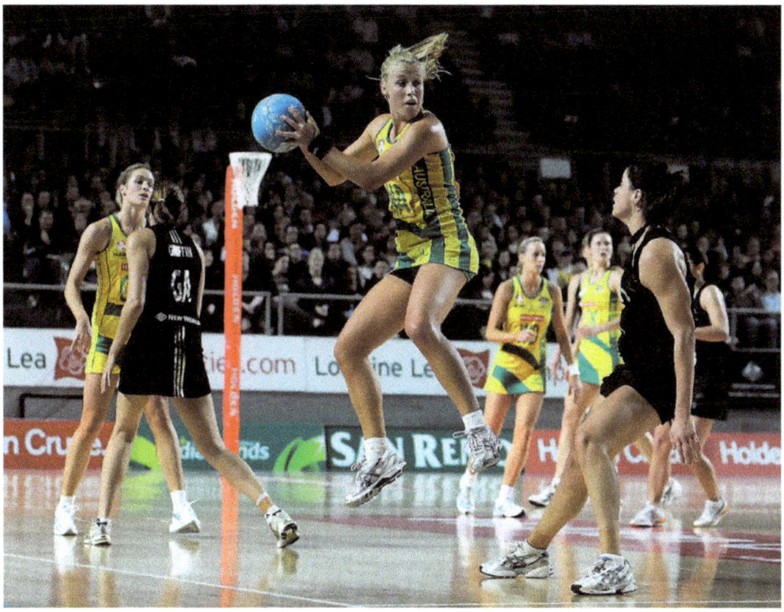

34.4.1 ACL-RSI Scale Development

Items developed for the scale were centred on three psychological responses identified by the literature as associated with returning to sport: *emotions*, *confidence*, and *risk appraisal* (see Table 34.1). To develop items in the emotions category, an extensive search of the literature identified fear of reinjury [16, 22, 23, 29], frustration [22, 23, 28, 29], nervousness, and tension [12, 29] as commonly reported emotions experienced by athletes during rehabilitation and the commencement of sport. Five items (items 1–5) were therefore developed to measure these emotions.

Sport confidence typically refers to the amount of confidence the athlete has in their ability to perform well at their sport. However, in the case of ACL reconstruction, it may also relate to the amount of confidence the athlete has in their knee function. Five items (items 6–10) were therefore generated to cover these two aspects of sports confidence. Three (items 6–8) were developed to target the athlete's confidence in their knee function and two (items 9–10) were developed to measure athletes' confidence in their overall ability to perform well at their sport. Two items (items 11–12) were included to investigate the cognitive risk appraisal of the athlete to reinjury. The second of these, item 12, was suggested by a patient group during pilot testing of the scale for relevance.

The ACL-RSI scale was completed by 220 athletes who had undergone ACL reconstruction between 8 and 22 months (mean = 12 months) previously. The scale was found to have high internal consistency (Cronbach's alpha = 0.96), and a principal component analysis confirmed the presence of one underlying factor that accounted for 67.8 % of the total variance. It is important to note that although the scale was designed around three constructs, these constructs were all highly related, and a single score between 0 and 100 is calculated for the scale where higher values indicate a more positive psychological response (see Table 34.1).

To validate the scale, the development sample was further divided into the following groups: (1) athletes who had returned to full completion, (2) training only, (3) not yet returned but planning to, and (4) given up sport. Athletes who had returned to full competition scored significantly higher than the other three groups, and athletes who had given up sport scored significantly lower [31].

Table 34.1 ACL-RSI items

Scale item	Order in scale
Emotions:	
1. Are you nervous about playing your sport?	3
2. Do you find it frustrating to have to consider your knee with respect to your sport?[a]	6
3. Do you feel relaxed about playing your sport?[b]	12
4. Are you fearful of reinjuring your knee by playing your sport?	7
5. Are you afraid of accidentally injuring your knee by playing your sport?	9
Confidence in performance:	
6. Are you confident that your knee will not give way by playing your sport?	4
7. Are you confident that you could play your sport without concern for your knee?	5
8. Are your confident about your knee holding up under pressure?	8
9. Are you confident that you can perform at your previous level of sports participation?	1
10. Are you confident about your ability to perform well at your sport?	11
Risk appraisal:	
11. Do you think you are likely to reinjure your knee by participating in your sport?	2
12. Do thoughts of having to go through surgery and rehabilitation again prevent you from playing your sport?	10

Each item is scored on a 0–100 scale and scores from the 12 items are summed and averaged to obtain a single score (0–100). Higher scores indicate a more positive psychological response

[a]Item 2 was from the Quality of Life Outcome Measure for Chronic ACL Deficiency (ACL-QOL) scale [22]

[b]Item 3 measures "tension" with the positive antonym relaxed used to get a balance between positively and negatively worded items

34.4.2 Can Return to Sport Be Predicted?

An important goal of injury rehabilitation is to be able to predict which athletes may benefit from psychological counselling or intervention so that psychological recovery can occur in parallel with physical recovery. It is therefore relevant to know whether the psychological responses that athletes experience during the rehabilitation period are related to sports resumption.

Two large-scale studies have been conducted which have shown that the ACL-RSI scale can be used to predict return to sports outcomes. The first enrolled 100 athletes who completed the ACL-RSI at 3, 6, and 12 months after undergoing ACL reconstruction surgery [19]. At 12 months, 51 % of the athletes had returned to competitive sports. Scores on the ACL-RSI at 6 months were significantly lower in the athletes who did not successfully return to their competition sport at 12 months compared to the athletes who did. Therefore, an athlete's readiness to return to sport at 6 months after ACL reconstruction surgery was related to whether or not they actually returned at 12 months. This result suggested that it may be possible to identify athletes at risk of not returning to competitive sport due to psychological reasons during rehabilitation.

The second and larger study of 187 patients administered a battery of psychological assessments, including the ACL-RSI scale, before ACL reconstruction surgery, as well as at 4 and 12 months after surgery [5]. At 12 months, only 56 athletes (31 %) had returned to their previous level of sports participation, consistent with earlier findings [8] and despite scoring well on standard outcome measures. Three variables, psychological readiness to return to sport, the participant's estimate of the number of months it would take to return to sport, and locus of control, predicted returning to sport by 12 months after surgery. Psychological readiness, as measured by the ACL-RSI, was the only variable to be predictive of return to sport at both preoperative and 4-month measurements. Therefore this study showed that even before the participants underwent surgery, their psychological responses were associated with their chances of returning to the pre-injury level 12 months later. The results of this study further suggested that a score of less than 56 points on the ACL-RSI may indicate an increased risk of not returning to the pre-injury level and may help clinicians to identify at-risk athletes.

The above cohort was subsequently followed at 2 years to specifically see whether those who had not returned by 12 months made a later return [6]. The group included 122 competitive- and recreational-level athletes who had not attempted sport at 12 months. Ninety-one per cent of athletes reported having returned to some form of sport. At 2 years after surgery, 66 % were still playing sport, with 41 % playing at their previous level and 25 % playing at a lower level. Thus, most of the athletes who were not playing sport at 1 year had returned to some form of sport within 2 years.

However, only approximately 40 % of athletes were still playing their sport at 2 years. When sport participation data was categorised by the type of sport, basketball had the highest return rate with 50 % of athletes playing at 2 years, followed by netball (41 %), Australian rules (37 %), and then soccer (26 %). It appears that the sustained participation rates for those athletes who do not return within the first 12 months postoperatively are low. Once again, a more positive psychological response was associated with participation in the pre-injury sport at 2 years.

Fact Box 5
The ACL-RSI scale is a useful tool for identifying athletes who may have difficulty returning to sport after ACL injury due to psychological reasons.

Overall, the ACL-RSI scale appears to be a useful tool for screening and identifying athletes who may have difficulty with the resumption of sport after ACL injury due to psychological reasons. The scale is currently available in English [31], Swedish [18], French [9], and German [24] versions, with other translations currently under way.

34.4.3 Do Returning Athletes Play with Fear?

Fear of reinjury has been identified as a primary reason cited by athletes who do not return to their pre-injury sport [17]. Ardern et al. [2] investigated whether fear of reinjury was still a consideration in athletes who made a successful return to their sport. A cohort of 209 athletes answered a series of questions regarding the behavioural manifestations of fear, such as playing with hesitation and being wary of injury-provoking situations. Overall, the results showed that athletes who had successfully returned to their pre-injury sport generally participated without fear of reinjury. Males who had earlier surgery (<3 months after injury) were found to participate in their pre-injury sport with the least amount of fear. This was consistent with previous work, which showed that during rehabilitation, males report being more influenced by powerful others, such as trained professionals (doctors, physiotherapists) and team-mates compared with females. This may be protective against any negative psychological impact associated with returning to sport after this surgery [32].

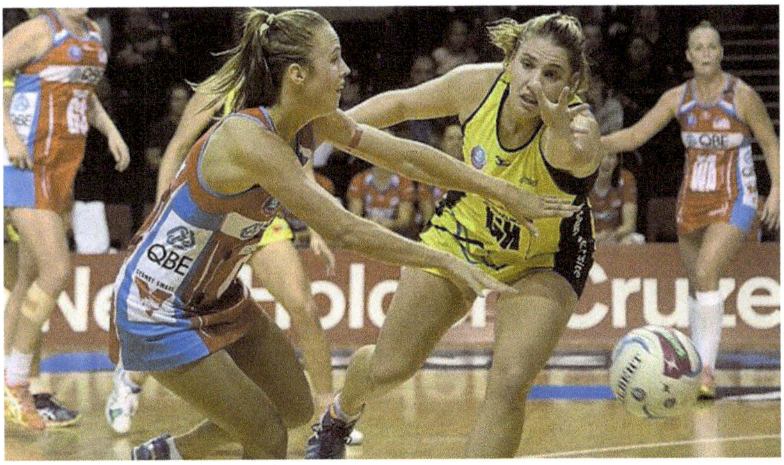

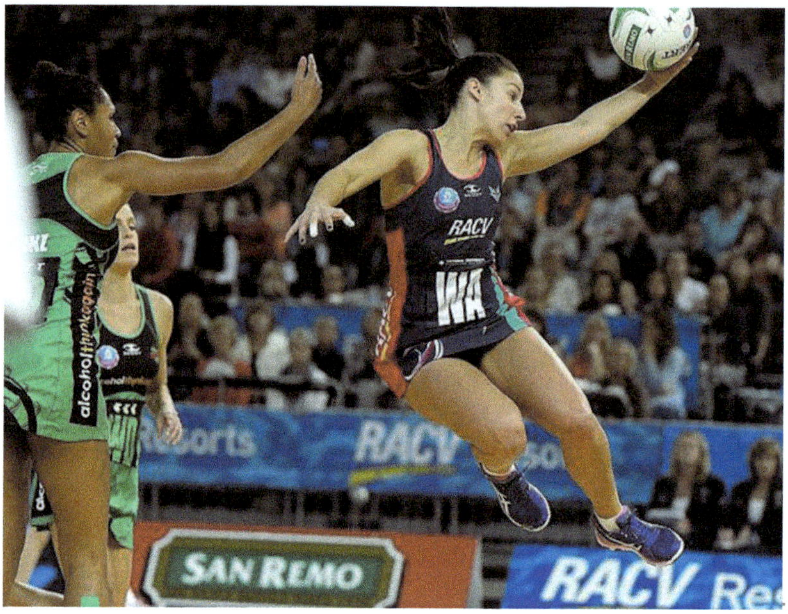

Conclusion

The rates of return to pre-injury sport following ACL reconstruction vary. In the experience of one research group in Melbourne, Australia, most patients eventually attempt a return. However, only approximately one-third resume and continue to play their pre-injury sport in the longer term. Rates appear to be higher in professional sports people, at least for Australian rules football. For the most part, the surgery has been successful in terms of restoring knee stability and function. There are many factors involved in the return to play decision-making process, and many athletes decide not to return for reasons other than their knee. Others may wish to return but find that psychological barriers are too great to overcome. Overall, returning to sport reflects an important participation outcome in this surgical group and should continue to be monitored in the longer term, as making a return to sport remains an important consideration for patients considering whether to undergo an ACL reconstruction in the first place.

References

1. Ardern CL, Osterberg A, Tagesson S, Gauffin H, Webster KE, Kvist J (2014) The impact of psychological readiness to return to sport and recreational activities after anterior cruciate ligament reconstruction. Br J Sports Med 48(22):1613–1619. doi:10.1136/bjsports-2014-093842
2. Ardern CL, Taylor NF, Feller JA, Webster KE (2012) Fear of re-injury in people who have returned to sport following anterior cruciate ligament reconstruction surgery. J Sci Med Sport 15(6):488–495
3. Ardern CL, Taylor NF, Feller JA, Webster KE (2012) Return-to-sport outcomes at 2 to 7 years after anterior cruciate ligament reconstruction surgery. Am J Sports Med 40(1):41–48. doi:10.1177/0363546511422999
4. Ardern CL, Taylor NF, Feller JA, Webster KE (2014) Fifty-five per cent return to competitive sport following anterior cruciate ligament reconstruction surgery: an updated systematic review and meta-analysis including aspects of physical functioning and contextual factors. Br J Sports Med 48(21):1543–1552. doi:10.1136/bjsports-2013-093398
5. Ardern CL, Taylor NF, Feller JA, Whitehead TS, Webster KE (2013) Psychological responses matter in returning to preinjury level of sport after anterior cruciate ligament reconstruction surgery. Am J Sports Med 41(7):1549–1558. doi:10.1177/0363546513489284

6. Ardern CL, Taylor NF, Feller JA, Whitehead TS, Webster KE (2015) Sports participation 2 years after anterior cruciate ligament reconstruction in athletes who had not returned to sport at 1 year: a prospective follow-up of physical function and psychological factors in 122 athletes. Am J Sports Med 43(4):848–856. doi:10.1177/0363546514563282
7. Ardern CL, Webster KE, Taylor NF, Feller JA (2011) Return to sport following anterior cruciate ligament reconstruction surgery: a systematic review and meta-analysis of the state of play. Br J Sports Med 45(7):596–606. doi:10.1136/bjsm.2010.076364
8. Ardern CL, Webster KE, Taylor NF, Feller JA (2011) Return to the preinjury level of competitive sport after anterior cruciate ligament reconstruction surgery: two-thirds of patients have not returned by 12 months after surgery. Am J Sports Med 39(3):538–543. doi:10.1177/0363546510384798
9. Bohu Y, Klouche S, Lefevre N, Webster K, Herman S (2015) Translation, cross-cultural adaptation and validation of the French version of the Anterior Cruciate Ligament-Return to Sport after Injury (ACL-RSI) scale. Knee Surg Sports Traumatol Arthrosc 23(4): 1192–1196
10. Bourke HE, Gordon DJ, Salmon LJ, Waller A, Linklater J, Pinczewski LA (2012) The outcome at 15 years of endoscopic anterior cruciate ligament reconstruction using hamstring tendon autograft for 'isolated' anterior cruciate ligament rupture. J Bone Joint Surg 94B(5):630–637
11. Bourke HE, Salmon LJ, Waller A, Patterson V, Pinczewski LA (2012) Survival of the anterior cruciate ligament graft and the contralateral ACL at a minimum of 15 years. Am J Sports Med 40(9): 1985–1992
12. Chan CS, Grossman HY (1988) Psychological effects of running loss on consistent runners. Percept Mot Skills 66(3):875–883
13. Feller JA, Anand B, Webster KE, Whitehead TS, Norsworthy CJ (2014) Return to sport outcomes after revision anterior cruciate ligament reconstruction. Biennial meeting of the Anterior Cruciate Ligament Study Group. Paper presented at the Biennial meeting of the Anterior Cruciate Ligament Study Group, Cape Town
14. Feller JA, Webster KE, Steinfort P (2003) Return to Australian Rules football following ACL reconstruction. Paper presented at the Football Australasia: controversies in 2003 Melbourne
15. Hui C, Salmon LJ, Kok A, Maeno S, Linklater J, Pinczewski LA (2011) Fifteen-year outcome of endoscopic anterior cruciate ligament reconstruction with patellar tendon autograft for "isolated" anterior cruciate ligament tear. Am J Sports Med 39(1):89–98. doi:10.1177/0363546510379975
16. Johnston LH, Carroll D (1998) The context of emotional responses to athletic injury: a qualitative analysis. J Sport Rehabil 7(3):206–220
17. Kvist J, Ek A, Sporrstedt K, Good L (2005) Fear of re-injury: a hindrance for returning to sports after anterior cruciate ligament reconstruction. Knee Surg Sports Traumatol Arthrosc 13(5):393–397
18. Kvist J, Osterberg A, Gauffin H, Tagesson S, Webster K, Ardern C (2013) Translation and measurement properties of the Swedish version of ACL-Return to Sports after Injury questionnaire. Scand J Med Sci Sports 23(5):568–575. doi:10.1111/j.1600-0838.2011.01438.x
19. Langford JL, Webster KE, Feller JA (2009) A prospective longitudinal study to assess psychological changes following anterior cruciate ligament reconstruction surgery. Br J Sports Med 43(5):377–381. doi:10.1136/bjsm.2007.044818
20. Leys T, Salmon LJ, Waller A, Linklater J, Pinczewski LA (2012) Clinical results and risk factors for reinjury 15 years after anterior cruciate ligament reconstruction: a prospective study of hamstring and patellar tendon grafts. Am J Sports Med 40(3):595–605
21. Liptak MG, Angel KR (2007) Outcome of anterior cruciate ligament injuries in an elite sporting population. A retrospective review of Australian Rules footballers. Paper presented at the 6th Biennial Conference of the International Society of Arthroscopy, Knee Surgery and Orthopaedic Sports Medicine Florence
22. Mohtadi N (1998) Development and validation of the quality of life outcome measure (questionnaire) for chronic anterior cruciate ligament deficiency. Am J Sports Med 26(3):350–359
23. Morrey MA, Stuart MJ, Smith AM, Wiese-Bjornstal DM (1999) A longitudinal examination of athletes' emotional and cognitive responses to anterior cruciate ligament injury. Clin J Sport Med 9(2):63–69
24. Müller U, Schmidt M, Krüger-Franke M, Rosemeyer B (2014) Die ACL–Return to Sport after Injury Skala als wichtiger Parameter bei der Beurteilung Rückkehr zum Sport Level I und II nach Rekonstruktion des vorderen Kreuzbands (deutsche Version). Sport Orthop Traumatol 30:135–144
25. Pinczewski LA, Lyman J, Salmon LJ, Russell V, Roe J, Linklater J (2007) A 10-year comparison of anterior cruciate ligament reconstructions with hamstring tendon and patellar tendon autograft. A controlled prospective trial. Am J Sports Med 35(4):564–574
26. Pinczewski LA, Deehan DJ, Salmon LJ, Russell VJ, Clingeleffer A (2002) A five-year comparison of patellar tendon versus four-strand hamstring tendon autograft for arthroscopic reconstruction of the anterior cruciate ligament. Am J Sports Med 30(4):523–536
27. Salmon LJ, Refshauge KM, Russell VJ, Roe JP, Linklater J, Pinczewski LA (2006) Gender differences in outcome after anterior cruciate ligament reconstruction with hamstring tendon autograft. Am J Sports Med 34(4):621–629
28. Smith AM, Scott SG, O'Fallon WM, Young ML (1990) Emotional responses of athletes to injury. Mayo Clin Proc 65(1):38–50

29. Smith AM, Stuart MJ, Wiese-Bjornstal DM, Milliner EK, O'Fallon WM, Crowson CS (1993) Competitive athletes: preinjury and postinjury mood state and self-esteem. Mayo Clin Proc 68(10):939–947
30. Trojani C, Sbihi A, Djian P, Potel JF, Hulet C, Jouve F, Bussiere C, Ehkirch FP, Burdin G, Dubrana F, Beaufils P, Franceschi JP, Chassaing V, Colombet P, Neyret P (2011) Causes for failure of ACL reconstruction and influence of meniscectomies after revision. Knee Surg Sports Traumatol Arthrosc Off J ESSKA 19(2):196–201. doi:10.1007/s00167-010-1201-6
31. Webster KE, Feller JA, Lambros C (2008) Development and preliminary validation of a scale to measure the psychological impact of returning to sport following anterior cruciate ligament reconstruction surgery. Phys Ther Sport 9(1):9–15
32. Webster KE, Langford J, Feller JA (2005) Psychological impact of anterior cruciate ligament reconstruction: an examination of gender differences. In: (ISSP) ISoSP (ed) Promoting health and performance for life. Proceedings of the 11th World Congress of Sport Psychology, Sydney

Return to Sport following ACL Reconstruction: The MOON Experience

35

Kirk McCullough, Evan Stout, and Kurt Spindler

Contents

K. McCullough, MD
Orthopaedic & Sports Medicine Clinic of Kansas City, 3651 College Blvd. Suite 100A, Leawood, KS 66211, USA

E. Stout, MD
JSP Health Network, 1500 S Main St, Fort Worth, TX 76104, USA

K. Spindler, MD (✉)
Cleveland Clinic Sports Health Center, Mail Code SH02, 5555 Transportation Blvd., Garfield Heights, OH 44125, USA
e-mail: spindlk@ccf.org

35.1 Introduction

Anterior cruciate ligament (ACL) tears are the most common ligamentous knee injury requiring surgical reconstruction for athletes at all levels of play. These injuries represent not only a season ending event but can oftentimes be career-ending injury for athletes regardless of sport participation. While the goal of ACL reconstruction is to stabilize and restore the biomechanics of the knee, the ultimate immediate outcome of interest to an athlete is successful return to competitive play. This requires not only a technically sound surgical reconstruction but also an extensive and detailed rehabilitation program focused not only in recovering physical function but also overcoming an athlete's fear of reinjury.

For most athletes return to play after injury is of utmost concern and a frequent cause of psychological stress and fear. Considering this, return to play at either the same or higher level should arguably be considered one of the primary outcomes in defining a successful recovery from injury for a competitive athlete. Appreciating the paramount importance of returning to play after an ACL reconstruction, a thorough understanding of available outcome data on return to play for athletes in various sports aids the medical provider in counseling athletes, coaches, and team management regarding timing of return to play and how future level of performance may be affected.

V. Musahl et al. (eds.), *Rotatory Knee Instability*, DOI 10.1007/978-3-319-32070-0_35

35.2 Summary of the MOON Group

In an effort to better define prognosis and predictors of ACL reconstruction, seven institutions (Cleveland Clinic Foundation, Vanderbilt Orthopaedic Institute, The Ohio State University, University of Iowa, Washington University, Hospital for Special Surgery, and University of Colorado) enrolled over 3,500 ACL reconstruction patients into a database to establish the largest prospective longitudinal ACL reconstruction cohort in the United States. This cohort group has been since known as the Multicenter Orthopaedic Outcomes Network (MOON) group.

To evaluate perioperative demographics and postoperative outcomes, each of these ACL reconstruction patients completed a questionnaire documenting a variety of factors including injury mechanism, patient-based outcome measures, history of previous knee surgery, and activity level before their surgery. For each surgery, surgeons completed a form documenting examination under anesthesia, status and treatment of meniscal and articular cartilage injuries, and details of ACL reconstruction and rehabilitation milestones.

In the prospective longitudinal cohort design of the MOON group, a series of five validated outcome measures were collected at baseline (within 2 weeks of surgery) and again at follow-up (at a minimum of 2 years, 6 years, and 10 years after ACL reconstruction). The patient-reported outcome measures used were administered in the following sequence: the Knee Injury and Osteoarthritis Outcome Score (KOOS, five subscales), the Western Ontario and McMaster Universities (WOMAC) Osteoarthritis Index, the Marx activity rating scale, the Medical Outcomes Study 36-Item Short Form, and the International Knee Documentation Committee subjective knee evaluation form.

The KOOS evaluates both short- and long-term effects of knee injuries in athletes and the potential for the development of osteoarthritis. The five subscale measures include pain, symptoms, activities of daily living, sports and recreation function, and knee-related quality of life. The most responsive subscale of the KOOS is the knee-related quality of life.

The WOMAC is the most frequently used patient-reported outcome measure specific for osteoarthritis of the lower extremity. The WOMAC is completely contained within the KOOS subscales of pain, symptoms, and activities of daily living.

The Marx activity rating scale is a four-question assessment evaluating the patient's ability to run, cut, decelerate, and pivot. This scale evaluates the level of symptoms and disability of the patient in relation to his or her activity level. The patient is asked about the components of physical function that are common to different sporting activities. Each one of the above activities is scored on a scale from 0 (performing the task 1 time per month) to 4 (performing the task 4 times per week) for a total of 16 points. The score has been shown to positively correlate with patient activity and returning to pivoting sports and to correlate inversely with age.

The Medical Outcomes Study 36-Item Short Form is the most frequently used general health outcome measure, and it has an important role in health policy development as well as clinical practice and research. This scale may be used to compare musculoskeletal and non-musculoskeletal diseases and conditions across the medical spectrum.

The International Knee Documentation Committee is a simplistic knee-specific patient-reported outcome measure designed by the American Orthopaedic Society of Sports Medicine in 1999. It consists of 18 questions and assesses any knee condition.

This prospective, longitudinal population cohort has provided higher-level evidence for physicians to use in discussion with an individual patient about their prognosis, treatment options, and lifestyle choices that affect the knee. Specifically, it has identified important data on return to play after ACL reconstruction. Recently data on return to play in football and soccer athletes within the MOON group have been published.

35.3 Return to Play in Football After ACLR

ACL injuries are one of the most common knee injuries in American football players after medial collateral ligament sprains and patella/patellar tendon injuries [5]. Nearly 8 % of participants at the National Football League's (NFL) Invitational Camp (also known as the NFL Scouting Combine) have a history of ACL injury, making ACL reconstruction the third most commonly performed surgical procedure on these athletes [1].

McCullough et al. reported on return to play in high school and college level football athletes from the MOON cohort [4]. The primary goal of the study was determine the return to play rate in these athletes after ACL reconstruction. Additionally, they investigated the relationship between patient-reported outcome scores and both patients return to play and perception of return to performance.

A total of 147 eligible football players (68 high school and 28 collegiate) were included in the study. Of the 68 high school athletes, 43 returned to playing football for a return to play rate of 63 %. The return to play rate among collegiate athletes was found to be similar but slightly higher with a 69 % return rate (18/26).

Return to play was also evaluated by player position, specifically between "skilled" and "nonskilled" positions. Positions included in the skilled group were quarterbacks, running backs, wide receivers, defensive backs, and special team players. The return to play rate between the two groups was not found to be statistically significant with a skilled return rate of 41 % and nonskilled rate of 50 %.

Fact Box 1: Return to Football After ACLR

- Return to play rate of high school athletes after ACL reconstruction – 63 %.
- Return to play rate of collegiate athletes after ACL reconstruction – 69 %.
- Player position did not have a statistically significant effect on the ability to return to play.

The most common reason for not returning to play was reported to be other interests, which included lost interest in the sport, interest in another sport(s) besides football, or other life interests (e.g., job, school, family, etc.). Other remaining reasons given for not returning to play that were performance related include fear, physical symptoms, and loss of speed or strength. Interestingly, fear was the second most common with 50 % of high school and 53 % collegiate athletes citing this reason for not returning to play.

Fact Box 2: Reasons for Not Returning to Football Play After ACLR

- 2/3 of all athletes listed "other interests" as reasons for not returning to play.
- ~50 % of all athletes identified fear as a major or contributing factor to not returning to play.
- 1/3 of all athletes cited physical symptoms or loss of speed and strength as reasons for not returning to play.

This finding speaks to the critical psychological component of recovery and return to play after ACL reconstruction that is often overlooked by the treatment team. It is important for the surgeon, therapist, trainer, coach, parents, and others to understand the psychological element to the patient's recovery as most athletes are not mentally prepared for injury and the extensive rehabilitation that follows. This fear of reinjury is an often underestimated component of recovery and likely plays a critical role in preventing athletes from returning to their sport or prior level of performance.

The other performance-related reasons for not returning to play, including physical symptoms and loss of speed or strength, were also relatively common, reported by 33 % of high school and 24 % of college football players. This was confirmed by the comparison of patient-reported outcome scores of three groups in the cohort: those who did not return to play, those who returned but at a lower level of performance, and those who returned at their previous level. In collegiate athletes, statistically significant differences were found between patients who did not return to play and those who did at the same performance level in IKDC, Marx activity scale, and KOOS knee-related quality of life scores. In high school athletes, differences between the three groups in IKDC, KOOS, and Marx activity scores did not reach statistical significance.

ACL injury and subsequent surgical reconstruction is a significant event in the life and career of American football players at any level. Our understanding of the anatomy of the ACL, the optimal technique for its reconstruction, and ideal protocol for postoperative rehabilitation has greatly improved over the past decade. Despite this, the literature has consistently shown a return to play rate range from 44 to 80 %, with a significant proportion of returning athletes experiencing a reduction in performance. It is critical for the surgeon to understand the psychological component of ACL injury and rehabilitation to assist the patient in overcoming the fear that keeps a significant portion of athletes from returning to play or returning at a decreased level of performance. Furthermore, a knowledge of the data on return to play helps the surgeon appropriately manage patient expectations postoperatively by understanding that despite a technically successful procedure, not all athletes return to their sport.

35.4 Return to Play in Soccer After ACLR

ACL rupture is also a very common and potentially serious injury in both male and female soccer players. These injuries have been associated with a delayed return to play and may be career ending. Using the MOON cohort data, Brophy et al. investigated return to play in male and female soccer athletes [2].

Specific risk factors including age, gender, side of injury (dominant versus nondominant limb), and graft choice were investigated in relation to return to play.

A total of 100 soccer athletes were identified from the group (55 male and 45 female) with a mean age of 24.2 years of age. The majority of the athletes were treated with bone-patellar tendon-bone autograft (69 %), followed by hamstring autograft (28 %).

The overall return to play rate in the cohort was 72 %, slightly higher than the return to play rate in the American football cohort. Of the male soccer players, 76 % returned to play, while 67 % of the female athletes returned to play. The average time to return was 12.2 ± 14.3 months postoperatively. A high percentage (85 %) of those who returned to soccer resumed at the same level of competition or higher. There was no significant difference in the time to return between male and female players. Evaluation of the identified risk factors demonstrated only age and gender as significant predictors of initial return to play. Specifically, females and athletes over the age of 30 were less likely to return to play. At the latest follow-up however, age, gender, and graft choice did not predict long-term return to play. At this follow-up interval of 7.2 ± 0.9 years, it was found that only 35 % of soccer players were still playing their sport (male, 38 %; female, 31 %), with only 46 % of these athletes reporting play at the same or higher level of competition as before their injury.

Fact Box 3: Return to Soccer After ACLR

- Seventy-two percent of athletes returned to soccer at an average of 12.2 ± 14.3 months after surgery.
- Eighty-five percent of those returning to play returned to the same or higher level of play.
- Age over 30 and female gender are significant risk predictors of return to play.
- No difference was found in return to play rate based on involvement of the dominant or nondominant leg.
- Females are more likely to undergo additional ACL surgery compared to males (20 % versus 5.5 %).
- Athletes with ACL reconstruction of the nondominant limb had a higher future rate of contralateral ACL reconstruction than those who underwent ACL reconstruction on their dominant limb (16 versus 3.5 %).
- Choice of graft has no significant effect on return to play.

The data from this study provide surgeons with important return to play information specific to soccer athletes after ACL reconstruction.

First, the initial return to play rate is high but decreases over time. Second, younger male players are more likely to successfully return to play. This becomes important outcome information for providers taking care of older and/or female soccer players. It is important for these patients to be counseled accordingly, especially if return to play is a primary motivator for surgical reconstruction. Additionally, females were less likely to attribute their ACL injury as the reason for not returning to the sport (25 %) as opposed to males where this was the primary reason. Finally, there is a high rate of subsequent ACL surgery, especially on the contralateral limb in the female cohort. Soccer athletes who injure their nondominant limb are at an increased risk of contralateral ACL rupture in the future. This helpful information promotes awareness of the need for specific counseling in this high-risk population, including the use of ACL injury prevention programs.

35.5 Meniscal and Cartilage Lesions in ACLR Athletes

It is not uncommon for athletes with ACL injuries to also sustain meniscal tears and articular cartilage lesions. Cox et al. found in reviewing 1307 athletes in the MOON cohort group, 46 % had lateral meniscal tears and 38 % medial meniscal tears [3]. Articular cartilage lesions by location were as follows: medial femoral condyle (25 %), lateral femoral condyle (20 %), medial tibial plateau (6 %), lateral tibial plateau (12 %), patella (20 %), and trochlea (9 %).

Cartilage Lesions in ACLR Facts

Incidence of meniscal tears in ACL injury	
Medial meniscus – 38 %	
Lateral meniscus – 46 %	
Articular lesions by location:	
Medial femoral condyle – 25 %	Lateral femoral condyle – 20 %
Medial tibial plateau – 6 %	Lateral tibial plateau – 12 %
Patella – 20 %	Trochlea – 9 %

Previous literature has suggested that meniscal and chondral injuries increase the incidence of post-traumatic osteoarthritis and clinically worse outcomes as measured by KOOS and IDKC scores. Little clinical data has been available on the effect that associated meniscal and chondral injuries have on return to play in athletes with ACL injuries. It has been suggested that concomitant chondral injuries would predict worse outcomes in athletes after ACL reconstruction.

Cox et al. prospectively evaluated return to play using the Marx activity rating scale in this patient cohort [3, 4]. Meniscal and articular cartilage injury was found to not be significant predictors of activity level and return to play at 2 and 6 years after ACL reconstruction with the exception of grade 4 cartilage injury to the medial femoral condyle. Athletes who had grade 4 chondromalacia at the time of ACL reconstruction experienced a significant decline in activity level as demonstrated by a significantly lower Marx score. Furthermore, older age (over 35), female gender, higher BMI, current smokers, lower education level, revision surgery, and lower baseline Marx scores predicted lower postoperative activity scores and return to play as well.

Fact Box 4: Return to Play After ACLR with Cartilage Lesion

- Grade 4 chondromalacia of the medial femoral condyle at the time of ACLR is a predictor of lower activity level, Marx scores, and return to play.
- Age over 35, female gender, BMI over 28, tobacco use, lower education level, revision surgery, and lower baseline Marx scores are negative predictors of lower Marx scores and return to play.

Conclusion

ACL injury and subsequent surgical reconstruction represents a significant potential career-altering event in the life of an athlete. Successful return to play has long been a primary outcome measure for a successful recovery in the competitive athlete. Historically there has been a focused interest on improving our understanding of the anatomy of the ACL and the technical aspects of the reconstructive procedure to improve the ability of athletes to return to their respective sport. However, recent literature, especially the outcomes from the MOON cohort studies, has provided specific data on return to play rates and important associated risk factors, and that other psychological factors such as fear must be adequately addressed. Understanding this data on return to play allows the medical provider to appropriately and accurately manage the expectations of the injured athlete and maximize the ability of the athlete to safely return to competitive play.

References

1. Brophy RH, Barnes R, Rodeo SA, Warren RF (2007) Prevalence of musculoskeletal disorders at the NFL combine--trends from 1987 to 2000. Med Sci Sports Exerc 39(1):22–27. doi:10.1249/01.mss.0000241637.52231.18
2. Brophy RH, Schmitz L, Wright RW, Dunn WR, Parker RD, Andrish JT, McCarty EC, Spindler KP (2012) Return to play and future ACL injury risk after ACL reconstruction in soccer athletes from the Multicenter Orthopaedic Outcomes Network (MOON) group. Am J Sports Med 40(11):2517–2522. doi:10.1177/0363546512459476
3. Cox CL, Huston LJ, Dunn WR, Reinke EK, Nwosu SK, Parker RD, Wright RW, Kaeding CC, Marx RG, Amendola A, McCarty EC, Spindler KP (2014) Are articular cartilage lesions and meniscus tears predictive of IKDC, KOOS, and Marx activity level outcomes after anterior cruciate ligament reconstruction? A 6-year multicenter cohort study. Am J Sports Med 42(5):1058–1067. doi:10.1177/0363546514525910
4. McCullough KA, Phelps KD, Spindler KP, Matava MJ, Dunn WR, Parker RD, Group M, Reinke EK (2012) Return to high school- and college-level football after anterior cruciate ligament reconstruction: a Multicenter Orthopaedic Outcomes Network (MOON) cohort study. Am J Sports Med 40(11):2523–2529. doi:10.1177/0363546512456836
5. Swenson DM, Collins CL, Best TM, Flanigan DC, Fields SK, Comstock RD (2013) Epidemiology of knee injuries among U.S. high school athletes, 2005/2006–2010/2011. Med Sci Sports Exerc 45(3):462–469. doi:10.1249/MSS.0b013e318277acca

Part VII

Future Directions

Quantifying the Forces During the Pivot Shift Test

36

Yuichi Hoshino

Contents

Y. Hoshino, MD, PhD
Department of Orthopaedic Surgery,
Kobe Kaisei Hospital, Kobe, Japan
e-mail: you.1.hoshino@gmail.com

36.1 Introduction

Although the movement of the knee during the pivot shift has improved in clarity as a result of motion capture technology [2, 3, 12, 14], the force required for eliciting the pivot shift remains largely unknown, especially from a quantitative perspective. The testing maneuver for the pivot shift test has substantial variety [21, 32, 33], and the force applied to the knee during the pivot shift test is inherently different between different techniques. Knowledge about what kind and how much of the force is applied to the knee during the pivot shift test would contribute to establishing a universally standardized pivot shift test (Fact Box 1) technique and to provide an evaluation that is as objective as possible in combination with the measurement technologies, such as an electromagnetic system [12, 22], image analysis by digital camera [13] or iPad [15], an accelerometer [20, 26], and a navigation system [16, 23, 25]. Further advancement of biomechanical research has the potential to achieve quantification of the forces during the pivot shift test in the near future, but the previous knowledge about the forces related to the pivot shift should be summarized for the progress of such biomechanics research.

V. Musahl et al. (eds.), *Rotatory Knee Instability*, DOI 10.1007/978-3-319-32070-0_36

Fact Box 1

There are three components of the force necessary to elicit the pivot shift.

1. *Valgus stress*: The most important force requisite to induce the pivot shift. Without the valgus force, the pivot shift does not occur [2, 17, 28, 29]. Ninety percent of clinicians intentionally apply the valgus force during the pivot shift test [21].
2. *Internal/external rotational stress*: These two opposite torques are required for each phase of the pivot shift. Moderate internal rotational stress is preferable to highlight the dislocation phase [18], whereas external rotational stress enhance the reduction movement [2, 29]. Application of this rotational torque in the clinical exam is also mixed; 57.6 % of clinicians applies internal rotational stress, and 24.2 % does external rotational stress [21].
3. *Axial compressive force*: Axial compressive force makes tibial anterior translation due to posteriorly tilted tibial plateau [7]. A large compressive force is considered to cause the ACL injury [8, 19]. Although valgus stress spontaneously induces compressive force on the lateral compartment, 60.7 % of clinicians intentionally apply compressive force during the pivot shift test [21].

36.2 The Forces to Induce the Pivot Shift

The pivot shift phenomenon occurs at the time of an ACL injury and is also a common symptom of knee instability due to ACL insufficiency. This instability can be reproduced by the pivot shift test [1, 6, 27, 35]. The in vivo mechanical stress at the time of ACL injury has been examined using video motion analysis with estimation of ground reaction force [19]. According to the report from Koga et al. [19], valgus loading is a contributing factor in the ACL injury mechanism. Although internal rotation followed by sudden external rotation of the tibia was observed at the time of injury [19], internal/external rotational loading was still unclear in that study.

When it comes to the pivot shift test as a clinical exam, it should be noted that the pivot shift phenomenon consists of two phases, which are dislocation and reduction of the lateral compartment [1, 6]. Different types and magnitudes of the force are assumed to be applied to the knee for each dislocation and reduction phase of the pivot shift.

Most in vitro biomechanics studies that examine the force applied for the pivot shift have focused on the dislocation phase of the pivot shift [17, 28]. Citak et al. [4] reported using a mechanized pivot shifter that the anterior tibial translation produced by 1 kg of valgus force was 6–7 mm in both the medial and lateral compartments, but additional incremental 1 kg increases in valgus force up to 5 kg induced only 1 mm or less of anterior tibial translation [4]. The magnitude of the pivot shift dislocation is not necessarily load dependent, and a moderate amount of valgus force is enough to provoke a significant level of pivot shift dislocation [4].

Robotic technology has been utilized to conduct knee laxity testing related to ligament injuries because of its ability to measure full 6° of freedom knee kinematics while both controlling and monitoring the force [5, 36, 37]. Kanamori et al. [17] compared knee kinematics under two different stress conditions using the robotic system; only internal rotational stress and a combined valgus and internal rotational force. They found that there was only a small difference in the rotational angle under both rotational stress, but a significant amount of the anterior tibial translation was demonstrated under a combined rotational stress, which they termed a simulated pivot shift test [17]. Thereafter, they tested the effect of the internal rotational torque on the anterior tibial translation and revealed that a minimal amount of the internal rotational force substantially enhanced the anterior tibial translation produced by the valgus force [18]. Based on those experiments, a combined rotatory load of

5-Nm internal tibial torque and 10-Nm valgus torque, called a "simulated pivot shift test," has been established and widely used as a gold standard for robotic experiments to examine ACL injury/reconstruction [9, 38] (Fact Box 2). Valgus stress with a minimum amount of internal rotational loading could maximize the dislocation of the lateral compartment, but the exact amount of those forces is still undetermined.

On the other hand, the reduction movement of the pivot shift phenomenon has rarely been investigated. Matsumoto reported in his cadaveric experiment that resection of the iliotibial band causes the pivot shift reduction movement to disappear [29]. Bull et al. [2] made a cadaveric knee model, which could reproduce the pivot shift reduction [2]. In the experiment, while an average of 30 N in iliotibial tract loads and 7 Nm in valgus force was needed to induce the pivot shift phenomenon, the balance between the valgus stress and the iliotibial tract forces were highly varied between specimens. These two applied forces were meticulously adjusted in each knee to elicit the pivot shift reduction [2]. External rotational force by the iliotibial band should be applied on top of the valgus stress to reproduce the reduction phase of the pivot shift and seems to be highly varied among individuals.

The force required for the pivot shift phenomenon is not single and constant. Based on those previous in vitro studies, the force required to generate the dislocation phase of the pivot shift includes a valgus force with a minimal internal rotational loading, whereas the following reduction phase necessitates external rotational loading on top of the valgus stress that comes from iliotibial band. Nonetheless, the quantification of those forces is not yet fully understood.

Fact Box 2

A simulated pivot shift test was defined as a combined internal tibial torque and valgus torque [17]. The coupled anterior tibial translation against a simulated pivot shift test load has often been used in previous studies to assess rotational laxity in several types of ACL injured/reconstruction models, including (representative examples):

- Comparison between single-bundle and double-bundle ACL reconstructions [38, 39]
- Comparison between different tunnel placements of single-bundle ACL reconstruction [24, 30]
- Comparison between different graft materials in the ACL reconstruction [10]

36.3 The Forces During the Pivot Shift Test

In vivo biomechanical analysis of the pivot shift test as a clinical examination has been conducted and as a result, the stress applied to the knee during the pivot shift test can be roughly estimated. A previous multicenter study [32] evaluating variations of the pivot shift test among 12 experienced international surgeons revealed that some surgeons applied external rotational stress to the knee during the pivot shift test, which exerted larger acceleration of the pivot shift reduction than other types of the pivot shift technique. Surgeons who applied fixed internal rotational stress provided the least acceleration [32] (Fig. 36.1). To accentuate the reduction phase of the pivot shift, the external rotational stress might be favorable, or, at least, internal rotational stress that is applied to make a dislocation of the pivot shift should be released to obtain a clear reduction of the pivot shift.

The applied force should be individualized. Mechanized pivot shift test provided better repeatability than a manually performed pivot shift test by applying a constant force to the knee, but manual performance of the pivot shift test exerted larger pivot shift movement than mechanized [31]. Adjustment of the force by the surgeon based on his/her experience and feeling is still better in terms of eliciting the pivot shift than a consistent amount of the applied force at a given moment. Individualized force in each knee to maximize the pivot shift might be determined

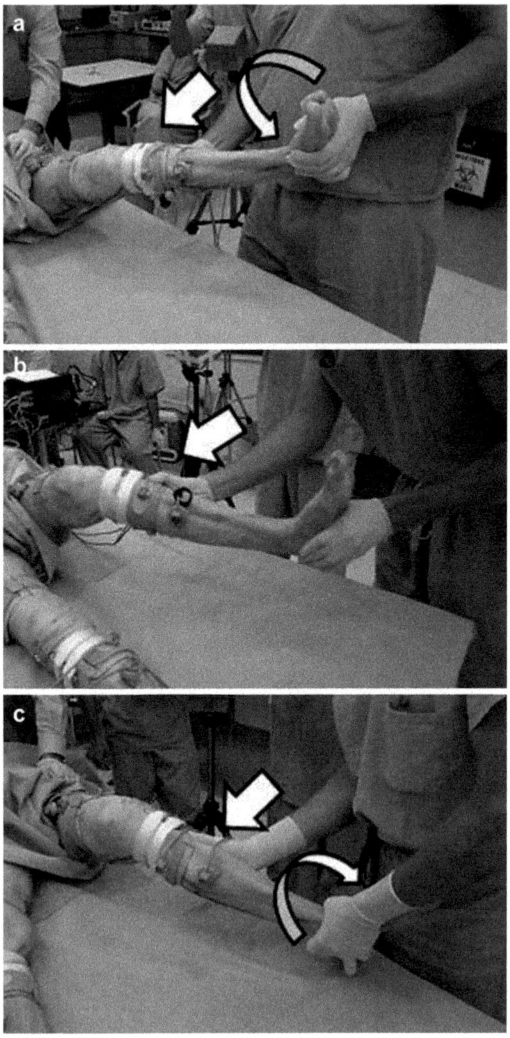

Fig. 36.1 Variation of the pivot shift test maneuver. Arrows indicate the directions of the applied force. Valgus stress is utilized in common. (**a**) Valgus stress is applied with an internal rotational stress. (**b**) Valgus stress is applied without axial rotational stress. (**c**) Valgus stress is applied with an external rotational stress

based on knee laxity, size, and condyle shape; its automated determination and application could possibly be achieved by the advancement of the biomechanics technology.

36.4 Future Work

Although the pivot shift test remains the most critical examination related to ACL injury and treatment, its clinical significance remains a focus of improvement, in part by exploring the forces during the pivot shift test.

The exact amount of the applied force during a pivot shift test performed clinically should be measured. Visual estimation of the applied force was conducted for 12 different surgeons, and the testing maneuver could be categorized based on the applied force, i.e., fixed internal rotation type, motion-allowing type, fixed external rotation type, and dislocation type [32]. However, the actual force applied to the knee during the pivot shift test remains unknown. It would be very informative if a force sensor, attachable to the knee and/or the examiner's hands, could be used to record the force during the actual pivot shift test. The mechanized pivot shifter was reported to be more consistent than the clinically performed pivot shift test, but the magnitude of the pivot shift elicited by the mechanized pivot shifter was not as large as that of the clinical pivot shift test [31]. The information about how much force is applied during a normal clinical pivot shift test would enhance the ability of the mechanized pivot shifter to provoke the pivot shift. Also, if the appropriate level of the force applied by experienced surgeons is revealed, the force would be utilized to educate less experienced clinicians, which could lead to better clinical pivot shift test performance and better consistency of the clinical pivot shift test among different surgeons.

The difference between the force during the pivot shift test and that at the time of ACL injury should be acknowledged. Although the pivot shift test reproduces the abnormal knee motion similar to the actual giving way of the knee, the motion and the applied force during the pivot shift test is supposed to be much smaller than those at the time of the giving way during in vivo jumping and landing activities. Similar to the fact that the force during the pivot shift test is still unknown, the exact mechanism of the ACL injury has not yet been fully characterized [8, 11, 19, 34]. Proper evaluation of both forces for the pivot shift test and the actual in vivo giving way of the knee are warranted to understand the limitations and the possibilities of the pivot shift test.

Conclusion

Valgus stress is requisite for the pivot shift test, while axial rotational loading should not be consistent through the pivot shift test. Internal rotational stress may accentuate the dislocation phase of the pivot shift, while external rotational stress in combination with the tension of the iliotibial band may enhance the reduction phase. The ideal amount of forces remains unknown, especially from a quantitative perspective.

References

1. Bull AMJ, Amis AA (1998) The pivot-shift phenomenon: a clinical and biomechanical perspective. Knee 5(3):141–158
2. Bull AM, Andersen HN, Basso O et al (1999) Incidence and mechanism of the pivot shift. An in vitro study. Clin Orthop Relat Res 363:219–231
3. Bull AM, Earnshaw PH, Smith A et al (2002) Intraoperative measurement of knee kinematics in reconstruction of the anterior cruciate ligament. J Bone Joint Surg Br 84(7):1075–1081
4. Citak M, O'Loughlin PF, Citak M et al (2012) Influence of the valgus force during knee flexion in neutral rotation. Knee Surg Sports Traumatol Arthrosc 20(8):1571–1574
5. Fujie H, Mabuchi K, Woo SL-Y et al (1993) The use of robotics technology to study human joint kinematics: a new methodology. J Biomech Eng 115:211–217
6. Galway HR, MacIntosh DL (1980) The lateral pivot shift: a symptom and sign of anterior cruciate ligament insufficiency. Clin Orthop Relat Res 147:45–50
7. Giffin JR, Vogrin TM, Zantop T et al (2004) Effects of increasing tibial slope on the biomechanics of the knee. Am J Sports Med 32(2):376–382
8. Hashemi J, Breighner R, Chandrashekar N et al (2011) Hip extension, knee flexion paradox: a new mechanism for non-contact ACL injury. J Biomech 44(4):577–585
9. Herbort M, Lenschow S, Fu FH et al (2010) ACL mismatch reconstructions: influence of different tunnel placement strategies in single-bundle ACL reconstructions on the knee kinematics. Knee Surg Sports Traumatol Arthrosc 18(11):1551–1558
10. Herbort M, Tecklenburg K, Zantop T et al (2013) Single-bundle anterior cruciate ligament reconstruction: a biomechanical cadaveric study of a rectangular quadriceps and bone--patellar tendon--bone graft configuration versus a round hamstring graft. Arthroscopy 29(12):1981–1990
11. Hewett TE, Torg JS, Boden BP (2009) Video analysis of trunk and knee motion during non-contact anterior cruciate ligament injury in female athletes: lateral trunk and knee abduction motion are combined components of the injury mechanism. Br J Sports Med 43(6):417–422
12. Hoshino Y, Kuroda R, Nagamune K et al (2007) In vivo measurement of the pivot-shift test in the anterior cruciate ligament-deficient knee using an electromagnetic device. Am J Sports Med 35(7):1098–1104
13. Hoshino Y, Araujo P, Irrgang JJ et al (2012) An image analysis method to quantify the lateral pivot shift test. Knee Surg Sports Traumatol Arthrosc 20(4):703–707
14. Hoshino Y, Kuroda R, Nagamune K et al (2012) Optimal measurement of clinical rotational test for evaluating anterior cruciate ligament insufficiency. Knee Surg Sports Traumatol Arthrosc 20(7): 1323–1330
15. Hoshino Y, Araujo P, Ahlden M et al (2013) Quantitative evaluation of the pivot shift by image analysis using the iPad. Knee Surg Sports Traumatol Arthrosc 21(4):975–980
16. Ishibashi Y, Tsuda E, Yamamoto Y et al (2009) Navigation evaluation of the pivot-shift phenomenon during double-bundle anterior cruciate ligament reconstruction: is the posterolateral bundle more important? Arthroscopy 25(5):488–495
17. Kanamori A, Woo SL, Ma CB et al (2000) The forces in the anterior cruciate ligament and knee kinematics during a simulated pivot shift test: a human cadaveric study using robotic technology. Arthroscopy 16(6):633–639
18. Kanamori A, Zeminski J, Rudy TW et al (2002) The effect of axial tibial torque on the function of the anterior cruciate ligament: a biomechanical study of a simulated pivot shift test. Arthroscopy 18(4):394–398
19. Koga H, Nakamae A, Shima Y et al (2010) Mechanisms for noncontact anterior cruciate ligament injuries: knee joint kinematics in 10 injury situations from female team handball and basketball. Am J Sports Med 38(11):2218–2225
20. Kopf S, Kauert R, Halfpaap J et al (2012) A new quantitative method for pivot shift grading. Knee Surg Sports Traumatol Arthrosc 20(4):718–723
21. Kuroda R, Hoshino Y, Kubo S et al (2012) Similarities and differences of diagnostic manual tests for anterior cruciate ligament insufficiency: a global survey and kinematics assessment. Am J Sports Med 40(1):91–99
22. Labbe DR, de Guise JA, Mezghani N et al (2010) Feature selection using a principal component analysis of the kinematics of the pivot shift phenomenon. J Biomech 43(16):3080–3084
23. Lane CG, Warren RF, Stanford FC et al (2008) In vivo analysis of the pivot shift phenomenon during computer navigated ACL reconstruction. Knee Surg Sports Traumatol Arthrosc 16(5):487–492
24. Loh JC, Fukuda Y, Tsuda E, et al (2003) Knee stability and graft function following anterior cruciate ligament reconstruction: comparison between 11 o'clock and 10 o'clock femoral tunnel placement. 2002 Richard O'Connor Award paper. Arthroscopy 19(3):297–304
25. Lopomo N, Zaffagnini S, Bignozzi S et al (2010) Pivot-shift test: analysis and quantification of knee

laxity parameters using a navigation system. J Orthop Res 28(2):164–169
26. Lopomo N, Signorelli C, Bonanzinga T et al (2012) Quantitative assessment of pivot-shift using inertial sensors. Knee Surg Sports Traumatol Arthrosc 20(4):713–717
27. Losee RE (1983) Concepts of the pivot shift. Clin Orthop Relat Res 172:45–51
28. Markolf KL, Park S, Jackson SR et al (2008) Simulated pivot-shift testing with single and double-bundle anterior cruciate ligament reconstructions. J Bone Joint Surg Am 90(8):1681–1689
29. Matsumoto H (1990) Mechanism of the pivot shift. J Bone Joint Surg Br 72(5):816–821
30. Musahl V, Plakseychuk A, VanScyoc A et al (2005) Varying femoral tunnels between the anatomical footprint and isometric positions: effect on kinematics of the anterior cruciate ligament-reconstructed knee. Am J Sports Med 33(5):712–718
31. Musahl V, Voos J, O'Loughlin PF et al (2010) Mechanized pivot shift test achieves greater accuracy than manual pivot shift test. Knee Surg Sports Traumatol Arthrosc 18(9):1208–1213
32. Musahl V, Hoshino Y, Ahlden M et al (2012) The pivot shift: a global user guide. Knee Surg Sports Traumatol Arthrosc 20(4):724–731
33. Noyes FR, Grood ES, Cummings JF et al (1991) An analysis of the pivot shift phenomenon. The knee motions and subluxations induced by different examiners. Am J Sports Med 19(2):148–155
34. Quatman CE, Hewett TE (2009) The anterior cruciate ligament injury controversy: is "valgus collapse" a sex-specific mechanism? Br J Sports Med 43(5): 328–335
35. Slocum DB, James SL, Larson RL et al (1976) Clinical test for anterolateral rotary instability of the knee. Clin Orthop Relat Res 118:63–69
36. Woo SL, Chan SS, Yamaji T (1997) Biomechanics of knee ligament healing, repair and reconstruction. J Biomech 30(5):431–439
37. Woo SL, Fisher MB (2009) Evaluation of knee stability with use of a robotic system. J Bone Joint Surg Am 91(Suppl 1):78–84
38. Yagi M, Wong EK, Kanamori A et al (2002) Biomechanical analysis of an anatomic anterior cruciate ligament reconstruction. Am J Sports Med 30(5):660–666
39. Yamamoto Y, Hsu WH, Woo SL et al (2004) Knee stability and graft function after anterior cruciate ligament reconstruction: a comparison of a lateral and an anatomical femoral tunnel placement. Am J Sports Med 32(8):1825–1832

How Can We Identify Copers?

37

Amy J.H. Arundale and Lynn Snyder-Mackler

Contents

A.J.H. Arundale
Biomechanics and Movement Science Program, University of Delaware, Newark, DE, USA

L. Snyder-Mackler (✉)
Biomechanics and Movement Science Program, University of Delaware, Newark, DE, USA

Department of Physical Therapy, University of Delaware, Newark, DE, USA
e-mail: smack@udel.edu

37.1 Introduction

Anterior cruciate ligament (ACL) reconstruction is generally considered standard of practice in the United States for young, active individuals early after ACL injuries [33, 36]. Athletes are often educated that ACL reconstruction will decrease static knee joint laxity, minimize further damage to the menisci and articular cartilage, and facilitate their return to preinjury level of sport [1, 33, 36]. However, not all athletes will return to sport following ACL reconstruction [2] and those who do have a high risk of second ACL injury and osteoarthritis development [3, 38, 39]. But research has clearly established that some individuals are able to return to high-level sports participation without ACL reconstruction [4, 8, 14–16, 20, 24–26, 29, 35] and with no difference in radiographic outcomes to athletes after ACL reconstruction [5, 19]. How can those who can return to activity without ACL reconstruction be identified? This chapter will examine the demographic, biomechanical, and functional differences between those who are able to return to their preinjury level of activity and those who are not, discuss the development of a screening algorithm which has been used to distinguish between these two groups, review the outcomes of screening, and provide current screening and treatment recommendations.

Clearly defining copers and non-copers is crucial to an accurate discussion. Copers are defined as athletes who are able to asymptomatically

V. Musahl et al. (eds.), *Rotatory Knee Instability*, DOI 10.1007/978-3-319-32070-0_37

return to their preinjury level of activity [44]. This definition sometimes also stipulates that these athletes are able to maintain their preinjury level of activity for one year following ACL injury [35, 44]. Non-copers are defined as athletes who have knee instability or episodes of giving way with activities of daily living or who are unsuccessful in returning to their preinjury level of activity. A third category of athletes is also present in some discussions. Adapters are athletes who have modified their lifestyle to avoid activities that could cause episodes of giving way or instability [9].

37.2 Differences Between Copers and Non-copers

There are differences between athletes initially classified as copers and non-copers in demographics, gait biomechanics, and functional measures. Demographically potential copers tend to be younger, more active, and have a higher preinjury level of activity than non-copers [32]. One study found that females with noncontact injuries were more likely to be non-copers [27]; however, neither sex nor age are clear predictors of whether an athlete may require ACL reconstruction in the future [10].

Copers and non-copers have a different response to ACL injury biomechanically. Non-copers demonstrate a hallmark "stiffening strategy" during both walking and jogging [41]. Non-copers walk with decreased knee flexion on their involved limb from initial contact throughout loading response compared to their uninvolved limb as well as bilaterally compared to copers and controls [41]. This "stiffening strategy" also involves increased muscular co-contraction around the knee compared to copers and controls [41]. Both copers and non-copers demonstrate decreased peak vertical ground reaction force compared to controls and decreased knee extensor power absorption on their involved limbs compared to their uninvolved. Although both groups demonstrate decreased power absorption, copers and non-copers differ in their strategy to transfer their support moment. Where copers transfer their support moment to the ankle, non-copers transfer their support moment to the hip, in what is viewed as a less successful strategy [41]. In general, copers demonstrate kinetics similar to controls, but kinematics similar to non-copers [45]. When copers, non-copers, and adapters are identified retrospectively, based only on their return to preinjury level of sport, copers seem to recover their cadence, step length, and step velocity faster after ACL injury than adapters and non-copers. In the 6 months following ACL injury, copers develop a walking cadence, step length, and velocity that are slightly higher than that of controls, where adapters walk similarly to controls, and non-copers never reach the cadence, step length, or velocity of controls [4].

Work in the early 2000s indicated that non-copers were less specific than copers and controls in the firing of their vastus lateralis during target-matching tasks. These findings were related to other work indicating that non-copers fired their quadriceps at inappropriate times, potentially promoting episodes of giving way [46]. More recent findings have indicated that non-copers have less refined use of their rectus femoris and lateral hamstrings during target-matching tasks, potentially relating to the correlation between slower hamstring activity and episodes giving way [32]. These target-matching task results may be reflected in walking gait, as the earlier activation, longer duration, and delayed peak activity of the gastrocnemius and hamstring muscles seen in non-copers [41].

There are conflicting reports on whether differences in quadriceps strength between copers and non-copers exist when tested isometrically at 90° of knee flexion [23]. However, there is a difference in the quadriceps strength profiles of copers and non-copers. Using isokinetic strength testing at 10° increments from 0 to 90° of knee flexion, non-copers have significantly greater quadriceps strength asymmetries at angles less than 40° and greater than 60° of knee flexion [11]. Multiple studies and systematic reviews have confirmed there are no differences between copers and non-copers in the static tibiofemoral laxity [10, 23, 27, 37, 42, 44]. Copers do have higher Knee Outcome Survey Activities of Daily Living and Sports Scale

Table 37.1 SURF classification developed by Daniel et al. [8]

Difference between limbs in KT-1000 arthrometer measurement	Hours of preinjury level I or II sports participation per year		
	<50 h	50–199 h	>=200 h
<5 mm	Low	Low	Moderate
5–7 mm	Low	Moderate	High
>7 mm	Moderate	High	High

scores, Lysholm scores, higher global ratings of perceived knee function [9, 23, 25], and lower levels of movement-related fear than non-copers [21]. There is no difference, though, between the two groups in International Knee Documentation Committee form[1] score [9, 23, 25]. As increased knee joint laxity prohibits an athlete from scoring in the highest categories on the International Knee Documentation Committee form, it is reasonable to expect that the form would not be able to distinguish between copers and non-copers [22, 28]. Nevertheless, the strength and self-report measures together indicate that copers have better knee function and less fear following ACL injury compared to non-copers.

37.3 Development of Decision-Making Algorithm

In 1994, Daniel et al. published a study following 292 patients for approximately 5 years following knee hemarthrosis, assessing tibiofemoral joint laxity, occupation, recreation, and operative or nonoperative injury management among other outcomes [8]. From this cohort, 236 individuals had greater than 3 mm difference in knee joint laxity between limbs, 191 of whom had no surgery in the first 90 days after injury. Beyond 90 days, only 46 required ACL reconstruction, leaving 147 that the authors deemed to be copers. From their findings, Daniel et al. developed a surgical risk factor classification system, or SURF classification, for assessing the need for meniscal or ACL surgery >90 days after injury based on preinjury hours of participation in level I and II sports and the difference between limbs with the KT-1000 arthrometer measurement (Table 37.1) [8].

In a prospective study, the SURF system was unsuccessful in identifying which individuals would go on to require ACL reconstruction, particularly those classified as moderate or high risk [15]. Within a few years, both Snyder-Mackler et al. and Eastlack et al. published findings indicating that there was no difference between copers and non-copers in static knee joint laxity [9, 44]. Eastlack et al. found that by using limb symmetry from single-legged crossover hop testing, quadriceps strength, global rating of knee function score, and Knee Outcomes Survey Sports score, they could retrospectively identify copers and non-copers with 97 % sensitivity and 92 % specificity [9].

The following year, in 2000, Fitzgerald et al. [16] published what is now one of the most cited papers on the subject of identifying copers and non-copers, "A decision-making scheme for returning patients to high-level activity with nonoperative treatment after anterior cruciate ligament rupture." Setting out to identify athletes who could return to their preinjury level of sport in the short term, this algorithm was designed to be conservative. Athletes with concomitant ligamentous injuries were excluded due to the risk of instability, and repairable meniscal injuries and chondral defects were excluded in the case that an episode of giving

[1] It is important to make the clear distinction between the International Knee Documentation Committee form and the International Knee Documentation Committee 2000 Subjective Knee form. The International Knee Documentation Committee form includes both self-report and physical examination findings, particularly ligament and joint assessment, rating the knee as either normal, nearly normal, abnormal, or severely abnormal. The International Knee Documentation Committee 2000 Subjective Knee form, is purely a self-report measure regarding knee function. Eastlack et al. and Snyder-Mackler et al. found no difference between copers and non-copers on the International Knee Documentation Committee form.

way did further damage to what was originally a repairable injury [24]. A maximum of one episode of giving way, particularly during activities of daily living, was a strict exclusion criteria as individuals who experienced instability during basic tasks would likely not be safe with higher level athletic movements [24].

The Fitzgerald et al. algorithm (hereafter referred to as the Fitzgerald screening algorithm) recommended that physical therapy be initiated immediately following ACL injury in order to address primary impairments [16]. When an athlete had no pain, minimal joint effusion, full range of motion, and was able to hop on their involved limb, they were screened and categorized [16]. Athletes were excluded if they were not successful in resolving their initial impairments within one month of injury as it was thought that athletes with faster symptom resolution were more likely to be successful in returning quickly to sport [24]. Shortly after the initial algorithm was published, greater than 70 % quadriceps strength was added to the prerequisites for an athlete to be screened [18]. Fitzgerald et al. found that athletes who had one or fewer episodes of giving way, a score >= 60 % on the global rating of knee function scale, a score >= 80 % on the Knee Outcomes Survey Activities of Daily Living scale, and >= 80 % limb symmetry on the six-meter timed hop had a significantly higher likelihood of returning to their preinjury level of activity (Fact Box 1) [16]. An athlete had to pass all four criteria to be classified as a coper, and the screening was only performed once. If identified as a potential coper, athletes in the Fitzgerald et al. study would proceed with further rehabilitation, attempt nonoperative management, and return to sport. Non-copers and those excluded from screening were referred for surgical management [16, 24]. Of the 93 athletes screened by Fitzgerald et al., 39 were identified as potential copers. Of those potential copers, 28 attempted nonoperative management, and 22 (79 %) were able to return to their preinjury level of activity approximately eight weeks after their ACL injury [16].

Fact Box 1

Fitzgerald Screening Algorithm [16, 18]

Athletes included if:

- Have no repairable meniscal injuries or chondral defects.
- Have no grade II or greater concomitant ligamentous injuries.
- Impairments (pain, range of motion, joint effusion, gait asymmetry, able to hop on involved limb) are resolved within 1 month of ACL injury.
- Have >= 70 % quadriceps strength limb symmetry at time of screening.

Athletes are classified as a coper if they have:

- >= 60 % global rating of perceived knee function score
- >= 80 % Knee Outcome Survey Activities of Daily Living Scale score
- >= 80 % Six-meter timed single-legged hop limb symmetry index
- ≤ One episode of giving way

37.4 Outcomes of Screening

The Fitzgerald screening algorithm has subsequently been referenced and used in numerous studies since its publication [6, 7, 10, 11, 13, 14, 23–26, 29, 31, 32, 34, 35, 40–42, 46]. It has been inaccurately interpreted, and in one such case, a clarification was published [7] due to the importance of using all of the inclusion and screening criteria rather than only using episodes of giving way. Further, in order to truly compare outcomes, consistency is crucial.

Hurd et al. [26] found that using the Fitzgerald screening algorithm, 72 % of athletes who were originally identified as copers successfully returned to their preinjury level of sport. Only six percent of athletes failed rehabilitation following screening and prior to attempting return to sport, and six percent became adapters. Upon follow-up, 40 % of copers who returned to their preinjury level of sport continued to play without ACL reconstruction [26]. The results of this study indicated that, in the short term, a high percentage of athletes were able to return to their preinjury level of sport, and while a majority of those athletes did eventually go on to have ACL reconstruction, there was a small group who remained active without surgery [26].

Moksnes et al. [35] also used the Fitzgerald screening algorithm to examine outcomes one year after ACL injury. In this study, the authors did not exclude athletes if they had a quadriceps strength limb symmetry < 70 % or if initial impairment resolution took longer than one month. The authors categorized the subjects as either potential copers or potential non-copers; then unlike Fitzgerald et al. who only provided rehabilitation to copers [16], Moksnes et al. provided all athletes with further rehabilitation [35]. At follow-up one year after ACL injury, the authors categorized athletes as true copers if they returned and maintained their preinjury level of activity or true non-copers if they had not returned to preinjury level of sport or had experienced episodes of giving way. Fifteen true copers were identified from a group of 25 potential copers. Of greater interest, 19 of 27 potential non-copers were able to become true copers after further rehabilitation. In all, 69 % of the cohort was treated non-operatively and able to return to their preinjury level of sport [35]. The finding that with further rehabilitation some of the athletes classified as potential non-copers are able to become true copers makes a large impact on clinical practice. These findings indicate that with the use of progressive strength training and perturbation training (techniques that will be discussed later in the chapter), non-copers are able to return to their preinjury level of sport and subsequently that their decision to undergo operative or nonoperative management can be delayed.

At a cursory glance, the Moksnes et al. results might seem to signify that the Fitzgerald screening algorithm is inaccurate in identifying copers and non-copers, but in fact these studies complement each other with their differing purposes and implications. The Fitzgerald screening algorithm aimed to identify athletes who could quickly return to sport. Fitzgerald et al. screened athletes four weeks after ACL injury, provided rehabilitation to only copers, and encouraged a quick return to play with a short-term follow-up. In contrast, Moksnes et al. aimed to examine outcomes of all athletes at one year, particularly the potential non-copers. Moksnes et al. screened athletes almost three months after ACL injury and did not follow up until one year. The Fitzgerald screening algorithm indicates short term and quick return to play; for example, a coper could finish physical therapy to get back in time for an important game. Moksnes et al. indicate that potential non-copers should undergo progressive strengthening and perturbation training, a potentially slower and extended rehabilitation course, allowing them the possibility to become a true coper and return to their preinjury level of sport without surgical intervention.

In contrast to the Fitzgerald screening algorithm, Kostogiannis et al. [30] examined the long-term outcomes of individuals with ACL injuries seen in their clinic from 1985 to 1989 with ACL injuries. These athletes were treated arthroscopically to confirm their ACL injury and to treat any concomitant injuries, then advised to avoid all contact sports and reduce their activity. Athletes were randomized to either a home-based exercise group or physical therapy, but 69 % of the home-based exercise group was eventually moved to the physical therapy group due to decreased range of motion and atrophy. Three years after ACL injury, 40 of the 100 athletes had returned to their preinjury level of activity, and 67 were able to successfully avoid ACL reconstruction 15 years later. The authors concluded that the majority of athletes do not require operative treatment, but could do so only with a decrease in activity and avoidance of all contact sports. Rather than successfully identifying copers, Kostogiannis et al. successfully created adapters, as those who returned to their preinjury level of sport did so against the direction of the researchers. The important point of this study, though, is that supervised physical therapy following ACL injury is essential and that with counseling and rehabilitation, return to preinjury level of sport is possible without operative management.

Fact Box 2
- Athletes after combined progressive strengthening and perturbation training are five times more likely to return to their preinjury level of sport than those who are trained with progressive strengthening alone [16].
- Athletes after perturbation training walk with increased knee flexion angles during stance, reduced muscular co-contraction around the knee, and improved coupling between the quadriceps and the hamstrings and soleus to enhance the dynamic stability of the knee [6].

37.5 Current Recommendations

The Fitzgerald screening algorithm remains widely used for identifying copers who can return to sport quickly. Further functional measures may complement the algorithm in identifying athletes who are able to return to sport without ACL reconstruction after rehabilitation. Eitzen et al. [13] found that age, preinjury activity level, episodes of giving way, Knee Outcome Survey Activities of Daily Living Scale score, International Knee Documentation Committee 2000 Subjective Knee form (IKDC) score, six-meter timed hop test limb symmetry, and quadriceps strength limb symmetry accounted for 43 % of the variance in whether or not an athlete was able to avoid ACL reconstruction in the 15 months after ACL injury. The authors also found that this predictive value increased to 47 % after ten sessions of progressive strengthening and perturbation training using a model that included age, preinjury activity level, episodes of giving way, IKDC score, pain rated on a visual analog scale, and the six-meter timed hop test limb symmetry [13]. Even though episodes of giving way and static knee joint laxity are the most commonly used criteria in surgical decision-making in the absences of the Fitzgerald screening algorithm, episodes of giving way explained only 3 % of the variance in whether or not an athlete required surgery, and there was no difference in static laxity between those who were operatively and non-operatively managed [13].

Fact Box 3
Recommendations for rehabilitation following ACL injury:
- Immediately following injury: Assessed by surgeon and initiate physical therapy.
- Weeks 1–4: Physical therapy addressing joint effusion, range of motion, pain, gait, and strength impairments.
  - End of Week 4: If minimal joint effusion, no pain, full range of motion, and able to hop on one leg without pain, then use Fitzgerald screening algorithm [16] to assess if athlete is a potential coper. Regardless of whether the athlete meets the screening requirements or not, a discussion between athlete, surgeon, and physical therapist should occur on the athlete's progress, if they are ready for screening, the results of screening, and operative vs nonoperative management.
- If screened as a potential coper:
  - Weeks 5–9: Perturbation and strength training [17]. This track is designed to help the athlete return quickly to sport. Upon completion of perturbation training, an athlete must have >90 % quadriceps strength limb symmetry index, >90 % limb symmetry on all four single-legged hop tests, and >90 % scores on the Knee Outcome Survey Activities of Daily Living Scale and

global rating of perceived knee function score as well as receive clearance from their surgeon before they may return to sport.

- If screened as a potential non-coper or does not meet screening requirements at week 4:
  - Weeks 5+: Continue with physical therapy to address deficits. This track is designed to help an athlete return to sport but on a longer time line. When an athlete is ready, use perturbation training and progressive strengthening to improve their strength and neuromuscular control [14]. At conclusion of therapy, athlete should achieve the same return to sport criteria discussed above prior to returning to sport.

More than the screening algorithms, rehabilitation is truly what allows an athlete to be a coper. Progressive strength training (Fig. 37.1) and a neuromuscular reeducation technique, called perturbation training (Fig. 37.2), are integral to the success of non-operative management [6, 13, 14, 18, 24–26, 31, 34, 35]. Fitzgerald et al. [17] randomized 26 copers to either a progressive strengthening or a strengthening and perturbation training group. Eleven of the twelve athletes in the perturbation group successfully returned to their preinjury level of sport, but only seven of the fourteen in the progressive strengthening group were successfully able to return. Athletes after perturbation training are almost five times (positive likelihood ratio 4.88) more likely to return to their preinjury level of sport compared to athletes who only receive strength training [17]. Perturbation training is safe for ACL-deficient athletes if they meet the Fitzgerald screening algorithm inclusion criteria. Only 4 % of athletes develop effusion during plyometric activities (Fig. 37.3) causing only a need to decrease the frequency of their rehabilitation sessions[14]. Progressive strengthening and perturbation training improve single-legged hop test distances and speeds, increase self-report of function, and bolster involved limb quadriceps peak torque values to the level of dominant limb normative values [14]. Biomechanically, athletes after perturbation training walk with increased knee flexion angles during stance, reduced muscular co-contraction around the knee, and improved coupling between the quadriceps and the hamstrings and soleus to enhance the dynamic stability of the knee [6]. All of these findings indicate that progressive strengthening and perturbation training are necessary in order to facilitate normalized gait, dynamic knee stability, and nonoperative return to preinjury level of sport (Fact Box 2).

Fact Box 4

- The decision to pursue operative or nonoperative management should not occur immediately after ACL injury. This decision should not be made at a minimum until a patient has gone through physical therapy to resolve initial impairments and screening.
- There is no difference in clinical outcomes between athletes who have surgery immediately following ACL injury and those who delay surgery, indicating that there is no additional risk associated with extended rehabilitation following ACL injury [43].
- There is no difference in return to sport rates [20], knee function, or osteoarthritis development between athletes who undergo ACL reconstruction and those who opt for nonoperative management [5, 19].
- *Take home message*: Non-operative management is a decision that can be changed; ACL reconstruction is a final decision with huge implications. It is crucial that we educate our patients accurately on all the benefits and risks regarding operative and nonoperative management of ACL injuries.

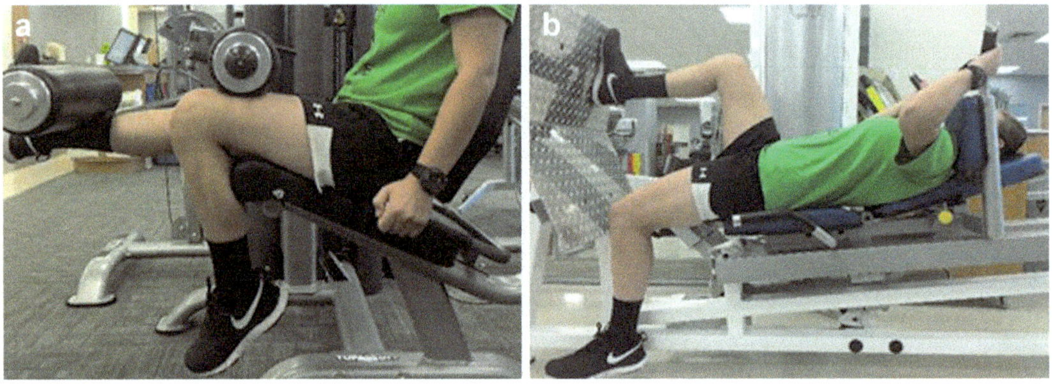

Fig. 37.1 Examples of progressive strength-training exercises. (**a**) Unilateral knee extension. (**b**) Unilateral leg press

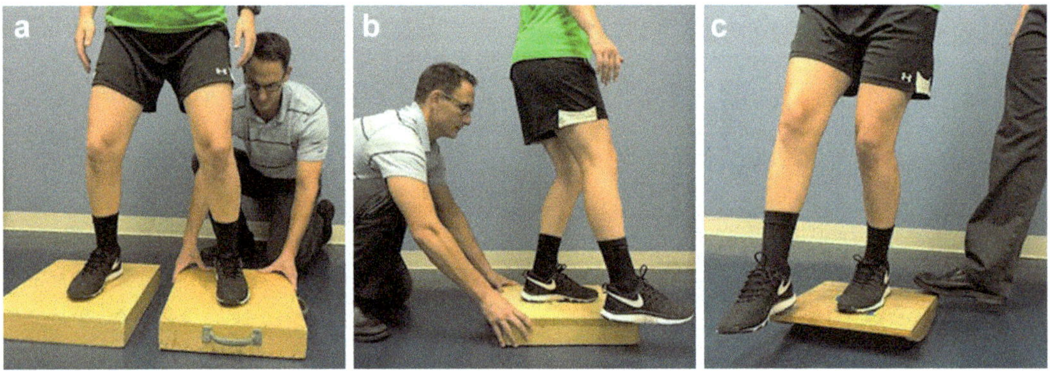

Fig. 37.2 Perturbation training. (**a**) Bilateral roller-board perturbation, (**b**) unilateral roller-board perturbation, and (**c**) unilateral rockerboard perturbation (See Fitzgerald et al. [16] or Eitzen et al.. [14] for a detailed description of perturbation training, progressive strength training, progression guidelines, and details of rehabilitation)

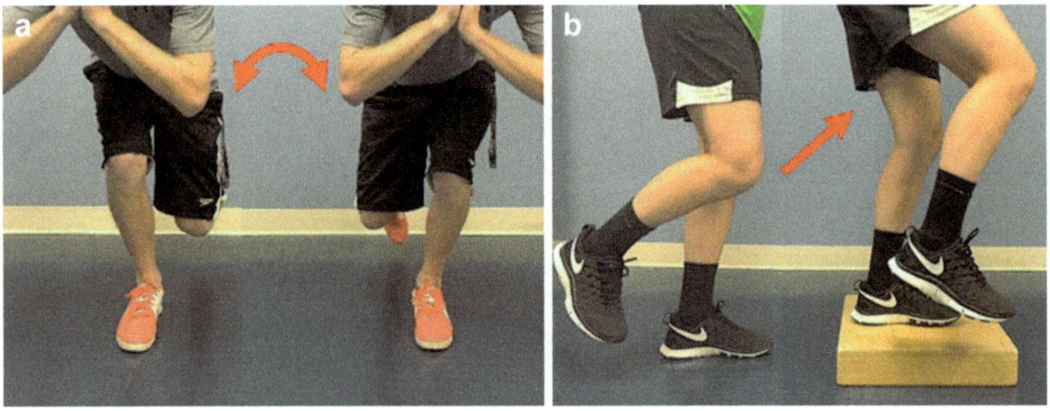

Fig. 37.3 Examples of plyometric exercises. (**a**)"Speed skaters" – starting on one leg, hop sideways and land on the other leg, with a soft, bent-knee landing. Repeat hopping back to the starting leg. (**b**) Single leg hop up – on a single leg hop up onto a *box*. *Box* size can be progressed to increase difficulty

Conclusion

This chapter has clearly demonstrated that some athletes following rehabilitation are able to return to their preinjury level of sport following ACL injury. Screening algorithms can identify athletes who are able to be copers both in the short and long term. Athletes should receive physical therapy immediately after ACL injury to resolve pain, range of motion, effusion, gait, and strength impairments (Fact Box 3). This care is crucial as it will influence a patient's outcomes regardless of whether they have surgery [12]. The decision to pursue operative or nonoperative management should not happen immediately following the ACL injury. A recent meta-analysis found no difference in clinical outcomes (including IKDC score, patient satisfaction, return to preinjury level of sport, static knee joint laxity, range of motion, incidence of arthrofibrosis, chondral injury, patellofemoral pain or joint crepitus, meniscal injury, or thromboembolic complications) between athletes who had surgery within three weeks of their ACL injury and those who had surgery greater than six weeks after ACL injury [43]. Outcomes of operative and non-operative ACL injury management do not necessarily favor surgery. ACL reconstruction does, in most cases, decreases static knee joint laxity [37], but a recent systematic review found that only 65 % of all athletes return to their preinjury level of sport and only 55 % return to competition after ACL reconstruction [2]. Such return to sport rates are very similar to those of non-operatively managed athletes discussed earlier in this chapter [14, 16, 26, 35] and supportive of Grindem et al. who found no significant difference between operative and non-operatively managed athletes returning to level I or higher level II sports in their first year after ACL injury [20]. In 2005, a *Cochrane Review* found there was insufficient evidence to recommend ACL reconstruction over non-operative management, and recent randomized control trials have found no difference between the two treatment methods with regard to knee function, but more importantly, no difference between the two treatments with regard to osteoarthritis development at 5 [19] and 14 years [5] following ACL injury. This evidence suggests that it is in the athletes' best interest to go through rehabilitation before making a treatment decision. An athlete who is screened one month after ACL injury and identified as a coper may be able to return for that last game of their season with rehabilitation. An athlete who is screened initially as a non-coper with progressive strengthening and perturbation training may be able to establish dynamic knee stability and return to their preinjury level of sport on a longer time frame. Not all athletes will be able to return to their preinjury level of sport non-operatively [24, 25], but even with operative management, they still may not be able to return [2] with the added higher risk and likely worse outcomes of a second ACL injury [36]. Thus, with all the benefits of rehabilitation, is it not worth counseling our athletes to be screened and go through physical therapy before they make the operative versus nonoperative decision? After all, the decision to go through rehabilitation and nonoperative management isn't final, the decision for ACL reconstruction is! (Fact Box 4).

References

1. Andernord D, Karlsson J, Musahl V, Bhandari M, Fu FH, Samuelsson K (2013) Timing of surgery of the anterior cruciate ligament. Arthroscopy 29(11): 1863–1871
2. Ardern CL, Taylor NF, Feller JA, Webster KE (2014) Fifty-five percent return to competitive sport following anterior cruciate ligament reconstruction surgery: an updated systematic review and meta-analysis including aspects of physical functioning and contextual factors. Br J Sports Med 48(21):1543–1552
3. Borchers JR, Kaeding CC, Pedroza AD et al (2011) Intra-articular findings in primary and revision anterior cruciate ligament reconstruction surgery a comparison of the MOON and MARS study groups. Am J Sports Med 39(9):1889–1893
4. Button K, van Deursen R, Price P (2006) Classification of functional recovery of anterior cruciate ligament

copers, non-copers, and adapters. Br J Sports Med 40(10):853–859
5. Chalmers PN, Mall NA, Moric M et al (2014) Does ACL reconstruction alter natural history? J Bone Joint Surg 96(4):292–300
6. Chmielewski TL, Rudolph KS, Snyder-Mackler L (2002) Development of dynamic knee stability after acute ACL injury. J Electromyogr Kinesiol 12(4):267–274
7. Chmielewski TL, Snyder-Mackler L (2007) Appropriate interpretation and application of a clinical classification scheme to describe dynamic knee stability after ACL injury. J Neurophysiol 98(1):557
8. Daniel DM, Stone ML, Dobson BE, Fithian DC, Rossman DJ, Kaufman KR (1994) Fate of the ACL-injured patient: a prospective outcome study. Am J Sports Med 22(5):632–644
9. Eastlack ME, Axe M, Snyder-Mackler L (1999) Laxity, instability, and functional outcome after ACL injury: copers versus noncopers. Med Sci Sports Exerc 31(2):210–215
10. Eggerding V, Meuffels DE, Bierma-Zeinstra SM, Verhaar JA, Reijman M (2015) Factors related to the need for surgical reconstruction after anterior cruciate ligament rupture: a systematic review of the literature. J Orthop Sports Phys Ther 45(1):37–44
11. Eitzen I, Eitzen T, Holm I, Snyder-Mackler L, Risberg M (2010) Anterior cruciate ligament deficient potential copers and non-copers reveal different isokinetic quadriceps strength profiles in the early stage after injury. Am J Sports Med 38(3):586–593
12. Eitzen I, Holm I, Risberg MA (2009) Preoperative quadriceps strength is a significant predictor of knee function two years after anterior cruciate ligament reconstruction. Br J Sports Med 43(5):371–376
13. Eitzen I, Moksnes H, Snyder-Mackler L, Engebretsen L, Risberg MA (2010) Functional tests should be accentuated more in the decision for ACL reconstruction. Knee Surg Sports Traumatol Arthrosc 18(11):1517–1525
14. Eitzen I, Moksnes H, Snyder-Mackler L, Risberg MA (2010) A progressive 5-week exercise therapy program leads to significant improvement in knee function early after anterior cruciate ligament injury. J Orthop Sports Phys Ther 40(11):705–721
15. Fithian DC, Paxton EW, Stone ML et al (2005) Prospective trial of a treatment algorithm for the management of the anterior cruciate ligament–injured knee. Am J Sports Med 33(3):335–346
16. Fitzgerald G, Axe M, Snyder-Mackler L (2000) A decision-making scheme for returning patients to high-level activity with nonoperative treatment after anterior cruciate ligament rupture. Knee Surg Sports Traumatol Arthrosc 8(2):76–82
17. Fitzgerald GK, Axe MJ, Snyder-Mackler L (2000) The efficacy of perturbation training in nonoperative anterior cruciate ligament rehabilitation programs for physically active individuals. Phys Ther 80(2):128–140
18. Fitzgerald GK, Axe MJ, Snyder-Mackler L (2000) Proposed practice guidelines for nonoperative anterior cruciate ligament rehabilitation of physically active individuals. J Orthop Sports Phys Ther 30(4):194–203
19. Frobell RB, Roos HP, Roos EM, Roemer FW, Ranstam J, Lohmander LS (2013) Treatment for acute anterior cruciate ligament tear: five year outcome of randomised trial. BMJ 346:f232
20. Grindem H, Eitzen I, Engebretsen L, Snyder-Mackler L, Risberg MA (2014) Nonsurgical or surgical treatment of ACL injuries: knee function, sports participation, and knee reinjury. J Bone Joint Surg 96(15): 1233–1241
21. Hartigan EH, Lynch AD, Logerstedt DS, Chmielewski TL, Snyder-Mackler L (2013) Kinesiophobia after anterior cruciate ligament rupture and reconstruction: noncopers versus potential copers. J Orthop Sports Phys Ther 43(11):821–832
22. Hefti E, Müller W, Jakob R, Stäubli H-U (1993) Evaluation of knee ligament injuries with the IKDC form. Knee Surg Sports Traumatol Arthrosc 1(3–4): 226–234
23. Herrington L, Fowler E (2006) A systematic literature review to investigate if we identify those patients who can cope with anterior cruciate ligament deficiency. Knee 13(4):260–265
24. Hurd W, Axe M, Snyder-Mackler L (2009) Management of the athlete with acute anterior cruciate ligament deficiency. Sports Health 1(1):39–46
25. Hurd WJ, Axe MJ, Snyder-Mackler L (2008) A 10-year prospective trial of a patient management algorithm and screening examination for highly active individuals with anterior cruciate ligament injury part 2, determinants of dynamic knee stability. Am J Sports Med 36(1):48–56
26. Hurd WJ, Axe MJ, Snyder-Mackler L (2008) A 10-year prospective trial of a patient management algorithm and screening examination for highly active individuals with anterior cruciate ligament injury: part 1, outcomes. Am J Sports Med 36(1):40–47
27. Hurd WJ, Axe MJ, Snyder-Mackler L (2008) Influence of age, gender, and injury mechanism on the development of dynamic knee stability after acute ACL rupture. J Orthop Sports Phys Ther 38(2):36–41
28. Irrgang JJ, Anderson AF, Boland AL et al (2001) Development and validation of the international knee documentation committee subjective knee form. Am J Sports Med 29(5):600–613
29. Kaplan Y (2011) Identifying individuals with an anterior cruciate ligament-deficient knee as copers and noncopers: a narrative literature review. J Orthop Sports Phys Ther 41(10):758–766
30. Kostogiannis I, Ageberg E, Neuman P, Dahlberg L, Fridén T, Roos H (2007) Activity level and subjective knee function 15 years after anterior cruciate ligament injury: a prospective, longitudinal study of nonreconstructed patients. Am J Sports Med 35(7):1135–1143
31. Lewek MD, Chmielewski TL, Risberg MA, Snyder-Mackler L (2003) Dynamic knee stability after anterior cruciate ligament rupture. Exerc Sport Sci Rev 31(4):195–200
32. MacLeod TD, Snyder-Mackler L, Buchanan TS (2014) Differences in neuromuscular control and quadriceps morphology between potential copers and

noncopers following anterior cruciate ligament injury. J Orthop Sports Phys Ther 44(2):76–84
33. Marx RG, Jones EC, Angel M, Wickiewicz TL, Warren RF (2003) Beliefs and attitudes of members of the American Academy of Orthopaedic Surgeons regarding the treatment of anterior cruciate ligament injury. Arthroscopy 19(7):762–770
34. Moksnes H, Risberg MA (2009) Performance-based functional evaluation of non-operative and operative treatment after anterior cruciate ligament injury. Scand J Med Sci Sports 19(3):345–355
35. Moksnes H, Snyder-Mackler L, Risberg MA (2008) Individuals with an anterior cruciate ligament-deficient knee classified as noncopers may be candidates for nonsurgical rehabilitation. J Orthop Sports Phys Ther 38(10):586–595
36. Myklebust G, Bahr R (2005) Return to play guidelines after anterior cruciate ligament surgery. Br J Sports Med 39(3):127–131
37. Neuman P, Kostogiannis I, Fridén T, Roos H, Dahlberg L, Englund M (2012) Knee laxity after complete anterior cruciate ligament tear: a prospective study over 15 years. Scand J Med Sci Sports 22(2):156–163
38. Paterno MV, Rauh MJ, Schmitt LC, Ford KR, Hewett TE (2012) Incidence of contralateral and ipsilateral anterior cruciate ligament (ACL) injury after primary ACL reconstruction and return to sport. Clin J Sport Med 22(2):116–121
39. Paterno MV, Rauh MJ, Schmitt LC, Ford KR, Hewett TE (2014) Incidence of second ACL injuries 2 years after primary ACL reconstruction and return to sport. Am J Sports Med 42(7):1567–1573
40. Risberg MA, Moksnes H, Storevold A, Holm I, Snyder-Mackler L (2009) Rehabilitation after anterior cruciate ligament injury influences joint loading during walking but not hopping. Br J Sports Med 43(6):423–428
41. Rudolph KS, Axe MJ, Buchanan TS, Scholz JP, Snyder-Mackler L (2001) Dynamic stability in the anterior cruciate ligament deficient knee. Knee Surg Sports Traumatol Arthrosc 9(2):62–71
42. Rudolph KS, Eastlack ME, Axe MJ, Snyder-Mackler L (1998) 1998 Basmajian student award paper: movement patterns after anterior cruciate ligament injury: a comparison of patients who compensate well for the injury and those who require operative stabilization. J Electromyogr Kinesiol 8(6):349–362
43. Smith TO, Davies L, Hing CB (2010) Early versus delayed surgery for anterior cruciate ligament reconstruction: a systematic review and meta-analysis. Knee Surg Sports Traumatol Arthrosc 18(3):304–311
44. Snyder-Mackler L, Fitzgerald GK, Bartolozzi AR, Ciccotti MG (1997) The relationship between passive joint laxity and functional outcome after anterior cruciate ligament injury. Am J Sports Med 25(2): 191–195
45. Williams GN, Chmielewski T, Rudolph KS, Buchanan TS, Snyder-Mackler L (2001) Dynamic knee stability: current theory and implications for clinicians and scientists. J Orthop Sports Phys Ther 31(10): 546–566
46. Williams GN, Snyder-Mackler L, Barrance PJ, Buchanan TS (2005) Quadriceps femoris muscle morphology and function after ACL injury: a differential response in copers versus non-copers. J Biomech 38(4):685–693

Experience with Computer Navigation: Present and Future

38

James Robinson and Philippe Colombet

Contents

J. Robinson, FRCS(Orth), MS (✉)
Department of Musculoskeletal Surgery, Avon Orthopaedic Centre, Bristol, UK
e-mail: jrrobinson@doctors.org.uk

P. Colombet, MD
Clinque du Sport, Bordeaux-Merignac, Mérignac, France

The ability to accurately quantify knee stability is valuable for both the diagnosis of instability patterns and the evaluation of ligament reconstructions. Several measurement devices have been developed to objectively assess knee stability (e.g. KT-1000®, MEDmetric, San Diego, CA and Rolimeter®, Aircast Europe, Neubeuern, Germany). These have allowed the measurement of isolated uniplanar motions such as anterior tibial translation or internal/external tibial rotation. The pivot-shift test is however a complex three-dimensional motion about a helical axis. Although, when viewed in the axial plane, the motion can be shown to comprise of anteroposterior tibial translation with coupled internal/external tibial rotation (a coupled movement is one that occurs automatically in response to a displacement applied in another degree of freedom of the knee [3]), the measurement of these more complex multiplanar motions has remained elusive. Electromagnetic tracking devices (e.g. the Flock of Birds®, Ascension Technology Corporation, Burlington, VT) offer potential but their use is limited as accuracy may be influenced by magnetic fields or ferromagnetic objects within their range, rendering their use problematic in the operating room [5].

The use of computer-assisted navigation in ACL surgery dates back to the 1990s [8, 14]. Initially systems were designed to aid the precision of bone tunnel placement [30] however, the ability to precisely quantify 6 degree-of-freedom (6-DOF) kinematics, enabling the objective

V. Musahl et al. (eds.), *Rotatory Knee Instability*, DOI 10.1007/978-3-319-32070-0_38

measurement of the pivot shift and coupled rotations/translations both in the laboratory and in the clinical settings became increasingly apparent [6, 29]. Intraoperative-navigated measurement of uniplanar motions has shown good intra-observer repeatability with other measurement devices (such as Rolimeter® or KT 1000® [25, 35]), and the navigated analysis of pivot shift correlates reasonably well with clinical pivot-shift grading [3, 4, 21].

38.1 Current Navigation Technology for the Use with Ligament Reconstruction

Navigation systems may be "image based" requiring anatomical reference data acquired either from preoperative computerised tomography [9], intraoperative fluoroscopy [18, 32] or radiographs [34]. "Image-free" systems require no preoperative imaging, but rely on the registration of anatomical reference points. The system softwre uses these points in a three-dimensional registration algorithm to adapt a standard knee model to match the patient's individual knee morphology. Active optoelectronic systems use an infrared camera to track the motion of reference arrays, rigidly fixed to the patient's anatomy that emits an infrared signal. Passive optoelectronic systems are the most widely used. The reference arrays are equipped with markers that simply reflect an infrared signal which is both generated and detected by the camera. Arrays can also be attached to probes and instruments so that their relative position can be recognised by the computer. The position in space of the markers is calculated approximately 60 times per second. Markers can also be mounted on probes, guides and even drills so that their position relative to the rigid body arrays can be displayed to the surgeon on a digital display in real time. Systems have been shown to have a high degree of measurement accuracy, in the range of ±0.1 mm for linear measurements and ±0.1° for angular measurements [6, 29].

In this chapter, we describe our current experience with the Surgetics station (PRAXIM Medivision, La Tronche, France) hardware. This is a passive optical, open-platform, image-free system that allows knee alignment and kinematics to be measured in addition to guiding tunnel positions. The Surgetics ACL Logics KOALA software (PRAXIM Medivision, La Tronche, France) may be used for navigating several different reconstruction procedures including ACL, MCL, LCL and lateral extra-articular pasty (LEAP). The Cartesian coordinate system is constructed from knee flexion/extension kinematic data, and surface landmarks are acquired using a pointer equipped with a navigation array. The surgeon uses a foot switch and a touchscreen to control the system.

38.2 Intraoperative Measurement of Knee Laxity

For the system to accurately measure tibiofemoral joint kinematics, the infrared optical sensor (camera) on the Surgetics station detects the relative positions of two rigid bodies, each with three disposable passive markers fixed onto the tibia and femur. The rigid body navigation arrays are must be rigidly fixed to the tibia and femur to ensure accuracy. This may be achieved with the use of bi-cortical Schanz screws with an external fixator-type attachment securing the array. The system used by the authors utilises a single specifically designed fixation nail that is triangular in cross section. A small (approx. 5 mm) skin incision is made to place the femoral rigid body at the junction of the middle and distal one-thirds of the femur. The triangular nail is placed percutaneously after drilling a 2.7-mm unicortical pilot hole. It is important to avoid transfixing the quadriceps tendon as this may lead to rapid loosening of the fixation with knee flexion/extension. The tibial rigid body is similarly fixed to the anteromedial face of the tibia. During hamstring autograft ACL reconstruction, the tibial rigid body is usually fixed through hamstring harvest incision. Both rigid bodies are carefully oriented towards the optical sensor, so they may be visualised during clinical laxity test-

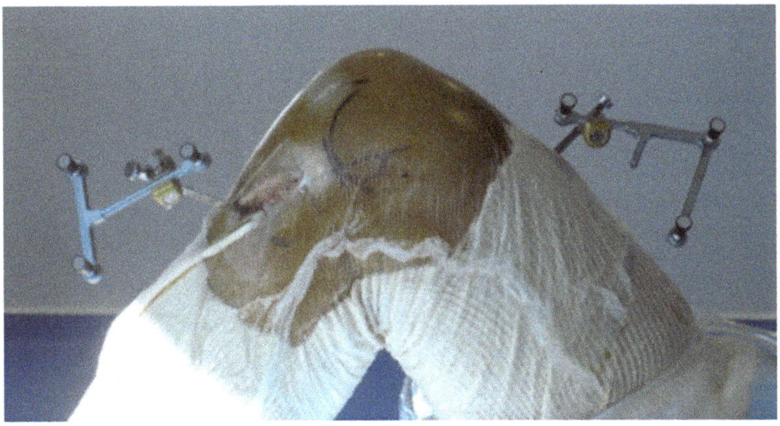

Fig. 38.1 The tibial (*T*) and femoral (*F*) passive optical navigation arrays are securely fixed to their respective bones using a unicortical triangular nails (as shown) or with an external fixator-type connectors and Schanz screws

ing, particularly the pivot-shift manoeuvre. The correct placement of navigation rigid bodies is critical as once positioned they cannot be moved. Care must be taken that they do not obstruct the passage of arthroscopic instruments through the portals or impede bone tunnel drilling (Fig. 38.1).

Fact Box 1

Passive rigid body arrays are rigidly fixed to bone. Anatomic reference points are digitised defining three orthogonal reference vectors about which 6-DOF kinematics are computed. Kinematic measurements may be made with high degree of accuracy: ±0.1 mm for linear measurements and ±0.1° for rotations.

A navigation probe, equipped with passive optical markers, is used to digitise specific anatomical landmarks: the centre of the medial tibial plateau and the centre of the lateral tibial plateau, the tips of the tibial spines, a point on the tibia just anterior to the centre of the intermeniscal ligament (all acquired arthroscopically) and tips of the medial and lateral malleoli (acquired percutaneously). The craniocaudal axis of the tibia is defined by a line passing through the ankle centre (the midpoint between the two malleoli) and the midpoint between the two tibial spines. These two positions are tracked during knee flexion/extension, and the midsagittal plane of the knee is defined as that containing the mean square of the cloud of points created by the tibia and ankle centres. The mediolateral vector of the tibia is defined as orthogonal to the midsagittal plane in the extended knee (0°). The anteroposterior vector is defined as being orthogonal to the tibial craniocaudal axis and the medial-lateral vector. These three orthogonal vectors (medial lateral, craniocaudal and anteroposterior) create the reference by which 6 degree-of-freedom kinematics may be computed by the navigation system, allowing the analysis of knee kinematics and laxity (in terms of translations and rotations).

Detailed information is therefore available to the surgeon as to the effect of the reconstruction on stabilising the knee. The laxity tests the surgeon wishes to perform, e.g. the internal/external rotation, varus/valgus laxity, anterior and posterior drawer, Lachman and pivot-shift tests, are selected from the navigation software's preoperative menu. During anterior-posterior laxity testing, tibial anterior translation is measured by tracking the positions of the centres of the medial and lateral tibial condyles projected onto the axial plane of the tibia relative to the femoral rigid body. For anterior drawer testing at 90° knee flexion (anterior drawer rest) and at 20° knee flexion (Lachman test), the navigation system measures anterior tibial translation and also measures the coupled internal tibial rotation that occurs. Similarly during posterior drawer testing at 90° and 20° flexion, coupled external tibial rotation may be measured (Fig. 38.2). In addition the navigated laxity examination is useful in determining

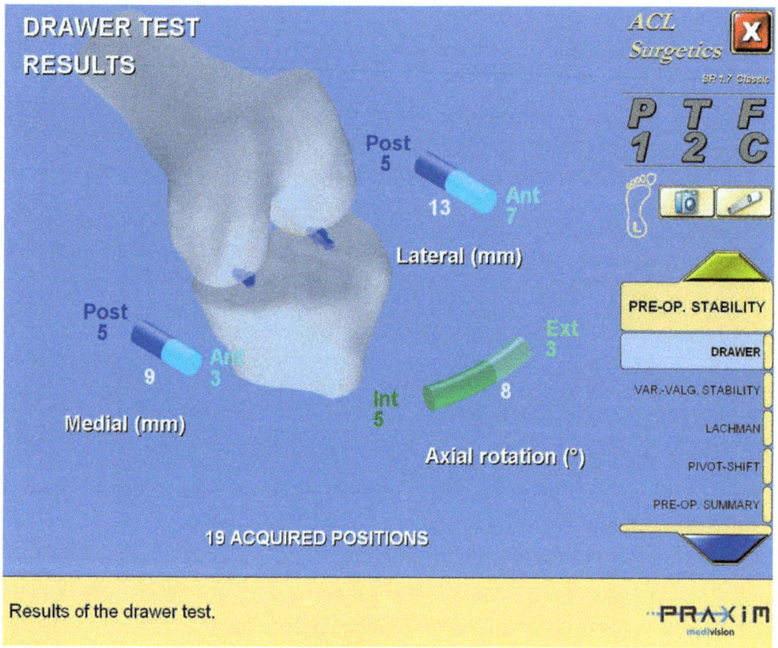

Fig. 38.2 An example screenshot from the navigation display taken intraoperatively following anteroposterior drawer testing. The anterior translation of the medial and lateral tibial condyles (3 mm and 7 mm, respectively) and coupled tibial internal rotation (5°) are shown

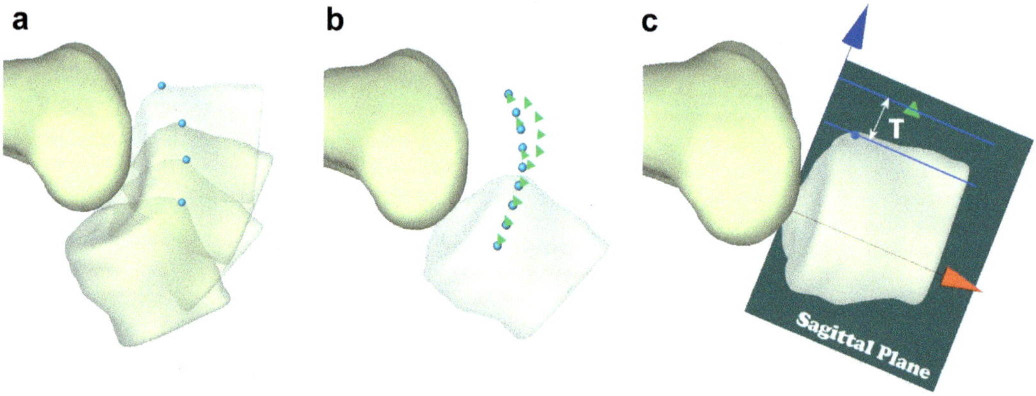

Fig. 38.3 (**a**) The motion of a digitised point on the anterior tibia was tracked in the midsagittal plane during passive flexion/extension (*circles*) and (**b**) during the pivot shift (*triangles*). (**c**) The maximum distance between these two trajectories defined the anterior translation (*T*) during the pivot shift

the "neutral" resting position of the knee which may be recorded so that the knee can be reproducibly returned to the same position of flexion and internal / external rotation for subsequent tests.

The Surgetics navigation system measures tibial translation during the pivot-shift test by tracking a digitised point on the tibia and comparing its motion path, in the midsagittal plane, with the motion of the same point during passive flexion/extension of the knee (Fig. 38.3). Tibial rotation that occurs during the pivot manoeuvre is measured by tracking the anterior vector of the tibia in the axial plane. Lane et al. [21] noted a good correlation between clinical pivot-shift test grade and tibial translation and rotation measured by the navigation and in addition characterised the P-shaped track of motion path of the digitised point on the anterior tibia during the pivot manoeuvre, showing this to have the closest correlation with pivot-shift test grade ($R^2 \geq 0.97$).

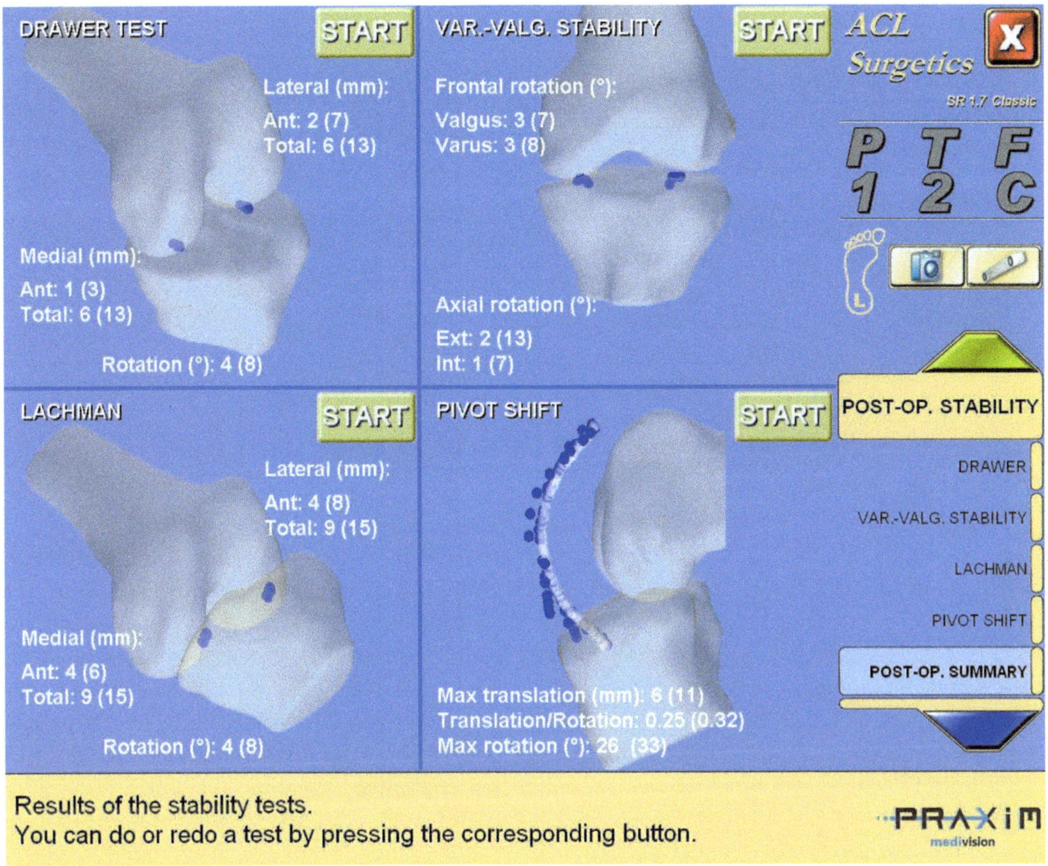

Fig. 38.4 Navigation screenshot showing postoperative laxity results following combined ACL/MCL reconstruction

The use of navigation in sports medicine is not restricted to ACL reconstruction. It may also be used for planning and performing reconstructions of peripheral ligament structures. Navigated medial collateral ligament (MCL) reconstruction, for example, assists the identification of optimum none tunnel positions: a point on the tibia at the attachment of the superficial MCL is defined and digitised; the computer then is able to produce an isometry map around the medial epicondyle of the femur to assist optimum placement of the femoral tunnel for graft isometry and assess control of both rotation laxity and anteromedial rotation that may result from combined MCL and ALC instability [20] (Fig. 38.4). Similarly for lateral extra-articular plasty (LEAP), the software may be used to determine the femoral tunnel position based on an isometry map.

38.3 Clinical Experience

For over a decade, we have utilised the computer-assisted navigation for both *in vitro* and *in vivo* laxity analysis to assess ACL reconstruction and associated surgery. Clinical, intraoperative navigation laxity testing has been performed for single-bundle (SB) ACL reconstruction and double-bundle (DB) ACL reconstruction and revision ACL reconstruction with and without lateral extra-articular palsy (±LEAP). The clinical results of the preoperative and postoperative laxity analysis for primary ACL reconstruction are shown in Table 38.1. For single-bundle ACL reconstruction, a four-strand hamstrings graft was used, fixed on the femoral side with an Endobutton CL® Smith and Nephew, Andover, MA) and with a bioabsorbable interference screw on the tibial

Table 38.1 Table showing navigated laxity test results for primary ACL reconstruction

Laxity test		Pre-op ($n = 183$)	Post-op single-bundle ACL reconstruction ($n = 162$)	Post-op double-bundle ACL reconstruction ($n = 21$)
Anterior drawer (90°)	Translation medial compartment (mm)	8.6 ± 2.5	1.6	0.6 ± 0.5
	Translation lateral compartment (mm)	12.9 ± 3.1	5.8	4.8 ± 1.3
	Coupled internal tibial rotation (°)	9.12 ± 4	8.5	7.2 ± 1.8
Lachman (20°)	Translation medial compartment (mm)	14.3 ± 4.2	2.3 ± 1.5	2.1 ± 1.1
	Translation lateral compartment (mm)	18.0 ± 4.4	3.1 ± 2.2	3.2 ± 1.4
	Coupled internal tibial rotation (°)	12.8 ± 4.8	2.7 ± 2.2	2.2 ± 1.6

side (BioRCI®, Smith and Nephew, Andover, MA). Double-bundle reconstructions were performed using a four-tunnel technique, using doubled or tripled semi-tendinosus autograft for the AM bundle and doubled or tripled gracilis autograft for the PL bundle. Grafts were fixed using Endobutton fixation devices on the femoral side and BioRCI screws on the tibial side.

It is accepted that pivot laxity remains the best indicator of a patient's subjective instability [19]. It is well recognised that rotational stability following ACL reconstruction may not be fully restored [12, 22, 24, 33] and that up to 30 % of patients may have a residual "pivot glide". Intraoperative-navigated laxity testing has demonstrated that single-bundle ACL reconstruction variably controls pivot-shift laxity (Fig. 38.5). Analysis of pre- and postoperative pivot-shift data showed that both double- and single-bundle ACL reconstructions reduced the translation and rotation occurring during the pivot shift. Translation was reduced by a mean of 12.3 mm in the SB group and 12.4 mm in the DB group. Rotation was reduced by 15.5° in the SB group and by 16.3° in the DB group. It must be noted that the groups were not comparative. Double-bundle reconstruction was utilised for patients with a higher degree of pivot-shift laxity (mean preoperative rotation occurring during the pivot-shift test was 25° in the SB group compared with 29.3° in the DB group) following a clinical study that was devised to investigate the effect of sequential reconstructions of the anteromedial (AM) and posterolateral (PL) bundles of the ACL on controlling the tibial rotation and translation occurring with the anterior drawer, Lachman and pivot-shift tests [31]. In this study two reconstruction protocols were used in 16 patients undergoing four-tunnel, double-bundle ACL reconstruction, creating the conditions where each bundle acted alone and combined with the other, so that the effects of each bundle could be assessed. The AM bundle was found to be the primary restraint to anterior laxity during the anterior drawer test reducing tibial translation by 67 %. The PL bundle was more important during the Lachman test reducing tibial translation by 73 %. The coupled internal rotation was reduced from 5.1° in ACL-deficient knees to 1.7° by isolated PL bundle reconstruction. The PL bundle was also important in controlling the tibial rotational laxity during the pivot shift, with isolated PL bundle reconstruction providing 14 % more reduction than isolated AM bundle reconstruction. This work suggested that for intra-articular ACL reconstruction the PL bundle was important in controlling the rotational component of the pivot shift and anterior laxity towards knee extension.

The role of lateral extra-articular pasty (LEAP) to augment intra-articular ACL reconstruction and improve control of pivot instability remains controversial. Although a recent systematic review of the literature [13] found that ACL

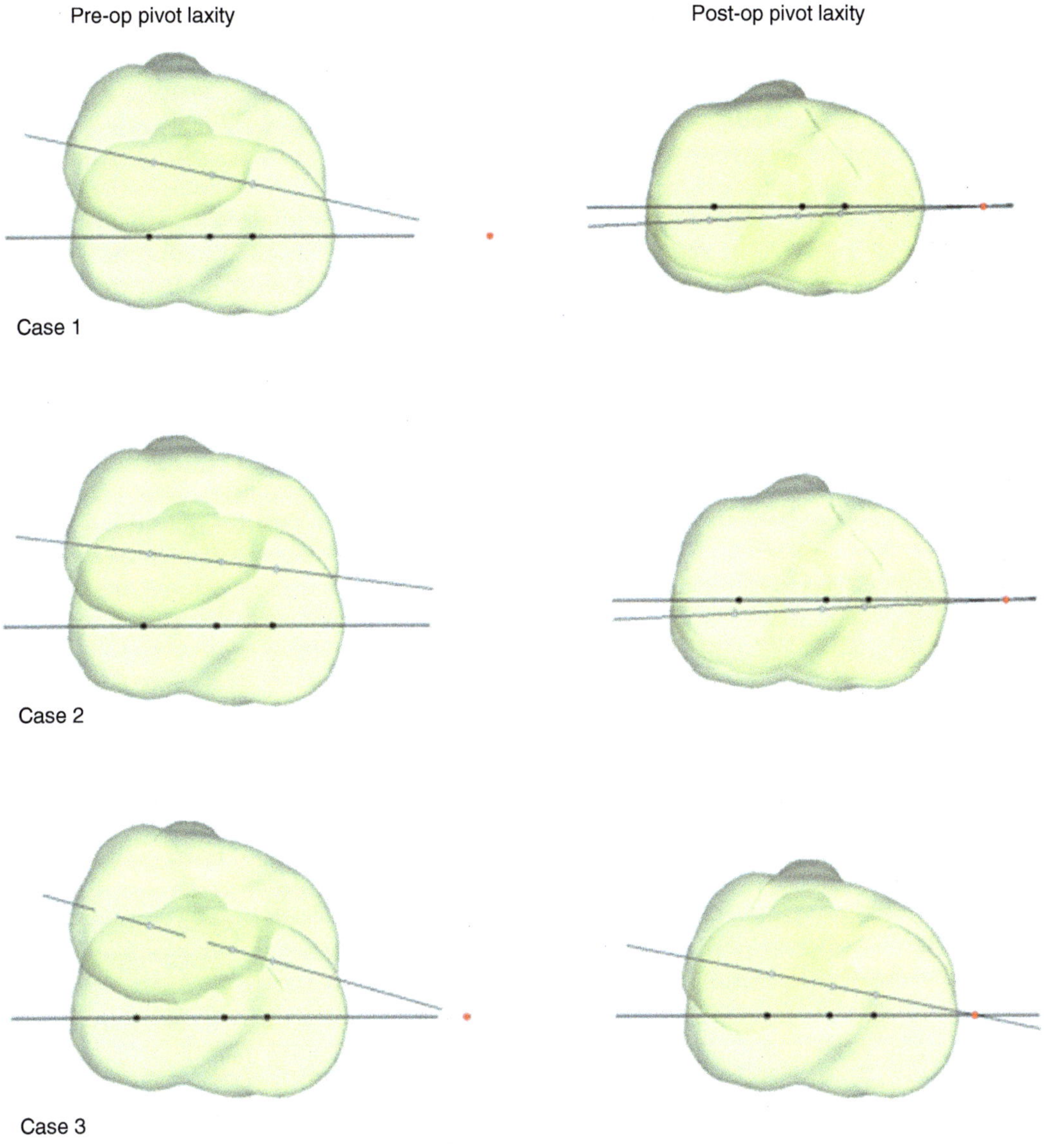

Fig. 38.5 Figure showing the maximum displacement of the tibial plateau during the pivot-shift test before and after ACL reconstruction in three individuals. Laxity appears to be well restored in *cases 1 and 2*. However, in *case 3* significant laxity persists

reconstruction combined with LEAP showed a significant improvement in control of pivot laxity over isolated ACL reconstruction, it was noted that studies lacked sufficient validity, sample size, methodological consistency and the was little standardisation of reconstruction procedures, rehabilitation protocols and outcome measures. The PRAXIM Surgetics navigation system has been used to assess the effect of a combined LEAP procedure on the control of rotational laxity in patients undergoing revision ACL reconstruction [7]. Twenty patients underwent navigated revision anterior cruciate ligament reconstruction with the addition of a percutaneous lateral extra-articular tenodesis. The navigation system was used to guide tunnel positioning in order to optimise the isometry of the LEAP. It was found that addition of the lateral tenodesis reduced coupled internal rotation ($P = .003$) occurring with the anterior drawer test and maximum internal rotation at 90° of flexion; however, although there was a trend towards improved control of rotation during the pivot-shift test, this did not reach statistical significance [6]. Isometry mapping has also demonstrated the importance of the femoral attachment location for LEAP, particularly if the reconstruction is taken *superficial* to the fibular collateral ligament (Fig. 38.6). The graft should be attached just proximal and posterior to the lateral epicondyle so that it remains isometric during knee flexion. Attachment of the extra-articular palsy anterior or distal to the epicondyle will result in an unfavourable tightening of the graft with progressive knee flexion.

The tibial translation and rotation that occurs during the pivot shift may be expressed as a ratio of translation to rotation (T/R). We have found for ACL-deficient patients mean preoperative tibial translation during the pivot shift = 18 ± 4 mm and tibial rotation during the pivot shift = 25 ± 7°, thus T/R = 0.52. This ratio may, however, vary between 0.25 and 0.86 with lower values indicating a higher degree of tibial rotation compared to translation, and conversely higher values indicate more translation than rotation. Pearle et al. [29] demonstrated that tibial rotation and displacement of the lateral compartment correlated closely with pivot-shift test grade. Recent studies have shown that the structures at the lateral aspect of the knee, particularly the ITB, have a much more significant role in the restraint of internal tibial rotation and the pivot shift than the ACL [17]·. The ACL and, in particular, its direct fibres are the primary restraint to anterior tibial translation at all angles of knee flexion [16]. The use of navigation to analyse the pivot shift may allow the surgeon to better understand the effect of different reconstructions on pivot laxity. It might, for example, be used to objectively determine whether routine single-bundle ACL reconstruction may be insufficient to fully control the rotational laxity in patients with high degrees of lateral compartment displacement and rotation during the pivot-shift test, indicating that additional surgery such as LEAP or DB reconstruction may be required to improve laxity control.

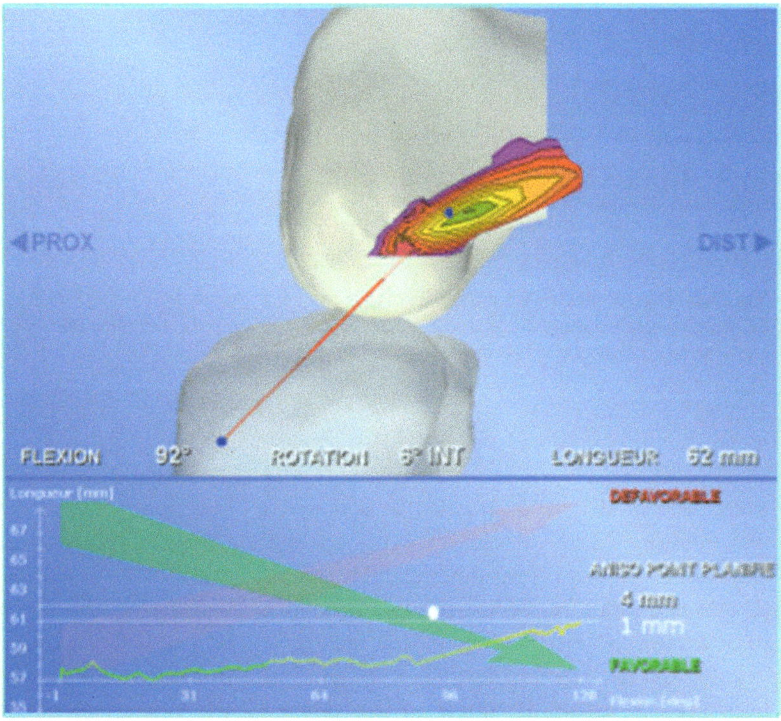

Fig. 38.6 The navigation computer display screen during a LEAP procedure. An "isometry map" is projected onto a digital image of the lateral femoral condyle, aiding selection of femoral tunnel position. Green indicates most isometric (<1 mm of length change), yellow less isometric and red the least isometric. The "isometry profile" (the distance between selected femoral and tibial attachment points through the range of knee flexion) is shown below. In this case a graft that is isometric between 0° and 90° but tightening slightly in deep flexion

Fact Box 2

A ratio of pivot translation to pivot rotation of <0.5 typically indicates increased lateral compartment displacement and may suggest the need for reconstructive techniques to improve the control of rotation (e.g. double-bundle ACL reconstruction and lateral extra-articular plasty).

38.4 Critical Analysis of the Present State of Navigation Laxity Measurement and the Future

Current computer-assisted navigation systems are a powerful tool in the accurate assessment of knee stability. In addition to the accurate measurement of 6 degree-of-freedom knee kinematics allowing objective assessment of reconstructions, navigation also allows exact determination and documentation of tunnel positions allowing studies to be made comparable. However, there are significant limitations to current technology. There is a need to invasively insert rigid body navigation arrays and measurement of laxity is only possible preoperatively and at time zero post intervention. In addition, side-to-side comparison with the contralateral limb is not possible. Complications related to navigation rigid body pin sites are rare but include acute fractures [15], stress fractures [28], superficial wound infections and osteomyelitis [1]. Thus our use of navigated laxity measurement is now limited to the use in clinical- and laboratory-based research studies.

Currently navigated laxity testing is not instrumented, and it is necessary to try to manually apply similar forces during pre-and postoperative testing to obtain comparable data. Therefore standardisation of navigated clinical laxity testing remains problematic, and whilst it is possible to use instruments such as a sterilised KT 1000® to apply known loads, these bulky instruments may interfere with the placement of the navigation rigid bodies. The interoperator variability of the pivot-shift test is known [27]. It remains particularly difficult to standardise the pivot-shift test clinically, and performing a pivot-shift test with consistent loading conditions is challenging (Fig. 38.7). Although it has been shown that the pivot shift may be simulated with combined valgus and internal rotation torques as the knee is flexed [10], systems to standardise pivot-shift application in the clinical setting exist but remain rudimentary, cumbersome and impractical for routine clinical use [26].

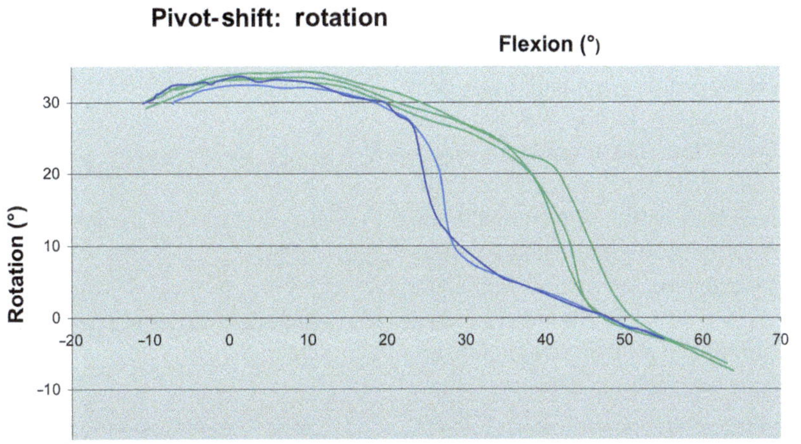

Fig. 38.7 Showing the intra-observer differences between the pivot-shift tests performed by the two authors JR (*blue*) and PC (*green*) on the same knee intraoperatively. All pivot-shift tests show a rapid reduction of the applied internal tibial rotation. There is good intra-observer reliability, between tests; however, the angle at which the reduction occurs is different between observers. The amount of external tibial rotation occurring as the knee reduces is, however, similar

The rigid body optical markers also suffer from "line-of-sight" problems that can be bothersome during surgery, particularly when performing navigated laxity tests. We have found spherical reflective markers have better visibility to the infrared camera than flat disc markers and are also less likely to be affected by arthroscopic irrigation fluid. Much work into improving navigation markers is still required, and certainly one of the key new advances will be a method of attaching navigation markers without the need for invasive bony fixation.

38.5 Future Directions

From the early days of computer-assisted navigation, there have been huge advances in motion-sensing technology. Gyroscopes, accelerometers and magnetometers are now incorporated into everyday devices such as smart phones and tablets. Studies have shown that non-invasive accelerometers may be used to accurately diagnose and grade pathological pivot laxity associated with ACL injury [2, 11, 23]. However, accelerometers remain limited in their ability to accurately quantify rotational and translational displacements. It is likely that accurate measurement of knee laxity by navigation systems will develop in two directions. Firstly, prototypes of ultra-sophisticated non-invasive systems are in development. These combine several technologies (accelerometers, gyroscopes and magnetometers) enabling not only qualitative assessment of subluxation such as that occurring with the pivot-shift test, but in addition, allow quantitative motion analysis of rotations and translations with a high level of precision (submillimetric). Lacking the need to fix rigid body arrays to bone, these newer, noninvasive systems will allow for objective laxity analysis in the office, during surgery and at subsequent postoperative follow-up. Current rigid body navigation systems only allow for intraoperative measurements; thus the efficacy of surgical reconstruction may only be assessed at time zero. As result, we have only a limited understanding as to the evolution of postoperatively knee laxity after ligament reconstruction. Whilst still in their prototype stages of development, these new systems offer exciting possibilities as powerful diagnostic tools and may prove invaluable in broadening our understanding of how knee laxity evolves and how different graft types, fixation and physical therapy regimes act to stabilise the knee over time.

Secondly, novel systems are in development, similar to those already in use in industry, that utilise virtual modelling and simulate rigid body analysis. Complex virtual models of the knee have been created [11] (Fig. 38.8) that have been defined by the geometric parameters of bony morphology and with the effect of ligament muscles and tendons, characterised by their linear stiffness, insertions and generated forces. Using rigid body simulation techniques, data from previous experiments into the effects of various loading conditions on knee kinematics (both *in vivo* and *in vitro*) has been added to the virtual model. The prototype system allows the virtual model to be individualised from patient CT or MRI data. Anatomical reference points are then digitised and the patient undergoes laxity examination. The data from the digitised ligament laxity tests is then analysed by the system comparing it with the virtual model to determine what lesions are implicated in producing the pattern of laxity and to suggest which structures may require reconstruction. This type of system will be particularly helpful in assessing laxity in secondary restraints and might be used interoperatively to virtually test different repair/reconstruction strategies and fine-tuning bone tunnel placement to optimise results.

Fact Box 3

Current navigation technology	Future navigation technology
Invasive:	Noninvasive:
Difficult to assess side-to-side laxity	Easy side-to-side measurement of laxity
Time zero data at time of surgery only	Data comparable with virtual model
Accurate	Accurate
Arrays may obstruct surgery	Easy to use in surgery and in the office

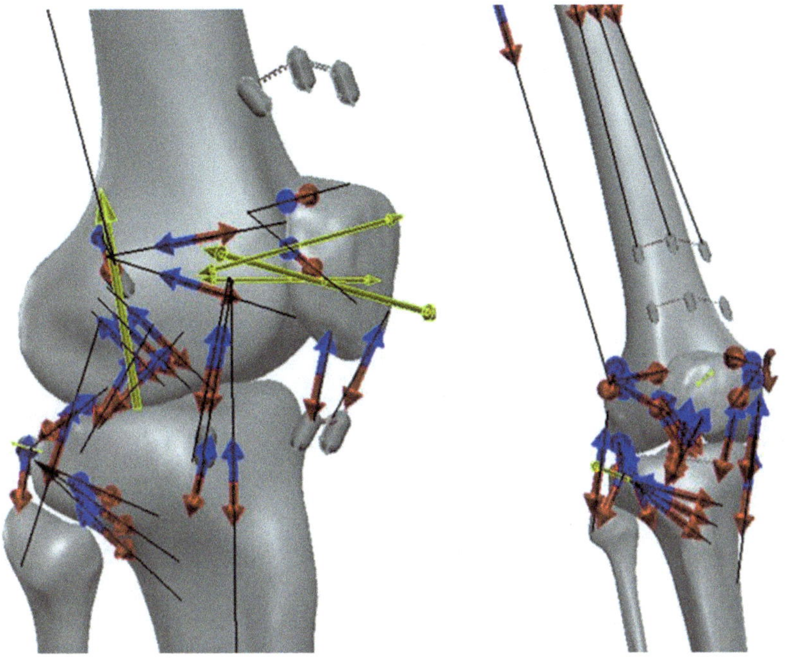

Fig. 38.8 Showing the action (*blue*) and reaction (*red*) force vectors occurring in various ligament bundles, tendons and muscles during active knee flexion. Joint contact forces are shown in *yellow*. Prototype navigation systems exist which compare a noninvasive, digitised laxity examination with the virtual model to suggest which structures are deficient and possible reconstruction strategies (Kindly reproduced from Laurent Geais' Thesis 2014)

Conclusion

Navigation is a powerful tool to assess knee laxity and to evaluate the effect of surgical reconstruction at time zero. Whilst present technology is somewhat time consuming and invasive, the technology offers exciting possibilities. Navigated stability measurement may allow surgeons to determine, intraoperatively, whether further surgical intervention is required if persistent laxity is detected after reconstruction. In addition, in the future, it may be possible to perform a navigated laxity evaluation and model the effect of different reconstruction strategies by simulation.

References

1. Berning ET, Fowler RM (2011) Thermal damage and tracker-pin track infection in computer-navigated total knee arthroplasty. J Arthroplasty 26(6):977.e21–977.e24
2. Borgstrom PH, Markolf KL, Wang Y et al (2015) Use of inertial sensors to predict pivot shift grade and diagnose an ACL injury during pre-operative testing. Am J Sports Med 43:857–864
3. Bull AM, Amis AA (1998) The pivot shift phenomenon: a clinical and biomechanical perspective. Knee 5:141–158
4. Bull AM, Andersen HN, Basso O, Targett J, Amis AA (1999) Incidence and mechanism of the pivot shift: an in vitro study. Clin Orthop Relat Res 363:219–231
5. Bull AM, Earnshaw PH, Smith A, Katchburian MV, Hassan AN, Amis AA (2002) Intraoperative measurement of knee kinematics in reconstruction of the anterior cruciate ligament. J Bone Joint Surg Br 84:1075–1081
6. Colombet P, Robinson J, Christel P, Franceschi J, Djian P (2007) Using navigation to measure rotation kinematics during ACL reconstruction: a cadaveric pilot study. Clin Orthop Relat Res 454:59–65
7. Colombet P (2011) Knee laxity control in revision anterior cruciate ligament reconstruction versus anterior cruciate ligament reconstruction and lateral tenodesis: clinical assessment using computer-assisted navigation. Am J Sports Med 39:1248–1254
8. Dessenne V, Lavallee S, Julliard R, Orti R, Martelli S, Cinquin P (1995) Computer-assisted knee anterior cruciate ligament reconstruction: first clinical tests. J Image Guid Surg 1:59–64
9. Ellermann A, Sielbold R (2004) ACL-reconstruction with the Navitrack system: critical analysis of navigation in ACL-surgery, in Navigation and robotics in total joint and spine surgery. Steihl J, Konermann W, Haaker R (eds). Springer, New York, pp 423–429

10. Engebretsen L, Wijdicks C, Anderson C, Westerhaus B, LaPrade R (2012) Evaluation of a simulated pivot shift test: a biomechanical study. Knee Surg Sports Traumatol Arthrosc 20:698–702
11. Geais L (2011) Characterization of the knee kinematics : identify the effects of different parameters on the knee kinematics using a model. ÉCOLE DOCTORALE ED415 Laboratoire de mécanique des structures et des systèmes couplés (EA3196) Conservatoire National des Arts et Métiers, Paris
12. Georgoulis AD, Papadonikolakis A, Papageorgiou CD, Mitsou A, Stergiou N (2003) Three-dimensional tibiofemoral kinematics of the anterior cruciate ligament–deficient and reconstructed knee during walking. Am J Sports Med 31(1):75–79
13. Hewison CE, Tran MN, Kaniki N, Remtulla A, Bryant D, Getgood A (2015) Lateral extra-articular tenodesis reduces rotational laxity when combined with anterior cruciate ligament reconstruction: a systematic review of the literature. Arthroscopy 31:2022–2034
14. Julliard R, Lavallee S, Dessenne V (1998) Computer assisted reconstruction of the anterior cruciate ligament. Clin Orthop Relat Res 354:57–64
15. Jung KA, Lee SC, Ahn NK et al (2011) Delayed femoral fracture through a tracker pin site after navigated total knee arthroplasty. J Arthroplasty 26(3):505.e9–505.e11
16. Kawaguchi Y, Kondo E, Takeda R, Akita K, Yasuda K, Amis AA (2015) The role of fibers in the femoral attachment of the anterior cruciate ligament in resisting tibial displacement. Arthroscopy 31(3):435–444
17. Kittl C, El Daou H, Athwal K, Gupte C, Weiler A, WIlliams A, Amis A (2015) The role of the anterolateral structures and the ACL in controlling internal rotational knee laxity ISAKOS
18. Klos TV, Habets RJ, Banks AZ, Banks SA, Devilee RJ, Cook FF (1998) Computer assistance in arthroscopic anterior cruciate ligament reconstruction. Clin Orthop Relat Res 354:65–69
19. Kocher M, Steadman JR, Briggs KK, Sterett WI, Hawkins RJ (2004) Relationships between objective assessment of ligament stability and subjective assessment of symptoms and function after anterior cruciate ligament reconstruction. Am J Sports Med 32:629–634
20. Kurimura M, Matsumoto H, Fujikawa K, Toyama Y (2004) Factors for the presence of anteromedial rotatory instability of the knee. J Orthop Sci 9(4):380–385
21. Lane CG, Warren RF, Stanford FC, Kendoff D, Pearle AD (2008) In vivo analysis of the pivot shift phenomenon during computer navigated ACL reconstruction. Knee Surg Sports Traumatol Arthrosc 16(5):487–492
22. Lie D, Bull AMJ, Amis AA (2007) Persistence of the mini pivot shift after anatomically placed anterior cruciate ligament reconstruction. Clin Orthop Relat Res 457:203–209
23. Lopomo N, Zaffagnini S, Signorelli C et al (2012) An original clinical methodology for non-invasive assessment of pivot shift test. Comput Methods Biomech Biomed Engin 15:1323–1328
24. Mae T, Shino K, Miyama T et al (2001) Single- versus two-femoral socket anterior cruciate ligament reconstruction technique: biomechanical analysis using a robotic simulator. Arthroscopy 17(7):708–716
25. Monaco E, Maestri B, Labianca L, Speranza A, Ferretti A (2011) Instrumented measurements of knee laxity: KT1000 vs navigation. J Bone Joint Surg Br 93-B(SUPP II):175
26. Musahl V, Voos J, O'Loughlin P, Stueber V, Kendoff D, Pearle A (2010) Mechanized pivot shift test achieves greater accuracy than manual pivot shift test. Knee Surg Sports Traumatol Arthrosc 18:1208–1213
27. Noyes FR, Grood ES, Cummings JF, Wrobble RR (1991) An analysis of the pivot shift phenomenon. The knee motions and subluxations induced by different examiners. Am J Sports Med 19(2):148–255
28. Ostendorf C, Fuchs B, Koch P (2006) Femoral stress fracture after computer navigated total knee arthroplasty. Knee 13(5):397–399
29. Pearle AD, Solomon DJ, Wanich T, Moreau-Gaudry A, Granchi CC, Wickiewicz TL et al (2007) Reliability of navigated knee stability examination: a cadaveric evaluation. Am J Sports Med 35:1315–1320
30. Picard F, DiGioia AM, Moody J, Martinek V, Fu FH, Rytel M, Nikou C, LaBarca RS, Jaramaz B (2001) Accuracy in tunnel placement for ACL reconstruction. Comparison of traditional arthroscopic and computer-assisted navigation techniques. Comput Aided Surg 6(5):279–289
31. Robinson J, Carrat L, Granchi C, Colombet P (2007) Influence of anterior cruciate ligament bundles on knee kinematics: clinical assessment using computer-assisted navigation. Am J Sports Med 35:2006–2013
32. Shafizadeh S, Huber H, Grote S, Hoeher J, Paffrath T, Tiling T, Bouillon B (2005) Principles of fluoroscopic-based navigation in anterior cruciate ligament reconstruction. Oper Tech Orthop 15:70–75
33. Tashman S, Collon D, Anderson K, Kolowich P, Anderst W (2004) Abnormal rotational knee motion during running after anterior cruciate ligament reconstruction. Am J Sports Med 32(4):975–983
34. Wiese M, Rosenthal A, Bernsmann K (2004) Clinical experience using the SurgiGATE system, In: Navigation and robotics in total joint and spine surgery. Steihl J, Konermann W, Haaker R (eds). New York.
35. Zaffagnini S, Bignozzi S, Martelli S, Imakiire N, Lopomo N, Marcacci M (2006) New intraoperative protocol for kinematic evaluation of ACL reconstruction: preliminary results. Knee Surg Sports Traumatol Arthrosc 14(9):811–816

How Do We Eliminate Risk Factors for ACL Injury?

39

Alexander E. Weber, Bernard R. Bach Jr., and Asheesh Bedi

Contents

A.E. Weber, MD (✉) • B.R. Bach Jr.
Division of Sports Medicine,
Department of Orthopaedic Surgery,
Rush University Medical Center,
166 West Harrison Street,
Chicago, IL 60612, USA
e-mail: Weber.ae@gmail.com

A. Bedi
Division of Sports Medicine, MedSport,
Department of Orthopaedic Surgery,
University of Michigan, Ann Arbor, MI, USA

39.1 Introduction

Injury to the anterior cruciate ligament (ACL) is one of the most common sports-related injuries throughout the world. These injuries affect all athletes, from childhood to middle-aged, and across all skill levels, from recreational to professional. Approximately 300,000 ACL injuries are sustained in the United States each year [19]. These injuries present significant burdens on patients, including lost time in sports participation or work, further meniscal and chondral damage to the affected knee due to instability, and ultimately the development of knee osteoarthritis (OA) [2, 20, 55]. The chance of OA in the affected knee is approximately 50% at 10 years following injury regardless of reconstruction status [55]. Injury to the ACL also has a significant cost burden on society. ACL injuries have become a public health concern given the consequences of ACL injury at both the individual and societal levels.

In addition to the aforementioned concerns, there has been a heightened awareness of ACL injury due to rapid increase in competitive sports participation at even younger ages. As sports participation has rapidly increased, so too has the number of ACL injuries, particularly in younger patients with more to lose at the personal level and more to contribute at the societal level. The increased frequency and burden of injury has led to a special interest in the identification of risk factors and prevention strategies to decrease the

V. Musahl et al. (eds.), *Rotatory Knee Instability*, DOI 10.1007/978-3-319-32070-0_39

incidence of ACL injury. The purpose of this chapter is to review ACL mechanism of injury, risk factors with an emphasis on modifiable risk factors, and prevention strategies for athletes at risk.

39.2 Mechanism of Injury

The vast majority of ACL injuries (approximately 75%) are noncontact in nature [5]. While the exact mechanism of noncontact injury is often debated, most noncontact ACL injuries are deceleration moments on the affected knee [7]. This can be in the form of landing from a jump, slowing to cut, or change in direction [44]. The body position of ACL injury following a jump landing involves hip and knee extension with knee valgus and tibial internal rotation. This combination associated with foot pronation may put the ACL at greatest risk [7]. Additionally, muscle imbalance and poor trunk control have also been implicated in noncontact ACL injury [22]. Most recently, restriction in adjacent joint range of motion, such as decreased hip range of motion, has been implicated as a potential cause for ACL injury [4].

39.3 Risk Factors

Numerous risk factors have been associated with ACL injury [1, 18, 24, 29, 46, 47]. Classification systems have been developed for these injury risk factors. Often employed classifications are intrinsic versus extrinsic or modifiable and nonmodifiable. Intrinsic, nonmodifiable risk factors include such things as gender, femoral notch width, tibial slope, genetic predisposition, and history of prior ACL injury. Females are known to have a higher risk of noncontact ACL injury when compared with males participating in similar sports [40]. Intrinsic modifiable risk factors include body mass index (BMI), neuromuscular deficits, hormonal status, and biomechanical deficiencies. Extrinsic modifiable risk factors include shoe/equipment choice, playing conditions, level of competition, and sport of participation [46, 47] (Table 39.1).

Table 39.1 Risk factors for ACL injury

Nonmodifiable	Modifiable
Intrinsic 1. Female gender 2. Previous ACL injury 3. Genetic predisposition 4. Extremity alignment 5. General ligamentous laxity 6. Femoral notch size 7. ACL volume 8. Posterior tibial slope	Intrinsic 1. BMI 2. Hormonal status 3. Neuromuscular control 4. Biomechanical deficits 5. Fatigue level
	Extrinsic 1. Sports type 2. Level of competition 3. Footwear 4. Playing surface 5. Weather conditions

ACL anterior cruciate ligament, *BMI* body mass index

39.4 Modifiable Risk Factors

There are many anatomic risk factors for ACL injury, which are nonmodifiable without surgical intervention such as knee recurvatum, increased tibial slope, reduced femoral notch width, decreased ACL volume, and shallow tibial plateau depth [11, 12, 27, 46, 47]. However, a modifiable anatomic risk factor for ACL injury is increased BMI [16]. Evans and colleagues have linked increased BMI to increased risk of noncontact ACL injury [16].

Modifiable neuromuscular and biomechanical risk factors for ACL injury include the landing, pivoting, and cutting techniques [46]. Proper techniques can be learned and may be linked to a reduction in the incidence of ACL tear. ACL-injured athletes tend to land with increased knee abduction moments and ground reactive forces [23]. In jump landing and cutting tasks, females exhibit greater hip and knee extension, knee valgus, and quadriceps activity as compared to hamstring activity. In addition to the lower extremity neuromuscular and biomechanical modifiable risk factors, weakness in core strength is also associated with increased risk of ACL injury [19]. Females have a higher risk of trunk malposition, which predicted ACL injury risk in studies conducted by Zazulak and colleagues [53, 54]. More broadly, muscle fatigue from long workouts or athletic activity may be associated with a breakdown in neuromuscular control and proper biomechanics [9, 19]. Neurocognitive performance based on reaction time, visual memory, and verbal memory may also contribute to the risk of noncontact ACL injury [50].

Hormonal status at time of sports participation has been linked to risk of ACL injury [6, 41, 42, 45, 52]. However, the data are mixed as to the phase of the menstrual cycle that is most risky for sports participation. The early and late follicular preovulatory stage has been implicated as the most at-risk portion of the menstrual cycle by some authors, while others have also evaluated the effects of menstrual cycle stage on ACL tear risk and found that the luteal or postovulatory phase was the most at-risk portion of the cycle [6, 18, 42]. Despite the associations between hormonal status and ACL injury risk, there is currently no consensus on how to apply this information practically to sports participation.

There are also a number of modifiable environmental factors that may contribute to ACL injury risk; however, how to apply knowledge of these modifiable risk factors is still largely undetermined. The type of footwear an athlete wears may place them at increased risk of ACL injury if the footwear increases the torsional resistance with the corresponding playing surface [26]. The playing surface may also affect risk of ACL injury. Surfaces that increase torsional resistance have also been implicated in injury risk. Women's handball players had a higher risk of injury with synthetic indoor surfaces as compared to wooden floors (lower torsional resistance) [35]. In terms of outdoor playing surfaces, grass appears to be safer for athletes than synthetic turf in terms of ACL injury risk [13, 38]. Lastly, weather conditions impact risk of ACL injury. Cold weather and high rain conditions may be protective for ACL injuries [37, 39].

Additional modifiable extrinsic factors include the type of sport and the level of competition. Competition has a higher ACL injury risk associated with it than does practice in handball-related ACL injuries [31]. Certain sports also have a higher risk of noncontact ACL injury that likely reflects the increased cutting and pivoting maneuvers, such as handball, downhill skiing, gymnastics, football, soccer, basketball, volleyball, and lacrosse [40, 41].

Fact Box 1

Proper jump landing techniques

Proper techniques	Sample exercises
1. Land softly with deep knee and hip flexion	A. Double leg squat B. Jump squat
2. Land with knees in line with toes	B. Jump squat C. Forward lunge
3. Land with toes pointing forward	B. Jump squat D. Forward-back hop
4. Land with feet shoulder width apart	B. Jump squat E. Box jump
5. Land with engaged core/gluteus muscle groups	B. Jump squat E. Box jump F. Multidirectional jumps

39.5 Prevention Strategies

Elimination of modifiable risk factors has been the focus of a number of noncontact ACL injury prevention programs [30, 34, 49]. There has been increasing interest in this area of research; however, few studies have attempted randomized controlled trials [25, 36, 48, 51]. The effective programs target neuromuscular and biomechanical deficits with an effort on improving modifiable weaknesses in each athlete [34]. To date, there have been a number of programs which have demonstrated successful reduction in noncontact ACL injuries; however, there is no gold

Table 39.2 Summary of effective components of an ACL injury prevention program

Prevention program component	Example of activity
Warm-up	Dynamic stretching
Balance training	Perturbation-enhanced proprioceptive exercises with wobble board or half ball
Plyometrics	Jump and jump landing training
Strength training	Core and lower extremity closed chain exercises

standard prevention program in the literature [21, 25, 28, 34]. Despite the lack of consensus on the most advantageous prevention program, there are similarities in each successful program, which will be outlined in this section (Table 39.2).

The most successful ACL injury prevention programs take on a multifaceted approach. The key components include stretching, strengthening, aerobic conditioning, plyometrics, proprioception, and balance training. The key tasks enveloped in these programs include education and biofeedback of proper body mechanics during cutting movements and proper jump landing techniques [1, 3]. Techniques of proper landing include soft landing on the forefoot with appropriate trunk, hip, and knee flexion. Knee valgus position should be avoided and landing on both feet should be encouraged. Appropriate feedback can come from a partner athlete or a member of the coaching staff. Additional self-feedback with use of mirrors or video has also been shown to be beneficial in injury prevention [15, 21]. The timing of program initiation has also been shown to impact the effectiveness of the prevention strategy. Successful ACL injury prevention programs start in the preseason (at least 6 weeks prior to competition) and are combined with an in-season maintenance program [1, 3].

Strengthening of the lower extremities and core is an important component of any ACL injury prevention strategy. Lower extremity muscle targets include the hamstrings, gluteus maximus, and abductor musculature. Hamstring strengthening ultimately increased the hamstring to quadriceps ratio, which may prevent potential ACL injury caused by anterior tibial translation [1, 14]. Strengthening of the gluteus maximus and gluteus medius reduces femoral rotation and knee valgus during landing and cutting activities [53]. Planks, bridges, and single-leg squats are core exercises that should be incorporated into a prevention program in order to correct lateral displacement of the trunk during jump landing and cutting activities [53, 54]. The level of difficulty can be increased from flat-ground exercise to perturbation-enhanced core strengthening with the use of a wobble board or similar devices. The use of perturbation-enhanced strengthening has demonstrated a significant risk reduction in male soccer players [10].

Plyometric training is also an important component of any successful ACL injury prevention program. Plyometrics should include single-leg exercises to aid in nullifying leg strength discrepancies and dual-leg exercises to promote proper jump landing and cutting techniques. Implementation of plyometrics into a prevention strategy has been shown to decrease landing forces, decrease hip adduction and abduction moments, and increase lower extremity power [1]. Hewett and colleagues also found a decreased incidence of serious knee injuries in female athletes using a prevention strategy that included plyometrics [21].

The results of such prevention strategies have been mixed; however, more recent meta-analyses and systematic reviews have attempted to quantify the reduction in ACL injury risk following a prevention program. Sadoghi et al. performed a systematic review of the available literature on ACL injury prevention programs and concluded that such programs provide a risk reduction of 52 % in female athletes and 85 % in male athletes [43]. A more recent meta-analysis of ACL injury prevention with neuromuscular training and educational intervention corroborated the findings of Sadoghi and colleagues by demonstrating an overall 50 % reduction in ACL injury rates with a prevention program [17]. Specifically looking at the highest risk athletes, female adolescents, Noyes and Barber-Westin found that neuromuscular retraining intervention programs significantly reduced the noncontact ACL injury rates [34]. In the systematic review by Noyes and Barber-Westin, the number of athletes needed to train in order to prevent a single ACL injury ranged from 70 to 98 athletes; however, the relative risk reduction on the entire athlete population ranged from 75 to 100% [34]. A similar but prior study by Noyes et al. also demonstrated that some prevention programs not only reduce injury risk but may increase athletic performance as well [33].

In addition to focusing on the modifiable intrinsic factors in ACL injury prevention programs, the modifiable extrinsic factors should also be considered. Athletes, coaches, and parents should be aware of the playing surfaces, playing conditions, and footwear that may increase the risk of ACL injury. Hardwood rather than synthetic floors should be used for indoor sports when appropriate. Grass fields rather than synthetic turf should be played upon when the option is available. Strategies should be in place to avoid excessive heat and dryness when possible. Young athletes should be discouraged from participation in cleats with longer and higher volume of spikes. Lastly, prophylactic knee bracing should be avoided in healthy athletes attempting to avoid ACL injury, as the literature does not support the routine use of knee bracing to prevent ACL injury [8, 32].

Conclusion

Noncontact injury to the ACL is common and often affects young athletes involved in jumping and cutting sports. The results of ACL injury can be far-reaching with implications for the athlete, society, and healthcare system. Anatomic risk factors such as decreased notch width, decreased ACL volume, increased lateral tibial slope, and knee laxity have all been demonstrated to increase the risk of ACL injury. Presently, there is no evidence to suggest prophylactic intervention to surgically correct any of the anatomic risk factors; however, in cases of ACL reconstruction, the surgeon should be aware of these factors as ACL volume, notch width, and tibial slope may be addressed. In all athletes modifiable risk factors associated with ACL injury should be identified and corrected. Prevention programs initiated in the preseason and maintained throughout the competitive season can reduce the risk of noncontact ACL injuries. Successful prevention programs should

Fact Box 2

Sample prevention strategy for male and female athletes

Components	Exercises	Duration
1. Dynamic warm-up	Jogging Dynamic stretching Light sport-specific drills Running, sprinting	5–10 min 1–17 exercises
2. Plyometrics	Box jumps Ladders Single-leg hops Multidirectional hops	5–15 min 1–7 exercises
3. Balance	Balance mat training Balance ball	5–10 min 3–5 exercises
4. Strengthening	Core Back Gluteus Hamstring Quadriceps	10–20 min 2–10 exercises
5. Agility	Ladders Sport-specific drills Line hops Multidirectional hops	5–30 min 2–4 exercises with repetition
6. Flexibility	Stretching (static or dynamic) Partnered and individual Muscle activation	5–15 min 1–6 exercises

include stretching, strengthening, plyometrics, and balance components. Education and feedback should be provided to the athletes in terms of jump landing and cutting techniques. Prevention programs that are initiated prior to the season may be most successful at reducing the risk of ACL injuries.

References

1. Acevedo RJ, Rivera-Vega A, Miranda G, Micheo W (2014) Anterior cruciate ligament injury: identification of risk factors and prevention strategies. Curr Sports Med Rep 13(3):186–191. doi:10.1249/JSR.0000000000000053
2. Ait Si Selmi T, Fithian D, Neyret P (2006) The evolution of osteoarthritis in 103 patients with ACL reconstruction at 17 years follow-up. Knee 13(5):353–358. doi:10.1016/j.knee.2006.02.014
3. Alentorn-Geli E, Myer GD, Silvers HJ, Samitier G, Romero D, Lazaro-Haro C, Cugat R (2009) Prevention of non-contact anterior cruciate ligament injuries in soccer players. Part 2: a review of prevention programs aimed to modify risk factors and to reduce injury rates. Knee Surg Sports Traumatol Arthrosc 17(8):859–879. doi:10.1007/s00167-009-0823-z
4. Bedi A, Warren RF, Wojtys EM, Oh YK, Ashton-Miller JA, Oltean H, Kelly BT (2014) Restriction in hip internal rotation is associated with an increased risk of ACL injury. Knee Surg Sports Traumatol Arthrosc. doi:10.1007/s00167-014-3299-4
5. Beynnon BD, Johnson RJ, Abate JA, Fleming BC, Nichols CE (2005) Treatment of anterior cruciate ligament injuries, part I. Am J Sports Med 33(10):1579–1602. doi:10.1177/0363546505279913
6. Beynnon BD, Johnson RJ, Braun S, Sargent M, Bernstein IM, Skelly JM, Vacek PM (2006) The relationship between menstrual cycle phase and anterior cruciate ligament injury: a case–control study of recreational alpine skiers. Am J Sports Med 34(5):757–764. doi:10.1177/0363546505282624
7. Boden BP, Dean GS, Feagin JA Jr, Garrett WE Jr (2000) Mechanisms of anterior cruciate ligament injury. Orthopedics 23(6):573–578
8. Bodendorfer BM, Anoushiravani AA, Feeley BT, Gallo RA (2013) Anterior cruciate ligament bracing: evidence in providing stability and preventing injury or graft re-rupture. Phys Sportsmed 41(3):92–102. doi:10.3810/psm.2013.09.2020
9. Borotikar BS, Newcomer R, Koppes R, McLean SG (2008) Combined effects of fatigue and decision making on female lower limb landing postures: central and peripheral contributions to ACL injury risk. Clin Biomech (Bristol, Avon) 23(1):81–92. doi:10.1016/j.clinbiomech.2007.08.008
10. Caraffa A, Cerulli G, Projetti M, Aisa G, Rizzo A (1996) Prevention of anterior cruciate ligament injuries in soccer. A prospective controlled study of proprioceptive training. Knee Surg Sports Traumatol Arthrosc 4(1):19–21
11. Chaudhari AM, Zelman EA, Flanigan DC, Kaeding CC, Nagaraja HN (2009) Anterior cruciate ligament-injured subjects have smaller anterior cruciate ligaments than matched controls: a magnetic resonance imaging study. Am J Sports Med 37(7):1282–1287. doi:10.1177/0363546509332256
12. Dienst M, Schneider G, Altmeyer K, Voelkering K, Georg T, Kramann B, Kohn D (2007) Correlation of intercondylar notch cross sections to the ACL size: a high resolution MR tomographic in vivo analysis. Arch Orthop Trauma Surg 127(4):253–260. doi:10.1007/s00402-006-0177-7
13. Drakos MC, Hillstrom H, Voos JE, Miller AN, Kraszewski AP, Wickiewicz TL, Warren RF, Allen AA, O'Brien SJ (2010) The effect of the shoe-surface interface in the development of anterior cruciate ligament strain. J Biomech Eng 132(1):011003. doi:10.1115/1.4000118
14. Ebben WP (2009) Hamstring activation during lower body resistance training exercises. Int J Sports Physiol Perform 4(1):84–96
15. Ettlinger CF, Johnson RJ, Shealy JE (1995) A method to help reduce the risk of serious knee sprains incurred in alpine skiing. Am J Sports Med 23(5):531–537
16. Evans KN, Kilcoyne KG, Dickens JF, Rue JP, Giuliani J, Gwinn D, Wilckens JH (2012) Predisposing risk factors for non-contact ACL injuries in military subjects. Knee Surg Sports Traumatol Arthrosc 20(8):1554–1559. doi:10.1007/s00167-011-1755-y
17. Gagnier JJ, Morgenstern H, Chess L (2013) Interventions designed to prevent anterior cruciate ligament injuries in adolescents and adults: a systematic review and meta-analysis. Am J Sports Med 41(8):1952–1962. doi:10.1177/0363546512458227
18. Griffin LY, Agel J, Albohm MJ, Arendt EA, Dick RW, Garrett WE, Garrick JG, Hewett TE, Huston L, Ireland ML, Johnson RJ, Kibler WB, Lephart S, Lewis JL, Lindenfeld TN, Mandelbaum BR, Marchak P, Teitz CC, Wojtys EM (2000) Noncontact anterior cruciate ligament injuries: risk factors and prevention strategies. J Am Acad Orthop Surg 8(3):141–150
19. Griffin LY, Albohm MJ, Arendt EA, Bahr R, Beynnon BD, Demaio M, Dick RW, Engebretsen L, Garrett WE Jr, Hannafin JA, Hewett TE, Huston LJ, Ireland ML, Johnson RJ, Lephart S, Mandelbaum BR, Mann BJ, Marks PH, Marshall SW, Myklebust G, Noyes FR, Powers C, Shields C Jr, Shultz SJ, Silvers H, Slauterbeck J, Taylor DC, Teitz CC, Wojtys EM, Yu B (2006) Understanding and preventing noncontact anterior cruciate ligament injuries: a review of the Hunt Valley II meeting, January 2005. Am J Sports Med 34(9):1512–1532. doi:10.1177/0363546506286866
20. Hanypsiak BT, Spindler KP, Rothrock CR, Calabrese GJ, Richmond B, Herrenbruck TM, Parker RD (2008)

Twelve-year follow-up on anterior cruciate ligament reconstruction: long-term outcomes of prospectively studied osseous and articular injuries. Am J Sports Med 36(4):671–677. doi:10.1177/0363546508315468
21. Hewett TE, Lindenfeld TN, Riccobene JV, Noyes FR (1999) The effect of neuromuscular training on the incidence of knee injury in female athletes. A prospective study. Am J Sports Med 27(6):699–706
22. Hewett TE, Myer GD (2011) The mechanistic connection between the trunk, hip, knee, and anterior cruciate ligament injury. Exerc Sport Sci Rev 39(4):161–166. doi:10.1097/JES.0b013e3182297439
23. Hewett TE, Myer GD, Ford KR, Heidt RS Jr, Colosimo AJ, McLean SG, van den Bogert AJ, Paterno MV, Succop P (2005) Biomechanical measures of neuromuscular control and valgus loading of the knee predict anterior cruciate ligament injury risk in female athletes: a prospective study. Am J Sports Med 33(4):492–501. doi:10.1177/0363546504269591
24. Huston LJ, Greenfield ML, Wojtys EM (2000) Anterior cruciate ligament injuries in the female athlete. Potential risk factors. Clin Orthop Relat Res 372:50–63
25. LaBella CR, Huxford MR, Grissom J, Kim KY, Peng J, Christoffel KK (2011) Effect of neuromuscular warm-up on injuries in female soccer and basketball athletes in urban public high schools: cluster randomized controlled trial. Arch Pediatr Adolesc Med 165(11): 1033–1040. doi:10.1001/archpediatrics.2011.168
26. Lambson RB, Barnhill BS, Higgins RW (1996) Football cleat design and its effect on anterior cruciate ligament injuries. A three-year prospective study. Am J Sports Med 24(2):155–159
27. Loudon JK, Jenkins W, Loudon KL (1996) The relationship between static posture and ACL injury in female athletes. J Orthop Sports Phys Ther 24(2):91–97. doi:10.2519/jospt.1996.24.2.91
28. Mandelbaum BR, Silvers HJ, Watanabe DS, Knarr JF, Thomas SD, Griffin LY, Kirkendall DT, Garrett W Jr (2005) Effectiveness of a neuromuscular and proprioceptive training program in preventing anterior cruciate ligament injuries in female athletes: 2-year follow-up. Am J Sports Med 33(7):1003–1010. doi:10.1177/0363546504272261
29. McLean SG, Beaulieu ML (2010) Complex integrative morphological and mechanical contributions to ACL injury risk. Exerc Sport Sci Rev 38(4):192–200. doi:10.1097/JES.0b013e3181f450b4
30. Myer GD, Sugimoto D, Thomas S, Hewett TE (2013) The influence of age on the effectiveness of neuromuscular training to reduce anterior cruciate ligament injury in female athletes: a meta-analysis. Am J Sports Med 41(1):203–215. doi:10.1177/0363546512460637
31. Myklebust G, Maehlum S, Holm I, Bahr R (1998) A prospective cohort study of anterior cruciate ligament injuries in elite Norwegian team handball. Scand J Med Sci Sports 8(3):149–153
32. Najibi S, Albright JP (2005) The use of knee braces, part 1: prophylactic knee braces in contact sports. Am J Sports Med 33(4):602–611. doi:10.1177/0363546505275128
33. Noyes FR, Barber Westin SD (2012) Anterior cruciate ligament injury prevention training in female athletes: a systematic review of injury reduction and results of athletic performance tests. Sports Health 4(1):36–46. doi:10.1177/1941738111430203
34. Noyes FR, Barber-Westin SD (2014) Neuromuscular retraining intervention programs: do they reduce noncontact anterior cruciate ligament injury rates in adolescent female athletes? Arthroscopy 30(2):245–255. doi:10.1016/j.arthro.2013.10.009
35. Olsen OE, Myklebust G, Engebretsen L, Holme I, Bahr R (2003) Relationship between floor type and risk of ACL injury in team handball. Scand J Med Sci Sports 13(5):299–304
36. Olsen OE, Myklebust G, Engebretsen L, Holme I, Bahr R (2005) Exercises to prevent lower limb injuries in youth sports: cluster randomised controlled trial. BMJ 330(7489):449. doi:10.1136/bmj.38330.632801.8F
37. Orchard J, Seward H, McGivern J, Hood S (1999) Rainfall, evaporation and the risk of non-contact anterior cruciate ligament injury in the Australian Football League. Med J Aust 170(7):304–306
38. Orchard JW, Chivers I, Aldous D, Bennell K, Seward H (2005) Rye grass is associated with fewer non-contact anterior cruciate ligament injuries than bermuda grass. Br J Sports Med 39(10):704–709. doi:10.1136/bjsm.2004.017756
39. Orchard JW, Powell JW (2003) Risk of knee and ankle sprains under various weather conditions in American football. Med Sci Sports Exerc 35(7):1118–1123. doi:10.1249/01.MSS.0000074563.61975.9B
40. Prodromos CC, Han Y, Rogowski J, Joyce B, Shi K (2007) A meta-analysis of the incidence of anterior cruciate ligament tears as a function of gender, sport, and a knee injury-reduction regimen. Arthroscopy 23(12):1320–1325 e1326. doi:10.1016/j.arthro.2007.07.003
41. Renstrom P, Ljungqvist A, Arendt E, Beynnon B, Fukubayashi T, Garrett W, Georgoulis T, Hewett TE, Johnson R, Krosshaug T, Mandelbaum B, Micheli L, Myklebust G, Roos E, Roos H, Schamasch P, Shultz S, Werner S, Wojtys E, Engebretsen L (2008) Non-contact ACL injuries in female athletes: an International Olympic Committee current concepts statement. Br J Sports Med 42(6):394–412. doi:10.1136/bjsm.2008.048934
42. Ruedl G, Ploner P, Linortner I, Schranz A, Fink C, Sommersacher R, Pocecco E, Nachbauer W, Burtscher M (2009) Are oral contraceptive use and menstrual cycle phase related to anterior cruciate ligament injury risk in female recreational skiers? Knee Surg Sports Traumatol Arthrosc 17(9):1065–1069. doi:10.1007/s00167-009-0786-0
43. Sadoghi P, von Keudell A, Vavken P (2012) Effectiveness of anterior cruciate ligament injury prevention training programs. J Bone Joint Surg Am 94(9):769–776. doi:10.2106/JBJS.K.00467
44. Shimokochi Y, Shultz SJ (2008) Mechanisms of noncontact anterior cruciate ligament injury. J Athl Train 43(4):396–408. doi:10.4085/1062-6050-43.4.396

45. Slauterbeck JR, Fuzie SF, Smith MP, Clark RJ, Xu K, Starch DW, Hardy DM (2002) The menstrual cycle, sex hormones, and anterior cruciate ligament injury. J Athl Train 37(3):275–278
46. Smith HC, Vacek P, Johnson RJ, Slauterbeck JR, Hashemi J, Shultz S, Beynnon BD (2012) Risk factors for anterior cruciate ligament injury: a review of the literature - part 1: neuromuscular and anatomic risk. Sports Health 4(1):69–78. doi:10.1177/1941738111428281
47. Smith HC, Vacek P, Johnson RJ, Slauterbeck JR, Hashemi J, Shultz S, Beynnon BD (2012) Risk factors for anterior cruciate ligament injury: a review of the literature-part 2: hormonal, genetic, cognitive function, previous injury, and extrinsic risk factors. Sports Health 4(2):155–161. doi:10.1177/1941738111428282
48. Steffen K, Myklebust G, Olsen OE, Holme I, Bahr R (2008) Preventing injuries in female youth football--a cluster-randomized controlled trial. Scand J Med Sci Sports 18(5):605–614. doi:10.1111/j.1600-0838.2007.00703.x
49. Sugimoto D, Myer GD, McKeon JM, Hewett TE (2012) Evaluation of the effectiveness of neuromuscular training to reduce anterior cruciate ligament injury in female athletes: a critical review of relative risk reduction and numbers-needed-to-treat analyses. Br J Sports Med 46(14):979–988. doi:10.1136/bjsports-2011-090895
50. Swanik CB, Covassin T, Stearne DJ, Schatz P (2007) The relationship between neurocognitive function and noncontact anterior cruciate ligament injuries. Am J Sports Med 35(6):943–948. doi:10.1177/0363546507299532
51. Walden M, Atroshi I, Magnusson H, Wagner P, Hagglund M (2012) Prevention of acute knee injuries in adolescent female football players: cluster randomised controlled trial. BMJ 344:e3042. doi:10.1136/bmj.e3042
52. Wojtys EM, Huston LJ, Boynton MD, Spindler KP, Lindenfeld TN (2002) The effect of the menstrual cycle on anterior cruciate ligament injuries in women as determined by hormone levels. Am J Sports Med 30(2):182–188
53. Zazulak BT, Hewett TE, Reeves NP, Goldberg B, Cholewicki J (2007) Deficits in neuromuscular control of the trunk predict knee injury risk: a prospective biomechanical-epidemiologic study. Am J Sports Med 35(7):1123–1130. doi:10.1177/0363546507301585
54. Zazulak BT, Hewett TE, Reeves NP, Goldberg B, Cholewicki J (2007) The effects of core proprioception on knee injury: a prospective biomechanical-epidemiological study. Am J Sports Med 35(3): 368–373. doi:10.1177/0363546506297909
55. Zebis MK, Andersen LL, Bencke J, Kjaer M, Aagaard P (2009) Identification of athletes at future risk of anterior cruciate ligament ruptures by neuromuscular screening. Am J Sports Med 37(10):1967–1973. doi:10.1177/0363546509335000

The Dynamic Interplay Between Active and Passive Knee Stability: Implications for Management of the High ACL Injury Risk Athlete

40

Ravi K. Grandhi, Dai Sugimoto, Mike Posthumus, Daniel Schneider, and Gregory D. Myer

Contents

R.K. Grandhi, MBA
Department of Pediatrics, University of Cincinnati, Cincinnati, OH, USA

College of Medicine, University of Cincinnati, Cincinnati, OH, USA

D. Sugimoto, PhD
Division of Sports Medicine, Department of Orthopaedics, Boston Children's Hospital, Boston, MA, USA

The Micheli Center for Sports Injury Prevention, Waltham, MA, USA

M. Posthumus, PhD
Division of Exercise Science and Sports Medicine, The University of Cape Town, Cape Town, South Africa

D. Schneider
College of Medicine, University of Cincinnati, Cincinnati, OH, USA

Division of Sports Medicine, Cincinnati Children's Hospital Medical Center, Cincinnati, OH, USA

G.D. Myer, PhD (✉)
Division of Sports Medicine, Cincinnati Children's Hospital Medical Center, Cincinnati, OH, USA

The Micheli Center for Sports Injury Prevention, Waltham, MA, USA
e-mail: greg.myer@cchmc.org

40.1 Introduction

The knee is composed of four major ligaments that provide passive restraint to the knee: the anterior cruciate ligament (ACL), posterior cruciate ligament (PCL), medial collateral ligament (MCL), and lateral collateral ligament (LCL) [62]. Together, these four major ligaments connect the femur to the tibia and fibula and help stabilize the knee joint, which allows the knee to flex and extend and rotate slightly both internally and externally.

The ACL plays an integral role in the stabilization of the knee joint, often preventing hyperextension injuries [62]. ACL injuries frequently occur during physical and sporting activities. Although several different interpretations exist, there are two main ACL injury mechanisms: contact (either a direct blow to the knee or contact to

V. Musahl et al. (eds.), *Rotatory Knee Instability*, DOI 10.1007/978-3-319-32070-0_40

other body parts) and noncontact [1, 4, 7, 60, 85]. Nearly 70 % of ACL injuries are a result of noncontact mechanisms [2, 6, 10]. The noncontact ACL injury occurs during cutting, an action where the athlete decelerates and then plants his/her foot into the ground. Other injuries occur when an athlete lands flat on his/her heels, which forces the tibia into the knee. This leads to greater ground reaction force (GRF) and often results in an ACL tear. Athletes who have injured their ACL report feeling that their knee gives out or that it "popped." Rotation is the movement of a joint along the longitudinal axis, and due to anatomical restraints, the knee has limited rotational movement. The combination of a "pop" during a rotational movement or rapid deceleration and early swelling is claimed to demonstrate a 90 % probability of rupture of the ACL [10]. The ACL and PCL play key roles in the limiting of movement. The severity of ACL injuries is determined based on the total number and degree of severity of structures damaged. The most severe manifestation of ACL injury is what is known as the "(O'Donoghue's) unhappy triad," which includes a medial meniscal and MCL tear, in combination with an ACL tear [11].

Females are at higher risk of noncontact ACL ruptures in comparison with their male counterparts [74, 91]. The cause of this discrepancy between the sexes is still unknown, but could be attributed to a combination of factors including: anatomy [13, 58, 94], hormones [54], genetics [42, 43, 70, 92, 98], muscular strength [27, 78], and training techniques [43]. Further, the onset of puberty in females may contribute to propensity of greater ACL injury risk in female athletes [7]. Knee laxity is increased in pubertal and postpubertal females, and estrogen and progesterone levels have been associated with anterior knee laxity [85]. Furthermore, it has previously been reported that body weight and body mass index (BMI) are risk factors for ACL ruptures in women, but not men [74].

The relative importance of differences between male and female ACL injury mechanisms has increased as female sports have increased in prevalence since the inception of Title IX of the Education Amendments Act in 1972. Across the United States in 2006, there was an estimated 350,000 ACL injuries [101] at an estimated cost of more than two billion [87]. Since then, this has only increased. The costs of ACL injury are not limited to surgical reconstruction, but include immediate postoperative rehabilitation and early onset of posttraumatic knee osteoarthritis (OA) care [39]. At least 50 % of women with an ACL injury will show significant pain, functional limitations, and radiographic signs of knee OA within 20 years of the first injury [24, 38]. One study investigated the status of knee OA after initial ACL injury in a cohort of female soccer players. In this study, 82 % of those who had an ACL injury demonstrated radiographic changes on their ACL-injured knee [38]. Additionally, 51 % showed radiographically observable knee OA signs [38]. Astonishingly, the mean age of the participants was 31 years old [38], and 75 % commented that their knee condition hinders their knee-related quality of life [38]. Similarly, another study reported a 71 % prevalence of moderate knee OA in 10–15 years following ACL reconstruction [64]. Therefore, identifying and providing preventive strategies can reduce the risk of unnecessary injury and surgeries, which can allow individuals to maintain a high level of physical activity throughout their lives.

Understanding some basic theories of causes in noncontact impact ACL injuries can provide greater understanding of the anatomy and physiology of injuries. There are two distinctive classifications as it relates to factors that might lead to an increased predisposition for ACL tears.

I. Passive factors:
   (a) Hormonal influences (leading to ligament laxity)
   (b) Genetics
   (c) Past medical history
   (d) Anatomy
II. Active factors:
   (a) Trunk and ligament relationship
   (b) Mechanical mechanism to lateral trunk motion and knee load
   (c) Quadriceps and neuromuscular training

An explanation of each of these factors will be addressed later in this chapter, along with a dis-

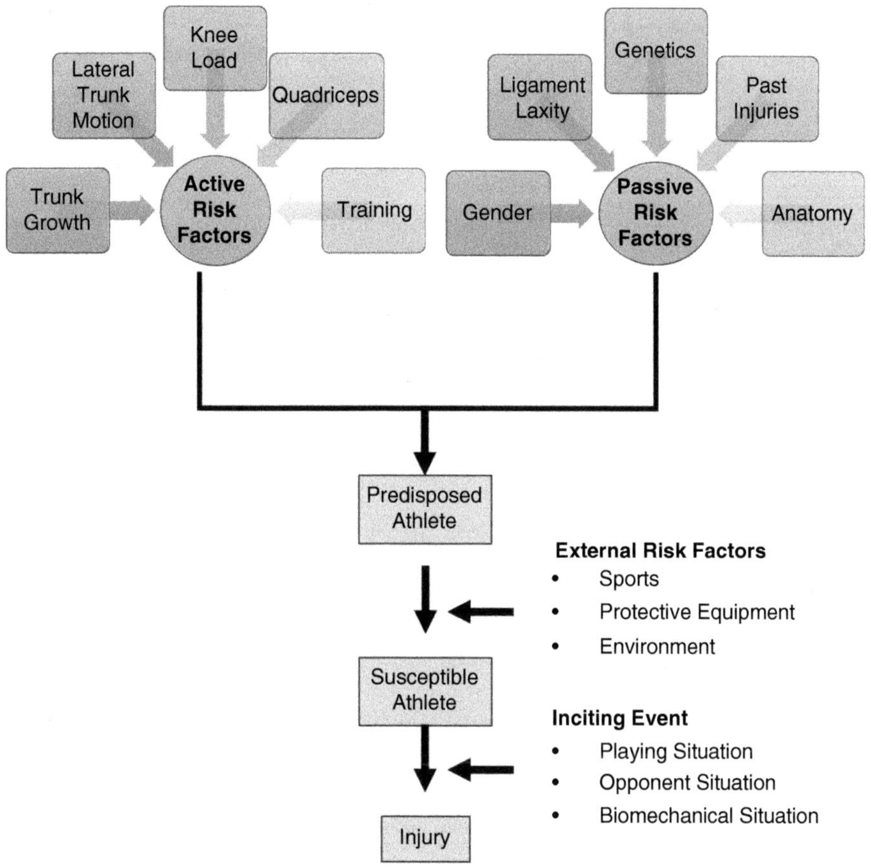

Fig. 40.1 A comprehensive overview of injury causation [55]

cussion of the interaction between passive and active factors. While the passive factors are truly innate, the active factors are modifiable, which may translate into ACL injury risk reduction (Fig. 40.1).

40.2 Passive Factors

The ACL provides a component of the passive restraint responsible for knee joint stability. Passive joint stability is based on intrinsic factors, which can be divided into those related to genetics and those related to the predominantly female hormones estrogen and progesterone, which can impact the ligament laxity [84]. The effects of hormones are additive with certain genetic factors, but genetic factors also occur with equal frequency in males and females. Past medical history (e.g., prior knee joint injury) also plays an important role and should be evaluated in the context of overall joint involvement.

40.2.1 Ligament Laxity

Most knee ligamentous injuries in women's sports occur via noncontact mechanisms [6, 8, 54]. Increased risk of ACL injury may occur when there are not sufficiently taut ligaments and tendons to stabilize the knee joint and absorb GRF. This results in a decreased joint stability [97]. While generalized joint laxity is not treated clinically, recent results indicate that increased general joint laxity greater than one standard deviation of the mean is associated with an increased risk of ACL injury [54]. From a case-control investigation within a cohort of 1500 athletes, there was a noted increased risk of injury with greater knee joint laxity [54]. This may lead to reduced dynamic knee stability during athletic maneuvers and may be associated with previously identified ACL injury risk factors [54]. These effects are most pronounced post puberty. During puberty, men and women experience increases in height and body mass along with hormonal changes. These changes may influence the status of joint laxity including the ligaments. Males demonstrate decreased joint flexibility and ligament laxity during puberty, while females show an increase [54]. Unlike females, males often also show a decrement in anterior-posterior knee laxity [54]. These joint laxity differences between adolescent male and female athletes are often associated with concomitant pubertal changes [54].

It is theorized that many of these changes are due to the steep rise in estrogen levels seen during puberty [8]. Quatman et al. [76] reported that 28 % of pubescent females exhibited knee hyperextension, while only 10 % of pubescent males demonstrated a similar trend. Others have noted similar findings as it relates to Tanner stages [98]. Sex hormones may exert their biologic effects on the ACL through the regulation of gene expression, especially many of the matrix metalloproteinase (MMP) genes [72]. *MMP3* and *MMP1* expression is higher in the ACL of women when compared with men [72]. However, more research is necessary to determine the exact variants associated with ACL ruptures.

40.2.2 Genetics

Recent findings on the relationship between genetics and injuries have highlighted the importance of collecting a family history as part of sports medicine hospital visits. Flynn et al. noted that a person with an ACL tear is twice as likely to have a relative who has an ACL tear [42]. Another study indicated that males who sustained an ACL injury are more likely to have a first-degree relative with an ACL tear compared to the males without ACL injury [42, 57]. More recently, specific genetic variants have been shown to associate with risk of ACL ruptures. Specific genes which have been implicated in the etiology of ACL ruptures include genes coding for structural proteins (*COL5A1*, *COL12Al*, *COL1A1*, *COL3A1*), genes coding for matrix regulators (MMP1, MMP3, MMP10, MMP12, TIMP1, TIMP2), genes coding for components of the angiogenesis-associated signaling pathway (*VEGFA*, KDR), and genes coding for proteoglycans (*ACAN*, *DCN*, *LUM*).

40.2.2.1 Structural Genes

The major structural components of ligaments are collagens, of which types I and V are the main constituents [71]. The first specific genetic variants that were associated with risk for ACL ruptures are located within the *COL1A1* and *COL5A1* genes [71, 73]. Both genes code for the alpha 1 chain of type I and type V collagen, respectively [71, 73]. Type I collagen constitutes 70–80 % of the dry mass and is responsible for the tensile strength of ligaments. Although a quantitatively minor collagen, type V collagen has a significant functional role. Type V intercalates into type I collagen where it regulates fibrillogenesis and is theorized to regulate lateral fibril growth. Specific genetic variants within the *COL12A1* and *COL3A1* genes are also associated with risk of ACL ruptures [72, 73]. The *COL12A1* gene encodes the alpha chain of type XII collagen, which is also involved in fibrillogenesis [73]. The *COL3A1* gene encodes for type III collagen, which, similarly to type V collagen, is also a minor fibrillar collagen and intercalates into the fibril with type I collagen [89].

The functional *COL1A1* Sp1 binding site polymorphism within the first intron of the gene was shown to associate with increased risk of ACL ruptures [31], cruciate ruptures, and shoulder dislocation in South African, Polish, and Swedish populations, respectively [16, 31, 71]. The T allele of this gene variant was shown to prevent ACL rupture. It is proposed that the T allele increases the expression of the a1 (1) chain and may produce a homotrimer consisting of three of the a1 (1) chains. This homotrimer formation may favorably change the tensile strength of the ligament. Further studies have also investigated additional variants within the

COL1A1 gene as potential risk factors for ACL ruptures. A haplotype (gene combination) of the Sp1 binding site polymorphism and gene variant rs1107946 was also shown to reduce the risk of ACL ruptures in Polish professional soccer players [16]. This haplotype was proposed to further enhance transcriptional activity of the *COL1A1* gene [29].

The *COL5A1* BstUI restriction fragment length polymorphism (RFLP) within the 3′-untranslated region (UTR) was implicated in the risk of ACL ruptures [73, 81]. The CC genotype has been shown to be significantly underrepresented in female patients with ACL ruptures, suggesting that this genotype is protective. This finding is in agreement with similar effects in other musculoskeletal soft tissue pathologies such as Achilles tendinopathy [40, 69], tennis elbow [3], and carpal tunnel syndrome [9]. Further, the *COL5A1* BstUI variant was also associated with a self-reported family history of ligament injuries in the female, but not male, participants [62]. It remains unknown why this variant only associates with risk of ACL rupture in females. One of the existing theories is that risk is mediated by a gene-hormone interaction [46, 72].

Similar to the *COL5A1 Bst*UI variant, the *COL12A1 Alu*I restriction fragment length polymorphism (RFLP) was also associated with risk of ACL ruptures in females. The AA genotype of *COL12A1* AluI RFLP [19] was associated with an increased risk of ACL rupture in female participants, both in a South African [72] and a Polish population [9]. The *COL3A1* rs1800255 variant was also associated with ACL ruptures in two independent studies of Polish soccer players [9] and Polish skiers [89]. In both studies, the AA genotype was significantly overrepresented in individuals who sustained ACL ruptures.

40.2.2.2 Extracellular Matrix Regulatory Genes

Regulators of degradation and remodeling of the extracellular matrix (ECM) are also critically important for the integrity and health of ligaments. The major regulators of the ECM include, but are not limited to, the family of matrix metalloproteinases (MMPs). The ECM of ligaments are principally regulated by the degradation family of at least 24 endopeptidases capable of degrading various components of the ECM. Disturbances to these regulatory genes may result in deregulation and thereby result in injury, such as ACL ruptures. Recently a cluster of genes, all located on chromosome 11q22, coding for MMP proteins, namely, *MMP1*, *MMP3*, *MMP10*, and *MMP12*, were associated with risk of ACL ruptures. This *MMP10-MMP1-MMP3-MMP12* gene cluster was significantly associated with an increased risk of ACL ruptures [92].

40.2.2.3 Signaling Genes

Angiogenic cytokines and growth factors, the angiogenesis-associated signaling cascade, have been implicated in ruptured ligaments and tendons and are believed to play a critical role in matrix remodeling following mechanical loading [5, 75]. Vascular endothelial growth factor (VEGF) is an essential regulator of angiogenesis and has been implicated in ligament injuries. The A isoform of VEGF (VEGFA), coded for by the *VEGFA* gene, is thought to have the highest angiogenic potency. VEGFA binds to the kinase insert domain receptor, coded for by the *KDR* gene. Recently, both the *VEGFA* and *KDR* genes were associated with ACL ruptures [77]. The CC genotype of the *VEGFA* rs699947 and the GG genotype of the *VEGFA* rs1570360 variant were overrepresented among individuals who had sustained an ACL rupture through a noncontact mechanism of injury [77]. The GA genotype of the *KDR* rs2071559 variant was overrepresented among females with ACL ruptures [77].

40.2.2.4 Proteoglycan Genes

Similar to structural proteins within ligaments and tendons, proteoglycans such as aggrecan, biglycan, decorin, fibromodulin, and lumican have important structural roles in ligaments and are also involved in fibrillogenesis [103]. Recently, the genes coding for aggrecan (*ACAN*), decorin (*DCN*), and lumican (*LUM*) were implicated in the etiology of ACL ruptures. The G allele of the ACAN rs1516797 variant was overrepresented in individuals with ACL ruptures, whereas the GG genotype of the *DCN* rs516155 variant was underrepresented among female individuals with ACL ruptures [41]. Further, haplotype analyses further implicated regions overlapping these two genes (*ACAN* and *DCN*), as well as the *LUM* gene [41].

Fact Box 1

- Structural proteins (*COL1A1*, *COL12A1*, *COL3A1*, and *COL5A1*), which are related to the construction of collagen, are directly associated with ACL injury.
- Proteoglycan genes (*ACAN*, *DCN*, *LUM*), which are involved in fibrillogenesis, were implicated in the etiology of ACL ruptures.
- Metalloproteinase (*MMP10-MMP1-MMP3-MMP12* gene cluster), which is associated with the construction of the extracellular matrix, is associated with an increased risk of ACL ruptures.
- Angiogenesis-associated signaling cascade (*VEGF* and *KDR*) has been implicated in ruptured ligaments and tendons and is believed to play a critical role in matrix remodeling following mechanical loading.

40.2.3 Past Injuries

A history of damage to the ACL makes individuals more susceptible to repeated injury. This can range from nonsurgically repaired minor, repetitive trauma to a previously surgically reconstructed ACL tear. A previous injury at a particular location can lead to overall tissue weakness and thus increased susceptibility to future injury. Subsequent ACL injury rate ranges between 2 and 19 % in the general population [22, 79, 102]. However, this rate increases to 24 [70]–29 % [97] in physically active adolescents. Additionally, compared with young athletes who never tore their ACL, those who have a past medical history of ACL injury have up to 15 times greater risk of subsequent ACL injury (age dependent) [70]. Another study reported a five times greater ACL re-tear rate compared to those who have never torn ACL in female soccer players [15]. Deficits in quadriceps strength and activation are also common after rehabilitation and return to sport [67]. Therefore, previous injury may play a significant role in the development of active risk factors for reinjury. The combination of having a past medical history of an ACL tear, along with the active and passive risk factors, will increase subsequent ACL tear significantly in physically active young athletes.

40.2.4 Anatomy

Anatomy is influenced by a number of factors, but independently also played a very important role in making individuals more susceptible to injury. In addition to the influence of genetics, anatomy evolves over time due to physical activity and the role of pubertal growth. Recently, specific variants have been highlighted that lead to increased susceptibility. These factors include intercondylar notch size, increased Q angle, skeletal growth, and body mass index relative to size.

40.2.4.1 Intercondylar Notch Size

The intercondylar notch size provides a way to identify the size of the cruciate ligaments that sit in the notch. However, it is the ACL size that is a factor for ACL injury, not the size of the notch. Domzalski et al. [13] retrospectively analyzed the MRI scans of 46 patients with ACL injuries and 44 patients with normal MRI findings. They found a significant ($p < 0.001$) difference in the mean value of the intercondylar notch width between normal knees (0.2691) and the ACL injury population (0.2415) [13]. A narrower intercondylar notch was found to be associated with the risk of ACL rupture in an immature population [13]. These findings were confirmed by Gormeli et al. [20]. Some studies have shown women having smaller notches than men which is likely related to concomitantly smaller ACLs [11, 55, 83, 88]. Moreover, there appears to be a positive genetic correlation in notch width. Siblings (and often sibling pairs) with injuries have significantly narrower notches than those with broader notches. This could partially explain the prevalence of ACL injuries in siblings [30]. When the notch is narrower, the space for ACL movement is more limited. Within this more restricted space, the condyles can pinch the ACL as the knee bends or straightens. It is theorized that pinching the ACL may lead to its rupture. Another variation of this same theory is that the narrow notch may cause the ACL to be shaved or thinned due to the friction and that this may predispose the ligament to rupture [94].

40.2.4.2 Increased Q Angle

The Q angle of the knee is a measurement of the angle between the quadriceps muscles and the patellar tendon [12]. The female pelvis is wider than the male pelvis, which increases the Q angle of the knee. The average Q angle in women is roughly 17° compared to only 10° in men [28]. Theoretically, this increases the pull of the quadriceps femoris muscle on the patella [45]. The patella/patellar tendon ratio should be nearly equal [100]. When the patellar tendon is too long, then a high-riding patella exists and may more easily be laterally displaced [100]. This causes increased stress at the knee and may result in other compensatory changes [14]. This also may cause increased foot pronation and flattening, especially in women [63]. The large Q angle concentrates more forces on the ACL for laxity restoration each time that the knee rotates especially with inward torque, predisposing it to a rupture [4].

40.2.4.3 Skeletal Growth

During peak growth (height and mass) velocity in pubertal athletes, the tibia and femur grow rapidly. Rapid growth leads to increased height of the center of mass, making muscular control of the trunk more challenging [51]. Moreover, increased body mass along with longer joint levers (extremities) creates greater forces that are more difficult to balance and dampen during athletic maneuvers. During this developmental period, male athletes show increased strength and power ("neuromuscular spurt") to meet the increased demands of growth and development [51]. However, female athletes do not demonstrate similar neuromuscular adaptations to match the increased demands [51].

In females, after the onset of puberty, there is a rapid increase in bone length and body mass without simultaneous increases in strength and recruitment of the musculature of the lower extremity posterior chain. Thus, there is a tendency for increased knee abduction moments (KAM) during landing tasks. If female athletes reach maturity without adaptations in core power and control to match whole-body increases in inertial load, their tendency is to demonstrate increased GRF and KAM during dynamic tasks [51, 52]. This makes them more susceptible to ACL rupture.

40.2.4.4 Body Mass Index Relative to Stature

Increased BMI relative to height has been reported to be a risk factor for ACL injuries, especially among female adolescent soccer players, college recreational athletes, and female army recruits [51, 66]. Women with a BMI greater than one standard deviation above the mean had a 3.5 times greater risk of ACL injury than those with lower BMI [95]. In female athletes older than 8 years, BMI was also a significant risk factor for increased knee injury risk [51]. When compared with a population of their peers, children with increased mass relative to their height had the potential for increased KAM. This plays a role in altered knee mechanics, which may increase the risk of ACL injuries in female athletes [51]. While body mass is, by nature, a passive etiology of ACL injury risk, it is a modifiable factor that could be targeted when necessary.

40.3 Active Factors

Active factors are related to how dynamic stabilizers such as muscles around the knee joint and proximal segments such as the hip and trunk provide knee stability relative to ACL. As an individual executes dynamic movements, different forces are placed on the extremities and often these forces may distribute stress on the ligaments. The combination of passive factors and dynamic forces may contribute to increased risk

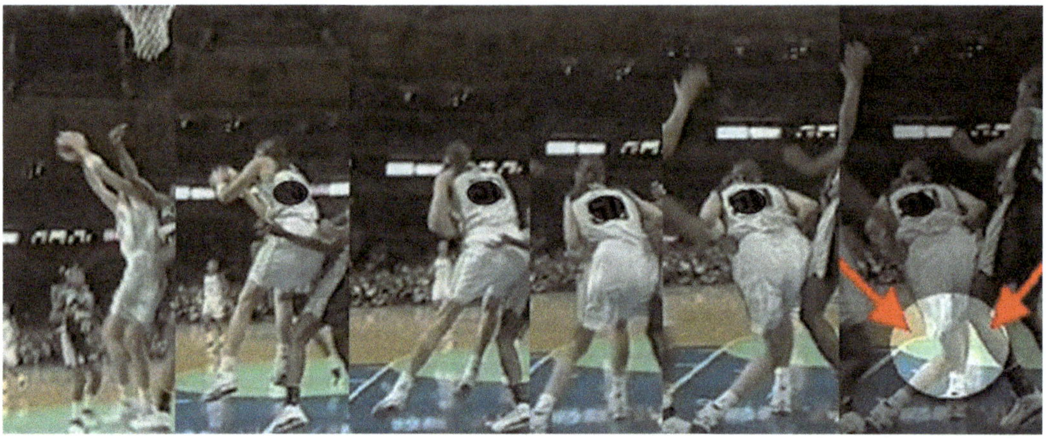

Fig. 40.2 Videographic depiction of an athlete with a kinematic pattern that is likely to demonstrate high knee abduction moment. The high knee abduction moment may indicate problems in the dynamic control of the knee. Those with high knee abduction moments combined with hip abduction moments are increasingly susceptible to ACL injury (Printed with permission from the *British Journal of Sports Medicine*. Credit: Myer et al. [51])

in certain individuals. It is theorized that this stress may result in increased injury risk for those with a preexisting predisposition to ACL rupture.

40.3.1 Trunk and Ligament Relationship

As athletes experience maturation, the trunk grows disproportionally compared to lower extremity musculatures such as the quadriceps and especially the hamstrings [48]. This causes a reduced level of neuromuscular and ligamentous control of dynamic knee joint stability because the supporting structure is not well developed relative to their growth. As a result, maturing athletes may not be able to sufficiently control lower extremity frontal plane motion during landing and cutting. Females often perform athletic movements with greater knee valgus angles and loads than males [17, 18]. As a result, there is a greater amount of stress placed on the ACL in dynamic movements because there is higher activation of the quadriceps despite the minimal knee flexion, hip flexion, greater hip adduction, and adductor movement [68]. Additionally, females typically land with their tibia rotated internally or externally as opposed to a neutral knee alignment [61]. Hewett et al. [27] reported that female athletes who exhibited excessive knee valgus moments during the early deceleration phase of a side-step cutting maneuver utilized a different lower extremity loading strategy than those who exhibited normal knee frontal plane moments. In particular, as discussed by Sigward and Powers [86], these subjects demonstrate a lower extremity pattern that includes greater laterally directed GRFs, increased hip abduction, hip internal rotation, and a more internally rotated foot progression angle. The most significant difference between those individuals who exhibited excessive valgus movement and those who do not was the lateral GRF, which was more than three times greater than those with normal knee frontal plane movements [86]. This suggests that these individuals contacted the ground differently. After accounting for the forces and moments acting at the foot segment, a laterally directed GRF would impose a laterally directed intersegmental force at the distal tibia. As a result of its long lever arm (the perpendicular distance from the center of mass of the tibia to the distal end of the tibia), a larger laterally directed force would create a greater valgus moment at the knee [86]. Additionally, it has been shown that knee flexion movement asymmetry predicts reinjury in athletes who had an ACL reconstruction [68] (Fig. 40.2).

Moreover, those same individuals with excessive knee valgus motion also had excessive hip abduction at the point of initial contact in cutting movement. This may suggest that these individuals were reaching out further with their foot at initial contact, possibly trying to facilitate the change in direction required of the cutting task [97]. Changing direction causes an overall alteration in posture, causing an imbalance between the inertial demands of the trunk and control and coordination to resist it. The causes of high knee loads and risky knee motions do not stem from the knee joint itself; rather, placing the knee in a vulnerable position might be a result of reduced control of body posture and trunk accelerations. The valgus movement at the knee is not visually observable, and the relative difference between safe knee positions and high-risk loads on the knee is just a few degrees [24, 34, 35]. Therefore, high-speed cameras and three-dimensional motion analysis image capture systems are often used to identify the dynamic knee loads associated with ACL injury risk [51]. A few studies have utilized video recordings of noncontact ACL injuries in female athletes. Video analysis indicated that when the body shifted over one leg, it was associated with high knee abduction or medial knee collapse [27]. Concurrently, increased lateral sway of the trunk may underlie medial collapse of the knee joint. Furthermore, trunk displacement and coronal plane knee loads both predict ACL injury risk in female athletes with high sensitivity and specificity up to 91 % of the time [24]. Thus, increased knee loading occurs through both neuromuscular and biochemical mechanisms related to increased trunk inertia and motion. Research has shown that neuromuscular control of the trunk and lower extremity can be improved with neuromuscular training [26]. This additional neuromuscular control has the potential to decrease the abduction load at the knee and decrease the risk of ACL injury.

The trunk and knee are coupled mechanistically and dynamically via the GRF lever arm, and a number of studies have reported the mechanical linkage between the proximal segment and knee joint kinematics. Hence, the ACL injury mechanism can be classified into two parts: the coronal plane components and the effects of lateral trunk motion on knee loads. The convergence of both these components makes females more susceptible to injury.

40.3.1.1 Coronal Plane Components of the ACL Injury Mechanism in Female Athletes

Coronal plane components focus mainly on the knee abduction load; knee abduction load has predicted ACL injury risk with 78 % sensitivity and 73 % specificity [24]. Female athletes demonstrate greater valgus knee movement primarily in the coronal plane. As a result, most ACL injuries in the female occur via noncontact mechanisms during landing and lateral pivoting [24]. Video analyses have highlighted this mechanism as including a combination of knee abduction, low knee flexion, lateral trunk motion causing the body to shift over one leg, and the plantar surface of the foot fixed flat on the surface, displaced away from the trunk [24].

When the trunk moves laterally (relative to the stance limb), the GRF vector will move slightly lateral to the side of the femoral head, which results in a greater lever arm relative to the knee joint center. This chain of events will trigger the potential knee abduction loading in combination with increased inertial acceleration of the trunk and thigh segments during dynamic movement. This knee load simultaneously increases the magnitude of vector force from ground reaction because of partial knee joint loading. It becomes essential to counteract the knee load with increasing reactive hip adductor torque to maintain upright stance and dissipate lower extremity forces. This can increase knee abduction movements, which are predictors of peak GRF and important parts of joint load. These movements cause pain in females and place knee ligaments in the high slope (load) segment of their force-length curve. Video analysis study suggests that the female trunk moves laterally toward the ACL-injured limb as the knee abducts. In order for the pelvis and trunk to maintain stance, the hip

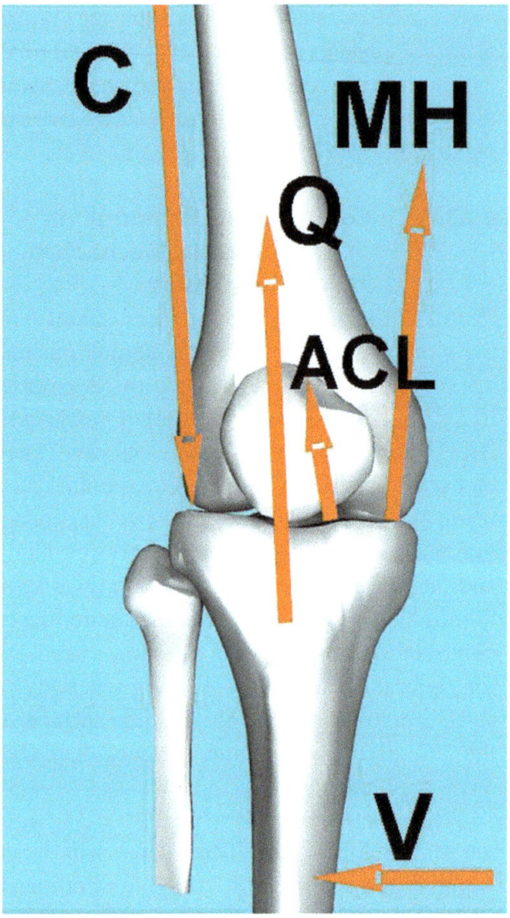

Fig. 40.3 Free-body diagram of the forces that act on the tibia. There is an equilibrium between the external valgus (*V*), articular contact force (*C*), quadriceps force (*Q*), medial hamstrings (*MH*), and anterior cruciate ligament (*ACL*). When there is external valgus loading, contact shifts to the lateral compartment. The moment is balanced with respect to the contact position and shows that Q and MH both help the ACL (and the MCL, not shown) stabilize the joint against valgus loading. Under a particular valgus load, any reduction in these muscular forces increases ligament loading (Printed with permission from the *Journal of Athletic Training*. Credit: Myer et al. [56])

adductors are activated to the lateral side; however, employment of this strategy during dynamic, high-load movements appear to be indicative of a viscous mechanical cycle, which may be an underlying mechanism of knee injury in female sports [24] (Fig. 40.3).

40.3.1.2 Mechanical Linkage Related to Lateral Trunk Motion and Knee Load in Female Athletes

Trunk position and knee external abduction movement (load) may be linked mechanically, since lateral flexion of the trunk creates abduction loads at the knee [23]. If trunk-mediated load influences the GRF to pass lateral to the head of the femur, then the knee is exposed to an external abduction torque [23]. As a result, a hip adductor must generate torque of equal magnitude to balance the external movement [23].

40.3.2 Quadriceps Dominance

Quadriceps dominance is an imbalance between knee extensor and flexor strength, recruitment, and coordination. Rapid growth occurs during puberty. With this growth comes a substantial increase in the movement of inertia of the limbs, which creates greater muscle strength to control the limbs during dynamic movements [67]. Vertical growth during the teenage years has a very different neuromuscular control profile for females than in males. Recent studies have shown that males experience a significant increase in neuromuscular strength and coordination as skeletal growth and maturation progress [24]. Further, as bone length and body mass increase, males demonstrate greater neuromuscular control of the knee joint compared with females, which allows them to better absorb loads because of the sufficient neuromuscular development [24]. This causes female knees to be exposed to greater GRF and high external knee abduction moments (load), which becomes especially significant in landing, pivoting, and deceleration [24].

Moreover, due to the hormonal changes that females undergo during puberty, the changes in lower limb strength are most evident during puberty. The quadriceps muscles are activated during an extensor movement to the knee prior to landing in order to prevent the knee from collapse upon landing. Round et al. [78] monitored changes in height, quadriceps strength, and testosterone level over the course of 4 years from 8 to 12 years of age that highlighted that boys and girls displayed similar increases in strength as they developed until one year prior to peak height velocity (PHV). This research demonstrated that there are clear gender differences in the rate of strength increases that were evident from 0 to 2 years PHV, whereby boys demonstrated an accelerated strength development and girls did not [78]. There was consistent increase in quadriceps strength in girls, which was proportional to the general increase in height and weight throughout the growth spurt [78]. In contrast, increased testosterone levels explained the greater increase in quadriceps strength displayed in boys [98]. Further studies have illustrated the development of isokinetic and isometric quadriceps strength after PHV and throughout puberty in boys, but not in girls. This may highlight the androgenic role of testosterone in promoting increased muscle mass and strength. Although estrogen has some androgenic properties, it is not as potent as testosterone. When normalized to body mass, boys showed an increase in strength of approximately 75 Nm/kg, whereas girls reported an increase of only 1–2 Nm/kg [98]. Therefore, despite a lack of statistical difference between genders, there is approximately 70–100 Nm of both absolute and relative torque, which could be considered clinically relevant [99].

The hamstring muscles also play a vital role during landing movements by impairing a posterior drawer force to the tibia, acting as a synergist to the ACL [93]. Many studies reporting changes in lower limb strength in girls throughout puberty focus on development of quadriceps strength, while only four studies [21, 40, 44, 96] investigated changes in hamstring strength through puberty in girls. Similar to changes in quadriceps strength, a significant increase in peak concentric and isometric hamstring muscle torque is typically displayed by males throughout puberty, while females do not express this increase [25]. Females also display weaker hamstring muscles relative to the quadriceps with age when compared with their male counterparts [25]. Further research has shown that females displayed an increase in quadriceps, but not hamstring, muscle strength with age. It is speculated that this decrease in hamstring strength relative to quadriceps strength with age may result in less protection of the ACL during dynamic movements, which may increase the risk of ACL injury in females [25].

In girls, there is a general consensus that muscle strength is continuously developing but the rate of the strength development is slower than the rate of skeletal growth compared with boys. The greater increase in quadriceps compared with hamstring muscle strength causes a greater reliance on the quadriceps and underutilization of the hamstrings. As a result, this reduced hamstring muscular torque is unable to act as an agonist to aid the ACL during dynamic movements such as landing.

40.4 Interplay of Active and Passive Control of the Knee

Dynamic knee stability is affected by both passive and active (neuromuscular) joint restraints, and interactions between both of these factors can influence dynamic control of the knee [54]. Some of the relationships between passive and active restraints may have their bases in genetics. Both structural and signaling genes have been linked to ACL injury, as mentioned above. While this evidence relates to the ligamentous structures of the knee, genetic makeup may play a role in determining one's neuromuscular characteristics. According to a recent review by Santos et al. [80], between 20 and 80 % of traits linked to physiological performance are highly associated with genetics. This evidence stretches back to 1973, when a study comparing neuromuscular characteristics of monozygotic and dizygotic twins reported high heritability indices for reflex and reaction time [33]. More recently, a 7-repeat allele in the dopamine D4 receptor gene has been implicated in those with longer reaction times [91].

Additionally, genetics influence fast-twitch muscle protein production via the ACTN3 gene, which encodes the protein α-actinin-3. The R577X polymorphism of this gene is associated with decreased production of fast-twitch muscle protein [80]. Athletes who are homozygous with two Rs, or normal alleles, produce greater power during anaerobic movements such as jumping and sprinting and also register increased peak quadriceps torque relative to those who are homozygous for the R577X polymorphism [32, 65, 99]. Interestingly, those with one or two normal (R) copies of the ACTN3 gene suffer fewer noncontact ankle injuries compared with R577X homozygotes [82].

These two specific genes serve as examples to illustrate how genetics may affect one's neuromuscular profile. Fortunately, dedicated neuromuscular training protocols can be initiated in athletes with deficits in these areas. Previous investigators have reported significant improvements in peroneus longus reaction time following a 6-week training program [37]. These improvements may give athletes more time to make necessary kinematic adjustments to reduce loads on the ACL during pivoting and cutting activities [37]. Strength deficits or imbalances are also risk factors that can be improved via neuromuscular training [49, 53]. Athletes may soon turn to gene sequencing in attempts to gain a competitive edge. As collaboration between the fields of genetics and sports medicine increases, clinicians may be able to add genetic information to their arsenal of tools used to identify at-risk individuals.

The potential exists for the coexistence of independent passive and active risk factors as well. For example, a female athlete with ligamentous laxity may develop quadriceps dominance during puberty and maturation. These neuromuscular changes could predispose this athlete to risky movement patterns that may place her already vulnerable ACL at increased risk for injury. The same notion can be applied for anatomical risk factors, such as small intercondylar notch width and small ACL. If this passive factor coexists with a weak trunk-stabilizing musculature that causes trunk dominance in an athlete, he/she would be at greater risk than if these factors existed singularly.

Athletes with a history of ACL injury can illustrate another scenario of the interplay of these factors. Previous injury and surgical reconstruction are not modifiable, but they can lead to both passive and active risk factors in athletes who return to sports. The kinematics and kinetics of the knee joint are compromised during ACL injury and are not fully restored by surgical reconstruction. Neuromuscular risk factors also develop following ACL injury, as graft tissue does not replace the proprioceptive functions of mechanoreceptors in the original ligament [36]. Additionally, quadriceps deficits and asymmetrical landing strategies are common after rehabilitation and return to sport [67]. When any of the aforementioned passive factors are observed in an athlete in combination with active factors, it is likely that a multiplicative effect exists that substantially increases the athlete's risk for ACL injury. Clinicians should therefore attempt to identify both categories of risk factors in athletes via the use of a variety of screening tools and techniques. By taking a holistic approach to screening athletes, at-risk individuals may be identified with high accuracy and subsequently enrolled in neuromuscular training programs to reduce the risk of injuries (Fig. 40.4).

40.5 Effects of Neuromuscular Training

ACL injuries are truly multifactorial not just based on the passive and active factors' theories presented in this chapter but also based on the environment and the activity levels of the individual. Much of the risk reduction can be mitigated via neuromuscular training starting at an early age [59], before the onset of symptoms. While many of the passive factors such as genetics, family histories, or gender cannot be modified, neuromuscular training will positively impact the dynamic forces that affect ACL tears.

The stability of the trunk is related to the hip's ability to control the trunk in response to forces

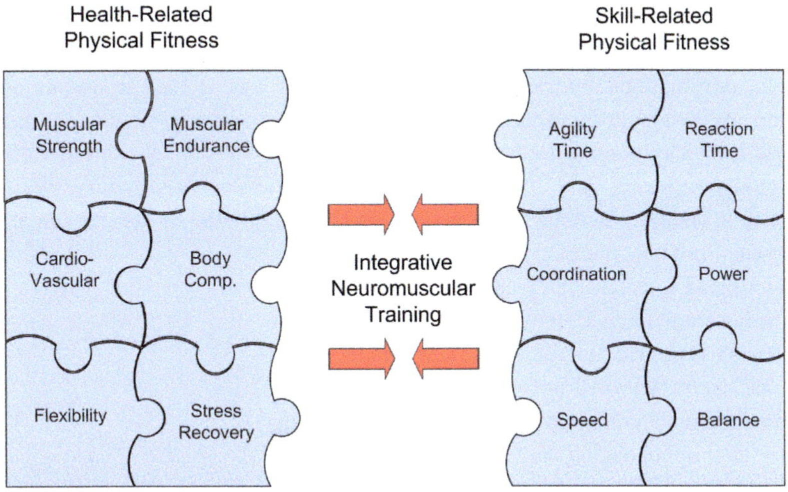

Fig. 40.4 The strategic importance of an integrative neuromuscular training to not only improve fitness but greater skill (Printed with permission from *Current Sports Medicine Reports*. Credit: Myer et al. [47])

generated from distal body segments and unexpected disturbances [24]. Deficits in proximal trunk neuromuscular control during dynamic movement may lead to uncontrolled lateral trunk motion, which may increase knee abduction motion and torque. This may lead to increased strain on the ACL and thus a propensity for injury. Neuromuscular control of the hip is required to control coronal plane trunk and pelvis motion, as hip adductor torque will counterbalance an external hip abduction movement created by a GRF lateral to the center of the femoral head.

Female athletes activate the hip musculature differently than the male subjects. Women adduct the hip more than men during both low- and high-intensity activities [24]. Increased hip adduction during dynamic motion and decreased hip abductor muscle recruitment can increase knee load and thus injury risk. During a landing or a squatting motion, females begin their descent in a more abducted knee position relative to males. They continue to remain in this position throughout the motion [24]. Ipsilateral trunk lean is a sign of weak hip abductors, because it moves the center of mass closer to the stance limb to reduce demand on the weak abductors.

When athletes land or cut on a single leg, the entire body must be balanced over one lower extremity. The trunk comprises greater than half of the body's mass. As a result, lateral trunk motion increases GRF and load. The body compensates with an equal and opposite force to counterbalance hip adductor torque. This increases the relative hip adductor-abductor torque ratio and most likely knee load, causing the individual to be more susceptible to injury [24]. Similarly, increased lateral trunk motion and change in direction of the GRF velocity augment the knee load of female athletes. Neuromuscular control of the hip, trunk, and knee is based on feedback control from the position and load of each segment. Dynamic stability of the knee is dependent on accurate sensory input and appropriate motor responses to rapid changes in body position. To maintain stability and performance, high levels of neuromuscular control are required during landing and cutting. Deficits in neuromuscular control of the trunk may contribute to lower extremity joint instability and injury. For example, abdominal muscle fatigue has a role in the etiology of hamstring injuries, and females have a greater body sway before injury compared to uninjured controls [24].

Neuromuscular control associated with the trunk segment and knee joint can predict ACL injury risk with very high sensitivity and specificity. It is therefore theorized that lateral trunk positioning creates high knee abduction torque (load). Trunk dominance suggests that males typically exhibit greater control of the trunk in performance situations as evidenced by greater activation of the internal oblique muscle. Leg dominance suggests that females exhibit greater kinematic leg asymmetry in knee valgus angles, hip abduction, and ankle abduction in performance situations. Future research needs to focus on utilizing neuromuscular training to prevent ACL injuries in all planes of motion.

Biomechanics and lower extremity strength can be altered in female subjects with neuromuscular training initiated during preadolescence [47], and a recent meta-analysis indicated that earlier implementation of neuromuscular training results in fewer ACL injuries in female athletes [59]. Neuromuscular power (i.e., rate of muscular recruitment and force generation, as evidenced by vertical jump height) can increase within 6 weeks of training [24]. Regular participation in sports is often not sufficient to increase power and a focused commitment to this type of training can reduce the risk of an ACL tear. Integrative neuromuscular training programs by trained professionals to develop fundamental motor skills rather than enhancing sports performance are the most beneficial [47]. Changes seen in female subjects may be greater than those in male subjects, since their baseline neuromuscular performance levels are lower [56]. Additionally, female athletes who were rated higher risk exhibited greater responses to alter the ACL risk movements compared to female athletes with low risk [50].

Despite strong training programs, it is nearly impossible to eliminate all sports-related injuries, but it is possible to reduce the number of acute injuries by 15–50% through adequate strength and conditioning practices [47]. It can be challenging to convince preadolescents to participate in prolonged periods of exercise; however, intermittent integrative neuromuscular training has been shown to be equally valuable to young athletes [47]. Similar challenges have existed trying to convince coaches to use their precious practice time for injury prevention. At the same time, adding this additional training program to the young athletes' already total exercise dose may increase the frequency of chronic repetitive stress fractures or other stress injuries due to overuse. As a result, this neuromuscular training should be a part of the total athlete training workload and adjusted accordingly during times of high demand. The exact amount of fitness to avoid stress injuries or other fatigue-related issues is often based on age and genetic makeup and can be quite variable among a given group of individuals. Healthcare providers, fitness specialists, and coaches need to be extremely cognizant of this to maximize the training and overall well-being of the individual [47].

Fact Box 2

- Passive risk factors include hormones, genetics, anatomy, and past medical history.
- Active risk factors include elevated GRF, excessive lateral trunk flexion angles, increased knee valgus loading patterns, and insufficient muscular development around the knee joint.
- Both categories may exist simultaneously in an athlete, placing him/her at greater risk than if one factor existed alone.
- Prior injury to the ACL can further propagate dynamic and passive deficits and may be related to the high risk of secondary ACL injury in athletes who return to sport.
- Neuromuscular training optimizes dynamic knee control and may be helpful for athletes to develop strategies that can overcome deficits in both dynamic and passive knee stability.

Conclusion

The knee joint consists of four major stabilizing ligaments, and the ACL plays a primary role to stabilize anterior-posterior translation on sagittal plane. In addition to its primary function, the ACL also stabilizes the knee joint in the coronal/frontal and horizontal planes. Risks of ACL rupture consist of both passive and active factors. The passive risk factors include hormonal influences, as well as genetics and anatomy, in addition to past medical history, and under the current medical practices, they are not modifiable to reduce the risk of ACL injury. In contrast, active risk factors are modifiable to a greater or lesser extent. Active and passive factors may coexist and place athletes at even greater risk than if they were affected by a sole risk factor. The effect of trunk movement, particularly lateral flexion, in conjunction with a chain of inertial movements including GRF, hip musculature activation, and knee loads on ACL injury, is considered the underlying mechanism of ACL injury. A mechanical connection between trunk motion and knee load, especially knee valgus movement, is reported from various laboratory-based biomechanical studies. Moreover, greater risk of ACL injury in females compared to males may stem from muscular strength development during puberty and PHV. From prepubescent to pubescent/maturation phases, males develop sufficient muscular strength in the quadriceps and hamstrings, which deliver a sufficient base of support. However, muscular development of females is less than that of their male counterparts. In order to facilitate the muscular development that delivers adequate support for the knee joint and especially the ACL during dynamic movements, neuromuscular training is proposed. The effect of neuromuscular training on ACL injury reduction in female athletes is well documented in recent meta-analyses. To optimize the effects of neuromuscular training, programs should be initiated at younger ages and provide additional training to coaches to help to mitigate the potentially negative effects of puberty.

Bibliography

1. Agel J, Arendt EA, Bershadsky B (2005) Anterior cruciate ligament injury in National Collegiate Athletic Association Basketball and Soccer: A 13-year review. Am J Sports Med 33(4):524–531
2. Agel J, Olson DE, Dick R et al (2007) Descriptive epidemiology of collegiate women's basketball injuries: National Collegiate Athletic Association Injury Surveillance System, 1988-1989 through 2003-2004. J Athl Train 42(2):202–210
3. Altinisik J, Meric G, Erduran M et al (2015) The BstUI and DpnII variants of the COL5A1 gene are associated with tennis elbow. Am J Sports Med 20(10):1784–1789
4. Arendt E, Dick R (1995) Knee injury patterns among men and women in collegiate basketball and soccer. NCAA data and review of literature. Am J Sports Me 23:694–701
5. Beye JA, Hart DA, Bray RC, Mcdougall JJ, Salo PT (2008) Injury-induced changes in mRNA levels differ widely between anterior cruciate ligament and medial collateral ligament. Am J Sports Med 36(7):1337–1346
6. Boden BP, Dean GS, Feagin JA, Garrett WE (2000) Mechanisms of anterior cruciate ligament injury. Orthopedics 23(6):573–578
7. Boden BP, Griffin L, Garett W (2000) Etiology and prevention of noncontact ACL injury. Phys Sportsmed 28(4):53–60
8. Boden BP, Sheehan FT, Torg JS, Hewett TE (2010) Noncontact anterior cruciate ligament injuries: mechanisms and risk factors. J Am Acad Orthop Surg 18(2):520–527
9. Burger M, de Wet H, Collins M (2015) The COL5A1 gene is associated with increased risk of carpal tunnel syndrome. Clin Rheumatol 34(4):767–774
10. Bytomski JR, Moorman C (2010) Oxford American Handbook of Sports Medicine. Oxford University Press, New York
11. Charlton WP, St. John TA, Ciccotti MG et al (2002) Differences in femoral notch anatomy between men and women: a magnetic resonance imaging study. Am J Sports Med 30:329–333
12. Cooney AD, Kazi Z, Caplan N, Newby M, Gibson ASC, Kader DF (2012) The relationship between quadriceps angle and tibial tuberosity–trochlear groove distance in patients with patellar instability. Knee Surg Sports Traumatol Arthrosc 20(12):2399–2404
13. Domzalski M, Grzelak P, Gabos P (2010) Risk factors for anterior cruciate ligament injury in skeletally immature patients: analysis of intercondylar notch width using magnetic resonance imaging. Int Orthop 34(5):703–707
14. Dugan SA (2005) Sports-related knee injuries in female athletes: what gives? Am J Phys Med Rehabil 84(2):122–130
15. Faude O, Junge A, Kindermann W et al (2006) Risk factors for injuries in elite female soccer players. Br J Sports Med 40(9):785–790
16. Ficek K, Ciezczyk P, Kaczmarczyk M et al (2013) Gene variants within the COL1A1 gene are associated with reduced anterior cruciate ligament injury in professional soccer players. J Sci Med Sport 16(5):396–400
17. Ford KR, Myer GD, Hewett TE (2003) Valgus knee motion during landing in high school female and male basketball players. Med Sci Sports Exerc 35:1745–1750
18. Ford KR, Myer GD, Toms HE, Hewett TE (2005) Gender differences in the kinematics of unanticipated cutting in young athletes. Med Sci Sports 37:124–129
19. Gerecke DR, Olson PF, Koch M et al (1997) Complete primary structure of two splice variants of

collagen XII, and assignment of alpha 1(XII) collagen (COL12A1), alpha 1(IX) collagen (COL9A1), and alpha 1(XIX) collagen (COL19A1) to human chromosome 6q12-q13. Genomics 41:236–242
20. Gormeli CA, Gormeli G, Ozturk YB, Ozdemir Z, Kahraman A (2014) The effect of the intercondylar notch width index on anterior cruciate ligament injuries a study on groups with unilateral and bilateral ACL injury. Orthop J Sports Med 2(11):supppl3
21. Heras Yague P, De La Fuente J (1998) Changes in height and motor performance relative to peak height velocity: a mixed-longitudinal study of Spanish boys and girls. Am J Hum Biol 10:647–660
22. Hettrich CM, Dunn WR, Reinke EK et al (2013) The rate of subsequent surgery and predictors after anterior cruciate ligament reconstruction: Two- and 6 year follow-up results from a multicenter cohort. Am J Sports Med 41(7):1534–1540
23. Hewett TE, Myer GD (2011) The mechanistic connection between the trunk, Hip, knee, and anterior cruciate ligament injury. Exerc Sport Sci Rev 39(4): 161–166
24. Hewett TE, Myer GD, Ford KR et al (2005) Biomechanical measures of neuromuscular control and valgus loading of the knee predict anterior cruciate ligament injury risk in female athletes: a prospective study. Am J Sports Med 33:492–501
25. Hewett TE, Myer GD, Zazulak BT (2008) Hamstrings to quadriceps peak torque ratios diverge between sexes with increasing isokinetic angular velocity. J Sci Med Sport 11(5):452–459
26. Hewett TE, Stroupe AL, Nance TA, Noyes FR (1996) Plyometric training in female athletes decreased impact forces and increased hamstring torques. Am J Sports Med 24:765–773
27. Hewett TE, Torg JS, Boden BP (2009) Video analysis of trunk knee motion during Non-contact anterior cruciate ligament injury in female athletes: lateral trunk and knee abduction motion are combined components of the injury mechanism. Br J Sports Med 43:417–422
28. Ireland ML (1996) Anterior cruciate ligament injuries in young female athletes: high risks call for new approaches. Your Patient Fitness 10(5):26–30
29. Jin H, Hof RJV, Albagha OM, Ralston SH (2009) Promoter and intron 1 polymorphisms of COL1A1 interact to regulate transcription and susceptibility to osteoporosis. Hum Mol Genet 18(15):2729–2738
30. Keays SL, Keays R, Newcombe PA (2016) Femoral intercondylar notch width size: a comparison between siblings with and without anterior cruciate ligament injuries. Knee Surg Sports Traumatol Arthrosc 24(3):672–679
31. Khoschnau S, Melhus H, Jacobson A et al (2008) Type I collagen alpha1 Sp1 polymorphism and the risk of cruciate ligament ruptures or shoulder dislocations. Am J Sports Med 36(12):2432–2436
32. Kikuchi N, Nakazato K, Min SK, Ueda D, Igawa S (2014) The ACTN3 R577X polymorphism is associated with muscle power in male Japanese athletes. J Strength Cond Res 28(7):1783–1789
33. Komi PV, Klissouras V, Karvinen E (1973) Genetic variation in neuromuscular performance. Int Z Angew Physiol 31(4):289–304
34. Krosshaug T, Nakamae A, Boden BP (2006) Mechanisms of anterior cruciate ligament injury in basketball: video analysis of 39 cases. Am J Sports Med 35(3):359–367
35. Krosshaug T, Bahr R (2005) A model-based image-matching technique for three-dimensional reconstruction of human motion from uncalibrated video sequences. J Biomech 38:919–929
36. Lee BI (2009) Min, KD, Choi, HS, et al. (2009) immunohistochemical study of mechanoreceptors in the tibial remnant of the ruptured anterior cruciate ligament in human knees. Knee Surg Sports Traumatol Arthrosc 17(9):1095–1101
37. Linford CW, Hopkins JT, Schulthies SS et al (2006) Effects of neuromuscular training on the reaction time and electromechanical delay of the peroneus longus muscle. Arch Phys Med Rehabil 87(3):395–401
38. Lohmander LS, Englund PM, Dahl LL, Roos EM (2007) The long-term consequence of anterior cruciate ligament and meniscus injuries: osteoarthritis. Am J Sports Med 35:1756–1769
39. Lohmander LS, Stenberg A, Englund M, Roos H (2004) High prevalence of knee osteoarthritis, pain, and functional limitations in female soccer players twelve years after anterior cruciate ligament injury. Arthritis Rheum 50(10):3145–3152
40. Loko J, Aule R, Sikkut T et al (2000) Motor performance status in 10 to 17-year-old Estonian girls. Scand J Med Sci Sport 10:109–113
41. Mannion S, Mtintsilana A, Posthumus M et al (2014) Genes encoding proteoglycans are associated with the risk of anterior cruciate ligament ruptures. Br J Sports Med 48(22):1640–1646
42. Martin R, Hugentobler J, Myer GD (2011) Is ACL injury all too familial for some patients? Sports Physiother 2:19–24
43. Mclean SG, Huang X, van den Bogert AJ (2005) Association between lower extremity posture at contact and peak when the tibia moves too far forward implications for ACL injury. Clin Biomech 20(8): 863–870
44. Merni F, Balboni M, Bargellini S et al (1981) Differences in males and females in joint movement range during growth. Med Sport 15:168–175
45. Mohammed J, Mohammed H, Abdinejad F, Hamid N (2007) Q-angle: an invaluable parameter for evaluation of anterior knee pain. Arch Iran Med 10(1): 24–26
46. Mokone GG, Schwellnus MP, Noakes TD, Collins M (2006) The COL5A1 gene and Achilles tendon pathology. Scand J Med Sci Sports 16(1):19–26
47. Myer GD, Faigenbaum AD, Ford KR et al (2011) When to initiate integrative neuromuscular training to reduce sports-related injuries and enhance health in youth? Curr Sports Med Rep 10(3):157–166
48. Myer GD, Ford KR, Barber KD et al (2009) The relationship of hamstrings and quadriceps strength to anterior cruciate ligament injury in female athletes. Clin J Sport Med 19(1):3–8

49. Myer GD, Ford KR, Brent JL, Hewett TE (2006) The effects of plyometric vs. dynamic stabilization and balance training on power, balance, and landing force in female athletes. J Strength Cond Res 20(2):345–353
50. Myer GD, Ford KR, Brent JL, Hewett TE (2007) Differential neuromuscular training effects on ACL injury risk factors in "high-risk" versus "low-risk" athletes. BMC Musculoskelet Disord 8(39):1–7
51. Myer GD, Ford KR, Khoury J et al (2011) Biomechanics laboratory-based prediction algorithm to identify female athletes with high knee loads that increase risk of ACL injury. Br J Sports Med 45:245–252
52. Myer GD, Ford KR, Khoury J, Succop P, Hewett TE (2010) Development and validation of a clinic-based prediction tool to identify female athletes at high risk for anterior cruciate ligament injury. Am J Sports Med 20(10):1–10
53. Myer GD, Ford KR, Palumbo JP, Hewett TE (2005) Neuromuscular training improves performance and lower-extremity biomechanics in female athletes. J Strength Cond Res 19(1):51–60
54. Myer GD, Ford KR, Paterno MV et al (2008) The effects of generalized joint laxity on risk of anterior cruciate ligament injury in young female athletes. Am J Sports Med 36(6):1073–1080
55. Myer GD, Ford KR, Stasi SLD et al (2015) High knee abduction moments are common risk factors for patellofemoral pain (PFP) and anterior cruciate ligament (ACL) injury in girls: Is PFP itself a predictor for subsequent ACL injury? Br J Sports Med 49:118–122
56. Myer GD, Ford KR, Hewett TE (2004) Rationale and Clinical Techniques for Anterior Cruciate Ligament Injury Prevention Among Female Athletes. J Athl Train 39(4):352–364
57. Myer GD, Heidt RS, Waits C et al (2013) Sex comparison of familial predisposition to anterior cruciate ligament injury. Knee Surg Sports Traumatol Arthrosc 22(2):387–391
58. Myer GD, Lloyd RS, Brent JL, Faigenbaum AD (2013) How young is too young to start training? ACSMs Health Fit J 17(5):14–23
59. Myer GD, Sugimoto D, Thomas S, Hewett TE (2013) The influence of age on the effectiveness of neuromuscular training to reduce anterior cruciate ligament injury in female athletes: a meta-analysis. Am J Sports Med 41(1):1–25
60. Myklebust G, Maehlum S, Engebretsen L et al (1997) Registration of cruciate ligament injuries in Norwegian top level team handball. A prospective study involving two seasons. Scand J Med Sci Sports 7:289–292
61. Nagano Y, Ida H, Akai M, Fukubayashi T (2007) Gender differences in knee kinematics and muscle activity during single limb drop landing. Knee 14:218–223
62. National Institute of Arthritis and Musculoskeletal and Skin Diseases (2013) Handout on health sports injuries. http://www.niams.nih.gov/Health_Info/Sports_Injuries/default.asp#ra_13. Accessed 25 Feb 2015
63. Nicholas JA, Hirshman EB (1995) The lower extremity and spine in sports medicine, vol 2. Mosby, St. Louis
64. Øiestad BE, Holm I, Engebretsen L, Risberg MA (2010) The association between radiographic knee osteoarthritis and knee symptoms, function and quality of life 10–15 years after anterior cruciate ligament reconstruction. Br J Sports Med 45(7):583–588
65. Orysiak J, Busko K, Michalski R et al (2014) Relationship between ACTN3 R577X polymorphism and maximal power output in elite Polish athletes. Medicina 50(5):303–308
66. Ostenberg A, Roos H (2000) Injury risk factors in female European football. A prospective study of 123 players during one season. Scand J Med Sci Sports 10:279–285
67. Otzel DM, Chow JW, Tillman MD (2015) Long-term deficits in quadriceps strength and activation following anterior cruciate ligament reconstruction. Phys Ther Sport 16(1):22–28
68. Pappas E, Carpas F (2012) Lower extremity kinematic asymmetry in males and female athletes performing jump-landing tasks. J Sci Med Sport 15:87–92
69. Paterno MV, Rauh MJ, Schmitt LC et al (2012) Incidence of contralateral and ipsilateral anterior cruciate ligament (ACL) injury after primary ACL reconstruction and return to sport. Clin J Sport Med 22(2):116–121
70. Paterno MV, Schmitt LC, Ford KR et al (2010) Biomechanical measures during landing and postural stability predict second anterior cruciate ligament injury after anterior cruciate ligament reconstruction and return to sport. Am J Sports Med 38:1968–1978
71. Posthumus M, September AV, Keegan M et al (2009) Genetic risk factors for anterior cruciate ligament ruptures: COL1A1 gene variant. Br J Sports Med 43(5):352–356
72. Posthumus M, September AV, O'Cuinneagain D et al (2009) The association between the COL12A1 gene and anterior cruciate ligament ruptures. Br J Sports Med 44(16):1160–1165
73. Posthumus M, September AV, O'Cuinneagain D et al (2009) The COL5A1 gene is associated with increased risk of anterior cruciate ligament ruptures in female participants. Am J Sports Med 37(11): 2234–2240
74. Prodromos CC, Han Y, Rogowski J, Joyce B, Shi K (2007) A meta analysis of the injury of anterior cruciate ligament tears as a function of gender, sport, and a knee injury-reduction regimen. Arthroscopy 23(12):1320–1325
75. Pufe T, Petersen W, Tillmann B, Mentlein R (2001) The angiogenic peptide vascular endothelial growth factor is expressed in fetal and ruptured tendons. Virchows Arch 439(4):579–585
76. Quatman CE, Ford KR, Myer GD et al (2008) The effects of gender and pubertal status on generalized joint laxity in young athletes. J Sci Med Sport 11(3):257–263

77. Rahim M, Gibbon A, Hobbs H et al (2014) The association of genes involved in the angiogenesis-associated signaling pathway with risk of anterior cruciate ligament rupture. J Orthop Res 32(12):1612–1618
78. Round JM, Jones DA, Honour JW et al (1999) Hormonal factors in the development of differences in strength between boys and girls during adolescence: a longitudinal study. Ann Hum Biol 26(1):49–62
79. Salmon L, Russell V, Musgrove T et al (2005) Incidence and risk factors for graft rupture and contralateral rupture after anterior cruciate ligament reconstruction. Arthroscopy 21(8):948–957
80. Santos CG, Pimentel-Coelho PM, Budowle B et al (2015) The heritable path of human physical performance: from single polymorphisms to the "next generation". Scand J Med Sci Sports (epub)
81. September AV, Cook J, Handley CJ et al (2009) Variants within the COL5A1 gene are associated with Achilles tendinopathy in two populations. Br J Sports Med 43(5):357–365
82. Shang X, Li Z, Cao X et al (2015) The association between the ACTN3 R577X polymorphism and noncontact acute ankle sprains. J Sports Sci 33(17): 1775–1779
83. Shelbourne KD, Davis TI, Klootwyk TE (1998) Relationship between intercondylar notch width of the femur and the incidence of anterior cruciate ligament tears: a prospective study. Am J Sports Med 26:402–408
84. Shultz SJ, Gansneder BM, Sander TC et al (2006) Absolute serum hormone levels predict the magnitude of change in anterior knee laxity across the menstrual cycle. J Orthop Res 24(2):124–131
85. Shultz SJ, Schmitz RJ, Nguyen AD (2008) Research retreat IV: ACL injuries–the gender bias: April 3-5, 2008 Greensboro. J Athl Train 43:530–531
86. Sigward S, Powers C (2007) Loading characteristics of females exhibiting excessive valgus movements during cutting. Clin Biomech 22:827–833
87. Silvers HJ, Mandelbaum BR (2007) Prevention of anterior cruciate ligament injury in the female athlete. Br J Sports Med 41(Suppl I):i52–i59
88. Souryal TO, Freeman TR (1993) Intercondylar notch size and anterior cruciate ligament injuries in athletes: a prospective study. Am J Sports Med 21(4):535–539
89. Stępień-Słodkowska M, Ficek K, Maciejewska-Karłowska A et al (2015) Overrepresentation of the COL3A1 AA genotype in Polish skiers with anterior cruciate ligament injury. Biol Sport 32(2):143–147
90. Stracciolini A, Casciano R, Friedman HL et al (2014) Pediatric sports injuries: a comparison of males versus females. Am J Sports Med 42(4):965–972
91. Szekely A, Balota DA, Duchek JM et al (2010) Genetic factors of reaction time performance: DRD4 7-repeat allele associated with slower responses. Genes Brain Behav 10(2):129–136
92. Tang Z, Yang L, Xue R et al (2009) Differential expression of matrix metalloproteinases and tissue inhibitors of metalloproteinases in anterior cruciate ligament and medial collateral ligament fibroblasts after a mechanical injury: involvement of the P65 subunit of NF-κB. Wound Repair Regen 17(5): 709–716
93. Taylor BT, Waxman JP, Richter SJ, Shultz SJ (2013) Evaluation of the effectiveness of anterior cruciate ligament injury prevention programme training components: a systematic review and meta-analysis. Br J Sports Med 49(2):79–87
94. Tillman MD, Smith KR, Bauer JA et al (2002) Differences in three intercondylar notch geometry indices between males and females: a cadaver study. Knee 9:41–46
95. Uhorchak JM, Scoville CR, Williams GN et al (2003) Risk factors associated with noncontact injury of the anterior cruciate ligament: a prospective four-year evaluation of 859 West Point cadets. Am J Sports Med 31:831–842
96. Vincent B, De Bock K, Ramaekers M et al (2007) ACTN3 (R577X) genotype is associated with fiber type distribution. Physiol Genomics 32(1):58–63
97. Volver A, Viru A, Viru M (2000) Improvement of motor abilities in pubertal girls. J Sports Med Phys Fitness 40(1):17–25
98. Webster KE, Feller JA, Leigh WB, Richmond AK (2014) Younger patients are at increased risk for graft rupture and contralateral injury after anterior cruciate ligament reconstruction. Am J Sports Med 42:641–647
99. Wild CY, Steele JR, Munro BJ (2012) Why do girls sustain more anterior cruciate ligament injuries than boys? A review of the changes in estrogen and musculoskeletal structure and function during puberty. Sports Med 42(9):733–749
100. Winkel D, Matthijs O, Phelps V, Vleeming A (1997) Diagnosis and treatment of the lower extremities: nonoperative orthopaedic medicine and manual therapy. Aspen, Gaithersburg
101. Wojtys EM, Brower AM (2010) Anterior cruciate ligament injuries in the prepubescent and adolescent athlete: clinical and research considerations. J Athl Train 45:509–512
102. Wright RW, Magnussen RA, Dunn WR, Spindler KP (2011) Ipsilateral graft and contralateral ACL rupture at five years or more following ACL reconstruction: a systematic review. J Bone Joint Surg Am 93(12):1159–1165
103. Young K, Samiric T, Feller J, Cook J (2011) Extracellular matrix content of ruptured anterior cruciate ligament tissue. Knee 18(4):242–246

Evidence-Based Medicine for Rotary Knee Instability

41

Kaitlyn L. Yin and Robert G. Marx

Contents

K.L. Yin • R.G. Marx, MD, MSc, FRCSC (✉)
Department of Orthopaedic Surgery,
Hospital for Special Surgery, 535 East 70th Street,
New York, NY 10021, USA
e-mail: marxr@hss.edu

41.1 Evidence-Based Medicine

The movement to incorporate evidence-based medicine (EBM) into clinical problem solving is relatively new. Since 1980, the use of current evidence from scientific literature to improve patient care has become more and more commonplace in clinical practice. EBM supplements physicians' individual experiences to inform patient care and provides statistical data and evidence to create medical guidelines and recommendations that improve patient outcomes [15].

Additionally, EBM aids in standardizing the care that patients receive. According to epidemiological data, the likelihood that a woman underwent a hysterectomy by age seventy varied from 20 to 70 % in different geographic areas in Maine [18]. Other surgeries, such as prostate surgery, heart bypass, and thyroid surgery, also showed wide variations in rates throughout the same geographical region [15].

Disagreements between physicians are not uncommon. One study sent surveys to 1100 orthopedic surgeons about rotator cuff surgeries and found variation in clinical and surgical decision-making [3]. Clinical agreement, defined as >80 % agreement among the respondents, was reached on only four out of nine clinical questions. There was no clinical agreement on the four hypothetical vignettes [3]. There are many variables present in the clinical setting that contribute to the variable care patients receive. EBM provides scientific evidence that can help control

V. Musahl et al. (eds.), *Rotatory Knee Instability*, DOI 10.1007/978-3-319-32070-0_41

for those variables and standardize the quality of care across patients.

However, although EBM is a useful supplement in clinical practice, its successful application relies on the physicians' clinical knowledge. The role of EBM is to give clinicians a foundation of scientific evidence from which to build their clinical decision-making. However, it is ultimately the clinician's decision whether evidence from certain studies applies to a specific patient's situation. EBM does not eliminate the role for clinical acumen but rather adds to it.

41.2 The Pivot Shift

The anterior cruciate ligament (ACL) works with lateral structures to stabilize the knee and prevent excessive anterior tibial translation [13]. The ACL also serves a role in preventing knee hyperextension and excessive tibial rotation [13]. When the ACL is torn, it may result in rotary instability of the femoral condyle that patients will describe as knee "giving way." For athletes, rotary knee laxity can preclude participation in sports that require cutting and sharp changes in direction, and even for nonathletes, intermittent episodes of knee "giving way" have a significant effect on patient satisfaction.

> **Fact Box 1**
> The pivot shift test measures rotary laxity. Typically, the clinician extends the patient's leg and applies a valgus force followed by gentle internal rotation and flexion with valgus. An ACL-deficient knee should demonstrate subluxation with subsequent reduction of the lateral tibial plateau.

The pivot shift diagnostic test evaluates the rotational instability of the knee. The clinician first extends the patient's leg, applying a valgus force. In the ACL-deficient knee, this maneuver results in an anterior subluxation of the lateral tibial plateau against the femoral condyle. The clinician then applies gentle internal rotation and flexion with valgus, and the knee should reduce around 15–30° of flexion [4]. The pivot shift's rotational subluxation and subsequent reduction can reproduce the feeling of "giving way" and can be predictive of patient outcomes, especially when performed postoperatively [12]. The pivot shift measures rotator laxity as opposed to other clinical tests for anterior cruciate ligament insufficiency such as the Lachman test, which measures anterior tibial translation [14].

Due to its complexity, pivot shift techniques vary based on surgeons' training and even region of practice [16]. Pivot shift grading is also subjective, and it is further complicated because patients have different baseline pivot shifts. The pivot shift test would benefit from standardization, suggesting a role for EBM. This chapter will focus on the evidence surrounding the use of the pivot shift test in clinical practice.

41.2.1 Pivot Shift Correlations with Patient Outcomes

The pivot shift offers valuable knowledge about the rotary stability of the knee, which correlates with patient satisfaction and outcomes. This is shown in a retrospective prognostic study by Leitze et al., who followed a cohort of 87 patients with an average follow-up of 9 years. The cohort was largely male (78 %) with an average age of 26 years at the time of surgery. Cases were chronic, and the time to surgery was 39 months on average [12]. Leitze et al. found that the presence of a positive pivot shift test was correlated with poor patient satisfaction ($p<0.01$) and measurable patient outcomes including the Losee score, HSS score, Feagin and Blake symptom and function scores (all $p<0.001$) [12]. Patients with positive postoperative pivot shifts were 14.4 times more likely to have unsatisfactory subjective outcomes, and laxity on the Lachman test alone did not correlate with a decline in patient satisfaction [12]. This study suggests that the use of the pivot shift is particularly valuable and practical among clinical tests for ACL laxity because it can predict functional status and outcomes.

Fact Box 2
In one study, patients with positive postoperative pivot shifts were 14.4 times more likely to have unsatisfactory subjective outcomes, while laxity on the Lachman test alone did not correlate with a decline in patient satisfaction [12].

These findings were replicated in other studies. The Jonsson et al. study evaluated 63 patients from a 68-patient cohort similar to the cohort in the Leitze et al. study (66 % male, average age 25 years, time to surgery 43 months) and found that a positive pivot shift 2 years postsurgery was correlated with decreased patient functional outcomes [6]. Kocher et al. also found significant correlations between pivot shift and patient satisfaction, giving way, difficulty cutting, sport participation, activity limitation, and overall knee function. In contrast, no significant correlations were found for the Lachman test or instrumented knee laxity and functional outcome [9].

Patients with severe pivot shifts (grades 2+ or 3+) in Kaplan et al.'s 52-patient large cohort were unable to return to unrestricted sports participation, while 29 of 37 patients with no pivot shift and 3 of 8 patients with 1+ pivot shift returned to unrestricted sports [7]. Finally, Ayeni et al. conducted a meta-analysis of randomized control trials about ACL reconstructions [1]. They included 65 papers, including the Leitze et al. and Jonsson et al. studies, with a total of 5061 patients. Forty-seven of these papers included the pivot shift test as an outcome, and 40/47 (80 %) demonstrated that the test correlated with patient's functional outcomes [1].

There is also some evidence that suggests a positive pivot shift may predict the development of osteoarthritis (OA). Neither Leitze et al. nor Jonsson et al. found correlations between pivot shift and radiographic evidence of OA [6, 12]. However, the latter study found that patients with a positive pivot shift 2 years after ACL reconstruction had a greater difference in bone scintigraphic uptake at 5–9 years post-op over the whole knee and in the lateral joint compartment ($p=0.03$ for both). Although there is no clear radiographic evidence of OA, increased scintigraphic uptake may precede radiographic signs of OA by several years [6]. Though the range of follow-up in the Leitze et al. study varied from 5 to 21 years, the average follow-up was 9 years, similar to the follow-up time in Jonsson et al.'s cohort. Perhaps a correlation would be found between positive pivot shift and radiographic OA onset with longer follow-up, and further research is needed.

41.2.2 Clinical Use of Pivot Shift Test

The pivot shift test is subjective, and its performance varies. The pivot test varies from surgeon to surgeon, and the forces applied during the pivot shift vary [10]. The test is difficult to standardize due to the multiple described ways to perform the examination, different forces applied in different directions, and confounding soft tissue contributions [10]. Moreover, the resultant grading of the shift adds further subjectivity to the process, and some patients naturally have some degree of joint laxity [10]. To compensate for this, surgeons should also perform a pivot shift test on the contralateral, non-injured leg to serve as a comparison [10].

Fact Box 3
The pivot shift test has been found to have a low sensitivity but a high specificity.

Another aspect of the pivot shift that should be considered is its sensitivity and specificity. Scholten et al.'s meta-analysis of 17 studies found pivot shift sensitivity was low ranging from 18 to 48 % [17]. Due to its low sensitivity, the pivot shift test should be performed in conjunction with other clinical tests, such as the Lachman test, which has a high sensitivity. The same study found that the Lachman test had a pooled sensitivity of 86 % (95 % CI 76–92 %). The pivot shift, however, had a higher specificity. Pivot shift specificity ranged from 97 to 99 %, while the

Lachman test's pooled specificity was 91 % (95 % CI 79–96 %) [17].

In another retrospective study of 147 patients, the Lachman test was positive in 98.6 % of patients with proven chronic ACL injuries, and the pivot shift was positive in 89.8 % [8]. Both tests were done under anesthesia, and the authors note that the pivot shift test may be less sensitive without anesthesia. This is demonstrated in another study that showed the pivot shift was positive in 35 % of knees with an ACL injury, and the number increased to 98 % with testing under anesthesia [2]. There was a smaller difference for the Lachman test. It was positive in 99 % of knees and 100 % under anesthesia [2]. This is a significant consideration because preoperative and postoperative evaluations are typically done in the clinical setting without anesthesia. As such, the clinician should accept and account for this limitation of the pivot shift.

Fact Box 4
The sensitivity of the pivot shift test increases when the patient is under anesthesia due to the absence of guarding.

The relationship between the pivot shift and Lachman test was further explored in a laboratory study by Markolf et al. Seventeen cadaver knees underwent pivot shift tests, and the anteroposterior (AP) knee laxities (mm), plateau displacement (mm), and tibial rotation (degrees) were all measured [14]. The measurements were taken under various knee conditions (intact, ACL-deficient, and post-ACL reconstruction) to simulate the progress of patients through ACL reconstruction. Markolf et al. found a weak correlation between absolute laxity and lateral tibial plateau displacement in ACL-deficient knees ($r^2=0.41$). Correlation between absolute laxity and tibial rotation was also weak ($r^2=0.34$). Markolf et al. found a stronger correlation when change in plateau displacement was plotted against change in laxity ($r^2=0.70$) in the 17 knees [14]. Tibial rotation also had a fair correlation with change in AP laxity in intact knees ($r^2=0.53$). Markolf et al. also gradually increased the laxity in individual knees and found that the pivot shift initially increased linearly with knee laxity up to an end point that falls before the point of ACL deficiency. After this end point, the slope decreases and flattens [14].

Although this is a laboratory study rather than clinical, it offers insight into the correlation between the pivot shift and Lachman test. There is a stronger correlation between the changes in AP laxity and changes in pivot shift than between the absolute values of those same measurements. Furthermore, when loosening the graft, the plateau displacement/tibial rotation largely stops increasing with laxity after a certain point. This evidence suggests that while the differences in laxity between the intact and ACL-deficient knees could predict differences in pivot shift, surgeons should be careful of using the pivot shift to distinguish between different types of ACL-deficient knees due to the observed weak correlation between absolute pivot shift magnitude and absolute laxity.

However, although correlations between the pivot shift and Lachman tests were reported, most of the reported correlations were not very large [14]. Clinical evidence indicates that using these tests together may not always be straightforward, and outcomes of the tests are not always consistent with each other. The majority of Leitze et al.'s patients who had positive 1–10 mm Lachman grades did not have concurrent positive pivot shifts [12]. For Lee et al., while the majority of patients had consistent pivot shift and Lachman tests, 13 of 137 patients demonstrated a negative Lachman and a positive pivot shift [11]. Clinical experience and knowledge together with evidence from the literature about these two tests can work together to aid decision-making.

41.3 Future Directions for Research

The development of a standardized technique would improve the pivot shift and promote its use in both research and clinical practice. Despite the difficulties, there has already been research aimed at standardizing the pivot shift. One group of researchers had 12 expert surgeons perform a pivot shift test on one cadaver leg and found that the techniques and clinical grading varied between them. The researchers then introduced a standardized technique that, while easily adopted by the surgeons, did not provide additional standardization of clinical grading [16]. Nonetheless, the authors recommended continued research toward development of a standardized pivot shift.

Another study coauthored by many of the same authors also looked at standardizing the pivot shift. Twelve expert surgeons performed pivot shifts on two cadaver legs, one with a low-grade pivot shift and one with a high-grade pivot shift. Electromagnetic tracking was used to measure anterior tibial translation and acceleration of the reduction during the pivot shift. There was no significant difference in anterior tibial translation between the surgeons' preferred technique and the standardized technique. However, there was less variation in acceleration. The increased consistency in acceleration supports the development and use of a standardized pivot shift test, though electromagnetic tracking is not currently widely used in a typical clinical setting [5].

There is awareness that the subjectivity and variability of the pivot shift test are limitations of this maneuver. Research toward developing a standardized pivot shift already exists, but no technique has yet been designated the "gold standard" of pivot shifts. The creation of a standardized pivot shift test, especially one that could be easily applied in the clinic, might be the next significant development in this field.

Conclusion

EBM does not replace clinical knowledge and experience. Rather, it supplements the physician's judgment with a foundation of evidence. EBM helps to standardize the treatments that patients receive to improve their outcomes. The pivot shift is a clinical diagnostic test for ACL deficiency, and its subjectivity and variability indicate a role for EBM in informing its use and application.

The pivot shift provides the clinician with valuable information, which supports its use in evaluating patients' knees post-ACL reconstruction surgery. However, there are also limitations to the pivot shift test. The main limitation is the differences in performance technique between surgeons that vary based on training. Patients also vary. Some may have some inherent degree of pivot shift, and a glide or positive shift is not necessarily indicative of ACL deficiency. Subjectivity even plays a role in the grading of the pivot shift. There has been research into creating a standardized pivot shift, but none has yet been developed and disseminated into general practice.

Despite these limitations, many studies in the literature point to the various merits of the pivot shift test. It measures the rotary instability of the knee, which significantly impacts patient satisfaction. Rotary instability contributes to the feeling of "giving way" that often prevents patients from returning to high levels of activity. Additionally, unlike other tests of ACL deficiency such as the Lachman test, the pivot shift has been shown to have a significant correlation with patients' functional outcomes, and there is some evidence that it correlates with possible future osteoarthritis development.

EBM helps clinicians to utilize the strengths of the pivot shift while being mindful of its limitations. Pivot shift should be used in conjunction with the Lachman test. The two tests measure different aspects of knee instability and can serve as complements. The Lachman test's high sensitivity can compensate for the pivot's low sensitivity, and the pivot shift can offer information on functional outcomes that the Lachman cannot predict. However, using these two tests together is not always a straightforward process, but evidence from the literature and the clinician's experience and judgment are ideally combined for optimal patient evaluation and management.

References

1. Ayeni OR, Chahal M, Tran MN, Sprague S (2012) Pivot shift as an outcome measure for ACL reconstruction: a systematic review. Knee Surg Sports Traumatol Arthrosc 20:767–777
2. Donaldson WF, Warren RF, Wickiewicz T (1985) A comparison of acute anterior cruciate ligament examinations. Initial versus examination under anesthesia. Am J Sports Med 13:5–10

3. Dunn WR, Schackman BR, Walsh C, Lyman S, Jones EC, Warren RF, Marx RG (2005) Variation in orthopaedic surgeons' perceptions about the indications for rotator cuff surgery. J Bone Joint Surg Am 87:1978–1984
4. Galway HR, MacIntosh DL (1980) The lateral pivot shift: a symptom and sign of anterior cruciate ligament insufficiency. Clin Orthop Relat Res 147:45–50
5. Hoshino Y, Araujo P, Ahlden M, Moore CG, Kuroda R, Zaffagnini S, Karlsson J, Fu FH, Musahl V (2012) Standardized pivot shift test improves measurement accuracy. Knee Surg Sports Traumatol Arthrosc 20: 732–736
6. Jonsson H, Riklund-Ahlström K, Lind J (2004) Positive pivot shift after ACL reconstruction predicts later osteoarthrosis: 63 patients followed 5-9 years after surgery. Acta Orthop Scand 75:594–599
7. Kaplan N, Wickiewicz TL, Warren RF (1990) Primary surgical treatment of anterior cruciate ligament ruptures. A long-term follow-up study. Am J Sports Med 18:354–358
8. Kim SJ, Kim HK (1995) Reliability of the anterior drawer test, the pivot shift test, and the Lachman test. Clin Orthop Relat Res 317:237–242
9. Kocher MS, Steadman JR, Briggs KK, Sterett WI, Hawkins RJ (2004) Relationships between objective assessment of ligament stability and subjective assessment of symptoms and function after anterior cruciate ligament reconstruction. Am J Sports Med 32: 629–634
10. Lane CG, Warren R, Pearle AD (2008) The pivot shift. J Am Acad Orthop Surg 16:679–688
11. Lee MC, Seong SC, Lee S, Chang CB, Park YK, Jo H, Kim CH (2007) Vertical femoral tunnel placement results in rotational knee laxity after anterior cruciate ligament reconstruction. Arthroscopy 23:771–778
12. Leitze Z, Losee RE, Jokl P, Johnson TR, Feagin JA (2005) Implications of the pivot shift in the ACL-deficient knee. Clin Orthop Relat Res 436:229–236
13. Liu-Ambrose T (2003) The anterior cruciate ligament and functional stability of the knee joint. BCMJ 45:495–499
14. Markolf KL, Jackson SR, McAllister DR (2010) Relationship between the pivot shift and Lachman tests: a cadaver study. J Bone Joint Surg Am 92:2067–2075
15. Meyer D (2004) Essential evidence-based medicine. Cambridge University Press, Cambridge
16. Musahl V, Hoshino Y, Ahlden M, Araujo P, Irrgang JJ, Zaffagnini S, Karlsson J, Fu FH (2012) The pivot shift: a global user guide. Knee Surg Sports Traumatol Arthrosc 20:724–731
17. Scholten RJPM, Opstelten W, van der Plas CG, Bijl D, Deville WLJM, Bouter LM (2003) Accuracy of physical diagnostic tests for assessing ruptures of the anterior cruciate ligament: a meta-analysis. J Fam Pract 52:689–694
18. Wennberg JE (1984) Dealing with medical practice variations: a proposal for action. Health Aff (Millwood) 3(2):6–32

Outcomes Based on Surgery and Rehabilitation

42

Stefano Zaffagnini, Tom Chao, Richard Joreitz, Nicola Lopomo, Cecilia Signorelli, and Volker Musahl

Contents

S. Zaffagnini (✉) • N. Lopomo • C. Signorelli
Laboratorio di Biomeccanica e Innovazione Tecnologica, Instituto Ortopedico Rizzoli, Via Di Barbiano 1/10, 40136 Bologna, Italy
e-mail: stefano.zaffagnini@unibo.it

T. Chao • R. Joreitz
Department of Orthopaedic Surgery, University of Pittsburgh Medical Center, 3200 Water Street, Pittsburgh, PA 15203, USA

V. Musahl
Department of Orthopaedic Surgery, UPMC Center for Sports Medicine, Pittsburgh, PA, USA

42.1 Introduction

Quantitative assessment of the outcomes of surgery and rehabilitation is evolving as a method to decrease the error rates in surgery and improve patient care. There are currently several quality steps taken towards understanding and improving the quantitative functional evaluation of the patients' conditions, but there remains a need for research efforts that could optimize such approaches.

In particular, anterior cruciate ligament (ACL) tears represent a common injury in the field of orthopaedics that demands considerable technical expertise by the surgeon as well as commitment to rehabilitation by the patient. The injury is a devastating event to the athlete, who is often forced to a long lay-off period during the recuperation interval (nearly 5–6 months). ACL reconstruction is currently the seventh most common surgical procedure in the United States [12]. During the period of 2000–2010, data generated specifically to ACL research have more than doubled [36].

The outcomes related to ACL reconstruction are by no means optimal. Almost two-thirds of patients are reported to be unable to return to preinjury level of performance [3] and as a consequence are counselled to undergo ACL reconstructive surgery [33]. Even after reconstructive surgery, the rate of return to sport at 12 months of follow-up is not so high. Moreover, in those patients who return to sport, there is a one in four chances for reinjury [19, 24].

V. Musahl et al. (eds.), *Rotatory Knee Instability*, DOI 10.1007/978-3-319-32070-0_42

Currently the accuracy of the surgeon's assessment of injury severity as well as recovery after surgical treatment is mainly based on the surgeon's sensibility in interpreting the clinical examination. However, as can be expected, this method does not have any element of standardization. The significance and role of any preoperative grading method lies in its ability to consistently support the decision-making process during diagnosis, surgical treatment and recovery phase after surgery. Moreover, an accurate diagnosis may be beneficial to provide patients with the correct information in order to help manage their expectations.

For the ACL-deficient patient, the need for careful determination of the condition of the injured knee reaches multiple levels in the treatment process. Preoperatively, the quantification of knee laxity level is critical during early evaluation of suspected ACL injury in order to determine if and what surgery is required. Intraoperatively, it is important to quantify the laxity level to immediately evaluate the recovery achieved during the surgery and identify the need to perform a secondary restraint procedure. Postoperatively, during the recovery processes, it is important to follow the laxity recovery in order to verify the healing process and rehabilitation course. Moreover, it is also clear that not only the surgical approach but also the rehabilitation phase plays a recognized role and needs to be carefully analysed in a systematic manner in order to achieve consistent results. Indeed, taking all these aspects together in respect to the assessment of the ACL-injured and ACL-reconstructed knee, it is necessary that a valid, reliable and quantitative evaluation can be performed at all stages of treatment.

The aim of the present chapter is to present measurement methods available for preoperative, intraoperative and postoperative quantitative functional evaluation (Fig. 42.1). In addition, the fundamental aspects of rehabilitation following ACL surgery will be described in detail in order to highlight this important area that guides the athlete towards a successful return to sporting activities.

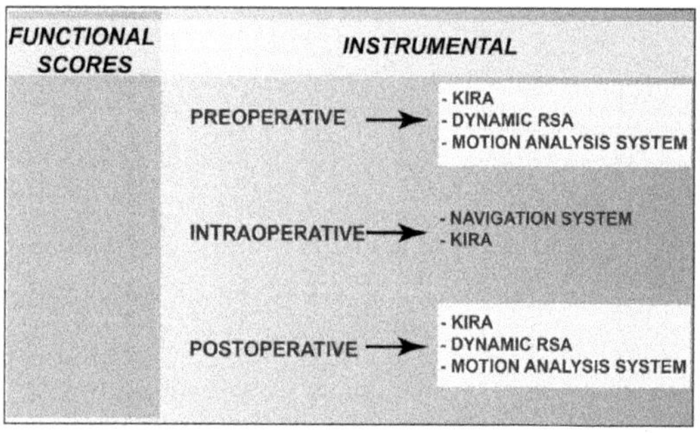

Fig. 42.1 Different approaches for quantitative functional evaluation of surgery and rehabilitation

42.2 Navigation System for Intraoperative Evaluation

Navigation systems allow precise measurements to be made intraoperatively in different planes in real time. With relation to the orthopaedic field, total knee arthroplasty (TKA) is probably the most well-known procedure to apply the use of navigation systems. The main goal of the navigation system in TKA is to improve the accuracy of bone resections, thereby correcting the alignment of the knee and optimizing the fit of the prosthetic implant. Analogously, during the first ACL-navigated reconstruction surgery, the navigation system was utilized to address tunnel placement for graft insertion. However, the purpose of the navigation system for ACL reconstruction quickly shifted towards measuring knee laxity in 3D conditions [22, 39, 45].

The reliability of the navigation system was demonstrated in 1997 by [39] who compared an image-free navigation system to robotic/UFS testing system in an in vitro study. The results demonstrated that the accuracy is in the range of ±0.1 mm for linear measurements and ±0.1° for angular measurements. Subsequently, the possibility to objectively quantify residual laxity and improve the evaluation of ACL reconstructive surgery was highlighted with the aid of this technology [32]. This study used the navigation system (BLU-IGS system) commercially distributed by Orthokey LLC (Lewes, DE, USA).

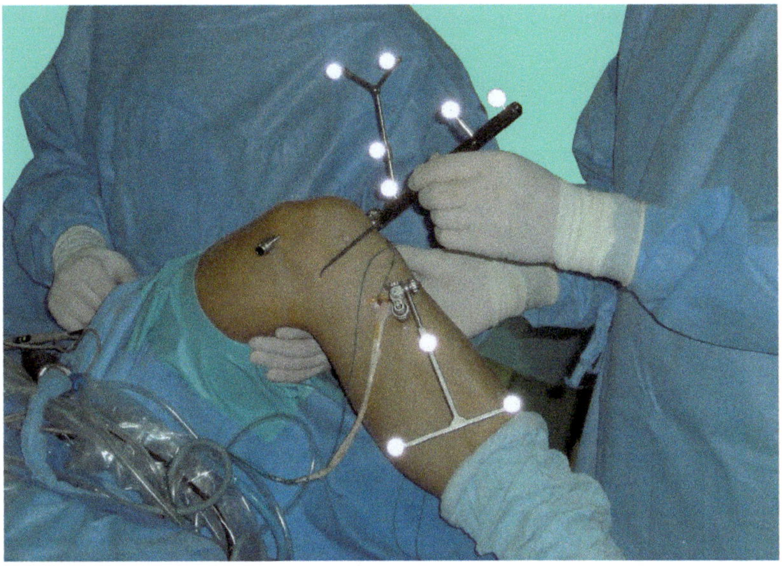

Fig. 42.2 Passive markers required by the navigation system for intraoperative laxity evaluation during ACL reconstructive surgery

For the purposes of navigational assessment of knee laxity, the clinical tests commonly performed are as follows: Lachman and anterior drawer tests for anterior-posterior laxity assessment, internal/external rotation test at 30° and 90° of knee flexion, varus/valgus stress tests at 0° and 30° of flexion (VV30) and the pivot shift test. The Lachman, anterior drawer, internal/external rotation and varus/valgus stress tests provide information regarding static laxity, while the pivot shift test provides information in terms of dynamic laxity of the examined knee.

The acquisition data is collected from the measurement of the position of passive reflecting spherical markers fixed on specific trackers (Fig. 42.2). A single marker position is defined with a 3D root mean square (RMS) volumetric accuracy of 0.35 mm and a 3D RMS volumetric repeatability of 0.2 mm (at 20 °C).

The main hardware and software features are:

- User-friendly interface focusing on essential information and specific results
- Real-time feedback of the computer-assisted procedure for knee laxity assessment
- Simplified 3D graphical display of data and results
- Quantitative description of the kinematic tests performed by the surgeon
- Real-time computation of clinical test results
- Flexibility in the order and number of kinematic acquisitions
- Fast elaboration and recording of data
- Flexible design suitable for different surgical techniques

An example of the interface observed during acquisition of navigational data is shown in Fig. 42.3.

No alteration of the normal surgical practice is needed in order to perform a navigated ACL reconstruction. Moreover, the surgical time is less than 10 min longer than the equivalent surgery without navigation [31]. The main advantage in using this system is to obtain a real-time quantification of the knee laxity during the entire surgical procedure, thus giving the surgeon the opportunity to immediately monitor the effect of the interventions administered on knee laxity.

Despite these attributes that contribute to the surgical precision during ACL reconstruction, there are some reservations that may deter from the use of navigation systems intraoperatively. Firstly, intraoperative navigational systems require the drilling of markers into the bone in

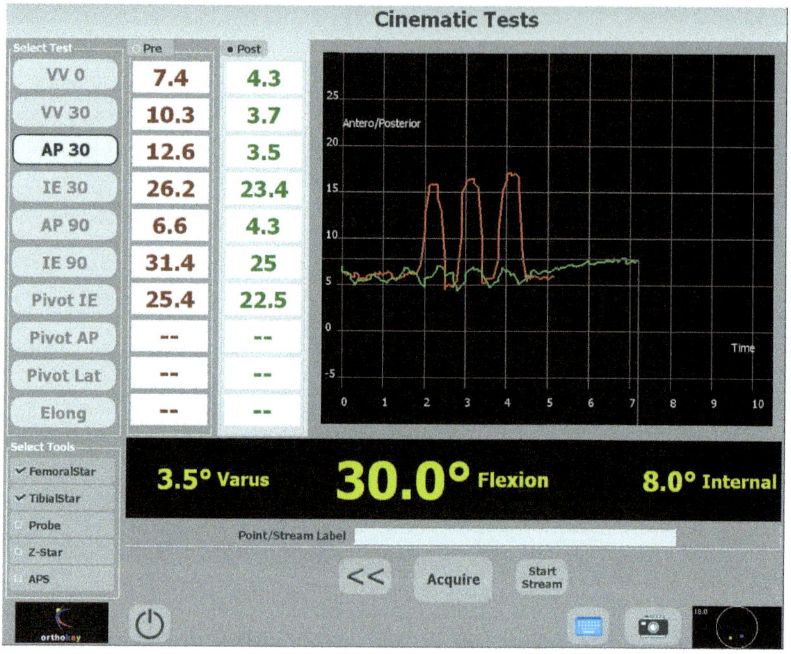

Fig. 42.3 Navigation system interface for intraoperative laxity evaluation

order to obtain information. While this may be considered a minor intervention, the idea of introducing further trauma into the bone may seem unnecessary in light of mandated reaming of bone tunnels that is required for ACL reconstruction. Secondly, another significant question concerning the use of these navigation systems is the reproducibility of knee laxity measurements. For example, while conducting in vivo assessments, the applied load is not standardized leading to variability in the calculation of measured knee laxity. This undoubtedly may affect the reliability of preoperative-to-postoperative comparisons in terms of the stability of the knee. Nevertheless, the reliability of the navigation system, both for static and dynamic assessments for knee laxity, has been demonstrated to be somewhat dependable [25, 28, 31]. Most of these reports have shown very good reliability for the pivot shift analysis (with a mean intra-tester ICC about 0.98) and an intra-tester repeatability of approximately 1 mm for the anterior drawer/Lachman, 1° for the varus/valgus stress test and 2° for the internal/external rotation stress test.

Over the course of the years, the use of navigation system for intraoperative ACL reconstruction evaluation has made it possible to quantitatively analyse many different aspects of the surgery [23]. For example, it has provided insight into the comparison of different surgical approaches [20, 46, 47] aided in determining the relationship between pre- and postoperative static and dynamic laxity level [26, 42], examined the effect of gender on surgery outcome [2], and produced information on the different contributions of the anteromedial and posterolateral bundle to knee laxity [22]. In the area of biomechanics, the application of the navigation system has allowed to quantify the effect of combined lesions in the ACL-deficient knee [5, 34].

It is apparent that the immediate feedback of intraoperative navigation has potential benefits in providing a real-time assessment of knee laxity during ACL reconstruction. Along with the current shift in paradigm towards anatomic ACL reconstruction, navigation provides an accessible tool to achieve the goals related to this concept.

Fact Box 1

- Intraoperative navigational technology is a highly accurate quantification technique that can measure translational and rotary movements in the range of

±0.1 mm for linear measurements and ±0.1° for angular measurements.
- The use of intraoperative navigation increases surgical time on average by only 10 min.
- Intraoperative navigation requires the use of static markers that are drilled into bony landmarks.

42.3 Systems for Preoperative and Postoperative Clinical Assessment

The diagnosis of an ACL injury is a process that includes information collected from a set of clinical tests such as the Lachman and pivot shift to confirm suspicions of injury. Often it is difficult to identify clinically significant laxity because of the small alterations in knee mechanics, as in the case with partial ligament injury. The detection of knee laxity may be improved calculations attained from computerized measurement systems.

42.3.1 System Based on Inertial Sensors

One of the first noninvasive systems based on inertial sensors validated for the clinical assessment of the pivot shift test was the KiRA (*Orthokey LLC, DE, USA*). KiRA is a medical device that can be utilized to analyse the severity of knee laxity, providing both real-time graphics and quantitative information about the pivot shift and Lachman tests. The device is a viable aid to the clinical examination, assisting in detecting and quantifying the grade of a suspected ACL injury.

During the routine knee examination, the KiRA can generate numerical values of the movement of the tibia in space and can be particularly useful for the assessment of the pivot shift test. The KiRA device is based on the concept that the pivot shift phenomenon can be measured by a dynamic parameter, such as 3D acceleration, and that the dynamic instability that may be detected by the pivot shift test is directly correlated with this value. The concept is supported by the analysis of the literature [27] that, as previously underlined, considers the velocity as well as the acceleration of the tibia during pivot shift test as a strong indicator of dynamic knee instability.

The sensors used with the KiRA each have a triaxial accelerometer and gyroscope embedded inside. These devices are able to communicate wirelessly to the software that is activated from common laptop computer. The sensor must be skin fixed on the tibial bone by the provided hypoallergenic strap. The device must be placed between the lateral aspect of the anterior tuberosity and the Gerdy's tubercle to achieve an optimal stability and minimize skin artefacts during the manoeuvre (Fig. 42.4).

The KiRA can also be used to quantify the grade of the Lachman examination. This application may be more essential to the treating surgeon, since the literature affirms that the Lachman test is the most sensitive test for the diagnosis of ACL injury and also the most common test performed by the surgeon to evaluate knee joint laxity [40]. In order to accurately quantify tibial translation while conducting the Lachman test, it is necessary to place the device against the distal aspect of the tibia. In addition, in order to minimize the interference from soft tissue artefact, the sensor must be fixed to a shin guard.

It is worth noting that the device may aid the surgeon in obtaining a rapid measurement of both dynamic and static knee laxity in the case of ACL injury without requiring excessive expenditure of costs and time. Furthermore, it may help to confirm the presence of laxity in circumstances in which only a partial ligament injury is encountered. The noninvasiveness, simplicity and portability of the tool have the advantage of accessibility of use in any clinical setting, whether academic or private, as well as allowing easy comparison of the mechanics of the injured to the contralateral joint. In the case of varying grades of pivot shift patterns, the findings may push the surgeon towards customizing the surgical approach to meet the demands of larger pivot shifts, such as adding an extra-articular tenodesis.

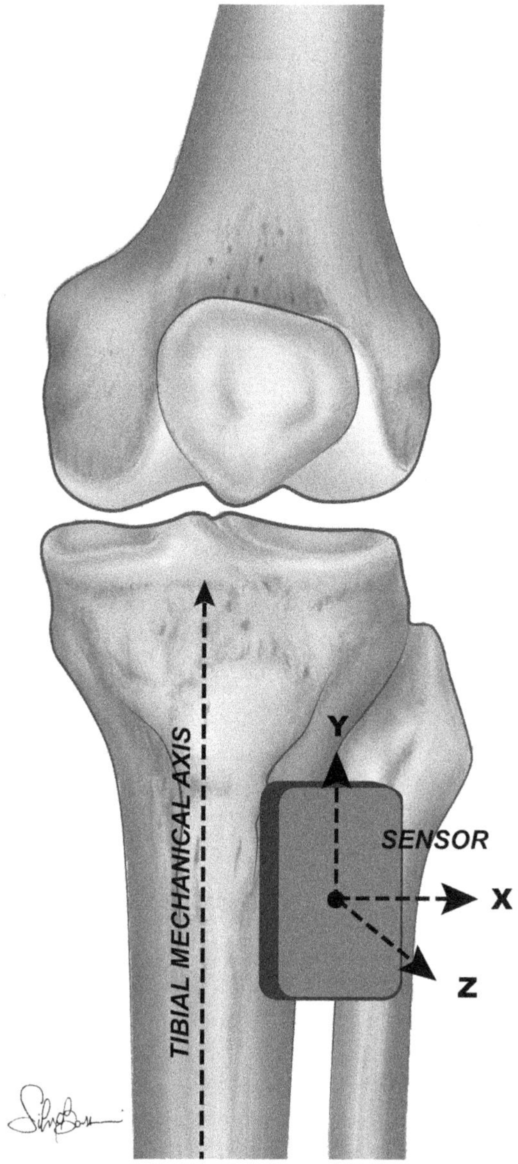

Fig. 42.4 Positioning of the KiRA (*Orthokey LLC, DE, USA*) device. *X, Y, Z* are the three axis along which the acceleration measurement is performed

The KiRA is not limited to the outpatient setting, but can be applied to the intraoperative theatre. For this specific purpose, the sensor needs to be enclosed in a specifically developed sterilizable box, which will then be affixed to the skin of the patient.

In recent years, several similar systems have been proposed to clinicians for the same purpose of quantifying dynamic knee stability with noninvasive tools. However, the KiRA device still represents one of the first reliable, inexpensive and simple methods to use as a quantitative aid for noninvasive evaluation of the knee suspected to have an ACL injury.

> **Fact Box 2**
> - The KiRA is an accelerometer that can quantify the speed of movements in a triaxial plane.
> - Both the Lachman exam and the pivot shift test can be assessed using the KiRA.
> - The portability of the KiRA allows for ease of use in the outpatient or operative setting.

42.3.2 Image Capture Software System

In objective quantification of the pivot shift test in routine, a clinical setting warrants methods that can easily and reliably measure rotatory laxity even in healthcare facilities with limited resources.

Tibial translation has been suggested to be a more realistic kinematic determinant of grade of the pivot shift grade than rotation [8]. This is highlighted in a study using a computer navigation system, which demonstrated that anterior translation of the lateral compartment of the knee correlates with the severity of the pivot shift test [7]. Image analysis techniques exploit this observation by directly quantifying the amount of tibial translation along the lateral aspect of the knee while the pivot shift test is being conducted. Utilizing a digital camera to record the video of the examination, the video must then be analysed by a linked software program one way such as ImageJ (National Institute of Health, Bethesda, MD, USA) [17]. The ImageJ software allows the user to display, edit and analyse images and is easily accessible to the scientific community free of charge [13, 21, 44]. However, analysis by the ImageJ software is time-consuming and is not applicable in routine clinical settings.

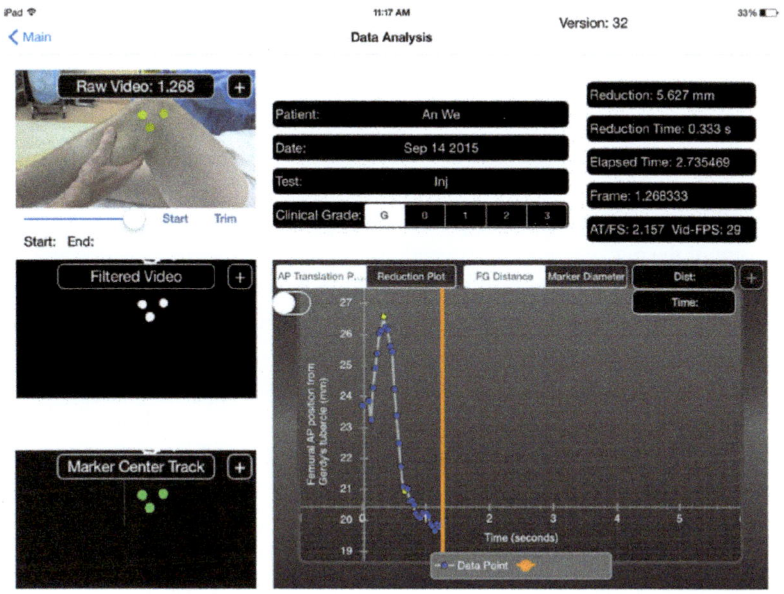

Fig. 42.5 Configuration of skin markers and display of software interface for PIVOT application for the iPad. A pivot shift test is performed in the photograph on the upper right with skin markers placed on the lateral femoral condyle, Gerdy's tubercle and the fibular head. Tracking of the skin markers as observed on the iPad interface is shown in the two *lower left boxes* prior to and during the performance of the pivot shift. The change in the anterior-posterior position of the femur in relation to Gerdy's tubercle is recorded as a function of time as observed in the *lower right image*. The velocity of the pivot shift or reduction is then calculated by subtracting the highest and lowest values along the graft and dividing this number by the time elapsed during the test. This is known as the reduction time. The information related to the test period is shown in the boxes above the *lower right image*

Recently, a software has been introduced that can be installed on a tablet computer such as the iPad and quantifies the pivot shift test by calculating lateral tibial compartment translation in nearly real time [35]. To improve visualization, circular markers are attached to the skin over three bony landmarks on the lateral side of the knee. The following landmarks were selected as they are easily identifiable: (1) lateral epicondyle of the knee, (2) Gerdy's tubercle and (3) the fibular head. In order to reduce background noise from the surroundings, the colour of the circular markers should contrast with the patients' skin, and a solid coloured background should be used.

During a test, the tablet's camera records the movement of the markers while the knee is being examined (Fig. 42.5). The software scans the images in real time and utilizes custom algorithms that shade the entire image except the markers by adjusting the brightness and contrast. The software then automatically tracks the movement of the markers and calculates the translation

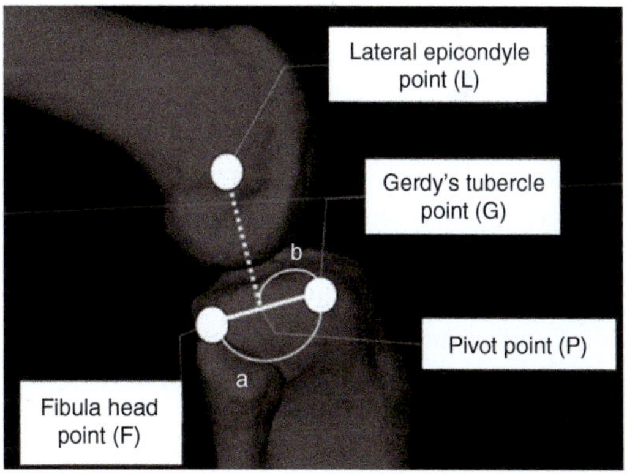

Fig. 42.6 Schematic for calculation of tibial movement using skin markers over the lateral epicondyle of the femur, fibular head and Gerdy's tubercle

of the pivot point defined by the intersection of the line between markers on the fibular head and Gerdy's tubercle with a perpendicular line crossing the femoral condyle marker (Fig. 42.6). After tracking the markers, the software provides a reduction plot that represents reduction of the tibia during pivot shift test. From this plot, the amount of translation can be determined by selecting the maximum and minimum points of the plot at the time of the reduction.

The validity of the software and its application has been investigated in controlled laboratory settings. The maximum error of the software in quantifying the movement of the markers was determined to be less than 6% at distances between 75 and 125 cm and a deviation angle of less than 45° [35]. The reliability of the PIVOT software in predicting the 3D bony motion during the pivot shift test has been evaluated in a cadaveric study utilizing an electromagnetic tracking system. It has been demonstrated that lateral compartment translation measured by the PIVOT software has a strong correlation with 3D bony motion with about three times higher translation in bony motion (Pearson correlation, 0.75–0.79; $p<0.05$). The intra-examiner reliability of the methodology was also demonstrated to be strong (intra-class correlation coefficient=0.70–0.82).

In ACL-injured patients, it was demonstrated that the PIVOT software can consistently detect and quantify lateral compartment translation [16]. The quantitative results from PIVOT software have also been validated by clinical grade of pivot shift test where incremental increase in lateral compartment translation measured by software was associated with increase in clinical grade of the pivot shift test [18].

Overall PIVOT software provides an easy, noninvasive and reliable tool to quantify the pivot shift test. This method allows clinicians who desire to obtain objective quantification of the pivot shift exam by providing the opportunity to do so portability, accurately and with data recording capabilities.

Fact Box 3

- Software analysis systems such as PIVOT provide instant feedback regarding tibial translation and rotation during the Lachman and pivot shift test.
- Measurements are calculated from the relationship of three markers strategically placed on the lateral femoral condyle, fibular head and Gerdy's tubercle.
- PIVOT readings demonstrate a high correlation with bony motion despite the fact that markers are placed on the skin.

42.3.3 Radiostereometry Analysis (RSA)

The radiostereometry analysis (RSA) was developed in 1973 to analyse the stability of bone-prostheses interfaces. Initially, it was based on a technique that required tantalum beads to be implanted into the prosthesis as well as the bone. The position of the beads from two radiographic projections could then give information regarding the movement of the studied anatomic structures and components in space, confirming suspected loosening of the prosthesis.

Over the recent years, the application of the RSA has evolved to study not only the micro-movements and microadjustments of the bone-prosthesis interface but also joint kinematics. The most well-known apparatus that achieves this purpose is the dynamic RSA. The dynamic RSA set-up is made of two x-ray tubes and two digital radiographic detectors (Fig. 42.7). The radiologic devices need to be highly synchronized to avoid motion artefacts and to increase accuracy. The radiographic detectors can be of two possible types: an image intensifier which allows more rapid capture of images (about 60 frames per seconds) at the expense of image quality or digital flat panels. The latter have the ability to produce higher-quality images at lower doses of radiation, but attain a much slower capture rate (8–15 frames per seconds). The typical accuracy of a dynamic RSA motion tracking is approximately 1 mm for translational movements and 1° for rotational movements.

In order to detect the movement of anatomic structures, the dynamic RSA does not require the use of tantalum beads as was the case with the original RSA technique. Instead, it utilizes a method known as model-based positioning. This method functions by constructing an external three-dimensional model of the analysed

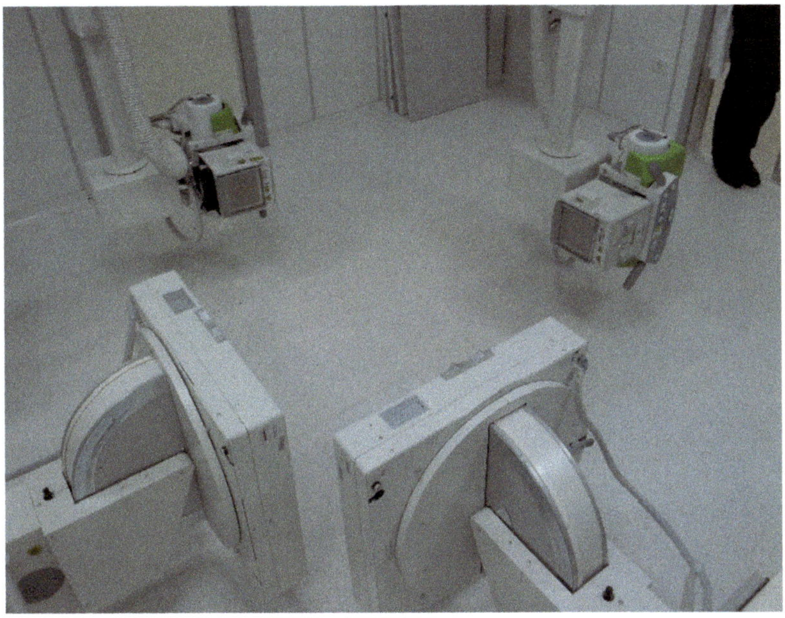

Fig. 42.7 Dynamic RSA set-up (BI-STAND DRX2, Cat Medical Systems spa)

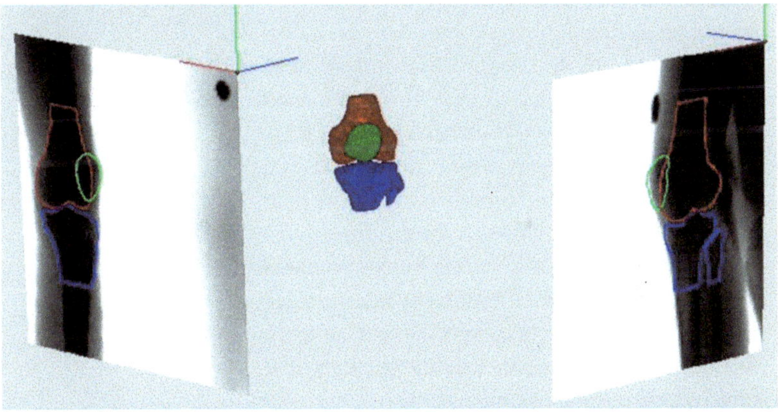

Fig. 42.8 Radiographic bone and bone model for RSA analysis

component (prosthesis or bone) with respect to the corresponding orthogonal radiographic projections taken prior to and after manipulation of the targeted joint (Fig. 42.8). Dedicated image processing and segmentation algorithms are then fed through software to optimize the computerized depiction of the anatomical models.

Model-based and dynamic RSA methods allow positional changes to be evaluated during real-time activities, making it possible to study the effect of ligamentous structures on the stability and mechanics of joints, such as is the case in ACL reconstruction.

Another notable advantage of dynamic RSA is its ability to track the three-dimensional movement of bones along with the interaction of the soft tissues that surround them. For this purpose, the base images are taken from MRI studies. The model-based algorithm that is generated from this data can then reproduce the position as well as the response of the soft tissues and bony structures during specific motor tasks. When combined with other applications, such as force platforms and electromyography, dynamic RSA can provide much information regarding joint stresses as well as the pattern of muscular group activation associated with certain movements. An example of dynamic RSA interpreting the joint reaction forces on the articular cartilage and menisci of the knee joint is shown in Fig. 42.9.

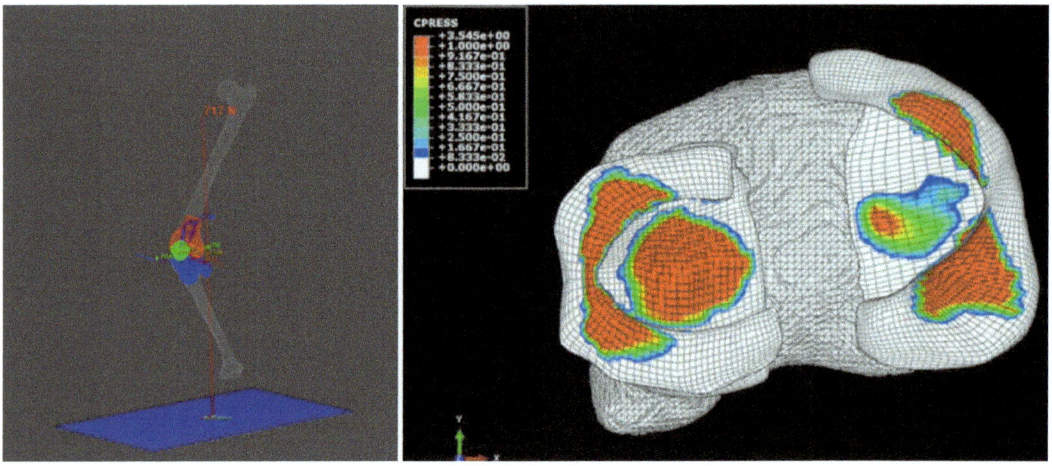

Fig. 42.9 Dynamic RSA data processing: bone position and ground reaction force (*on the left*). Finite element (FE) simulation of the stresses on the tibial cartilage and menisci (*on the right*)

After ACL reconstruction, information in terms of the joint mechanics and muscular control can be gathered during some common motor tasks such as level walking and ascent/descent of steps as well as a single-leg squat through the aid of dynamic RSA. Taken together, dynamic RSA is a highly accurate system that can explore in a noninvasive manner the biomechanics of a joint in motion in the setting of specific modifications. Moreover, direct tracking of the bony structures using radiographs may circumvent inaccuracies and motion artefacts that may be encountered with conventional motion capture systems that aim to accomplish the same purpose.

The dynamic RSA opens up further opportunities to acquire a deeper comprehension of the biomechanics of human joints. Future applications of this technique may add to the body of knowledge concerning ACL surgery through the comparison of different surgical approaches and the prediction of the development of osteoarthritis.

Fact Box 4

- Dynamic radiostereometry analysis (RSA) assesses motions in bony structures by reconstructing three-dimensional models from orthogonal radiographs taken during dynamic activity.
- The capabilities of dynamic RSA can be expanded to the analysis of soft tissue structures by using MRI images as the source data.
- By combining dynamic RSA with other analytical devices, such as force platforms and electromyograms, information regarding the distribution of joint contact forces and muscle activity can be studied in detail.

42.4 Full-Body Motion Analysis Systems

For all the technology that has been described to enhance the accuracy of ACL reconstruction, the fact remains that in order to limit the risk of reinjury, the evaluation of both biomechanical and neuromuscular aspects of the athlete need to be considered during the postoperative phase. Presently, there is a lack of clear criteria available to define when the athlete has achieved sufficient ability to advance to the next step in the rehabilitation phase after ACL reconstruction. In particular, it is unclear how to quantitatively assess where the athlete resides within their functional range during a specific stage in their rehabilitation [41].

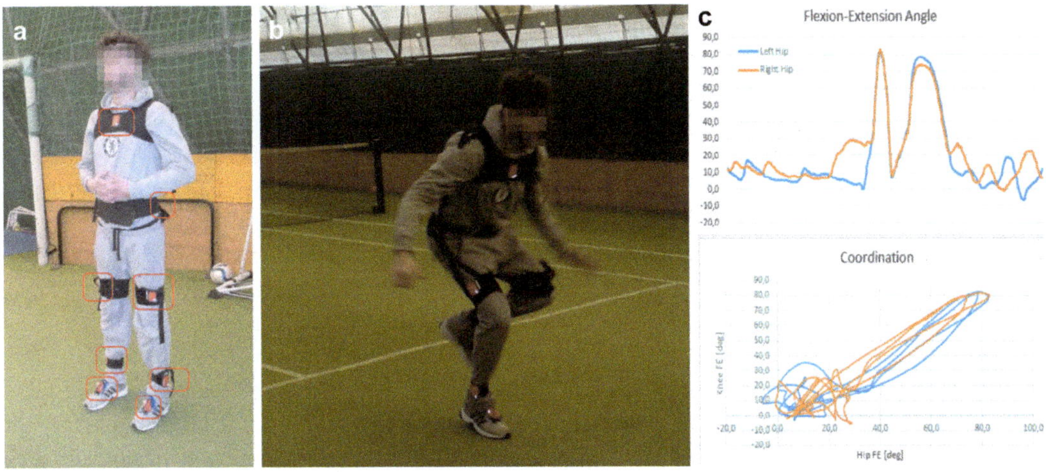

Fig. 42.10 (**a–c**) The Xsens system (Xsens Technologies, NL) used during field acquisition (Courtesy of Isokinetic, Bologna, Italy): (**a**) static calibration, (**b**) landing after a single-leg hop, (**c**) example of kinematic patterns (Courtesy of NCS Lab, Carpi, Italy)

Moreover, there are no standardized methods to provide a quantitative assessment about an athlete's performance during on-the-field rehabilitation tasks and specific motor gestures.

A solution to overcome this problem may be the use of a motor analysis system to perform on-the-field data acquisition. This particular kind of system would be based on the gait analysis systems that have been seen used in human motion laboratories. Currently, there are multiple motion analysis systems available, with the Xsens system (Xsens Technologies, NL) and the Microsoft Kinect Sensor (Microsoft Corp, Redmond, WA, USA) being the most technological advanced of their kind. These lightweight kinetic tracking devices communicate wirelessly with a local computer to generate data regarding the movement of the subject under study.

An example of its use in the scientific literature in the context of a validated clinical protocol is the project 'Outwalk', a system designed to analyse gait in children suffering from cerebral palsy [10]. This protocol helps to determine the 3D kinematics of individual body segments and can be used to isolate the interaction of certain joints, such as the thorax-pelvis complex. The product, in addition to the computed data, is shown in Fig. 42.10. Such a device can easily be translated to the monitoring of athletic rehabilitation. Some examples of motor tasks that can be studied for sport applications include the single-leg hop test, triple hop test, single-leg squat or jump/land. All of these manoeuvres have been used to judge in a subjective way the ability of the athlete to return to play.

The reliability of these devices for the assessment of rehabilitation parameter is currently underway. This technology would help to provide an objective measure to rehabilitation milestones. More specifically, it would allow the quantification of specific kinematic and temporal-spatial parameters, giving context to athletic performance acquired real time during the execution of the motor tasks. The potential afforded by this approach may further advance postoperative treatments that may then optimize the outcome of surgeries used to treat sport-related injuries such as ACL ruptures.

Fact Box 5

- Motion analysis systems offer the potential to provide more accurate objective feedback regarding rehabilitation stages following ACL reconstruction.
- A device of this kind, termed the 'Outwalk', has been used to describe the kinematics of cerebral palsy patients.

- The devices can be applied to analyse simple and complex athletic maneuvres such as single-leg hop test, triple hop test, single-leg squat or jump/land.

42.5 Rehabilitation After ACL Reconstruction

Returning to sports and avoiding knee joint instability associated with reinjury are key measures of success after anterior cruciate ligament reconstruction [29]. The clinical return to sport decision-making process emphasizes a highly structured set of objective tests, with associated criteria for progression between phases, which is recommended but commonly reported in the literature [6, 43].

Individuals progress through this rehabilitation programme in five phases. Phase 1 begins immediately after surgery and is centred on regaining range of motion, strength, patella mobility and flexibility and normalizing gait. Phases 2–5 encompass progressive return to running, agility training, jumping, hopping and cutting and assume clearance from the surgeon for running and agreement with the criteria established for advancement to subsequent stages. The objective tests and criteria to progress between phases focus on three areas to determine whether or not individuals are ready to attempt more demanding activities: (1) mastery of the current phase, (2) neuromuscular control and (3) quadriceps strength. Phases 2–5 involve working with a physical therapist to initiate new activities. Mastery is typically assessed through observation of the highest level of performance allowed in the progression. Failure to master the tasks of an individual phase is mediated with focused practice and instruction in respect to proper technique. The inclusion of activity mastery as a prerequisite for advancement to the next phase ensures that individuals take time to practise each skill and incorporate proper movement patterns during dynamic tasks even if their strength and neuromuscular control would allow them to progress in multiple phases.

Quadriceps strength should be measured as precisely and accurately as possible within the clinical setting due to its importance in the recovery of function and its propensity to be underrehabilitated. When available, isometric or isokinetic dynamometry should be used, as it isolates the quadriceps and provides reliable measures of strength without compensation. In cases where dynamometry is not available, a 1 repetition maximum (1-RM) on a knee extension machine [4, 37] or leg press machine [37] can be used to assess strength. The contralateral leg cannot assist in initiating the lift and cannot be on the floor or on the platform. For the 1-RM leg extension, the individual is positioned in 90° hip and knee flexion with the resistance pad placed proximally to the malleoli. The individual is instructed to extend their knee as smoothly as possible to 45° of knee flexion (early phases of rehabilitation) or full knee extension (after 4 months post-op) against the weight. The limb symmetry index is calculated as the 1 repetition maximum load of the involved limb divided by the 1 repetition maximum load of the uninvolved limb expressed as a percentage.

Movement patterns and stability are tested with three basic tests. The step and hold is a low level approximation where the individual steps from the uninjured limb onto the injured limb, at least the distance of the individual's normal stride length. Mastery of this exercise is when the patient demonstrates no loss of balance or excessive movement outside of the sagittal plane. The single-leg squat is performed to appropriate prescribed angle of knee flexion for ten repetitions to screen for deviations. Deviations are operationally defined as the use of compensatory patterns including loss of balance, contralateral hip drop, excessive femoral abduction or adduction, excessive femoral internal rotation or abnormal trunk movement. Progression to phases 3, 4 and 5 require the individual to complete the single-leg squat with additional weight to increase the challenge. The Y-balance test is a measure of stability between limbs [14].

When beginning to run, alternating periods of walking and jogging are implemented with progressive increases in distance [1]. A distance-based progression over a time-based progression is advocated in order to more accurately control the load experienced by the knee joint.

Basic agility drills include forward/backward shuttle running, side shuffling, carioca and "quick feet" drills using a ladder or hurdles in a forward and lateral direction. Deceleration with hip and knee flexion to absorb the load for direction changes is emphasized when running and preparing to change directions. Effort begins at approximately 50 % speed and continues at that level until the individual can complete the drills without hesitation or compensation during deceleration to change directions.

When beginning to jump, the individual begins with forward jumps and jumps onto a box. Cues are given to emphasize avoiding dynamic valgus, to exaggerate hip and knee flexion and to equally distribute weight on both extremities when loading into the jump and landing [11, 15, 30, 38]. When the individual demonstrates good form with forward jumps, they will progress with lateral jumps and rotational jumps. Hopping follows the same progression as jumping in phase 4 – single forward hops on the floor and onto a box – progressing to hops out of the sagittal plane and multiple hops.

For cutting activities, individuals should first practise running in an "S" pattern as shown in Fig. 42.10 and then progress to 45° cuts and then to sharper angle cuts. Pivoting should begin when the individual is competent with cutting at sharp angles. As with low level agility drills, confidence and performance dictate the speed of cutting and pivoting drills, and the individual should not progress to high level cutting and pivoting drills if they demonstrate compensation patterns or express decreased confidence at higher speeds [9]. Individuals should be able to tolerate controlled cutting and pivoting at full speed before practising unanticipated cutting and sport-specific movements.

Return to practise testing can occur when the individual can run and perform all agility and plyometric and sport-specific drills without any hesitation, compensatory patterns and complaints of increased pain or display any signs or symptoms of inflammation. The return to practise test includes a strength assessment, functional testing for symmetrical performance and functional testing for running situations. Individuals must demonstrate a 90 % quadriceps LSI to pass the return to sport test.

After clearance from the physical therapist and surgeon, patients may return to practise. Individuals typically begin practising with unopposed drills with sport-specific movements and general conditioning. When their unopposed performance is sufficient per the discretion of the coach and athletic trainer, individuals can begin controlled contact drills. Lastly, individuals can return to organized competitive practices in their respective sports. Individuals return to their physician for full return to competition clearance when they can practise at 100 % effort (with contact if applicable) and have no complaints of pain or signs and symptoms of inflammation.

Fact Box 6

- Return to sport following ACL reconstruction involves five individual phases of rehabilitation.
- Phase 1 of the return to sport programme typically concentrates on recovery of functional range of motion.
- Through phases 2–5, the athlete must demonstrate progressive competency in motion and agility tests, running, and cutting exercises.
- The three main criteria that are used to assess whether an athlete may safely progress to the next stage in therapy are mastery of the current phase, neuromuscular control and quadriceps strength.
- Assessment of quadriceps strength must be performed accurately due to the propensity for this muscle to be underrehabilitated.
- Return to practise requires a strength assessment, functional testing for symmetrical performance and functional testing for running situations.
- Return to full sport may be allowed when the athlete demonstrates ability to practise at 100 % effort.

Conclusion

Quantitative measurements of joint mechanics in the setting of ACL surgery offer the potential of maximizing surgical outcomes. These assessments can be done in the preoperative, intraoperative and postoperative phases. Information gathered from this technology can provide direct feedback regarding the stability of the knee after graft placement, as is the case with the measurement of the pivot shift using the KiRA or iPad system. Furthermore, subjective milestones in the course of rehabilitation after ACL reconstruction can be objectively quantified. In the future, these applications may lead to development of a standardized treatment algorithm for the ACL-injured patient with the goal of achieving maximum athletic potential while at the same time preventing post-traumatic OA for the patient.

References

1. Adams D, Logerstedt D, Hunter-Giordano A, Axe MJ, Snyder-Mackler L (2012) Current concepts for anterior cruciate ligament reconstruction: a criterion-based rehabilitation progression. J Orthop Sports Phys Ther 42(7):601–614
2. Aldrian S, Valentin P, Wondrasch B, Krusche-Mandi I, Ostermann RC, Platzer P, Hofbauer M (2014) Gender differences following computer-navigated single- and double-bundle anterior cruciate ligament reconstruction. Knee Surg Sports Traumatol Arthrosc 22(9): 2145–2152
3. Ardern CL, Taylor NF, Feller JA, Whitehead TS, Webster KE (2013) Psychological responses matter in returning to preinjury level of sport after anterior cruciate ligament reconstruction surgery. Am J Sports Med 41(7):1549–1558
4. Augustsson J, Thomee R, Karlsson J (2004) Ability of a new hop test to determine functional deficits after anterior cruciate ligament reconstruction. Knee Surg Sports Traumatol Arthrosc 12(5):350–356
5. Bonanzinga T, Signorelli C, Lopomo N, Grassi A, Neri MP, Filardo G, Zaffagnini S, Marcacci M (2015) Biomechanical effect of posterolateral corner sectioning after ACL injury and reconstruction. Knee Surg Sports Traumatol Arthrosc 23(10):2918–2924
6. Barber-Westin SD, Noyes FR (2011) Factors used to determine return to unrestricted sports activities after anterior cruciate ligament reconstruction. Arthroscopy 27(12):1697–1705
7. Bedi A, Musahl V, Lane C, Citak M, Warren RF, Pearle AD (2010) Lateral compartment translation predicts the grade of pivot shift: a cadaveric and clinical analysis. Knee Surg Sports Traumatol Arthrosc 18(9):1269–1276
8. Bull AM, Earnshaw PH, Smith A, Katchburian MV, Hassan AN, Amis AA (2002) Intraoperative measurement of knee kinematics in reconstruction of the anterior cruciate ligament. J Bone Joint Surg Br 84(7): 1075–1081
9. Chmielewski TL, Jones D, Day T, Tillman SM, Lentz TA, George SZ (2008) The association of pain and fear of movement/reinjury with function during anterior cruciate ligament reconstruction rehabilitation. J Orthop Sports Phys Ther 38(12):746–753
10. Cutti AG, Ferrari A, Garofalo P, Raggi M, Cappello A, Ferrari A (2010) 'Outwalk': a protocol for clinical gait analysis based on inertial and magnetic sensors. Med Biol Eng Comput 48(1):17–25
11. Di Stasi S, Myer GD, Hewett TE (2013) Neuromuscular training to target deficits associated with second anterior cruciate ligament injury. J Orthop Sports Phys Ther 43(11):777–792, A1–11
12. Fox JA, Pierce M, Bojchuk J, Hayden J, Bush-Joseph CA, Bach BR Jr (2004) Revision anterior cruciate ligament reconstruction with nonirradiated fresh-frozen patellar tendon allograft. Arthroscopy 20(8): 787–794
13. Fujii M, Sasaki Y, Araki D, Furumatsu T, Miyazawa S, Ozaki T, Linde-Rosen M, Smokinski P, Fu FH (2014) Evaluation of the semitendinosus tendon graft shift in the bone tunnel: an experimental study. Knee Surg Sports Traumatol Arthrosc. [Epub ahead of print]. DOI 10.1007/s00167-014-3461-z
14. Gribble PA, Hertel J, Plisky P (2012) Using the star excursion balance test to assess dynamic postural-control deficits and outcomes in lower extremity injury: a literature and systematic review. J Athl Train 47(3):339–351
15. Hewett TE, Di Stasi SL, Myer GD (2013) Current concepts for injury prevention in athletes after anterior cruciate ligament reconstruction. Am J Sports Med 41(1):216–224
16. Hoshino Y, Araujo P, Ahlden M, Samuelsson K, Muller B, Hofbauer M, Wolf MR, Irrgang JJ, Fu FH, Musahl V (2013) Quantitative evaluation of the pivot shift by image analysis using the iPad. Knee Surg Sports Traumatol Arthrosc 21(4):975–980
17. Hoshino Y, Araujo P, Irrgang JJ, Fu FH, Musahl V (2012) An image analysis method to quantify the lateral pivot shift test. Knee Surg Sports Traumatol Arthrosc 20(4):703–707
18. Hoshino Y, Musahl V, Irrgang JJ, Lopomo N, Zaffagnini S, Karlsson J, Kuroda R, Fu FH (2015) Quantitative evaluation of the Pivot shift test, relationship to clinical Pivot shift grade. American Orthopaedic Society for Sports Medicine, Orlando

19. Hui C, Salmon LJ, Kok A, Maeno S, Linklater J, Pinczewski LA (2011) Fifteen-year outcome of endoscopic anterior cruciate ligament reconstruction with patellar tendon autograft for "isolated" anterior cruciate ligament tear. Am J Sports Med 39(1):89–98
20. Imbert P, Belvedere C, Leardini A (2015) Knee laxity modifications after ACL rupture and surgical intra- and extra-articular reconstructions: intra-operative measures in reconstructed and healthy knees. Knee Surg Sports Traumatol Arthrosc. [Epub ahead of print]. DOI: 10.1007/s00167-015-3653-1
21. Iriuchishima T, Ryu K, Aizawa S, Fu FH (2014) The difference in centre position in the ACL femoral footprint inclusive and exclusive of the fan-like extension fibres. Knee Surg Sports Traumatol Arthrosc 24(1):254–259
22. Ishibashi Y, Tsuda E, Yamamoto Y, Tsukada H, Toh S (2009) Navigation evaluation of the pivot-shift phenomenon during double-bundle anterior cruciate ligament reconstruction: is the posterolateral bundle more important? Arthroscopy 25(5):488–495
23. Klos TV (2014) Computer-assisted anterior cruciate ligament reconstruction. Four generations of development and usage. Sports Med Arthrosc 22(4): 229–236
24. Leys T, Salmon L, Waller A, Linklater J, Pinczewski L (2012) Clinical results and risk factors for reinjury 15 years after anterior cruciate ligament reconstruction: a prospective study of hamstring and patellar tendon grafts. Am J Sports Med 40(3):595–605
25. Lopomo N, Bignozzi S, Martelli S et al (2009) Reliability of a navigation system for intra-operative evaluation of antero-posterior knee joint laxity. Comput Biol Med 39(3):280–285
26. Lopomo N, Signorelli C, Bonanzinga T, Marcheggiani-Muccioli GM, Neri MP, Visani A, Marcacci M, Zaffagnini S (2014) Can rotatory knee laxity be predicted in isolated anterior cruciate ligament surgery? Int Orthop 38(6):1167–1172
27. Lopomo N, Zaffagnini S, Amis AA (2013) Quantifying the pivot shift test: a systematic review. Knee Surg Sports Traumatol Arthrosc 21(4):767–783
28. Lopomo N, Zaffagnini S, Bignozzi S, Visani A, Marcacci M (2010) Pivot-shift test: analysis and quantification of knee laxity parameters using a navigation system. J Orthop Res 28(2):164–169
29. Lynch AD, Logerstedt DS, Grindem H, Eitzen I, Hicks GE, Axe MJ, Engebretsen L, Risberg MA, Snyder-Mackier L (2013) Consensus criteria for defining 'successful outcome' after ACL injury and reconstruction: a Delaware-Oslo ACL cohort investigation. Br J Sports Med 49(5):335–342
30. Mandelbaum BR, Silvers HJ, Watanabe DS, Knarr JF, Thomas SD, Griffin LY, Kirkendall DT, Garrett W (2005) Effectiveness of a neuromuscular and proprioceptive training program in preventing anterior cruciate ligament injuries in female athletes: 2-year follow-up. Am J Sports Med 33(7):1003–1010
31. Martelli S, Lopomo N, Bignozzi S, Zaffagnini S, Visani A (2007) Validation of a new protocol for navigated intraoperative assessment of knee kinematics. Comput Biol Med 37(6):872–878
32. Martelli S, Zaffagnini S, Falcioni B, Motta M (2001) Determination of an optimal kinematic protocol for computer-assisted evaluation of anterior cruciate ligament deficiency. Ann Biomed Eng 29(12):1112–1121
33. Marx RG, Jones EC, Angel M, Wickiewicz TL, Warren RF (2003) Beliefs and attitudes of members of the American Academy of Orthopaedic Surgeons regarding the treatment of anterior cruciate ligament injury. Arthroscopy 19(7):762–770
34. Monaco E, Ferretti A, Labianca L, Maestri B, Speranza A, Kelly MJ, D'Arrigo C (2012) Navigated knee kinematics after cutting of the ACL and its secondary restraint. Knee Surg Sports Traumatol Arthrosc 20(5): 870–877
35. Muller B, Hofbauer M, Rahnemai-Azar AA, Wolf M, Araki D, Hoshino Y, Araujo P, Debski RE, Irrgang JJ, Fu FH, Musahl V (2015) Development of computer tablet software for clinical quantification of lateral knee compartment translation during the pivot shift test. Comput Methods Biomech Biomed Engin 19(2):217–228
36. Musahl V, Hoshino Y, Becker R, Karlsson J (2012) Rotatory knee laxity and the pivot shift. Knee Surg Sports Traumatol Arthrosc 20(4):601–602
37. Neeter C, Gustavsson A, Thomee P, Augustsson J, Thomee R, Karlsson J (2006) Development of a strength test battery for evaluating leg muscle power after anterior cruciate ligament injury and reconstruction. Knee Surg Sports Traumatol Arthrosc 14(6): 571–580
38. Paterno MV, Schmitt LC, Ford KR, Rauh MJ, Myer GD, Huang B, Hewett TE (2010) Biomechanical measures during landing and postural stability predict second anterior cruciate ligament injury after anterior cruciate ligament reconstruction and return to sport. Am J Sports Med 38(10):1968–1978
39. Pearle AD, Solomon DJ, Wanich T, Moreau-Gaudry A, Granchi CC, Wickiewicz TL, Warren RF (2007) Reliability of navigated knee stability examination: a cadaveric evaluation. Am J Sports Med 35(8):1315–20
40. Prins M (2006) The Lachman test is the most sensitive and the pivot shift the most specific test for the diagnosis of ACL rupture. Aust J Physiother 52(1):66
41. Schmitt LC, Paterno MV, Hewett TT (2012) The impact of quadriceps femoris strength asymmetry on functional performance at return to sport following anterior cruciate ligament reconstruction. J Orthop Sports Phys Ther 42(9):750–759
42. Signorelli C, Bonanzinga T, Lopomo N, Marcheggiani-Muccioli GM, Bignozzi S, Filardo G, Zaffagnini S, Marcacci M (2013) Do pre-operative knee laxity values influence post-operative ones after anterior cruciate ligament reconstruction? Scand J Med Sci Sports 23(4):e219–e224
43. Thomee R, Kaplan Y, Kvist J, Myklebust G, Risberg MA, Theisen D, Tsepis E, Werner S, Wondrasch B, Witvruow E (2011) Muscle strength and hop performance criteria prior to return to sports after ACL

reconstruction. Knee Surg Sports Traumatol Arthrosc 19(11):1798–1805
44. Wang JH, Kim JG, Ahn JH, Lim HC, Hoshino Y, Fu FH (2012) Is femoral tunnel length correlated with the intercondylar notch and femoral condyle geometry after double-bundle anterior cruciate ligament reconstruction using the transportal technique? An in vivo computed tomography analysis. Arthroscopy 28(8): 1094–1103
45. Zaffagnini S, Bignozzi S, Martelli S, Imakiire N, Lopomo N, Marcacci M (2006) New intraoperative protocol for kinematic evaluation of ACL reconstruction: preliminary results. Knee Surg Sports Traumatol Arthrosc 14(9):811–816
46. Zaffagnini S, Marcheggiani Muccioli GM, Signorelli C, Lopomo N, Grassi A, Bonanzinga T, Nitri M, Marcacci M (2014) Anatomic and nonanatomic double-bundle anterior cruciate ligament reconstruction: an in vivo kinematic analysis. Am J Sports Med 42(3): 708–715
47. Zaffagnini S, Signorelli C, Lopomo N, Bonanzinga T, Marchegiiani-Muccioli GM, Bignozzi S, Visani A, Marcacci M (2012) Anatomic double-bundle and over-the-top single-bundle with additional extra-articular tenodesis: an in vivo quantitative assessment of knee laxity in two different ACL reconstructions. Knee Surg Sports Traumatol Arthrosc 20(1):153–159

CPI Antony Rowe
Chippenham, UK
2018-08-16 09:58